Active and Healthy Aging: Critical Approaches to Disease Management

Active and Healthy Aging: Critical Approaches to Disease Management

Editor: Freya Phillips

MURPHY & MOORE
www.murphy-moorepublishing.com

www.murphy-moorepublishing.com

MURPHY & MOORE

Cataloging-in-Publication Data

Active and healthy aging : critical approaches to disease management / edited by Freya Phillips.
p. cm.
Includes bibliographical references and index.
ISBN 978-1-63987-008-0
1. Older people--Health and hygiene. 2. Older people--Diseases--Treatment. 3. Older people--Medical care.
4. Aging. I. Phillips, Freya.
RA564.8 .A28 2022
362.198 97--dc23

Murphy & Moore Publishing,
1 Rockefeller Plaza,
New York City, NY 10020, USA

ISBN 978-1-63987-008-0 (Hardback)

Contents

Preface

It is often said that books are a boon to mankind. They document every progress and pass on the knowledge from one generation to the other. They play a crucial role in our lives. Thus I was both excited and nervous while editing this book. I was pleased by the thought of being able to make a mark but I was also nervous to do it right because the future of students depends upon it. Hence, I took a few months to research further into the discipline, revise my knowledge and also explore some more aspects. Post this process, I begun with the editing of this book.

Aging refers to the process of becoming older that is associated with changes in the physiological, biological, environmental, psychological and social processes. It increases the risk of diseases in human beings. There are various factors which can increase the rate of aging such as a compromised immune system and obesity. Biologically, it is a result of a wide range of cellular and molecular damage over time. Active and healthy aging is the process of improving the quality of life by optimizing opportunities related to health and safety. It involves the development and maintenance of the functional abilities in older age, which in turn facilitates well-being. This book brings forth some of the most innovative concepts and elucidates the unexplored aspects of active and healthy aging as well as disease management. The various studies that are constantly contributing towards advancing technologies to promote active and healthy aging are examined in detail. The topics covered in this book offer the readers new insights in this field.

I thank my publisher with all my heart for considering me worthy of this unparalleled opportunity and for showing unwavering faith in my skills. I would also like to thank the editorial team who worked closely with me at every step and contributed immensely towards the successful completion of this book. Last but not the least, I wish to thank my friends and colleagues for their support.

Editor

1

AMP-activated Protein Kinase Controls Exercise Training- and AICAR-induced Increases in SIRT3 and MnSOD

Josef Brandauer[1,2†], Marianne A. Andersen[1†], Holti Kellezi[1], Steve Risis[1], Christian Frøsig[3], Sara G. Vienberg[1] and Jonas T. Treebak[1]*

[1] Section of Integrative Physiology, The Novo Nordisk Foundation Center for Basic Metabolic Research, University of Copenhagen, Copenhagen, Denmark, [2] Department of Health Sciences, Gettysburg College, Gettysburg, PA, USA, [3] Section of Molecular Physiology, Department of Nutrition, Exercise and Sports, The August Krogh Centre, University of Copenhagen, Copenhagen, Denmark

Edited by:
Brian McDonagh,
University of Liverpool, UK

Reviewed by:
Han-Zhong Feng,
Wayne State University School of Medicine, USA
Bruno Bastide,
University of Lille Nord de France, University of Lille1, France
Qiang Tong,
Baylor College of Medicine, USA

***Correspondence:**
Jonas T. Treebak,
The Novo Nordisk Foundation Center for Basic Metabolic Research, Section of Integrative Physiology, University of Copenhagen, Blegdamsvej 3b, Building 6, 6th floor, DK2200 Copenhagen, Denmark
jttreebak@sund.ku.dk

† These authors have contributed equally to this work.

The mitochondrial protein deacetylase sirtuin (SIRT) 3 may mediate exercise training-induced increases in mitochondrial biogenesis and improvements in reactive oxygen species (ROS) handling. We determined the requirement of AMP-activated protein kinase (AMPK) for exercise training-induced increases in skeletal muscle abundance of SIRT3 and other mitochondrial proteins. Exercise training for 6.5 weeks increased SIRT3 ($p < 0.01$) and superoxide dismutase 2 (MnSOD; $p < 0.05$) protein abundance in quadriceps muscle of wild-type (WT; $n = 13$–15), but not AMPK α2 kinase dead (KD; $n = 12$–13) mice. We also observed a strong trend for increased MnSOD abundance in exercise-trained skeletal muscle of healthy humans ($p = 0.051$; $n = 6$). To further elucidate a role for AMPK in mediating these effects, we treated WT ($n = 7$–8) and AMPK α2 KD ($n = 7$–9) mice with 5-amino-1-β-D-ribofuranosyl-imidazole-4-carboxamide (AICAR). Four weeks of daily AICAR injections (500 mg/kg) resulted in AMPK-dependent increases in SIRT3 ($p < 0.05$) and MnSOD ($p < 0.01$) in WT, but not AMPK α2 KD mice. We also tested the effect of repeated AICAR treatment on mitochondrial protein levels in mice lacking the transcriptional coactivator peroxisome proliferator-activated receptor γ-coactivator 1α (PGC-1α KO; $n = 9$–10). Skeletal muscle SIRT3 and MnSOD protein abundance was reduced in sedentary PGC-1α KO mice ($p < 0.01$) and AICAR-induced increases in SIRT3 and MnSOD protein abundance was only observed in WT mice ($p < 0.05$). Finally, the acetylation status of SIRT3 target lysine residues on MnSOD (K122) or oligomycin-sensitivity conferring protein (OSCP; K139) was not altered in either mouse or human skeletal muscle in response to acute exercise. We propose an important role for AMPK in regulating mitochondrial function and ROS handling in skeletal muscle in response to exercise training.

Keywords: AMPK, SIRT3, MnSOD, SOD2, ROS, OSCP, exercise training, mitochondrial biogenesis

Introduction

Mitochondrial density and capacity for oxidative ATP synthesis in skeletal muscle are tightly linked to cellular energetic demands (Spina et al., 1996; Egan and Zierath, 2013). Protein deacetylases such as sirtuins (SIRTs) are important modulators of gene expression and protein activity and are involved in mitochondrial biogenesis. SIRT1 is mainly located in the nucleus and deacetylates the transcriptional coactivator, peroxisome proliferator-activated receptor γ-coactivator 1α (PGC-1α) (Nemoto et al., 2005), thereby increasing mitochondrial biogenesis (Puigserver et al., 1998) and improving mitochondrial function (Gerhart-Hines et al., 2007). PGC-1α also induces gene expression of the mitochondrial sirtuin SIRT3 (Schwer et al., 2002) in muscle cells and hepatocytes (Kong et al., 2010).

SIRT3 modulates mitochondrial gene expression and function. SIRT3-driven processes occur via a general deacetylation of mitochondrial proteins (Lombard et al., 2007), including key elements of the citric acid cycle and proteins involved in oxidative phosphorylation (Hallows et al., 2006; Schwer et al., 2006; Wu et al., 2013; Vassilopoulos et al., 2014), or reactive oxygen species (ROS) handling (Someya et al., 2010; Tseng et al., 2013). Thus, SIRT1 may increase SIRT3 expression via PGC-1α deacetylation to facilitate an increase in mitochondrial function and/or density.

Exercise training and caloric restriction (CR) induce mitochondrial biogenesis, but SIRT1-mediated adaptations to exercise and CR are blunted in AMP-activated protein kinase (AMPK)-deficient skeletal muscle (Cantó et al., 2010). AMPK is a heterotrimeric protein consisting of multiple catalytic (α1, α2) and regulatory (β1, β2, γ1, γ2, γ3) subunits. AMPK functions as a major sensor of cellular energy status and can be activated pharmacologically and in response to muscle contraction and CR (Koh et al., 2008). Importantly, AMPK directly phosphorylates PGC-1α (Jäger et al., 2007) which may result in SIRT1-mediated deacetylation and activation of PGC-1α (Cantó et al., 2009) and thus link cellular energy status, mitochondrial biogenesis, and ROS handling.

AMPK activation via 5-amino-1-β-D-ribofuranosyl-imidazole-4-carboxamide (AICAR) increases SIRT3 mRNA level in hepatocytes (Buler et al., 2014). While SIRT3 reduces oxidative stress induced by CR (Someya et al., 2010), AMPK partly coordinates the cellular response to CR (Shinmura et al., 2007), supporting the hypothesis that AMPK may regulate SIRT3.

Exercise training increases ROS processing in skeletal muscle (Parise et al., 2005) via a mechanism that is incompletely understood. A potential mitochondrial signaling cascade response involving SIRT3 and FOXO3A-dependent transcription of catalase and MnSOD has been proposed (Jacobs et al., 2008), but the role of this cascade in exercise-training induced adaptations is unknown. MnSOD and catalase govern the conversion of superoxide to water and oxygen in sequential steps (Reid, 2001). Activation of MnSOD is enhanced by SIRT3-dependent deacetylation at K122, enabling the cell to scavenge ROS (Tao et al., 2010). Other regulatory acetylation sites have also been reported (Qiu et al., 2010; Chen et al., 2011), but the importance for each of these sites in relation to different stimuli remains elusive.

In summary, activation of AMPK via exercise or pharmacological treatment may phosphorylate PGC-1α, increase SIRT3 protein expression, and enhance the ability of skeletal muscle to better handle ROS via deacetylation and activation of MnSOD. Whether this pathway is redundant or exclusively dependent on AMPK is unknown. Given the functional connection between AMPK activators and PGC-1α-dependent increases of SIRT3 abundance and its downstream targets, we determined the effects of exercise training and pharmacological AMPK activation via AICAR in mouse models overexpressing a kinase dead version of the catalytic α2 AMPK subunit dominant in skeletal muscle as well as in skeletal muscle of PGC-1α deficient mice.

Materials and Methods

Exercise Training—Humans

Skeletal muscle samples were obtained from young male subjects previously described in an earlier study (Frøsig et al., 2004). The exercise training study was performed in compliance with the Helsinki II Declaration, with approval from the local ethics committee (#KF 01-070/96). Exercise training consisted of 15 sessions of one-legged knee extensor endurance training over the course of 3 weeks. The duration of the exercise sessions started at 1 h per session and was gradually increased to 2 h per session for the final 5 sessions. Needle biopsies were obtained under local anesthesia (2% lidocaine) from the right and left *vastus lateralis* muscles before training and 15 h ($n = 8$) after the final exercise bout.

Acute Exercise—Humans

Vastus lateralis muscle samples were obtained from healthy young men before and after an acute bout of one-legged knee-extensor exercise. Selected data from this experiment have been published previously (Treebak et al., 2014). This study was approved by the local ethics committee (#KF 1277313) and complied with the Helsinki II Declaration. Seven subjects volunteered to perform an acute bout of one-legged knee-extensor exercise at 80% of peak work load for 1 h during the morning after an overnight fast. In the 1-h exercise bout, peak work load was increased to 100% for 5 min intervals after 15 min and again after 35 min. Needle biopsies from the right and left *vastus lateralis* muscle were obtained before (Pre) and immediately after (Post) exercise cessation as described (Treebak et al., 2014).

Animal Experiments

All animal experiments complied with the European Convention for the protection of Vertebrate Animals used for Experiments and Other Scientific Purposes (Council of Europe 123, Strasbourg, France, 1985) and were approved by the Danish Animal Experimental Inspectorate (#2012-15-2934-26 and #2012-15-2934-307).

Exercise Training—Mice

Female mice (9–15 weeks of age) overexpressing a kinase dead (KD) α2 AMPK subunit in skeletal muscle (Mu et al., 2001) or WT littermates underwent 6.5 weeks of endurance exercise training ($n = 12$–15/group). Selected data from these experiments have been published previously (Brandauer et al., 2013). Mice had free access to running wheels for voluntary running 7 days/week. Running distance was recorded using a cycle odometer (#BC1009, Sigma Sport®, Germany). WT and AMPK α2 KD mice performed similar amounts of voluntary running (Brandauer et al., 2013). In addition, mice were exercised 1 h/day at 16 m/min on a motorized treadmill (Exer-3/6, Columbus Instruments) on weekdays as described (Brandauer et al., 2013). The treadmill was horizontal the first week, and the incline was increased by 2.5° per week up to 10° where it remained for the duration of the study. The morning following the final exercise bout, mice were anesthetized by an intraperitoneal (i.p.) injection using Avertin (250 mg tribromoethanol/kg body weight). Quadriceps muscles were removed, snap-frozen in liquid nitrogen, and stored at −80°C until further analyses.

AICAR Treatment Studies

To determine whether AICAR-induced increases in SIRT3 and other mitochondrial proteins depend on AMPK, male AMPK α2 KD and WT mice (11–12 weeks of age) received a daily subcutaneous injection of 500 mg/kg body weight AICAR or 0.9% NaCl solution for 4 weeks ($n = 7$–8) as described (Brandauer et al., 2013). Mice were anesthetized via i.p. injection of Avertin (250 mg/kg body weight) 24 h following the last AICAR/vehicle treatment to avoid any confounding effects of the last AICAR/saline injection. Quadriceps muscle was obtained, snap-frozen in liquid N_2, and stored at −80°C. Samples from a previously published study of male and female whole-body PGC-1α KO and WT mice were also analyzed. The mice in this study were treated with AICAR under the same conditions as described above (Leick et al., 2009, 2010a). In order to determine the acute effect of a single injection of AICAR, we analyzed samples originating from a previous study (Leick et al., 2010a). Male and female PGC-1α KO mice and WT littermates ($n = 6$–8) were injected subcutaneously with a single dose of AICAR (500 mg/kg body weight) or saline. Quadriceps muscles were taken 4 h after the injection, snap-frozen in liquid N_2 and stored at −80°C.

Acute Exercise in Previously Trained or Untrained Mice

To assess the effects of acute exercise in trained and untrained mouse skeletal muscle, female C57BL/6JBom (Taconic, Denmark) mice (9–10 weeks of age) underwent 5.5 weeks of endurance exercise training ($n = 26$) or served as sedentary controls ($n = 24$). The training consisted of voluntary running with free access to wheel cages 7 days/week with running distance being recorded by a cycle odometer (#BC1009, Sigma Sport®, Germany). In addition, mice were exercised 1 h/day on weekdays with accelerating speeds from 8 to 18 m/min on a motorized treadmill (Exer-3/6, Columbus Instruments) or placed on a "mock" treadmill for the sedentary control group. The treadmill was horizontal the first week, and the incline was increased by 2.5° per week up to 10° at the final week to account for increased performance and to ensure a continuous training stimulus. Untrained control animals were acclimatized to treadmill running for 15–20 min with accelerating speeds from 8 to 18 m/min at a 5° incline for three consecutive days, with 1 day of rest prior to the acute exercise experiment. On the experimental day, both trained and sedentary control mice were divided into three groups: non-exercised controls ($n = 8$ sedentary, 9 trained), and mice performing either moderate-intensity ($n = 8$ sedentary, 8 trained) or high-intensity acute exercise ($n = 7$ sedentary, 8 trained), resulting in six experimental groups. Based on the recorded running distances of each mouse, mice were assigned to one of the three groups so that the average amount of training performed in the training period was similar between the three groups (i.e., 5.1 ± 0.6 km/day; mean ± SEM). Mice then performed an acute treadmill exercise bout for 1 h or served as sedentary controls. "Moderate intensity" was defined as 12 m/min at 0° incline, while "high intensity" was defined as 18 m/min with a 10° incline. Mice were euthanized by cervical dislocation immediately after the acute exercise bout. Quadriceps muscles were quickly removed, snap frozen in liquid nitrogen, and stored at -80° until further analysis.

Tissue Processing and Western Blot Analyses

All muscle samples were processed using steel bead homogenization (Tissue Lyser II, Qiagen) in ice-cold lysis buffer (pH 7.4; 10% glycerol; 1% IGEPAL; Hepes, 50 mM; NaCl, 150 mM; NaF, 10 mM; EDTA, 1 mM; EGTA, 1 mM; sodium pyrophosphate, 20 mM; sodium orthovanadate, 2 mM; sodium-pyrophosphate 1 mM; nicotinamide 5 mM; Thiamet G 4 μM and protease inhibitors (SigmaFast, Sigma Aldrich) according to manufacturer's instructions). Protein concentrations were determined using BCA assays (Thermo Scientific, #23223 and #23224). Equal amounts of protein were resolved by SDS-PAGE and transferred to polyvinylidene difluoride (PVDF) membranes (Millipore, Denmark) as described (Brandauer et al., 2013). Western blots were executed in a balanced design, with samples from all experimental conditions present on all gels, and identical internal control samples included on each blot. The internal control sample was prepared as a pool of all samples from a given experiment. All samples on individual gels were normalized to the internal control sample in order to permit comparison of samples resolved on separate gels. Following transfer, samples were subjected to immunoblot analysis to detect protein abundance using following antibodies against SIRT3 (Cell Signaling, #5490S), SIRT1 (Millipore, #07-131), MnSOD, (Millipore, #06-948), MnSOD K122 acetylation (kindly provided by Prof. David Gius, Northwestern University Feinberg School of Medicine, Chicago, Illinois; see Tao et al., 2010) and Catalase (R&D Systems, #AF3398). Protein abundance of the oxidative phosphorylation complexes was determined using antibodies against Complex I (NDUFB8, Invitrogen, #459210), Complex II (Fp subunit, Invitrogen, #459200), Complex III (Core subunit I, Invitrogen, #459140), Complex IV (Subunit I, Invitrogen, #459600), Complex V (i.e., F1F0 ATP synthase; oligomycin-sensitivity conferring protein [OSCP] subunit (Santa Cruz, #sc-74786), cytochrome C (BD Biosciences #556433) and OSCP K139 acetylation (kindly provided by Prof. David Gius). The specificity of the MnSOD K122 and OSCP K139 antibody used in this study has been verified (Tao et al., 2010; Vassilopoulos et al., 2014) and was confirmed by "split-blot" analyses, where samples prepared from the same mouse quadriceps muscle or human *vastus lateralis* muscle was resolved in three adjacent wells. After transfer to PVDF, the membrane was cut through the center well and the membrane halves were probed with the total MnSOD/OSCP or MnSOD K122/OSCP K139 antibodies, respectively. Complete alignment of the bands was confirmed (**Figure 7**).

Quantitative Polymerase Chain Reaction (qPCR)

qPCR was performed as described (Brandauer et al., 2013). RNA from quadriceps muscles was extracted using Trizol (Invitrogen, #15596-018) and reverse transcription was performed using iScript cDNA synthesis kit (BioRad, #170-8891). Real-time qPCR was performed using 2 µl of template cDNA, 300 nM of sense and antisense oligonucleotides and SYBR Green PCR Master Mix (AH Diagnostic, #600882) in a final volume of 10 µl. Fluorescence measurements and data analysis were performed on the CFX96 real time system (BioRad). Gene expression was determined using primer sequences: SIRT3 forward primer: 5′-TACAGAAATCAGTGCCCCGA-3′ and reverse primer: 5′-GGTGGACACAAGAACTGCTG-3′; MnSOD forward primer: 5′-ACTGAAGTTCAATGGTGGGG- 3′ and reverse primer: 5′-GCTTGATAGCCTCCAGCAAC- 3′ and normalized by input cDNA (Qubit ssDNA assay kit, Invitrogen, #Q10212).

Statistics

Statistical analyses were performed by either 2 × 2 analysis of variance (ANOVA), by 2 × 3 ANOVA, or by 2 × 2 repeated-measures ANOVA as appropriate. The Tukey test was used *post-hoc*. If statistical interactions were borderline significant ($0.05 < p < 0.1$) and the observed power was low (<0.5), individual *t*-tests were performed as noted in the description of the results. As incomplete sample sets are excluded from statistical analyses in repeated-measures ANOVA, statistical analyses performed on data from the human training study were only performed on 6 sets of samples. Statistical significance was set at $p < 0.05$. All data are reported as mean ± SEM.

Results

Exercise Training in Mice Increases SIRT3 and MnSOD in an AMPK-Dependent Manner

To verify the potency of the exercise training program and to assess the importance of AMPK on exercise-induced mitochondrial adaptations in skeletal muscle, we performed Western blot analyses on mitochondrial Complex I through V (OSCP) and cytochrome C on samples from WT and AMPK α2 KD mice that had completed 6.5 weeks of endurance exercise training. WT and AMPK α2 KD mice performed similarly in average distance run (Brandauer et al., 2013), average duration of exercise/day (WT, 140 ± 16 min/day; KD, 168 ± 29 min/day; $p = 0.38$) and average running speed (WT, 1.39 ± 0.04 km/h; KD, 1.27 ± 0.07 km/h, $p = 0.15$).

We found no interaction effects in any of the data sets presented in **Figures 1A–F**, likely due to low statistical power. However, if individual *t*-tests were performed between control and trained mice, we found significant ($p < 0.05$) increases in Complexes I, II, and IV protein abundance in the WT mice only. Collectively, these data suggest a regulatory role for AMPK in mediating the effects of endurance exercise training on mitochondrial protein expression.

Endurance exercise training increased SIRT3 protein abundance in skeletal muscle from WT, but not AMPK α2 KD mice ($p < 0.01$; $n = 12–15$) (**Figure 2A**). On the other hand, no statistical differences in SIRT3 mRNA levels were observed between genotypes or in response to exercise training (**Figure 2B**). Exercise training tended to increase skeletal muscle MnSOD protein levels in WT relative to KD mice (WT, 49%; AMPK α2 KD, 11%; genotype × treatment interaction effect, $p = 0.079$; observed power 0.294; **Figure 2C**). A *t*-test showed an exercise-induced increase in skeletal muscle MnSOD protein level in WT ($p < 0.05$), but not AMPK α2 KD mice. MnSOD mRNA levels were unchanged in response to exercise training in both genotypes (**Figure 2D**). Endurance exercise did not alter SIRT1 (**Figure 2E**) or catalase protein levels (**Figure 2F**). Thus, AMPK is required for upregulation of SIRT3 and MnSOD protein levels in response to exercise training.

Skeletal Muscle MnSOD Protein Abundance is Increased Following Endurance Exercise Training in Human Skeletal Muscle

We employed a model of one-legged endurance exercise training to study SIRT3 and MnSOD protein abundance in trained and untrained human skeletal muscle. A repeated-measures ANOVA revealed no significant changes in SIRT3 protein content following exercise training in humans ($n = 6$; **Figure 3A**). When samples were analyzed to determine MnSOD content, a borderline significant interaction effect (leg × intervention; $p = 0.051$, $n = 6$; observed power; 0.471; **Figure 3B**) was observed. A *t*-test comparing the control leg to the trained leg after the exercise intervention revealed MnSOD protein was increased in trained skeletal muscle ($p < 0.05$). Collectively, our data indicate that protein content of MnSOD is upregulated in response to exercise training in human skeletal muscle.

Repeated AMPK Activation by AICAR Increases SIRT3 and MnSOD Protein in an AMPK- and PGC-1α-Dependent Manner

To more directly confirm a role for AMPK in the regulation of skeletal muscle SIRT3 and MnSOD protein abundance, we treated WT and AMPK α2 KD mice with AICAR, a pharmacological AMPK activator. We performed Western blot analyses for proteins involved in oxidative phosphorylation to determine the efficacy of the AICAR treatment. Similarly to the results observed in the exercise training studies, any AICAR-induced increase in skeletal muscle abundance of oxidative phosphorylation complex proteins was blunted in AMPK α2 KD mice (**Figures 4A–F**). However, no significant interaction effects were found for Complex I-V, most likely due to low statistical power. When individual *t*-tests were performed, significant increases in protein content were found in the WT group for Complexes I, IV, and V. Treatment with AICAR increased

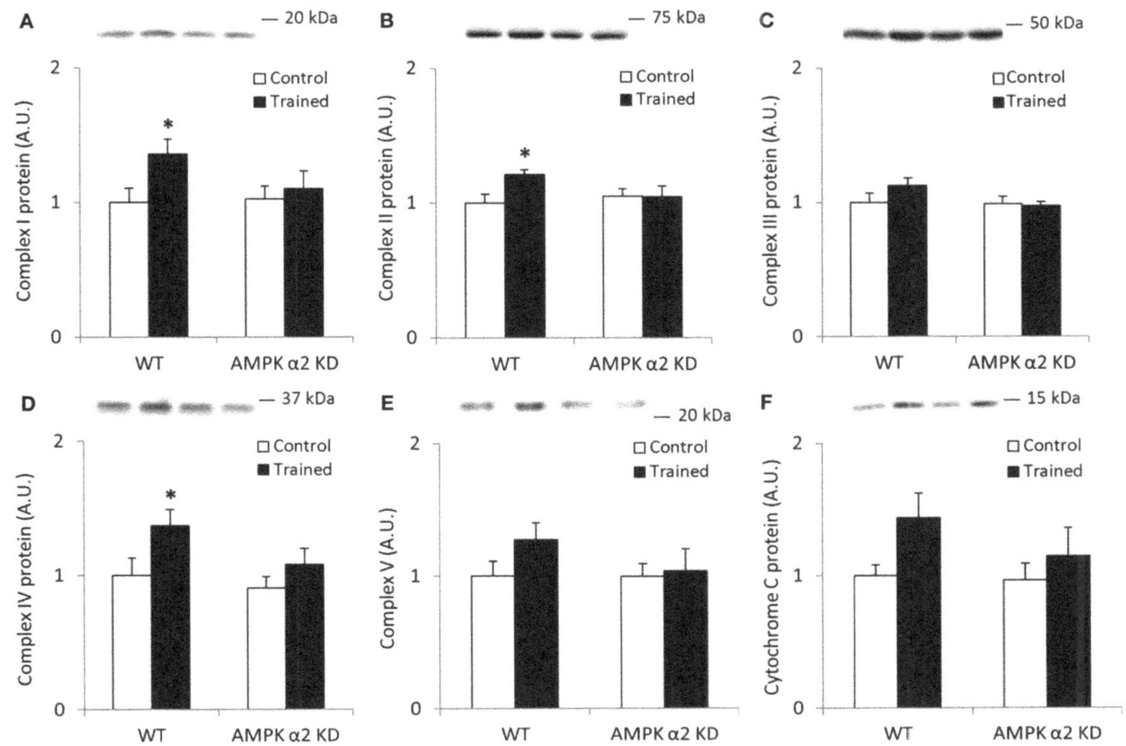

FIGURE 1 | Exercise training increase mitochondrial oxidative phosphorylation complexes in an AMPK α2-dependent manner. Protein levels of oxidative phosphorylation complexes, **(A)** Complex I, **(B)** Complex II, **(C)** Complex III, **(D)** Complex IV, **(E)** Complex V (oligomycin-sensitivity conferring protein subunit, OSCP), and **(F)** Cytochrome C were evaluated in quadriceps muscle of sedentary (control) or exercise trained female WT and AMPK α2 KD mice ($n = 13–15$). Values are mean ± SEM. *indicates vs. WT control ($p < 0.05$) analyzed by unpaired t-tests.

abundance of cytochrome C in the WT mice ($p < 0.01$) in an AMPK-dependent manner (treatment × genotype interaction effect $p < 0.05$), and protein levels were lower in AMPK α2 KD mice ($p < 0.01$; **Figure 4F**).

AICAR treatment resulted in AMPK α2-dependent increases in SIRT3 protein levels (treatment × genotype interaction effect $p < 0.05$; $n = 7–8$; **Figure 5A**) whereas mRNA expression increased independent of genotype ($p < 0.01$; **Figure 5B**). Likewise, MnSOD protein levels increased in an AMPK α2-dependent manner (treatment × genotype interaction effect $p < 0.05$; $n = 7–8$; **Figure 5C**) while MnSOD mRNA expression increased in response to AICAR independent of AMPK α2 ($p < 0.01$, $n = 6–8$; **Figure 5D**). Together, these data support the hypothesis that AMPK activation governs post-transcriptional regulation of SIRT3 and MnSOD protein levels. Repeated treatment with AICAR did not increase SIRT1 or catalase protein levels (**Figures 5E,F**).

We next assessed whether increases in SIRT3 and MnSOD following AICAR treatment depend on functional PGC-1α signaling. AICAR treatment increased skeletal muscle protein level of SIRT3 and MnSOD in WT, but not in PGC-1α KO mice (treatment × genotype interaction effect $p < 0.05$; $n = 9–10$; **Figures 6A,B**), and total protein of SIRT3 and MnSOD was generally reduced in control PGC-1α KO mice ($p < 0.01$; $n = 9–10$; **Figures 6A,B**). SIRT1 and catalase protein levels were similar in the WT and PGC-1α mice and remained unaltered in response to repeated AICAR treatment (**Figures 6C,D**). These data suggest that SIRT3 and MnSOD protein abundance is regulated in a signaling axis involving both AMPK and PGC-1α. In an attempt to establish indirect evidence that upregulation of SIRT3 and MnSOD protein with AICAR is mediated through transcriptional regulation of the SIRT3 and MnSOD genes by a PGC-1α-dependent mechanism, we measured mRNA levels of SIRT3 and MnSOD in PGC-1α KO animals treated repeatedly with AICAR over 4 weeks. Although mRNA levels of both SIRT3 and MnSOD were reduced in the PGC-1α KO animals, no increase with AICAR was detected in either genotype (**Figures 6E,F**). To determine whether an acute AICAR injection would increase mRNA levels of SIRT3 and MnSOD, we analyzed samples from PGC-1α KO and WT mice taken 4 h after a single injection of AICAR/saline (Leick et al., 2010a). As in the repeated-AICAR experiment, PGC-1α KO mice had lower mRNA levels of SIRT3 and MnSOD, but AICAR did not increase SIRT3 or MnSOD mRNA (**Figures 6G,H**).

Combined Effects of Endurance Exercise Training and Acute Exercise on Mitochondrial Protein Acetylation State in Mouse Quadriceps Muscle

SIRT3 is involved in the activation of MnSOD by deacetylating K122. Deacetylation of this residue would be expected

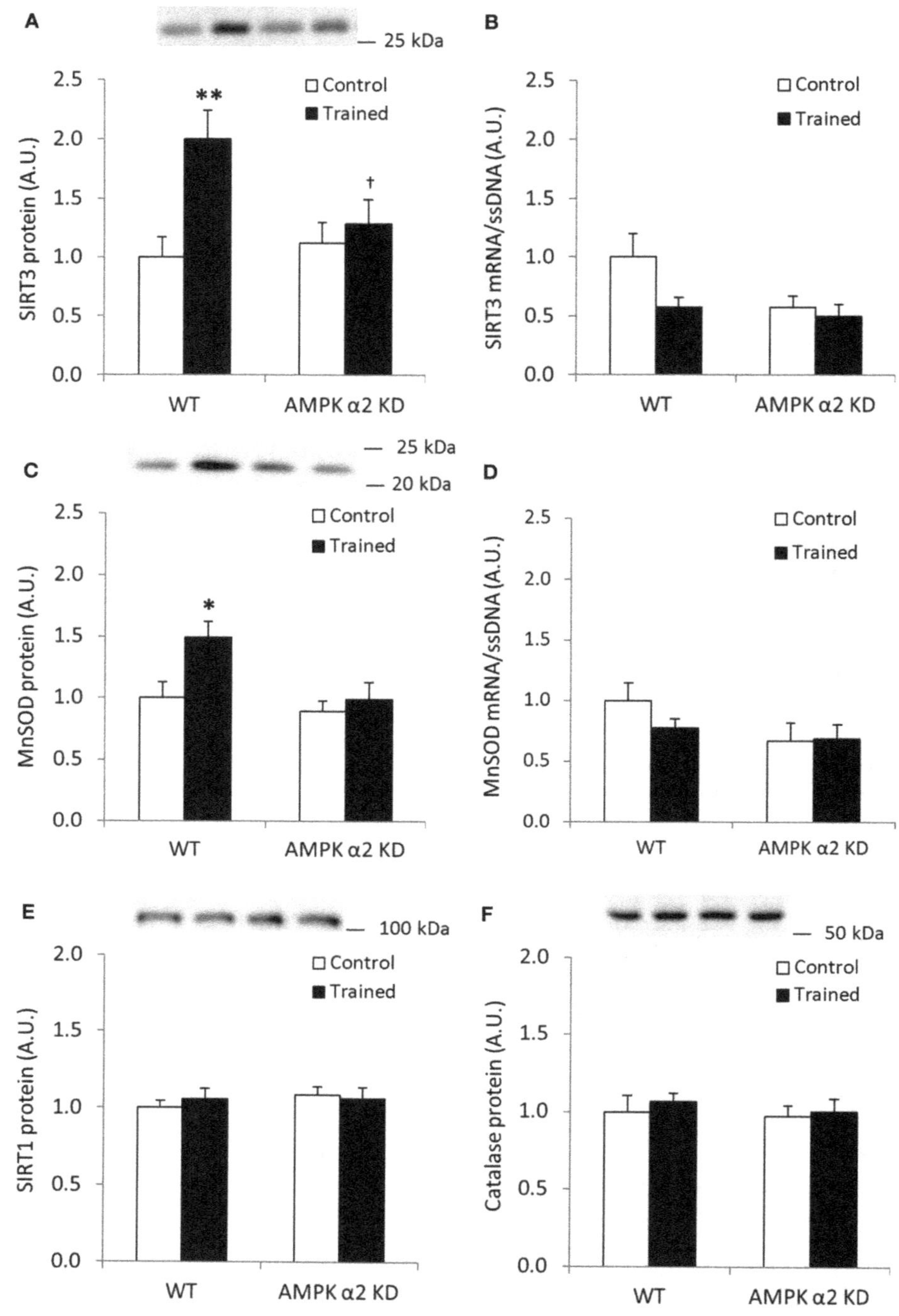

FIGURE 2 | Exercise training increases SIRT3 and MnSOD protein in mouse skeletal muscle in an AMPK α2-dependent manner. (A) SIRT3 protein, **(B)** SIRT3 mRNA ($n = 11$–14), **(C)** MnSOD protein, **(D)** MnSOD mRNA ($n = 11$–14), **(E)** SIRT1 protein, and **(F)** Catalase protein levels were measured in quadriceps muscle of control or exercised trained female WT and AMPK α2 KD mice ($n = 13$–15 for protein measurements). Quadriceps muscles were obtained the day after the final bout of exercise. Values are mean ± SEM. An interaction effect ($p < 0.05$; treatment × genotype) was present in **(A)**. * indicates vs. WT control ($p < 0.05$; analyzed by independent *t*-test), ** indicates vs. WT control ($p < 0.01$), and † indicates genotype effect within trained groups ($p < 0.05$).

to occur if superoxides are produced in mitochondria during exercise. To determine whether SIRT3-mediated deacetylation of mitochondrial proteins in skeletal muscle is dependent on training status, and whether acute exercise in sedentary and exercise trained muscle would lead to a differentiated acetylation response, C57BL/6JBom mice were exercise trained or

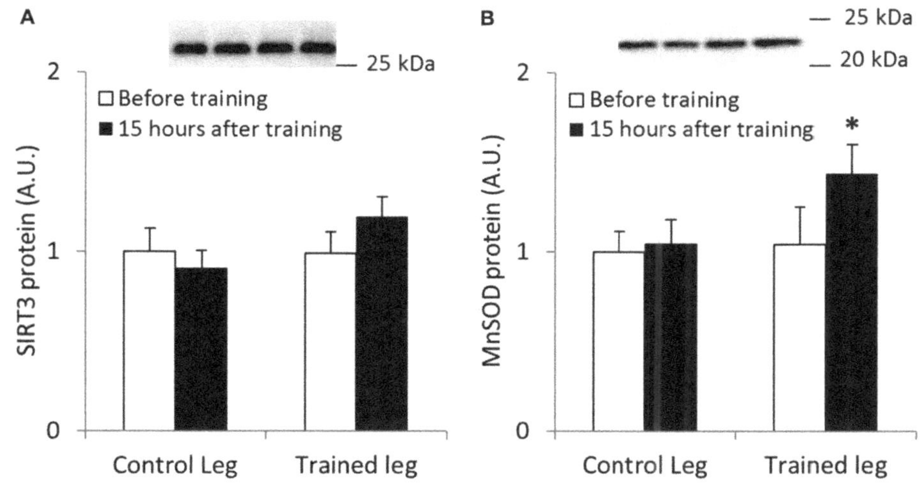

FIGURE 3 | One-legged knee-extensor endurance exercise training increases MnSOD protein levels in human *vastus lateralis* muscle. Male individuals performed 15 sessions of 1–2 h of one-legged knee extensor endurance exercise training over a period of 3 weeks. SIRT3 and MnSOD protein levels were measured from biopsies obtained before training and 15 h after the last bout of exercise ($n = 8$). **(A)** SIRT3 and **(B)** MnSOD protein levels. A borderline interaction effect of leg × intervention ($p = 0.051$) was found for MnSOD protein levels (observed power 0.471). * indicates vs. control leg after training ($p < 0.05$; paired *t*-test). Values are mean ± SEM. Statistical analyses were performed for $n = 6$ due to incomplete sample sets.

maintained as sedentary controls. On the day of tissue collection, mice were subjected to an acute 1-h bout of "moderate" or "high" intensity exercise or served as sedentary controls. Thus, using muscle samples from this experiment in addition to an antibody against acetylated K122 of MnSOD known to be important for MnSOD activity (Tao et al., 2010), the putative improved ability of trained muscle to handle ROS could be determined. To test the specificity of antibodies against total MnSOD and MnSOD K122 in skeletal muscle, we performed "split-blot" analyses and found bands from both antibodies to align in mouse and human skeletal muscle (**Figure 7A**). OSCP K139 antibody specificity has been previously validated (Vassilopoulos et al., 2014), and we further verified total OSCP and OSCP K139 specificity in skeletal muscle tissue by performing "split-blot" analyses and confirming that bands for OSCP and OSCP K139 align in human and mouse skeletal muscle (**Figure 7B**).

First, we confirmed that exercise training increases SIRT3 protein content in mouse quadriceps muscle (**Figure 8A**). Unexpectedly, 60 min of high-intensity acute exercise caused further increases in SIRT3 protein abundance in both previously sedentary and trained mice (**Figure 8A**). This increase in protein content was not accompanied by a parallel increase in SIRT3 mRNA in these samples relative to samples from any of the other groups (data not shown). Contrary to the AMPK α2 KD/WT exercise training study described above (**Figures 2E,F**), SIRT1 and catalase protein levels increased in response to exercise training. No additional change occurred in response to acute exercise (**Figures 8B,C**). Furthermore, MnSOD protein levels increased with exercise training (**Figure 8D**) to a similar degree as WT mice in the AMPK α2 KD/WT training study (**Figure 8D** vs. **Figure 2C**).

Although the importance of mitochondria as a source of superoxides during muscle contraction has been questioned (McArdle et al., 2004), we assessed acetylation level of MnSOD in response to exercise training and an acute bout of exercise. We detected increased acetylation of MnSOD K122 in the samples from exercise-trained animals, whereas acetylation levels were unaffected by acute exercise (**Figure 8E**). When MnSOD K122 acetylation status was normalized to total MnSOD protein abundance, acetylation status remained unchanged across conditions (**Figure 8F**).

We also tested the hypothesis that acetylation of OSCP on the K139 residue is a marker of cellular energy stress, and that exercised trained muscle would be less susceptible to exercise-induced changes in K139 acetylation. OSCP protein abundance increased with exercise training in mouse quadriceps muscle (**Figure 8G**), in addition to a pronounced increase in acetylation of OSCP K139 (**Figure 8H**). When OSCP acetylation level was normalized to total OSCP protein, K139 acetylation increased with exercise training (**Figure 8I**). Contrary to our hypothesis, OSCP K139 acetylation relative to total OSCP was unaffected by acute exercise (**Figures 8H,I**).

Acetylation Patterns in Human *Vastus Lateralis* with Acute Exercise

To compare the MnSOD and OSCP acetylation response obtained in exercised mouse quadriceps muscle with acutely exercised human skeletal muscle, we determined the acetylation level of these proteins in samples obtained from strenuously exercised *vastus lateralis* muscle of healthy young men. Acute exercise did not alter total protein abundance of either MnSOD or OSCP, nor did this intervention alter relative protein acetylation directly following exercise cessation (**Figures 9A–F**).

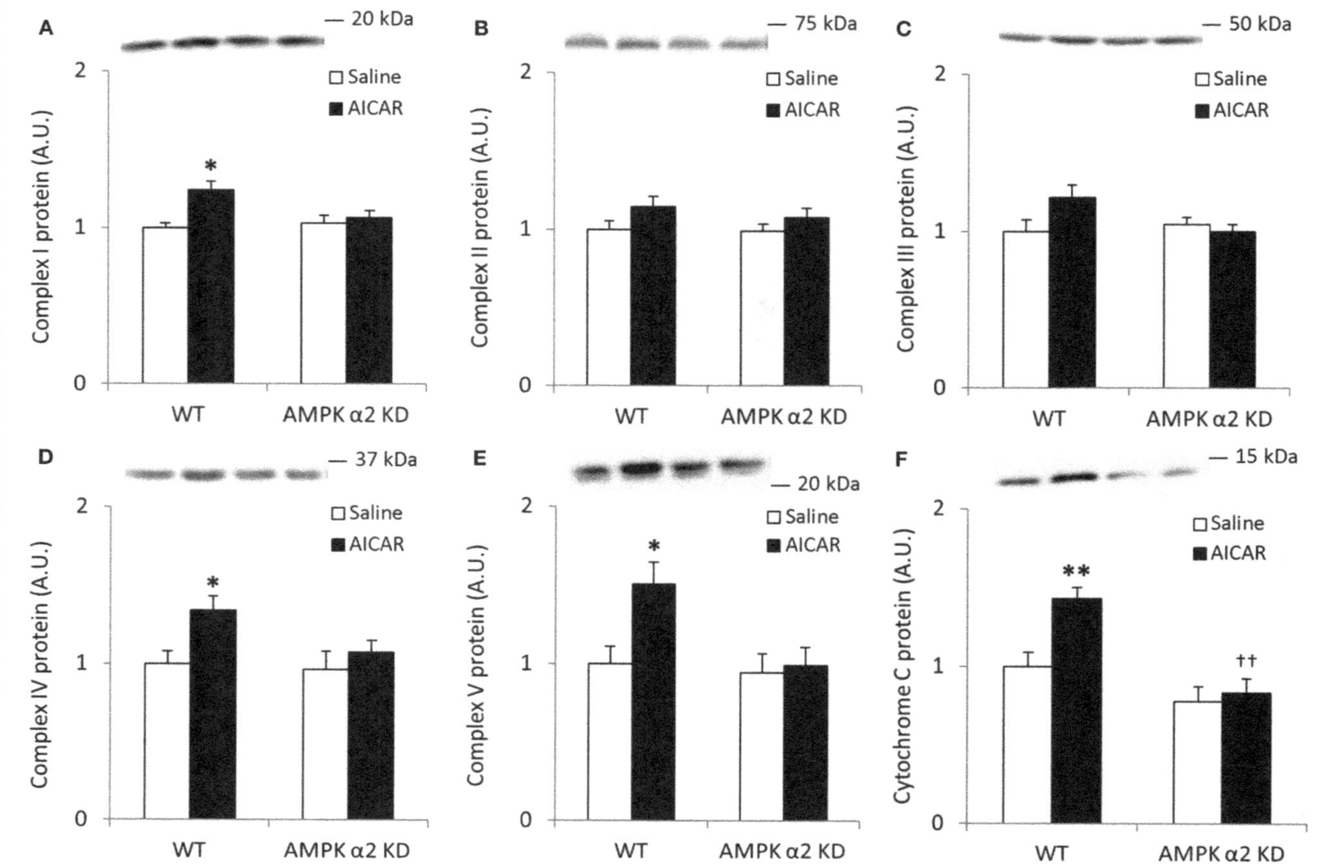

FIGURE 4 | Repeated treatment with AICAR increases abundance of mitochondrial electron transport chain proteins in an AMPK α2-dependent manner. WT and AMPK α2 KD male mice were given daily subcutaneous injections with AICAR (500 mg/kg body weight) or saline for 4 weeks. **(A–E)** Protein abundance of oxidative phosphorylation Complexes I–V and **(F)** Cytochrome C was measured in quadriceps muscle ($n = 7–8$). A significant interaction effect (treatment × genotype; $p < 0.05$) was observed for Cytochrome C. Values are mean ± SEM. * indicates vs. WT saline ($p < 0.05$) analyzed by *t*-tests, ** indicates vs. WT saline ($p < 0.01$), and †† indicates genotype effect within AICAR treated animals ($p < 0.01$).

Discussion

AMPK is a cellular "fuel gauge" that integrates and communicates disruptions in cellular energy charge to downstream targets (Hardie, 2011). One key signaling pathway by which AMPK exerts its effects is via the AMPK-PGC-1α-SIRT3 axis, which likely affects mitochondrial function and gene expression to adapt to metabolic changes (Hallows et al., 2006; Schwer et al., 2006; Someya et al., 2010; Tseng et al., 2013; Wu et al., 2013; Vassilopoulos et al., 2014). Here, we present evidence that AMPK is required for the increase in skeletal muscle SIRT3 and MnSOD protein abundance in addition to proteins in the mitochondrial respiratory complexes following exercise training and repeated AICAR treatment.

AMPK plays a critical role in mediating AICAR-induced increases in mitochondrial protein abundance (Jørgensen et al., 2007). The present study confirms these findings and provides additional evidence that AMPK is required to fully beget exercise training-induced increases in mitochondrial oxidative phosphorylation complexes. This observation is in line with recent data showing that exercise training-induced adaptations in skeletal muscle on mitochondrial Complexes I-V are dependent on the upstream AMPK kinase, LKB1 (Tanner et al., 2013). Other studies employing the same (Abbott and Turcotte, 2014) or similar mouse models of AMPK deficiency (Röckl et al., 2007) as in the present investigation did not detect AMPK-dependent defects in the ability to increase mitochondrial protein content. However, these studies only assessed citrate synthase activity and did not report the abundance of electron transport chain proteins.

The one-legged endurance exercise training model represents a well-controlled method to study contraction-mediated adaptations in *vastus lateralis* muscle in humans (Andersen et al., 1985; Frøsig et al., 2004). Despite a relatively small sample size, we found near-significant increases in skeletal muscle MnSOD protein level in the trained, but not untrained leg of healthy volunteers. Conversely, SIRT3 protein levels were not increased. This is in conflict with emerging evidence that SIRT3 expression is increased in exercise-trained human and rodent skeletal muscle (Lanza et al., 2008; Palacios et al., 2009). While an early cross-sectional study reported higher protein activity of MnSOD in

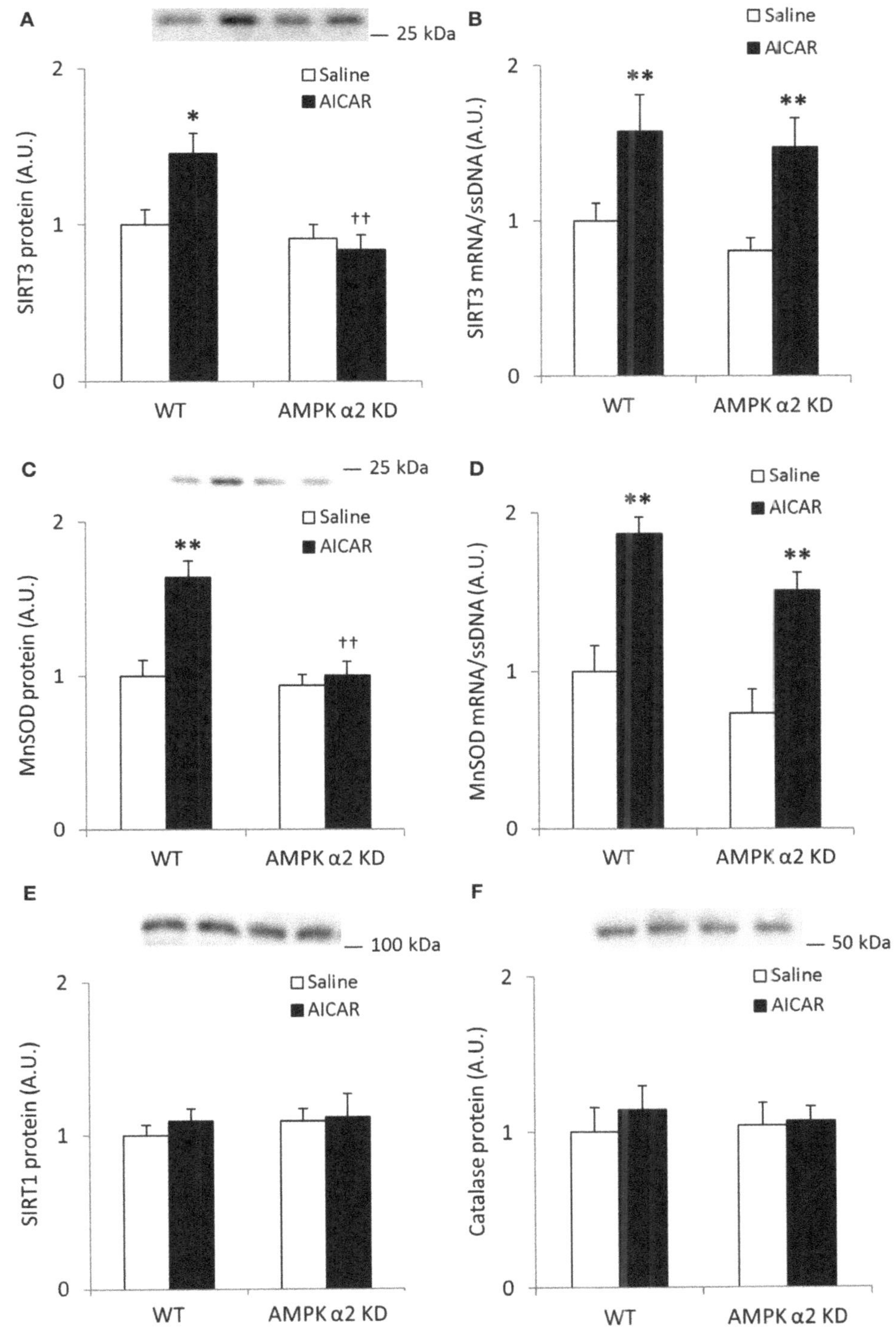

FIGURE 5 | Increases in quadriceps SIRT3 protein levels after repeated AICAR treatment are abolished in AMPK α2 KD mouse skeletal muscle. Levels of **(A)** SIRT3 protein, **(B)** SIRT3 mRNA, **(C)** MnSOD protein, **(D)** MnSOD mRNA, **(E)** SIRT1 protein, and **(F)** Catalase protein were determined in quadriceps muscle from WT and AMPK α2 KD male mice ($n = 7$–8) treated with daily subcutaneous injections of AICAR (500 mg/kg body weight) or saline for 4 weeks. Values are mean ± SEM. Interaction effects (treatment × genotype) were present in **(A)** ($p < 0.05$) and **(C)** ($p < 0.01$). * indicates vs. saline within genotype ($p < 0.05$), ** indicates vs. saline within genotype ($p < 0.01$), and †† indicates genotype effect within AICAR treated samples ($p < 0.01$).

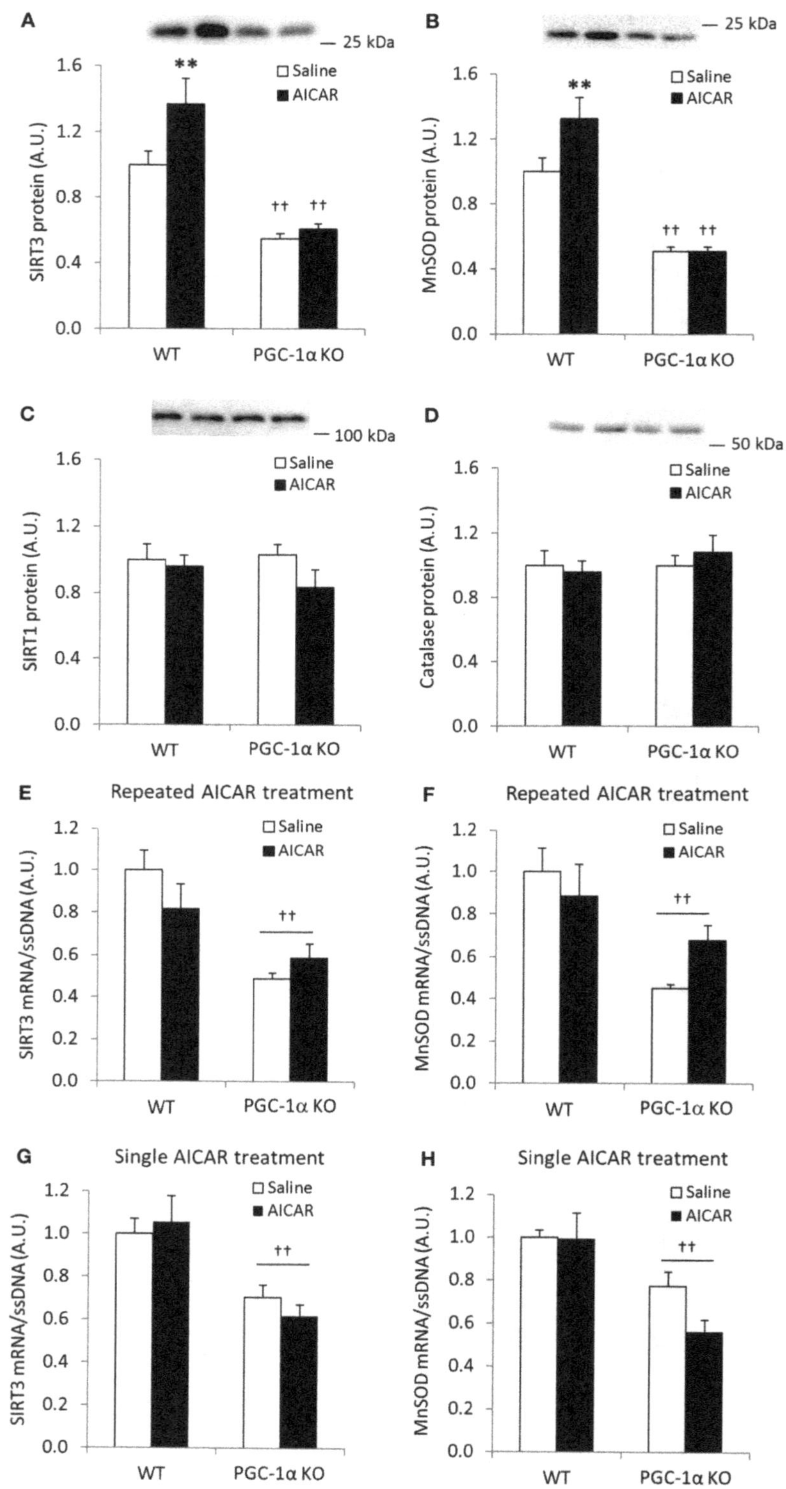

FIGURE 6 | AICAR-induced upregulation of SIRT3 and MnSOD protein in mouse skeletal muscle is dependent on PGC-1α. WT and PGC-1α KO mice received daily subcutaneous injection of AICAR (500 mg/kg body weight) or saline for 4 weeks. Quadriceps muscles were obtained the day after the last injection. **(A)** SIRT3 protein, **(B)** MnSOD protein, **(C)** SIRT1 protein, **(D)** Catalase protein, **(E)** SIRT3 mRNA, **(F)** MnSOD mRNA ($n = 9$–10). mRNA levels of **(G)** SIRT3 and **(H)** MnSOD were obtained from quadriceps muscles from WT and PGC-1α KO mice 4 h after a single injection of saline or AICAR (500 mg/kg body weight, $n = 6$–8). Values are mean ± SEM. Interaction effects (treatment × genotype) were present for data in **(A, C)** ($p < 0.05$), ** indicates vs. WT saline ($p < 0.01$), †† indicates genotype effect vs. WT ($p < 0.01$).

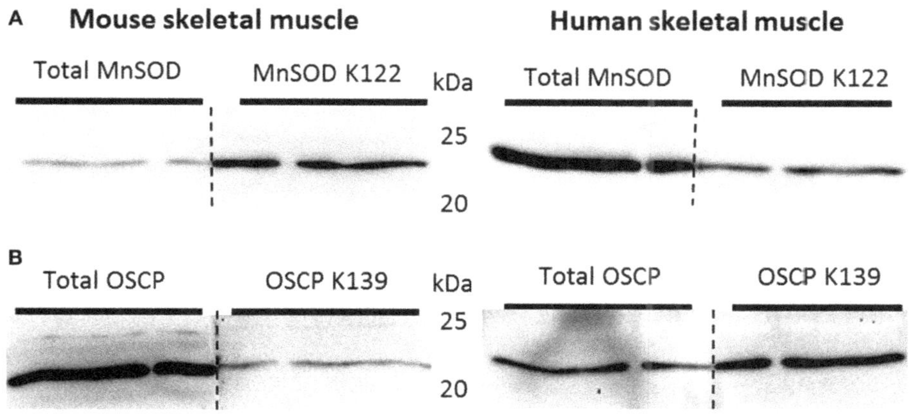

FIGURE 7 | Validation of antibodies targeting acetylated residues of MnSOD and OSCP. Validation of antibodies targeting **(A)** acetylated residue K122 of MnSOD and total MnSOD and **(B)** OSCP acetylation at residue K139 and total OSCP in mouse and human skeletal muscle by "split-blot" analysis.

skeletal muscle of individuals with high aerobic fitness (Jenkins et al., 1984), some longitudinal studies have called these findings into question (Tiidus et al., 1996; Tonkonogi et al., 2000).

In our study, SIRT3 or ROS defense protein abundance was unaltered by exercise training in AMPK α2 KD mice. These results are inconsistent with the notion that SIRT3 may be induced by exercise in an AMPK-independent manner (Gurd et al., 2012). While 7 days of chronic electrical stimulation increased SIRT3 level in rat hind limb muscles, AICAR treatment had no effect (Gurd et al., 2012). Apart from obvious species and protocol differences between the two studies, these findings could also suggest additional, possibly time-sensitive, regulatory mechanisms of SIRT3 protein levels.

Activation of SIRT1 via deletion of poly (ADP-ribose) polymerase-1 (PARP-1), a major NAD-consuming enzyme, increases mitochondrial content (Bai et al., 2011). In the present study, SIRT1 and catalase protein abundance was not consistently increased with exercise training, despite a substantive increase in skeletal muscle SIRT3 protein levels in WT mice. These findings corroborate earlier reports showing that SIRT1 expression is not strongly correlated with contraction-induced changes in mitochondrial protein abundance (Chabi et al., 2009; Ringholm et al., 2013). A proportionally larger increase in SIRT1 activity, rather than protein abundance, may explain the enhanced response to endurance training and AICAR in WT mice in our study. For example, high-intensity interval training increases overall SIRT1 activity, despite decreasing SIRT1 protein concentration in humans (Gurd et al., 2010). However, SIRT1 is an NAD-dependent sirtuin, and we have previously reported that AMPK α2 KD, PGC-1α KO, and corresponding WT littermates respond similarly in increasing protein abundance of nicotinamide phosphoribosyltransferase, the rate-limiting enzyme in NAD recycling, in response to exercise training (Brandauer et al., 2013). These data suggest that the differential response in mitochondrial protein abundance following exercise training is unrelated to SIRT1 activation via NAD. Interestingly, PARP-1 deletion leads to an activation of SIRT1, but not SIRT3, suggesting possible differences in sirtuin activation in different cellular compartments (Bai et al., 2011).

While SIRT3 and MnSOD protein abundance increased in response to exercise training in WT mice, SIRT3, and MnSOD mRNA levels were unaffected in both genotypes. On the other hand, repeated AICAR treatment increased SIRT3 and MnSOD protein levels in an AMPK α2-dependent manner, while mRNA levels of SIRT3 and MnSOD were increased in both WT and AMPK α2 KD mice. These data strongly suggest that AMPK is involved in post-transcriptional regulation of SIRT3 and MnSOD gene products with AICAR. Although previous studies have failed to demonstrate a role for AMPK α2 in regulating gene expression in mouse skeletal muscle after acute exercise (Jørgensen et al., 2005; Brandauer et al., 2013), we cannot rule out that AMPK could be important for promoting gene transcription of SIRT3 and MnSOD after exercise. Further studies are needed to clarify the differential effects of AICAR and exercise training on mRNA expression of these two genes.

We assessed the necessity of PGC-1α in mediating AICAR-induced increases in SIRT3 and MnSOD protein levels. While SIRT3 and MnSOD mRNA levels did not increase in WT or whole-body PGC-1α KO mice with either a single dose of AICAR or in response to repeated AICAR treatment, SIRT3 and MnSOD protein abundance with repeated AICAR treatment increased in WT mice but was abolished in PGC-1α KO mice. These mice also had drastically reduced SIRT3 and MnSOD protein abundance in untreated muscle, further underscoring the importance of PGC-1α in the maintenance of mitochondrial integrity. Although no data from exercise-trained PGC-1α KO muscle are presented here, exercise training restores muscle MnSOD concentration in a PGC-1α-independent manner in young mice (Geng et al., 2010), whereas the exercise training response on MnSOD protein levels has been found to be PGC-1α-dependent in old mice (Leick et al., 2010b; Olesen et al., 2013).

Our data on mitochondrial protein abundance should be interpreted in context with previously published literature on fiber type switching following exercise training or AICAR

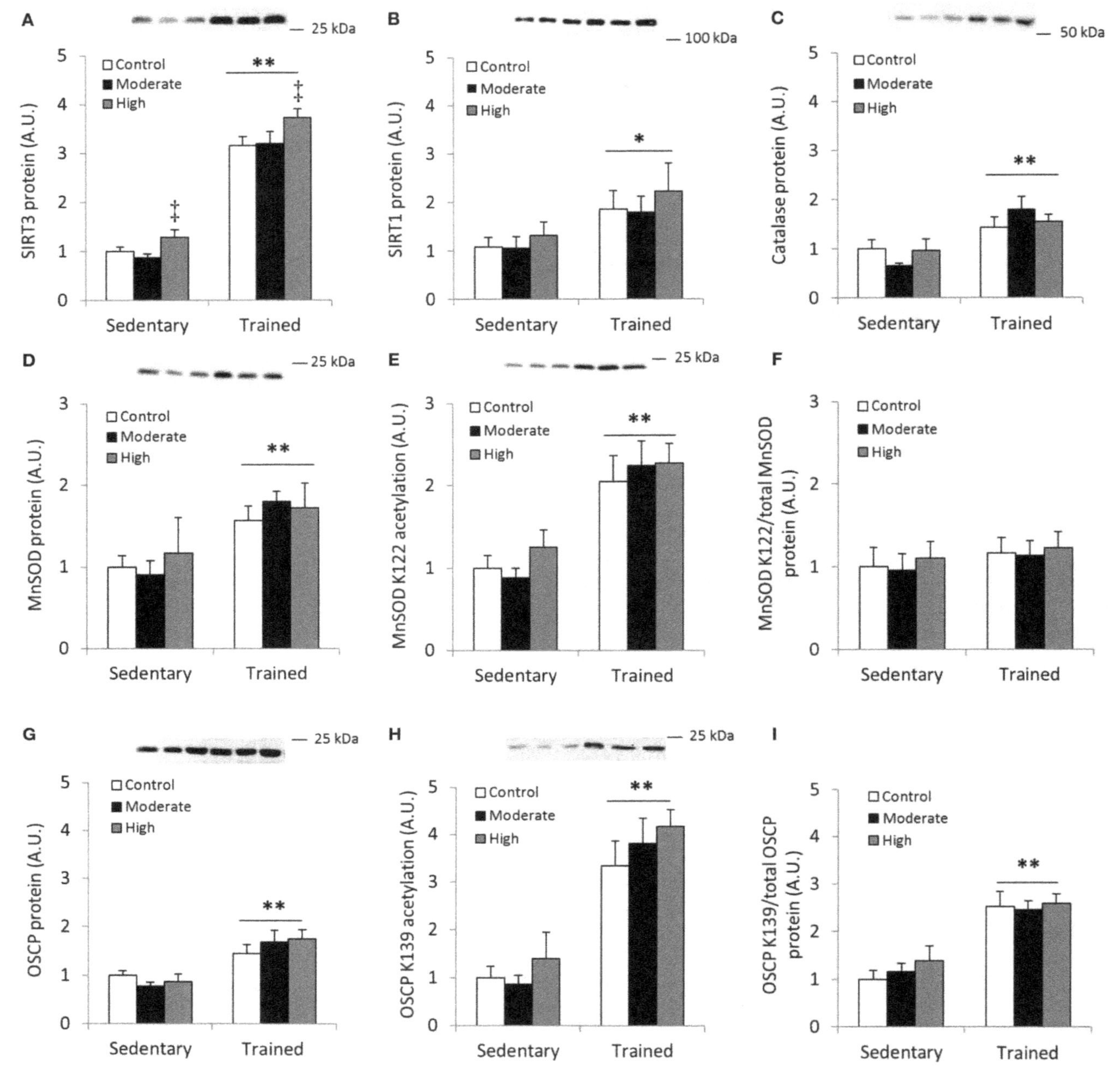

FIGURE 8 | Acute exercise does not result in deacetylation of MnSOD K122 or OSCP K139 in mouse skeletal muscle. C57BL/6JBom mice were exercise trained for 5.5 weeks ("Trained") or kept as sedentary controls ("Sedentary"). On the day of tissue collection, both groups were further divided into three groups that either rested ("Control") or performed 60 min of treadmill running at either 12 m/min (0° incline; "Moderate") or 18 m/min (10° incline; "High" intensity). **(A)** SIRT3, **(B)** SIRT1 and **(C)** Catalase protein abundance was measured in quadriceps muscles after 1 h of treadmill exercise. **(D)** Total MnSOD, **(E)** MnSOD K122 acetylation levels and **(F)** MnSOD K122 acetylation levels normalized to total MnSOD levels. **(G)** Protein levels of the Complex V subunit, F_1F_0 ATP synthase oligomycin-sensitivity conferring protein (OSCP), **(H)** OSCP K139 acetylation levels and **(I)** OSCP K139 acetylation/total OSCP. Values are mean ± SEM. $^{*/**}$ indicates main effect vs. sedentary ($p < 0.05/0.01$), ‡ main effect vs. control ($p < 0.01$), $n = 7$–9.

administration. AMPK and PGC-1α are vital regulators of cellular metabolic adaptations, and a functional AMPK α2 subunit appears to be required to fully realize training-induced IIb to IIa/x fiber type conversion (Röckl et al., 2007). Repeated AICAR treatment alone may be insufficient to change skeletal muscle fiber type (Bamford et al., 2003; Putman et al., 2003), although data from dystrophic mice indicates that AICAR may cause a phenotypic shift toward a more slow-twitch, oxidative

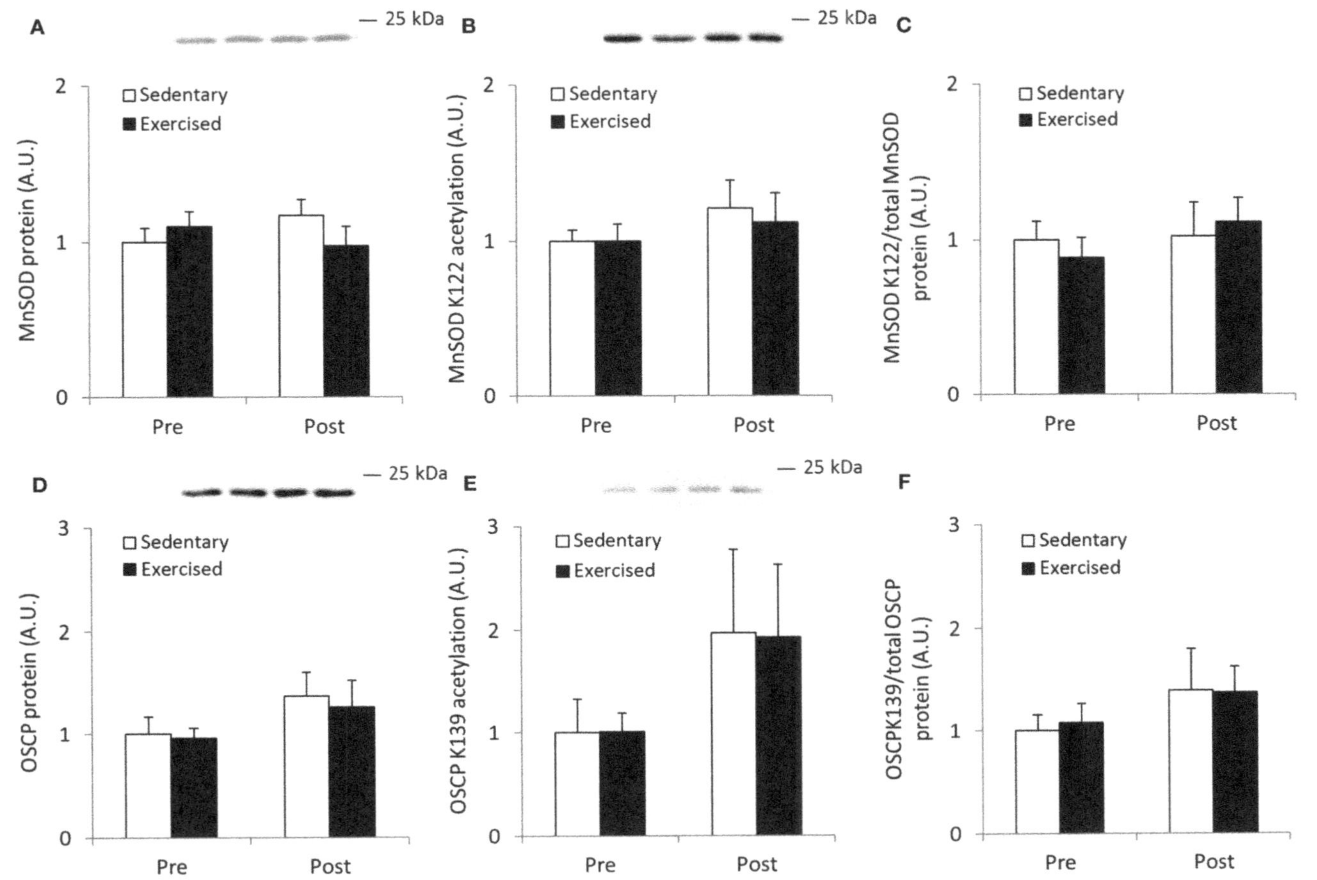

FIGURE 9 | Acetylation status of MnSOD K122 and OSCP K139 is unaffected by acute exercise in human skeletal muscle. Male subjects performed an acute bout (1 h) of one-legged extensor exercise at 80% peak work load after an over-night fast and *vastus lateralis* muscle biopsies from both legs were obtained before (Pre) and immediately after (Post) the exercise bout ($n = 7$). **(A)** MnSOD protein, **(B)** MnSOD K122 acetylation and **(C)** MnSOD K122 acetylation/MnSOD total protein abundance. **(D)** OSCP protein, **(E)** Acetylation status of OSCP K139 and **(F)** OSCP K139 normalized to total OSCP protein abundance. Values are mean ± SEM. No significant effects were observed.

fiber type under some circumstances (Ljubicic et al., 2011). PGC-1α is not only a major stimulator of mitochondrial biogenesis but also promotes type II to type I fiber type conversion (Lee et al., 2006), along with other factors such as calcineurin (Naya et al., 2000). Our data and these lines of evidence further support the notion that AMPK and PGC-1α are centrally important regulators of metabolic and contractile performance of mammalian skeletal muscle. However, the finding that AICAR treatment increases mitochondrial biogenesis, but may not necessarily change fiber type suggests that these processes may commonly occur in tandem but not be regulated by the same physiological stimuli.

SIRT3 is known to have deacetylase activity in the mitochondrion (Lombard et al., 2007). MnSOD activity is regulated through deacetylation via SIRT3 and plays an important role in handling and regulating ROS levels in mitochondria (Ahn et al., 2008; Tao et al., 2010). MnSOD has multiple acetylation sites (Rardin et al., 2013) where key lysine residues (e.g., K68 and K122) are deacetylated in response to exercise and cellular stress (Tao et al., 2010). To elucidate the interplay between aerobic fitness and stress induced by acute exercise, trained or untrained WT mice were subjected to an acute bout of "moderate" or "high"-intensity exercise, or assigned to a non-exercise control group. Despite the substantial increase in SIRT3 protein abundance, acetylation of regulatory lysine residue K122 of MnSOD or K139 of OSCP was not reduced in exercise-trained and/or acutely exercised mice at the various exercise intensities. Rather, when normalized to total protein levels, MnSOD K122 acetylation was unaltered between exercise trained and untrained mice, whereas acetylation status of K139 on OSCP was increased. This exercise training-induced increase in MnSOD implicates an enhanced cellular ROS handling capacity. However, our data on MnSOD and OSCP acetylation following acute exercise are not in obvious agreement with reported exercise-induced reductions in acetylation of these sites (Vassilopoulos et al., 2014). One difference between the two exercise protocols is that all mice in the present study completed the "moderate" and "high" intensity exercise bouts, while the exercise protocol in the previous study (Vassilopoulos et al., 2014) was exhaustive. Exhaustive exercise may be required to detect an appreciable deacetylation of MnSOD and OSCP at these lysine residues. The lack of exercise-induced changes in MnSOD and OSCP acetylation was compared with human skeletal muscle samples obtained in conjunction with a one-legged exercise protocol. Under these conditions, we also failed to observe a differential regulation of MnSOD K122 and OSCP K139 between the exercised and sedentary legs. Thus, the effects of acute exercise on MnSOD and OSCP deacetylation may vary across different experimental models and organisms. Further studies are warranted to determine the exact factors regulating SIRT3-regulated protein deacetylation with acute exercise.

The substantial increase in K139 acetylation we found after exercise training in mice may seem counterintuitive. One explanation for this observed increased OSCP acetylation could be that total cellular mitochondrial content is enhanced. Exercise training may thus have resulted in an ATP-generating potential that surpasses the actual need for ATP, leading to ATP synthase inhibition via OSCP acetylation. Another possibility is that lysine residues other than K139 on OSCP or lysines on other subunits of the ATP synthase are important for ATP synthase activity, and that acetylation status of these is changed in response to training.

The fact that concentrations of the mitochondrial SIRT3 protein were more than 3-fold higher in exercise-trained compared with untrained mice presents an intriguing observation. Why increased deacetylase protein concentration would result in unchanged or even increased acetylation levels in MnSOD or OSCP, respectively, is not immediately clear. In this context, a previous study reported that SIRT3 reduces mitochondrial protein synthesis via deacetylation of the ribosomal protein MRPL10 (Yang et al., 2010). Such an adaptation would induce an ATP-"sparing" effect that would preserve ATP pools for cross-bridge cycling and maintaining calcium homeostasis. In short, an acute increase in SIRT3 protein or activity is consistent with an inhibition of protein synthesis and other energetically costly processes by AMPK activation (Jensen et al., 2009; Hardie, 2011; White and Schenk, 2012).

In conclusion, we provide evidence for both AMPK and PGC-1α in regulating protein abundance of SIRT3 and MnSOD. These proteins are important for the regulation of mitochondrial adaptation and the handling of ROS, respectively. The interactive effects of acute and chronic exercise on MnSOD and OSCP acetylation status constitute an unexplored avenue, with implications for intensity- and duration-dependent mitochondrial adaptations that warrant further investigation.

Author Contributions

Experiments and analyses of samples in the present manuscript were conducted in Section of Integrated Physiology at the Novo Nordisk Foundation Center for Basic Metabolic Research, University of Copenhagen.

1. Conception and design of the experiments: JB, MAA, SGV, JTT.
2. Collection, analysis and interpretation of data: JB, MAA, HK, SR, CF, SGV, JTT.
3. Drafting the manuscript: JB, MAA, JTT.
4. Edited, revised and approved the final version of the manuscript: All.

Financial Support

Support for this study was provided by the Novo Nordisk Foundation Center for Basic Metabolic Research and the Novo Nordisk Foundation (Excellence Project Award) to JTT. JB was supported by a Research and Professional Development Grant by Gettysburg College.

Acknowledgments

The authors wish to acknowledge the following people from Section of Molecular Physiology, Department of Nutrition, Exercise and Sports, University of Copenhagen for generous access to human skeletal muscle samples: Prof. Jørgen F. P. Wojtaszewski, Prof. Erik A. Richter, Prof. Bente Kiens, Dr. Jonas M. Kristensen, and Dr. Christian Pehmøller. Prof. Henriette Pilegaard and Dr. Lotte Leick, Molecular Integrative Physiology, Department of Biology, University of Copenhagen, and Mr. Joachim Fentz, Section of Molecular Physiology, Department of Nutrition, Exercise and Sports, University of Copenhagen are acknowledged for providing generous access to samples from PGC-1α knockout mice. Marianne M. Andersen, Betina Bolmgren, and Christine B. Janssens are acknowledged for skilled technical expertise. Prof. Morris J. Birnbaum (Howard Hughes Medical Institute and University of Pennsylvania School of Medicine) and Prof. Bruce Spiegelman (Dana-Farber Cancer Institute, Harvard Medical School) are acknowledged for providing founder AMPK α2 KD and PGC-1α KO mice, respectively. Prof. David Gius (Northwestern University Feinberg School of Medicine, Chicago, Illinois, USA) is acknowledged for kindly providing antibodies targeting acetylated K122 of MnSOD and K139 of OSCP. Finally, the authors wish to thank Prof. Juleen R. Zierath (Department of Molecular Medicine, Karolinska Institutet) for helpful discussions during the manuscript preparation.

References

Abbott, M. J., and Turcotte, L. P. (2014). AMPK-α2 is involved in exercise training-induced adaptations in insulin-stimulated metabolism in skeletal muscle following high-fat diet. *J. Appl. Physiol.* 117, 869–879. doi: 10.1152/japplphysiol.01380.2013

Ahn, B.-H., Kim, H.-S., Song, S., Lee, I. H., Liu, J., Vassilopoulos, A., et al. (2008). A role for the mitochondrial deacetylase Sirt3 in regulating energy homeostasis. *Proc. Natl. Acad. Sci. U.S.A.* 105, 14447–14452. doi: 10.1073/pnas.0803790105

Andersen, P., Adams, R. P., Sjogaard, G., Thorboe, A., and Saltin, B. (1985). Dynamic knee extension as model for study of isolated exercising muscle in humans. *J. Appl. Physiol.* 59, 1647–1653.

Bai, P., Cantó, C., Oudart, H., Brunyánszki, A., Cen, Y., Thomas, C., et al. (2011). PARP-1 inhibition increases mitochondrial metabolism through SIRT1 activation. *Cell Metab.* 13, 461–468. doi: 10.1016/j.cmet.2011.03.004

Bamford, J. A., Lopaschuk, G. D., MacLean, I. M., Reinhart, M. L., Dixon, W. T., and Putman, C. T. (2003). Effects of chronic AICAR administration on the metabolic and contractile phenotypes of rat slow- and fast-twitch skeletal muscles. *Can. J. Physiol. Pharmacol.* 81, 1072–1082. doi: 10.1139/y03-110

Brandauer, J., Vienberg, S. G., Andersen, M. A., Ringholm, S., Risis, S., Larsen, P. S., et al. (2013). AMP-activated protein kinase regulates nicotinamide phosphoribosyl transferase expression in skeletal muscle. *J. Physiol.* 591(Pt 20), 5207–5220. doi: 10.1113/jphysiol.2013.259515

Buler, M., Aatsinki, S.-M., Izzi, V., Uusimaa, J., and Hakkola, J. (2014). SIRT5 is under the control of PGC-1α and AMPK and is involved in regulation of mitochondrial energy metabolism. *FASEB J.* 28, 3225–3237. doi: 10.1096/fj.13-245241

Cantó, C., Gerhart-Hines, Z., Feige, J. N., Lagouge, M., Noriega, L., Milne, J. C., et al. (2009). AMPK regulates energy expenditure by modulating NAD+ metabolism and SIRT1 activity. *Nature* 458, 1056–1060. doi: 10.1038/nature07813

Cantó, C., Jiang, L. Q., Deshmukh, A. S., Mataki, C., Coste, A., Lagouge, M., et al. (2010). Interdependence of AMPK and SIRT1 for metabolic adaptation to fasting and exercise in skeletal muscle. *Cell Metab.* 11, 213–219. doi: 10.1016/j.cmet.2010.02.006

Chabi, B., Adhihetty, P. J., O'Leary, M. F. N., Menzies, K. J., and Hood, D. A. (2009). Relationship between Sirt1 expression and mitochondrial proteins during conditions of chronic muscle use and disuse. *J. Appl. Physiol.* 107, 1730–1735. doi: 10.1152/japplphysiol.91451.2008

Chen, Y., Zhang, J., Lin, Y., Lei, Q., Guan, K.-L., Zhao, S., et al. (2011). Tumour suppressor SIRT3 deacetylates and activates manganese superoxide dismutase to scavenge ROS. *EMBO Rep.* 12, 534–541. doi: 10.1038/embor.2011.65

Egan, B., and Zierath, J. R. (2013). Exercise metabolism and the molecular regulation of skeletal muscle adaptation. *Cell Metab.* 17, 162–184. doi: 10.1016/j.cmet.2012.12.012

Frøsig, C., Jørgensen, S. B., Hardie, D. G., Richter, E. A., and Wojtaszewski, J. F. P. (2004). 5′-AMP-activated protein kinase activity and protein expression are regulated by endurance training in human skeletal muscle. *Am. J. Physiol. Endocrinol. Metab.* 286, E411–E417. doi: 10.1152/ajpendo.00317.2003

Geng, T., Li, P., Okutsu, M., Yin, X., Kwek, J., Zhang, M., et al. (2010). PGC-1alpha plays a functional role in exercise-induced mitochondrial biogenesis and angiogenesis but not fiber-type transformation in mouse skeletal muscle. *Am. J. Physiol. Cell Physiol.* 298, C572–C579. doi: 10.1152/ajpcell.00481.2009

Gerhart-Hines, Z., Rodgers, J. T., Bare, O., Lerin, C., Kim, S.-H., Mostoslavsky, R., et al. (2007). Metabolic control of muscle mitochondrial function and fatty acid oxidation through SIRT1/PGC-1alpha. *EMBO J.* 26, 1913–1923. doi: 10.1038/sj.emboj.7601633

Gurd, B. J., Holloway, G. P., Yoshida, Y., and Bonen, A. (2012). In mammalian muscle, SIRT3 is present in mitochondria and not in the nucleus; and SIRT3 is upregulated by chronic muscle contraction in an adenosine monophosphate-activated protein kinase-independent manner. *Metab. Clin. Exp.* 61, 733–741. doi: 10.1016/j.metabol.2011.09.016

Gurd, B. J., Perry, C. G. R., Heigenhauser, G. J. F., Spriet, L. L., and Bonen, A. (2010). High-intensity interval training increases SIRT1 activity in human skeletal muscle. *Appl. Physiol. Nutr. Metab.* 35, 350–357. doi: 10.1139/H10-030

Hallows, W. C., Lee, S., and Denu, J. M. (2006). Sirtuins deacetylate and activate mammalian acetyl-CoA synthetases. *Proc. Natl. Acad. Sci. U.S.A.* 103, 10230–10235. doi: 10.1073/pnas.0604392103

Hardie, D. G. (2011). Energy sensing by the AMP-activated protein kinase and its effects on muscle metabolism. *Proc. Nutr. Soc.* 70, 92–99. doi: 10.1017/S0029665110003915

Jacobs, K. M., Pennington, J. D., Bisht, K. S., Aykin-Burns, N., Kim, H.-S., Mishra, M., et al. (2008). SIRT3 interacts with the daf-16 homolog FOXO3a in the mitochondria, as well as increases FOXO3a dependent gene expression. *Int. J. Biol. Sci.* 4, 291–299.

Jäger, S., Handschin, C., St-Pierre, J., and Spiegelman, B. M. (2007). AMP-activated protein kinase (AMPK) action in skeletal muscle via direct phosphorylation of PGC-1alpha. *Proc. Natl. Acad. Sci. U.S.A.* 104, 12017–12022. doi: 10.1073/pnas.0705070104

Jenkins, R. R., Friedland, R., and Howald, H. (1984). The relationship of oxygen uptake to superoxide dismutase and catalase activity in human skeletal muscle. *Int. J. Sports Med.* 5, 11–14. doi: 10.1055/s-2008-1025872

Jensen, T. E., Wojtaszewski, J. F. P., and Richter, E. A. (2009). AMP-activated protein kinase in contraction regulation of skeletal muscle metabolism: necessary and/or sufficient? *Acta Physiol. (Oxf).* 196, 155–174. doi: 10.1111/j.1748-1716.2009.01979.x

Jørgensen, S. B., Treebak, J. T., Viollet, B., Schjerling, P., Vaulont, S., Wojtaszewski, J. F. P., et al. (2007). Role of AMPKalpha2 in basal, training-, and AICAR-induced GLUT4, hexokinase II, and mitochondrial protein expression in mouse muscle. *Am. J. Physiol. Endocrinol. Metab.* 292, E331–E339. doi: 10.1152/ajpendo.00243.2006

Jørgensen, S. B., Wojtaszewski, J. F. P., Viollet, B., Andreelli, F., Birk, J. B., Hellsten, Y., et al. (2005). Effects of alpha-AMPK knockout on exercise-induced gene activation in mouse skeletal muscle. *FASEB J.* 19, 1146–1148. doi: 10.1096/fj.04-3144fje

Koh, H.-J., Brandauer, J., and Goodyear, L. J. (2008). LKB1 and AMPK and the regulation of skeletal muscle metabolism. *Curr. Opin. Clin. Nutr. Metab. Care* 11, 227–232. doi: 10.1097/MCO.0b013e3282fb7b76

Kong, X., Wang, R., Xue, Y., Liu, X., Zhang, H., Chen, Y., et al. (2010). Sirtuin 3, a new target of PGC-1alpha, plays an important role in the suppression of ROS and mitochondrial biogenesis. *PLoS ONE* 5:e11707. doi: 10.1371/journal.pone.0011707

Lanza, I. R., Short, D. K., Short, K. R., Raghavakaimal, S., Basu, R., Joyner, M. J., et al. (2008). Endurance exercise as a countermeasure for aging. *Diabetes* 57, 2933–2942. doi: 10.2337/db08-0349

Lee, W. J., Kim, M., Park, H.-S., Kim, H. S., Jeon, M. J., Oh, K. S., et al. (2006). AMPK activation increases fatty acid oxidation in skeletal muscle by activating PPARalpha and PGC-1. *Biochem. Biophys. Res. Commun.* 340, 291–295. doi: 10.1016/j.bbrc.2005.12.011

Leick, L., Fentz, J., Biensø, R. S., Knudsen, J. G., Jeppesen, J., Kiens, B., et al. (2010a). PGC-1{alpha} is required for AICAR-induced expression of GLUT4 and mitochondrial proteins in mouse skeletal muscle. *Am. J. Physiol. Endocrinol. Metab.* 299, E456–E465. doi: 10.1152/ajpendo.00648.2009

Leick, L., Hellsten, Y., Fentz, J., Lyngby, S. S., Wojtaszewski, J. F. P., Hidalgo, J., et al. (2009). PGC-1alpha mediates exercise-induced skeletal muscle VEGF expression in mice. *Am. J. Physiol. Endocrinol. Metab.* 297, E92–E103. doi: 10.1152/ajpendo.00076.2009

Leick, L., Lyngby, S. S., Wojtaszewski, J. F. P., Wojtasewski, J. F. P., and Pilegaard, H. (2010b). PGC-1alpha is required for training-induced prevention of age-associated decline in mitochondrial enzymes in mouse skeletal muscle. *Exp. Gerontol.* 45, 336–342. doi: 10.1016/j.exger.2010.01.011

Ljubicic, V., Miura, P., Burt, M., Boudreault, L., Khogali, S., Lunde, J. A., et al. (2011). Chronic AMPK activation evokes the slow, oxidative myogenic program and triggers beneficial adaptations in mdx mouse skeletal muscle. *Hum. Mol. Genet.* 20, 3478–3493. doi: 10.1093/hmg/ddr265

Lombard, D. B., Alt, F. W., Cheng, H.-L., Bunkenborg, J., Streeper, R. S., Mostoslavsky, R., et al. (2007). Mammalian Sir2 homolog SIRT3 regulates global mitochondrial lysine acetylation. *Mol. Cell. Biol.* 27, 8807–8814. doi: 10.1128/MCB.01636-07

McArdle, A., van der Meulen, J., Close, G. L., Pattwell, D., Van Remmen, H., Huang, T. T., et al. (2004). Role of mitochondrial superoxide dismutase in contraction-induced generation of reactive oxygen species in skeletal muscle extracellular space. *Am. J. Physiol. Cell Physiol.* 286, C1152–C1158. doi: 10.1152/ajpcell.00322.2003

Mu, J., Brozinick, J. T. Jr., Valladares, O., Bucan, M., and Birnbaum, M. J. (2001). A role for AMP-activated protein kinase in contraction- and hypoxia-regulated glucose transport in skeletal muscle. *Mol. Cell* 7, 1085–1094. doi: 10.1016/S1097-2765(01)00251-9

Naya, F. J., Mercer, B., Shelton, J., Richardson, J. A., Williams, R. S., and Olson, E. N. (2000). Stimulation of slow skeletal muscle fiber gene expression by calcineurin *in vivo*. *J. Biol. Chem.* 275, 4545–4548. doi: 10.1074/jbc.275.7.4545

Nemoto, S., Fergusson, M. M., and Finkel, T. (2005). SIRT1 functionally interacts with the metabolic regulator and transcriptional coactivator PGC-1{alpha}. *J. Biol. Chem.* 280, 16456–16460. doi: 10.1074/jbc.M501485200

Olesen, J., Ringholm, S., Nielsen, M. M., Brandt, C. T., Pedersen, J. T., Halling, J. F., et al. (2013). Role of PGC-1α in exercise training- and resveratrol-induced prevention of age-associated inflammation. *Exp. Gerontol.* 48, 1274–1284. doi: 10.1016/j.exger.2013.07.015

Palacios, O. M., Carmona, J. J., Michan, S., Chen, K. Y., Manabe, Y. J. L. W. III., Goodyear, L. J., et al. (2009). Diet and exercise signals regulate SIRT3 and activate AMPK and PGC-1α in skeletal muscle. *Aging (Albany. NY)* 1, 771–783.

Parise, G., Phillips, S. M., Kaczor, J. J., and Tarnopolsky, M. A. (2005). Antioxidant enzyme activity is up-regulated after unilateral resistance exercise training in older adults. *Free Radic. Biol. Med.* 39, 289–295. doi: 10.1016/j.freeradbiomed.2005.03.024

Puigserver, P., Wu, Z., Park, C. W., Graves, R., Wright, M., and Spiegelman, B. M. (1998). A cold-inducible coactivator of nuclear receptors linked to adaptive thermogenesis. *Cell* 92, 829–839. doi: 10.1016/S0092-8674(00)81410-5

Putman, C. T., Kiricsi, M., Pearcey, J., MacLean, I. M., Bamford, J. A., Murdoch, G. K., et al. (2003). AMPK activation increases uncoupling protein-3 expression and mitochondrial enzyme activities in rat muscle without fibre type transitions. *J. Physiol.* 551, 169–178. doi: 10.1111/j.1469-7793.2003.00169.x

Qiu, X., Brown, K., Hirschey, M. D., Verdin, E., and Chen, D. (2010). Calorie restriction reduces oxidative stress by SIRT3-mediated SOD2 activation. *Cell Metab.* 12, 662–667. doi: 10.1016/j.cmet.2010.11.015

Rardin, M. J., Newman, J. C., Held, J. M., Cusack, M. P., Sorensen, D. J., Li, B., et al. (2013). Label-free quantitative proteomics of the lysine acetylome in mitochondria identifies substrates of SIRT3 in metabolic pathways. *Proc. Natl. Acad. Sci. U.S.A.* 110, 6601–6606. doi: 10.1073/pnas.1302961110

Reid, M. B. (2001). Invited review: redox modulation of skeletal muscle contraction: what we know and what we don't. *J. Appl. Physiol.* 90, 724–731.

Ringholm, S., Olesen, J., Pedersen, J. T., Brandt, C. T., Halling, J. F., Hellsten, Y., et al. (2013). Effect of lifelong resveratrol supplementation and exercise training on skeletal muscle oxidative capacity in aging mice; impact of PGC-1α. *Exp. Gerontol.* 48, 1311–1318. doi: 10.1016/j.exger.2013.08.012

Röckl, K. S. C., Hirshman, M. F., Brandauer, J., Fujii, N., Witters, L. A., and Goodyear, L. J. (2007). Skeletal muscle adaptation to exercise training: AMP-activated protein kinase mediates muscle fiber type shift. *Diabetes* 56, 2062–2069. doi: 10.2337/db07-0255

Schwer, B., Bunkenborg, J., Verdin, R. O., Andersen, J. S., and Verdin, E. (2006). Reversible lysine acetylation controls the activity of the mitochondrial enzyme acetyl-CoA synthetase 2. *Proc. Natl. Acad. Sci. U.S.A.* 103, 10224–10229. doi: 10.1073/pnas.0603968103

Schwer, B., North, B. J., Frye, R. A., Ott, M., and Verdin, E. (2002). The human silent information regulator (Sir)2 homologue hSIRT3 is a mitochondrial nicotinamide adenine dinucleotide-dependent deacetylase. *J. Cell Biol.* 158, 647–657. doi: 10.1083/jcb.200205057

Shinmura, K., Tamaki, K., Saito, K., Nakano, Y., Tobe, T., and Bolli, R. (2007). Cardioprotective effects of short-term caloric restriction are mediated by adiponectin via activation of AMP-activated protein kinase. *Circulation* 116, 2809–2817. doi: 10.1161/CIRCULATIONAHA.107.725697

Someya, S., Yu, W., Hallows, W. C., Xu, J., Vann, J. M., Leeuwenburgh, C., et al. (2010). Sirt3 mediates reduction of oxidative damage and prevention of age-related hearing loss under caloric restriction. *Cell* 143, 802–812. doi: 10.1016/j.cell.2010.10.002

Spina, R. J., Chi, M. M., Hopkins, M. G., Nemeth, P. M., Lowry, O. H., and Holloszy, J. O. (1996). Mitochondrial enzymes increase in muscle in response to 7-10 days of cycle exercise. *J Appl Physiol* 80, 2250–2254.

Tanner, C. B., Madsen, S. R., Hallowell, D. M., Goring, D. M. J., Moore, T. M., Hardman, S. E., et al. (2013). Mitochondrial and performance adaptations to exercise training in mice lacking skeletal muscle LKB1. *Am. J. Physiol. Endocrinol. Metab.* 305, E1018–E1029. doi: 10.1152/ajpendo.00227.2013

Tao, R., Coleman, M. C., Pennington, J. D., Ozden, O., Park, S.-H., Jiang, H., et al. (2010). Sirt3-mediated deacetylation of evolutionarily conserved lysine 122 regulates MnSOD activity in response to stress. *Mol. Cell* 40, 893–904. doi: 10.1016/j.molcel.2010.12.013

Tiidus, P. M., Pushkarenko, J., and Houston, M. E. (1996). Lack of antioxidant adaptation to short-term aerobic training in human muscle. *Am. J. Physiol. Regul. Integr. Comp. Physiol.* 271, R832–R836.

Tonkonogi, M., Walsh, B., Svensson, M., and Sahlin, K. (2000). Mitochondrial function and antioxidative defence in human muscle: effects of endurance training and oxidative stress. *J. Physiol.* 528, 379–388. doi: 10.1111/j.1469-7793.2000.00379.x

Treebak, J. T., Pehmøller, C., Kristensen, J. M., Kjøbsted, R., Birk, J. B., Schjerling, P., et al. (2014). Acute exercise and physiological insulin induce distinct phosphorylation signatures on TBC1D1 and TBC1D4 proteins in human skeletal muscle. *J. Physiol.* 592, 351–375. doi: 10.1113/jphysiol.2013.266338

Tseng, A. H. H., Shieh, S.-S., and Wang, D. L. (2013). SIRT3 deacetylates FOXO3 to protect mitochondria against oxidative damage. *Free Radic. Biol. Med.* 63, 222–234. doi: 10.1016/j.freeradbiomed.2013.05.002

Vassilopoulos, A., Pennington, J. D., Andresson, T., Rees, D. M., Bosley, A. D., Fearnley, I. M., et al. (2014). SIRT3 deacetylates ATP synthase F1 complex proteins in response to nutrient- and exercise-induced stress. *Antioxid. Redox Signal.* 21, 551–564. doi: 10.1089/ars.2013.5420

White, A. T., and Schenk, S. (2012). NAD+/NADH and skeletal muscle mitochondrial adaptations to exercise. *Am. J. Physiol. Endocrinol. Metab.* 303, E308–E321. doi: 10.1152/ajpendo.00054.2012

Wu, Y.-T., Lee, H.-C., Liao, C.-C., and Wei, Y.-H. (2013). Regulation of mitochondrial F(o)F(1)ATPase activity by Sirt3-catalyzed deacetylation and its deficiency in human cells harboring 4977bp deletion of mitochondrial DNA. *Biochim. Biophys. Acta* 1832, 216–227. doi: 10.1016/j.bbadis.2012.10.002

Yang, Y., Cimen, H., Han, M.-J., Shi, T., Deng, J.-H., Koc, H., et al. (2010). NAD+-dependent deacetylase SIRT3 regulates mitochondrial protein synthesis by deacetylation of the ribosomal protein MRPL10. *J. Biol. Chem.* 285, 7417–7429. doi: 10.1074/jbc.M109.053421

2

Video Games and other Online Activities may Improve Health in Ageing

Marios Kyriazis[1] and Elisavet Kiourti[2]*

[1] ELPIS Foundation for Indefinite Lifespans, Larnaca, Cyprus, [2] University of Cyprus, Nicosia, Cyprus

Keywords: hormesis, stress response, video games, information exposure, literacy practices

Edited by:
Helena Canhao,
Unidade EpiDoC, Epidemiologia de doenças crônicas, Portugal

Reviewed by:
Constança Paúl,
Universidade do Porto, Portugal
Sarah Damanti,
Università degli Studi di Milano, Italy

****Correspondence:***
Marios Kyriazis
drmarios@live.it

INTRODUCTION

Humans are highly adaptable organisms. Our environment is now increasingly more digital, and we need to assimilate a vast amount of information, much of which requires us to act (1). This has an impact on our neuronal stress response mechanisms, which are activated in order to minimize any disturbance to our homeostasis, or more precisely to our homoeodynamic space (2). Therefore, function is dynamically maintained within healthy limits.

In this paper, we propose that by exposing ourselves to informative, co-interactive digital platforms which are defined by a variety of "Information-that-requires-action in time and on demand," we are subjected to beneficial positive stress which upregulates neuronal function. This neuronal upregulation has a positive impact on the rest of the somatic repair processes which may reduce age-related degeneration (3). Beneficial positive stress is invoked when the information is important or significant, in the sense that it entices the organism to act, and thus adapt (i.e., reach a state which is functionally better compared to the previous one). When such information reaches the neuron, it acts as a cognitive stimulus which induces the neuron to upregulate its metabolism in order to process this new information (4). It has been argued that such exposure to novel digital information can influence our somatic repair processes through hormetic events (3). Hormesis is a widespread phenomenon in nature that is defined by a non-linear "low dose stimulation, high dose inhibition" principle. This means that exposure to a relatively weak stimulus may positively challenge the organism and upregulate the stress response. This results in health benefits, whereas an excessive, suboptimal, or prolonged exposure may result in damage and disease (5). Hormetic challenges (positive stress) may be used in order to reduce age-related dysfunction in general (6).

DISCUSSION

Video Games in Later Life

There is increasingly strong evidence that online video games have beneficial cognitive effects in older adults (7). For instance, video game training improves several aspects of cognitive functioning (8), such as reaction time, memory, and attention span, as well as general cognitive control and multitasking (9). Complex 3-D video games improve hippocampal-associated memory (10) and also physical parameters, such as postural balance and muscle strength (11), particularly those games that concentrate on strategy (12). Video games may also be useful in dementia (13). One way these activities may effect health enhancement is through a hormetic mechanism. In this case, the instigation of hormesis is based on a continual state of cognitive novelty, when one operates at the "outer edge of their comfort zone," performing mental activities that are "challenging but do-able." In practice, this translates as an activity that provokes rather than annoys, and it is pleasantly frustrating.

Cognitive Stimulation through Video Games

In the case of online video games, we find an example which is at the intersection where digital information, human brain, and human biology interact. Many thousands of players all over the world participate in virtual online worlds and interact with a variety of video game genres. Globally, gamers play competitively and cooperatively in their communities of practice (14, 15), in a way that is beyond just entertainment. Video games are complex digi-social microcosms which are constructed by social conventions and rules that may be different from actual world rules. For example, the rules may defy the physical law of gravitation and others, such as mortality and social conventions. These microcosms are carriers of complex layers of meaning, reflecting a certain set of ideologies about society and its power relationships. These virtual microcosms induce hormetic health benefits (16). It is not just a matter of being physically able to perform an action, but it is also an opportunity to interact with new kinds of text genres that require different literacy skills than the conventional ones encountered when we passively read a book. These new text genres are very relevant not only for the individual player but also for the rest of the team because the players can use the information to initiate actions which influence the behavior of other players. Players are becoming agents who provide meaning of the text within the game (17, 18). The linguistic interactions and overall performance of the player is also relevant, because these engage the player into debates with other players and thus strengthen social bonds. These social bonds may, again, break the rules of politeness (19) and open new horizons of performative and linguistic interactions which are, perhaps, totally new for the older person. New verbal and non-verbal expressions may develop in order to help increase the pleasure of playing the game. Imagination and simulation of an experience prepare the player to tackle problems in real life situations. Thus, the elements of novelty and creativity flourish. Strategic problem-solving (20), creative thinking, overlapping goal development, involvement with digital literacy practices (21), learning of new skills, and many other cognitive skills become the fruits of such game activities (22–25). Therefore, the aging player may develop skill sets and cognitive capabilities which could be very useful, even essential, in the course of their life. Examples of action- and goal-directed simulations of embodied experience video games include multiplayer games, like World of Warcraft, League of Legends, Minecraft, and Ikariam. The brain activities involved during the course of such games enhance cognition in multiple ways and are thus considered as hormetic. In addition to these, there exist other video games which are more oriented toward literary creativity with prose and poetry, such as the video game Elegy for a Dead World (26).

Internet and Health

Being cognitively stimulated in a virtual setting is shown to have several health benefits. For instance, playing online action video games affects the plasticity of sensorimotor regions in the gray matter, and improves connectivity between neurons, particularly those involved in attention and experience (27). Use of general video games for 1 h a day improves spatial memory, cognitive control, and complex verbal span (28). These cognitive benefits are not specific to action video games, but other active online experiences may also improve cognition. General use of the Internet has been studied in a variety of settings and initial results show health promoting effects (29) including an increase in life expectancy (30). For instance, a study in Taiwan found that internet use (broadband, wireless, or mobile) is positively associated with quality of life, self-esteem, and reduction in stress (31).

In addition, it was shown that higher levels of Internet use among older people are associated with lower levels of loneliness, improved social support and psychological well-being, and better life satisfaction (32). Web-based interventions which are specific to memory and cognition have a special role to play in cases of mild cognitive impairment and dementia (33).

How does online cognitive stimulation upregulate health? When a mildly stressful information from an online cognitive activity (i.e., information which requires a fast response and instant feedback, such in video games) reaches the neuron, it activates the neuronal stress response which facilitates adaptation to this stressful situation. Neurotransmitters and molecules involved in memory and in cognition are also involved. Such molecules include cyclic guanosine monophosphate, glutamate, leptin, and angiotensin IV. Another marker in hormesis is Heat Shock Proteins (HSP) which is expressed in cases of shock (challenge). Overexpression of HSP is neuroprotective (34).

The risk always exists that excessive use of the Internet, particularly in a way that is repetitive and non-meaningful, may lead to social isolation of the user. In this paper, we highlight the importance of the meaningfulness of information sharing, i.e., information that requires the user to act. In addition, despite concerns that use of online platforms may lead to social isolation, some researchers (35), report that it may, on the contrary, actually decrease loneliness and social isolation. However, older people may experience physical limitations such as arthritis, visual problems, etc. which may impede full use of online activities. The market needs to take into account these age-related limitations.

Cognitive Challenges May Impact on Physical Health

It is well accepted that physical exercise has cognitive benefits and that cognitive exercise has cognitive benefits [for example, Ref. (36)]. What is less well studied, but nevertheless important, is the *physical* benefits obtained through *cognitive* training. Some research exists in this respect. We know, for example, that while cognitive exercise may increase the speed of information processing (37), it can also improve certain physical health parameters in older people, including vitality, physical functioning, and bodily pain, as well as social and emotional functioning, and instrumental activities of daily living (38). This type of hormetically intense cognitive training not only improves physical functioning but its effects were found to persist for several years (39). A significant number of older people who followed a program of cognitive exercises rated their physical health and quality of life as excellent or very good (40). While clearly more research is needed in this respect, there could be some possible physical health benefits obtained through cognitive stimulation. The hormetic health benefits of cognitive challenges can be augmented by playing online video games or similar engaging activities.

There is growing evidence that these concepts are valid within human groups in the community. D'Orsi et al. (41) have shown that internet use was significantly associated with a lower risk of 10-year mortality, controlling for sex, age, education, cognitive function, functional impairment, and diabetes. In another study, d'Orsi et al. (42), found a specific association between increased use of internet and reduction of dementia risk. Therefore, we could speculate on the potential physical effects obtained through a combination of both physical and cognitive activities, while awaiting further corroboration.

CONCLUSION

The increasing presence of online environments, such as action video games and other digital media platforms that share similar characteristics, translate into opportunities for information sharing among the users. In several instances, this information is actually quite meaningful, in the sense that it incites the recipient to act, and it can thus be considered hormetic. We have argued elsewhere (16) that such information may act as a cognitive challenge that upregulates neuronal stress response pathways, the same way as other hormetic challenges and stressors that result in "positive stress" such as physical exercise, heat or cold exposure, radiation, and medication.

Thus, the main points of this paper are several. Cognitive challenges may act along universally encountered hormetic principles, in order to invoke the neuronal stress response. This, as a consequence, upregulates neuronal health and it is likely to result in cognitive health improvement in older people. One example of such cognitive challenge is interaction with online video games, although other challenging cognitive activities may carry similar benefits. We need to encourage increasing use of online action video games for older people.

AUTHOR CONTRIBUTIONS

Both contributors have contributed to the conception of the work; MK has discussed biologically related concepts and EK has worked on the acquisition of data and presentation of concepts relating to computer gaming. MK has drafted the work and both have revised it critically; both have agreed the corrections following peer review. Both approve the paper for publication of the content and agree to be accountable for all aspects of the work in ensuring that questions related to the accuracy or integrity of any part of the work are appropriately investigated and resolved.

FUNDING

No funding was available for this paper.

REFERENCES

1. Kyriazis M. Systems neuroscience in focus: from the human brain to the global brain? *Front Syst Neurosci* (2015) 9:7. doi:10.3389/fnsys.2015.00007
2. Demirovic D, Rattan SI. Establishing cellular stress response profiles as biomarkers of homeodynamics, health and hormesis. *Exp Gerontol* (2012) 48(1):94–8. doi:10.1016/j.exger.2012.02.005
3. Kyriazis M. Neurons vs germline: a war of hormetic tradeoffs. *Curr Aging Sci* (2017) 10(4):242–5. doi:10.2174/1874609810666170413123547
4. Kyriazis M. Reversal of informational entropy and the acquisition of germ-like immortality by somatic cells. *Curr Aging Sci* (2014) 7(1):9–16. doi:10.2174/1874609807666140521101102
5. Kim B, Brandli A, Mitrofanis J, Stone J, Purushothuman S, Johnstone DM. Remote tissue conditioning – an emerging approach for inducing body-wide protection against diseases of ageing. *Ageing Res Rev* (2017) 37:69–78. doi:10.1016/j.arr.2017.05.005
6. Rattan SI, Gonzalez-Dosal R, Nielsen ER, Kraft DC, Weibel J, Kahns S. Slowing down aging from within: mechanistic aspects of anti-aging hormetic effects of mild heat stress on human cells. *Acta Biochim Pol* (2004) 51(2):481–92.
7. De Schutter B, Vanden Abeele V. Towards a gerontoludic manifesto. *Anthropol Aging* (2015) 36(2):112–20. doi:10.5195/AA.2015.104
8. Toril P, Reales JM, Ballesteros S. Video game training enhances cognition of older adults: a meta-analytic study. *Psychol Aging* (2014) 29(3):706–16. doi:10.1037/a0037507
9. Anguera JA, Boccanfuso J, Rintoul JL, Al-Hashimi O, Faraji F, Janowich J, et al. Video game training enhances cognitive control in older adults. *Nature* (2013) 501(7465):97–101. doi:10.1038/nature12486
10. Clemenson GD, Stark CE. Virtual environmental enrichment through video games improves hippocampal-associated memory. *J Neurosci* (2015) 35(49):16116–25. doi:10.1523/JNEUROSCI.2580-15.2015
11. Lee Y, Choi W, Lee K, Song C, Lee S. Virtual reality training with three-dimensional video games improves postural balance and lower extremity strength in community-dwelling older adults. *J Aging Phys Act* (2017) 25(4):621–7. doi:10.1123/japa.2015-0271
12. Ray NR, O'Connell MA, Nashiro K, Smith ET, Qin S, Basak C. Evaluating the relationship between white matter integrity, cognition, and varieties of video game learning. *Restor Neurol Neurosci* (2017) 35(5):437–56. doi:10.3233/RNN-160716
13. Narme P. Benefits of game-based leisure activities in normal aging and dementia. *Geriatr Psychol Neuropsychiatr Vieil* (2016) 14(4):420–8. doi:10.1684/pnv.2016.0632
14. Wenger E. *Communities of Practice: Learning, Meaning, and Identity (Learning in Doing: Social, Cognitive and Computational Perspectives)*. Cambridge: Cambridge University Press (1998).
15. Wenger-Trayner E, Wenger-Trayner B. *Communities of Practice: A Brief Introduction*. (2015). Available from: http://wenger-trayner.com/wp-content/uploads/2015/04/07-Brief-introduction-to-communities-of-practice.pdf
16. Kyriazis M, Kiourti E. Chapter 27. Interactions with technology as a cognitive healthy ageing hormetic stimulus. In: Rattan S, Kyriazis M, editors. *The Science of Hormesis in Health and Longevity*. Amsterdam: Elsevier (2018).
17. Gee JP. *Good Video Games & Good Learning: Collected Essays on Video Games, Learning, and Literacy*. New York: P. Lang (2007).
18. Kiourti E. *(Dis)conneting Literacy Practices: A Critical Comparison of FPS Video Games and School*. Nicosia, Cyprus: University of Cyprus (2018).
19. Ensslin A. *The Language of Gaming*. New York: Palgrave Macmillan (2012).
20. Gee JP. *What Video Games Have to Teach Us About Learning and Literacy*. New York: Palgrave Macmillan (2003).
21. Steinkuehler C. Massively multiplayer online gaming as a constellation of literacy practices. *eLearning* (2007) 4(3):297–318. doi:10.2304/elea.2007.4.3.297
22. Clark A. *Being There: Putting Brain, Body, and World Together Again. 1997*. Cambridge, MA: MIT Press (1997).
23. Barsalou LW. Perceptual symbol systems. *Behav Brain Sci* (1999) 22:577–609. doi:10.1017/S0140525X99532147
24. Shaefer E. Blizzard entertainment's Diablo II. In: Grossman A, editor. *Postmortems from Game Developers: Insights from the Developers of Unreal*

Tournament, Black & White, Age of Empires, and Other Top-Selling Games. San Francisco: CMP Books (2004). p. 79–90.

25. McKenzie N. Searching for the intangible: commercial game designers wrestle with educational games. *Paper presented at the 2005 Games, Learning, and Society Conference.* Madison, WI (2005).
26. Khan J. *Review: Elegy for a Dead World.* (2014). Available from: https://www.hardcoregamer.com/2014/12/12/review-elegy-for-a-dead-world/122598/
27. Gong D, He H, Liu D, Ma W, Dong L, Luo C, et al. Enhanced functional connectivity and increased grey matter volume of insula related to action video game playing. *Sci Rep* (2015) 5:9763. doi:10.1038/srep09763
28. Oei AC, Patterson MD. Enhancing cognition with video games: a multiple game training study. *PLoS One* (2013) 8(3):e58546. doi:10.1371/journal.pone.0058546
29. Jones RB, Ashurst EJ, Atkey J, Duffy B. Older people going online: its value and before-after evaluation of volunteer support. *J Med Internet Res* (2015) 17(5):e122. doi:10.2196/jmir.3943
30. Alzaid A, Komal K, Al-Maraghi A, Alsulami M. Examining the relationship between the internet and life expectancy. *Paper Presented at the 24th International Business Information Management Association Conference – Crafting Global Competitive Economies: 2020 Vision Strategic Planning and Smart Implementation.* Milan, Italy (2014). p. 1142–51.
31. Te-Hsin L. Association between use of Internet services and quality of life in Taiwan. *J Data Sci* (2011) 9:83–92.
32. Heo J, Chun S, Lee S, Lee KH, Kim J. Internet use and well-being in older adults. *Cyberpsychol Behav Soc Netw* (2015) 18(5):268–72. doi:10.1089/cyber.2014.0549
33. LaMonica HM, English A, Hickie IB, Ip J, Ireland C, West S, et al. Examining Internet and eHealth practices and preferences: survey study of Australian older adults with subjective memory complaints, mild cognitive impairment, or dementia. *J Med Internet Res* (2017) 19(10):e358. doi:10.2196/jmir.7981
34. Ortega L, Calvillo M, Luna F, Pérez-Severiano F, Rubio-Osornio M, Guevara J, et al. 17-AAG improves cognitive process and increases heat shock protein response in a model lesion with Aβ25-35. *Neuropeptides* (2014) 48(4):221–32. doi:10.1016/j.npep.2014.04.006
35. Morahan-Martin J, Schumacher P. Loneliness and social uses of the Internet. *Comput Human Behav* (2003) 19:659–71. doi:10.1016/S0747-5632(03)00040-2
36. Ji Z, Li A, Feng T, Liu X, You Y, Meng F, et al. The benefits of Tai Chi and brisk walking for cognitive function and fitness in older adults. *PeerJ* (2017) 5:e3943. doi:10.7717/peerj.3943
37. Dye MWG, Green CS, Bavelier D. Increasing speed of processing with action video games. *Curr Dir Psychol Sci* (2009) 18(6):321–6. doi:10.1111/j.1467-8721.2009.01660.x
38. Wolinsky FD, Unverzagt FW, Smith DM, Jones R, Wright E, Tennstedt SL. The effects of the ACTIVE cognitive training trial on clinically relevant declines in health-related quality of life. *J Gerontol B Psychol Sci Soc Sci* (2006) 61(5):S281. doi:10.1093/geronb/61.5.S281
39. Rebok GW, Ball K, Guey LT, Jones RN, Kim HY, King JW, et al. Ten-year effects of the advanced cognitive training for independent and vital elderly cognitive training trial on cognition and everyday functioning in older adults. *J Am Geriatr Soc* (2014) 62(1):16–24. doi:10.1111/jgs.12607
40. Wolinsky FD, Mahncke H, Vander Weg MW, Martin R, Unverzagt FW, Ball KK, et al. Speed of processing training protects self-rated health in older adults: enduring effects observed in the multi-site ACTIVE randomized controlled trial. *Int Psychogeriatr* (2010) 22(3):470–8. doi:10.1017/S1041610209991281
41. D'Orsi E, Xavier AJ, Steptoe A, Oliveira C, Ramos LR, Orrell M, et al. Internet use and physical activity can improve 10-year survival of older adults: results from the English Longitudinal Study of Aging. *The 2015 Ageing Summit.* London (2015).
42. D'Orsi E, Xavier AJ, Rafnsson SB, Steptoe A, Hogervorst E, Orrell M. Is use of the internet in midlife associated with lower dementia incidence? Results from the English Longitudinal Study of Ageing. *Aging Ment Health* (2017) 10:1–9. doi:10.1080/13607863.2017.1360840

3

Selfie Aging Index: An Index for the Self-assessment of Healthy and Active Aging

Judite Gonçalves[1,2], Maria Isabel Gomes[3], Miguel Fonseca[3], Tomás Teodoro[4], Pedro Pita Barros[1] and Maria-Amália Botelho[4]*

[1] Nova Healthcare Initiative Research, Nova School of Business and Economics, Universidade Nova de Lisboa, Lisbon, Portugal, [2] School of Business and Management, Queen Mary University of London, London, United Kingdom, [3] Center for Mathematics and Applications, Faculty of Sciences and Technology, Universidade Nova de Lisboa, Lisbon, Portugal, [4] Chronic Diseases Research Center, Nova Medical School, Universidade Nova de Lisboa, Lisbon, Portugal

Edited by:
Giuseppe Liotta,
Università degli Studi di Roma Tor Vergata, Italy

Reviewed by:
Rosa Liperoti,
Università Cattolica del Sacro Cuore, Italy
Taro Kojima,
The University of Tokyo, Japan

***Correspondence:**
Judite Gonçalves
judite_goncalves@msn.com

Introduction: Governments across Europe want to promote healthy and active aging, as a matter of both public health and economic sustainability. Designing policies focused on the most vulnerable groups requires information at the individual level. However, a measure of healthy and active aging at the individual level does not yet exist.

Objectives: This paper develops the *Selfie Aging Index* (SAI), an individual-level index of healthy and active aging. The SAI is developed thinking about a tool that would allow each person to take a *selfie* of her aging status. Therefore, it is based entirely on self-assessed indicators. This paper also illustrates how the SAI may look like in practice.

Methods: The SAI is based on the Biopsychosocial Assessment Model (MAB), a tool for the multidimensional assessment of older adults along three domains: biological, psychological, and social. Indicators are selected and their weights determined based on an ordered probit model that relates the MAB indicators to self-assessed health, which proxies healthy and active aging. The ordered probit model predicts the SAI based on the estimated parameters. Finally, predictions are rescaled to the 0–1 interval. Data for the SAI development come from the Study of the Aging Profiles of the Portuguese Population and the Survey of Health, Aging, and Retirement in Europe.

Results: The selected indicators are BMI, having difficulties moving around indoors and performing the activities of daily living, feeling depressed, feeling nervous, lacking energy, time awareness score, marital status, having someone to confide in, education, type of job, exercise, and smoking status. The model also determines their weights.

Conclusion: Results shed light on various factors that contribute significantly to healthy and active aging. Two examples are mental health and exercise, which deserve more attention from individuals themselves, health-care professionals, and public health policy. The SAI has the potential to put the individual at the center of the healthy and active aging discussion, contribute to patient empowerment, and promote patient-centered care. It can become a useful instrument to monitor healthy and active aging for different actors, including individuals themselves, health-care professionals, and policy makers.

Keywords: Selfie Aging Index, healthy aging, active aging, aging index, multidimensional index, biopsychosocial assessment model, ordered probit model, self-assessed health

> I have enjoyed greatly the second blooming … suddenly you find – at the age of 50, say – that a whole new life has opened before you.
>
> Agatha Christie

INTRODUCTION

In 2016, people aged 55 and over (55+) accounted for 32% of the European Union's (EU) population, and people aged 65 and over (65+) for 19%. The EU countries with the oldest populations are Italy, Germany, Greece, and Portugal, where the 55+ represent 34–35% of the population and the 65+ represent 21–22% (own calculations based on Eurostat data). These numbers are expected to rise in the future, challenging EU governments to promote the healthy and active aging of their populations, as a matter of both public health and economic sustainability.

The concept of healthy and active aging was defined by the World Health Organization (WHO) as the process of optimizing opportunities for health to enhance quality of life as people age. The word "healthy" refers to physical, mental, and social well-being, while the word "active" refers to continuing participation in social, economic, cultural, spiritual, and civic affairs (1). It should be noted that some studies focus specifically on healthy aging or active aging alone. Other studies refer only to healthy aging or active aging but possibly mean both healthy and active aging.

To design policies to promote healthy and active aging, as well as to track their progress, measurement is crucial. With that in mind, the European Commission (EC) and the United Nations Economic Commission for Europe introduced the Active Aging Index (AAI) in 2012. The AAI is a multidimensional index that measures the level to which older people (55+) live independent lives, participate in the labor market and social activities as well as their capacity to actively age (2). As its name suggests, the AAI focuses specifically on active aging. It conceptualizes active aging as "the situation where people continue to participate in the formal labor market as well as engage in other unpaid productive activities and live healthy, independent, and secure lives as they age" (3). The AAI represents the first initiative to measure healthy and active aging. It has inspired the measurement of healthy and active aging around the world, which clearly shows the increasing interest in the aging phenomenon (4, 5).

The AAI provides a societal perspective of the aging phenomenon and is a useful tool for top-down policy design. However, it only allows for the comparison of average levels of active aging across countries. Designing policies focused on the most vulnerable groups requires information about the distributions of healthy and active aging within countries, as well as information about how healthy and active aging correlates with individual characteristics. To obtain such information, we need to measure healthy and active aging at the individual level. To that end, two recent studies develop individual-level indices of active aging based on the AAI conceptual framework (6, 7).

It is not clear that the AAI conceptual framework, developed to capture active aging at the aggregate level, is appropriate to measure active aging at the individual level. The four domains of the AAI are (1) employment, (2) participation in society, (3) independent, healthy, and secure living, and (4) capacity and enabling environment for active aging. At the individual level, these domains include indicators such as (1) being employed, (2) looking after grandchildren, (3) worrying about vandalism and crime, and (4) Internet use (7). Such indicators do not appear relevant for example in a study about older people's perceptions of active aging. According to that study, individuals associate active aging with maintaining physical health and functioning, leisure and social activities, mental functioning and activity, and social relationships and contacts (8). However, this apparent discrepancy does not imply that the AAI conceptual framework is inappropriate for an individual-level index. In fact, such discrepancy may simply reflect different perspectives of older people—the "insiders"—and researchers—the "outsiders"— as has been documented [e.g., Ref. (9)].

The AAI-based individual-level indices have other potential limitations. First, the expert group who developed the AAI chose the weights of the indicators, which implies value judgments. Second, in the individual-level indices all indicators are dichotomized. Such strategy does not take full advantage of the variations in the data.

Focusing specifically on healthy aging, Lara et al. (10) provide a list of measures that capture key features of healthy aging, grouped into five domains: physiological and metabolic health, physical capability, cognitive function, social well-being, and psychological well-being (e.g., cardiovascular function, strength, episodic memory, mental health, perceived social support). Kuh et al. (11) conceptualize healthy aging within a life-course framework, distinguishing between healthy biological aging and changes in psychological and social well-being, and provide a review of objective measures of physical capability (e.g., grip strength, walking speed). To our knowledge, healthy aging has not been operationalized in any multidimensional index.

This paper develops the *Selfie Aging Index* (SAI). The SAI is based on a conceptual framework that tries to capture both healthy and active aging at the individual level. Its underlying methodology allows the weights to be determined by the variations and correlations present in the data, avoiding value judgments. The SAI is also innovative in that it may be entirely self-assessed, thinking about future applications of the SAI as a tool for older people to track their aging status. Thus, clinical indicators or measurements that require unusual tools are not considered (e.g., cardiovascular function, grip strength). Finally, this paper also illustrates how the SAI can be used in practice. To the absolute value of the SAI, which allows individuals to keep track of their aging status over time, we add a relative component that allows individuals to compare themselves to their peers.

MATERIALS AND METHODS

Conceptual Framework

The SAI is based on the Biopsychosocial Assessment Model [MAB—*Modelo de Avaliação Biopsicosocial*, registered copyright No 4065/2007 (12)]. The MAB is a tool for the multidimensional assessment of older adults. It consists of several indicators grouped into three domains, for example ability to conduct daily activities such as bathing or eating (biological domain), feelings of depression or nervousness (psychological domain), and having someone to confide in (social domain). The full list of indicators is available in Table S1 in Supplementary Material. The domains and subdomains of the MAB capture the various elements of the conceptual definition of healthy and active aging of the WHO (see Introduction). Thus, the MAB seems suitable as a starting point to operationalize the measurement of healthy and active aging at the individual level. The MAB has been extensively validated and is currently used by the National Network of Continued Integrated Care (RNCCI—*Rede Nacional de Cuidados Continuados Integrados*) to characterize inpatients of the Portuguese health-care system (13). Unlike previous conceptual models, the MAB does not rely on clinical indicators or measurements that require unusual tools. This is appealing when we think about potential applications of the SAI as a tool for individuals to self-assess their aging status.

Statistical Method

To construct the SAI, we need to select a subset of the MAB indicators. The original MAB includes a long list of indicators (see Table S1 in Supplementary Material), which is incompatible with a simple self-assessment tool for older adults. We also need to determine the weights for the aggregation of the indicators into a single index. Estimating an ordered probit model allows us to do both things, while avoiding value judgments in the selection of indicators and their respective weights. Indicators are selected based on their statistical significance and contribution to model fit, and the weights are determined based on correlations between the indicators. Another advantage of the ordered probit model is that it easily deals with any type of indicator, continuous or categorical. Ordered probit models have been used to construct health indices, in order to have a single continuous variable to measure health status [e.g., Ref. (14)].[1] The idea behind this method is predicting a latent variable—the SAI—based on the MAB indicators. To do this, we use self-assessed health in the left hand-side of the ordered probit model [i.e., self-assessed health works as a kind of proxy for healthy and active aging, following, for example, Ref. (15, 16)]. The MAB indicators appear as right hand-side variables. Though self-assessed health consists in individuals' ratings of their health in a scale (e.g., very bad, bad, fair, good, very good), the ordered probit model predicts a continuous variable based on the estimated parameters. The last step in computing the SAI is rescaling that predicted variable to a more intuitive 0–1 interval. This is done using the theoretical limits of the latent variable, which can be computed as the predicted values when all MAB indicators are set at their least and most favorable values. In sum, the SAI score is obtained by plugging the individual's characteristics in the ordered probit model, obtaining the prediction in the latent scale, and rescaling it to the 0–1 interval.

Data

We use data from the Study of the Aging Profiles of the Portuguese Population [EPEPP—*Estudo do Perfil de Envelhecimento da População Portuguesa* (17–19)] and the Survey of Health, Aging and Retirement in Europe (SHARE; Wave 4 (20)). The EPEPP was conducted specifically to evaluate the aging status of Portuguese older adults based on an earlier version of the MAB. It was designed to be representative of the Portuguese population aged 55+ and covered about 2,700 individuals, interviewed in 2005–2006. The SHARE is a broader survey of European older adults that also contains most of the MAB indicators. It was designed to be representative of the 50+ population, but we only consider individuals aged 55+. The SHARE includes about 1,700 individuals aged 55+ in Portugal, interviewed in 2011.

There are some differences between the two datasets in self-assessed health and the MAB indicators. Self-assessed health has four levels in the EPEPP survey (bad/very bad, poor, fair, good/very good), and five levels in the SHARE survey (poor, fair, good, very good, excellent). In the EPEPP, health complaints are classified into complaints that affect or not mobility, complaints regarding eyesight, and complaints regarding hearing. In the SHARE, the long list of health conditions available allows for a much more detailed analysis of health complaints, including for example complaints about the musculoskeletal system or the respiratory system. A few MAB indicators are lacking in each dataset. The EPEPP does not include indicators of lack of interest or trouble sleeping, and the SHARE does not include waist measurement, variables related with falls, measures of mobility outdoors or climbing stairs, spatial awareness, or time alone in a 24-h period. Table S1 in Supplementary Material provides the link between the MAB indicators and the questions in the EPEPP and SHARE.[2]

Procedure

Given the differences between the EPEPP and SHARE surveys outlined above, the analyses of the two datasets are complementary. Estimating separate ordered probit models allows us to determine if the same MAB indicators appear relevant for healthy and active aging in both samples, providing external validity to our methodology. This is especially informative given that the EPEPP was conducted prior to the financial crisis and the SHARE was conducted after the crisis, i.e., the individuals in each sample faced different socioeconomic environments. Estimating separate models is the first stage in our procedure. All MAB indicators available in each survey are used. The original coding of the answers is maintained, in order to take full advantage of the information available. For example, the question "Over the past month, did you feel sad or depressed?" has four possible answers in the EPEPP survey ("No," "Little time," "Half of the time," and "Most of the time"), and two possible answers in the SHARE survey ("Yes" and "No").

In the second stage, the two datasets are combined. All MAB indicators available in both surveys are considered, except for health complaints (including complaints about the emotional status) because the corresponding questions are not posed in comparable ways (see Data and Table S1 in Supplementary Material). Combining the datasets requires recoding the answers to the questions that are posed in different ways in the two surveys. The new self-assessed health variable has three levels: poor/bad/very bad, fair, good/very good/excellent. Table S2 in

[1] Ryser V-A, Weaver F, and Gonçalves J (Forthcoming). Health-related inequalities in life satisfaction among the 50+ population in Europe: evidence from SHARE. *Swiss J Sociol.*

[2] Co-authors of this study are involved in the EPEPP study and the SHARE project in Portugal and have thorough knowledge of the datasets.

Supplementary Material presents the new coding for all variables. Combining the datasets increases the sample size substantially, enhancing statistical power.

In the third stage, the model estimated in the combined dataset is simplified by eliminating the MAB indicators that do not contribute to improve model fit. To do this, the indicators are progressively added to the model according to their contribution to the log-likelihood (i.e., stepwise regression). With each addition, we assess the likelihood ratio test, as well as Akaike's and the Bayesian Information Criteria (AIC, BIC). We consider that an indicator does not contribute to improve model fit if the null hypothesis of the likelihood ratio test is not rejected at the 10% significance level and the value of the AIC or the BIC increases.[3] The SAI is calculated based on the resulting simplified model.

Recoding the variables when combining the two datasets may introduce bias. Furthermore, the EPEPP and SHARE surveys were conducted several years apart under different socioeconomic environments, which may affect the relationships between the variables. To explore these potential issues, we estimate an ordered probit model, including interactions between the MAB indicators and a binary indicator of the observation's source (EPEPP or SHARE). Checking whether the associations between the MAB indicators and self-assessed health differ according to the source of data gives an indication of the extent of the problem. Given that one of the recoded variables is self-assessed health, we also test whether the estimated cutoffs significantly differ according to the dataset.

Validity Checks

To investigate the validity of the SAI, we assess its value as a predictor of several outcomes, namely the probability of having had a doctor visit and number of doctor visits over the previous 12 months, mental health (EURO-D depression scale), number of chronic conditions, and number of symptoms. The EURO-D depression scale varies between 0 (not depressed) and 12 (very depressed) and is essentially a count of 12 items, including for example feeling guilty about anything, having no hopes for the future, and lacking appetite. The number of chronic conditions is a count of up to ten conditions including for example hypertension, diabetes, and arthritis. The number of symptoms is a count of up to 12 symptoms including for example pain, incontinence, and fatigue. None of these outcomes is an indicator in the SAI. We regress each outcome on the SAI and evaluate the statistical significance of the associated coefficient as well as the R^2. The probability of having a doctor visit and the number of doctor visits are available in both surveys, but the remaining outcomes are available only in the SHARE.

The SAI in Practice

In order to illustrate how the SAI may look like in practice, we calculate SAI scores for several hypothetical individuals. The absolute value of the SAI may be used by individuals to monitor their aging status over time. To provide some context, we add a relative component that allows individuals to compare themselves to their peers. The individual SAI scores are displayed in the distribution of SAI scores of people aged ±2 years. The larger sample size of the combined dataset allows us to have a significantly larger pool of peers for each individual in the dataset.

[3]The likelihood ratio test is a statistical test used to compare the goodness of fit of two nested models. Under the null hypothesis, the simpler model is better, because it fits the data as well as the more complex one, but is more parsimonious. Lower values of the AIC and BIC indicate better model fit.

RESULTS

Estimation Results Using the EPEPP Sample

Results based on the EPEPP sample are presented in Table S3 in Supplementary Material. The MAB indicators with a statistically significant coefficient, at the 10% significance level or lower, are health complaints, obesity (captured by waist measurement), having fallen due to internal causes, such as fainting, having sequelae from falling that affect mobility, needing someone's help to perform the activities of daily living (ADLs), self-assessed emotional status, feeling depressed, feeling nervous, lacking energy, spending less than 8 h per day alone, having someone to confide in, exercising, and smoking status. Most of these variables have the expected associations with self-assessed health (i.e., the respective estimated coefficients have the expected signs). The remaining variables have no significant associations with self-assessed health. Looking at the magnitudes of the estimated coefficients, we can see that the variables with the largest associations with self-assessed health are complaints that do not affect mobility, self-assessed emotional status, feeling depressed most of the time, exercising more than 4 h per week, and smoking at present (coefficients larger than 0.3 in absolute value).

Estimation Results Using the SHARE Sample

Table S4 in Supplementary Material presents the results based on the SHARE sample. The MAB indicators that have a statistically significant association with self-assessed health are health complaints except for those regarding the urinary system, difficulties moving around indoors and performing the ADLs, being depressed, being nervous, having trouble sleeping, lacking energy, marital status, living with someone else, having someone to confide in, education, and exercising. All of these variables except for living with someone else have the expected associations with self-assessed health. The coefficients of the remaining variables are not statistically significant. The variables with the largest associations with self-assessed health are complaints about hearing, the circulatory system, and the musculoskeletal system, having difficulties moving around indoors, and being divorced.

Estimation Results Using the Combined Sample

Table 1 presents the results based on the combined dataset. Model 1 includes all MAB indicators available in both datasets. Model 2 excludes the indicators that do not contribute to improve the overall fit of the model. The excluded indicators are difficulties performing the instrumental activities of daily living (IADLs) and living with someone else, as well as age and gender. Including these variables in the model does not significantly increase the log-likelihood and the value of the AIC or the BIC increases, indicating worse fit (Table S5 in Supplementary Material).

We focus on the results of Model 2. The average marginal effects are shown in **Table 2**. For instance, on average and keeping all else constant, an obese person is seven percentage points less likely to report good, very good, or excellent health than a normal weight person. Having difficulties moving around indoors decreases the probability of reporting the highest level of health by nine percentage points. All three emotional status indicators have sizeable associations with self-assessed health. For example, feeling depressed decreases the likelihood of reporting good, very good, or excellent health by about ten percentage points. Having someone to confide in increases the probability of reporting the highest level of health by almost five percentage points. Engaging in moderate physical activities, such as going for a walk, contributes even more to the probability of reporting the highest level of health than engaging in more vigorous activities, such as sports (about nine and six percentage points, respectively). Taking into account the sample means and proportions, presented in Table S6 in Supplementary Material, all estimated associations are sizeable. Finally, on average individuals from the SHARE sample are more likely to report the highest level of health.

Including interactions between the MAB indicators and a binary indicator of the observation's source (EPEPP or SHARE) produces the results presented in Table S7 in Supplementary Material. Out of the 20 interaction terms, only 4 are statistically significant, indicating that most associations between the MAB indicators and self-assessed health do not depend on the source of data. If allowed to differ according to the data source, the cutoffs are also not significantly different at the 5% significance level (results available upon request).

TABLE 1 | Estimation results of the ordered probit model using the combined sample.

	Model 1	Model 2
	Coefficient (SE)	**Coefficient (SE)**
Gender: female	−0.072 (0.048)	
Age	−0.079** (0.036)	
Age^2	0.001** (0.000)	
BMI (ref: normal weight)		
Undernourished	−0.115 (0.244)	−0.115 (0.240)
Overweight	−0.114** (0.050)	−0.106** (0.049)
Obese	−0.268*** (0.055)	−0.250*** (0.054)
Difficulties moving around indoors	−0.340*** (0.108)	−0.322*** (0.105)
Number of difficulties in the activities of daily living	−0.127*** (0.022)	−0.139*** (0.021)
Number of difficulties in the instrumental activities of daily living	−0.032 (0.023)	
Depressed	−0.363*** (0.047)	−0.365*** (0.047)
Nervous	−0.209*** (0.044)	−0.206*** (0.043)
Lack of energy	−0.345*** (0.051)	−0.349*** (0.051)
Time awareness	0.069* (0.036)	0.069** (0.037)
Marital status (ref: widowed)		
Married	0.046 (0.074)	0.014 (0.055)
Single	−0.126 (0.109)	−0.094 (0.109)
Divorced/separated	0.229** (0.111)	0.210** (0.107)
Lives with someone else	−0.076 (0.077)	
Has someone to confide in	0.163** (0.077)	0.164* (0.076)
Years of education	0.064*** (0.018)	0.065*** (0.018)
Years of education^2	−0.001 (0.001)	−0.001 (0.001)
Type of job: manual work	−0.152*** (0.045)	−0.147*** (0.044)
Vigorous physical activities	0.186*** (0.045)	0.199*** (0.045)
Moderate physical activities	0.306*** (0.044)	0.309*** (0.043)
Smoking status (ref: non-smoker)		
Former smoker	0.034 (0.055)	0.055 (0.051)
Current smoker	0.226*** (0.052)	0.241*** (0.051)
SHARE	0.408*** (0.050)	0.427*** (0.048)
Cutoff 1	−3.204** (1.268)	−0.309* (0.169)
Cutoff 2	−1.586 (1.267)	−1.303*** (1.171)
Observations	3,606	3,643
Pseudo R^2	0.138	0.135

Robust SEs in parentheses.

, **, and * denote statistical significance at the 10, 5, and 1% significance levels.*

TABLE 2 | Marginal effects in Model 2.

	Probability of reporting		
	Poor, bad, or very bad health	**Fair health**	**Good, very good, or excellent health**
	Average marginal effect (SE)	**Average marginal effect (SE)**	**Average marginal effect (SE)**
BMI (ref: normal weight)			
Undernourished	0.029 (0.060)	0.004 (0.008)	−0.032 (0.067)
Overweight	0.027** (0.012)	0.003** (0.002)	−0.030** (0.014)
Obese	0.062*** (0.014)	0.008*** (0.002)	−0.070*** (0.015)
Difficulties moving around indoors	0.080*** (0.026)	0.010** (0.004)	−0.091*** (0.029)
Number of difficulties in the activities of daily living	0.035*** (0.005)	0.004*** (0.001)	−0.039*** (0.006)
Depressed	0.091*** (0.012)	0.012*** (0.003)	−0.103*** (0.013)
Nervous	0.051*** (0.011)	0.007*** (0.002)	−0.058*** (0.012)
Lack of energy	0.087*** (0.013)	0.011*** (0.003)	−0.098*** (0.014)
Time awareness	−0.017* (0.009)	−0.002* (0.001)	0.019* (0.010)
Marital status (ref: widowed)			
Married	−0.003 (0.014)	−0.000 (0.002)	0.004 (0.016)
Single	0.023 (0.027)	0.003 (0.004)	−0.026 (0.031)
Divorced/separated	−0.052* (0.027)	−0.007* (0.004)	0.059* (0.030)
Has someone to confide in	−0.041** (0.019)	−0.005* (0.003)	0.046** (0.022)
Years of education	−0.016*** (0.004)	−0.002*** (0.001)	0.018*** (0.005)
Years of education^2	0.000 (0.000)	0.000 (0.000)	−0.000 (0.000)
Type of job: manual work	0.037*** (0.011)	0.005*** (0.002)	−0.041*** (0.012)
Vigorous physical activities	−0.050*** (0.011)	−0.006*** (0.002)	0.056*** (0.013)
Moderate physical activities	−0.077*** (0.011)	−0.010*** (0.002)	0.087*** (0.012)
Smoking status (ref: non-smoker)			
Former smoker	−0.014 (0.013)	−0.002 (0.002)	0.015 (0.014)
Current smoker	−0.060*** (0.013)	−0.008*** (0.002)	0.068*** (0.014)
SHARE	−0.106*** (0.012)	−0.014*** (0.003)	0.120*** (0.013)

Robust standard errors in parentheses.

, **, and * denote statistical significance at the 10, 5, and 1% significance levels.*

Calculating the SAI

Selfie Aging Index scores for all individuals in the combined data-set are calculated based on Model 2. Figure S1 in Supplementary Material shows the distributions of the SAI according to selected individual characteristics. It is important to note that the distributions are unconditional, i.e., there is no adjustment for other characteristics.

Validity Checks

Table S8 in Supplementary Material shows the results from regressions of the probability of having a doctor visit, number of doctor visits, mental health, number of chronic conditions, and number of symptoms on the SAI score. The associations between the SAI score and each outcome considered are negative, as expected. The *t*-statistics associated with the SAI coefficients are considerably high, indicating statistical significance at any conventional significance level. The R^2s are also sizeable. These results reveal that the SAI is a strong predictor of the probability of having a doctor visit, number of doctor visits, mental health, number of chronic conditions, and number of symptoms.

DISCUSSION

Findings from the Ordered Probit Models

In general, the MAB indicators have the expected associations with self-assessed health. There are only a few exceptions. In the EPEPP model, having complaints about hearing has a positive estimated coefficient, and spending less than 8 h per day alone has a negative estimated coefficient. Spending less than 8 h per day alone may be capturing other unmeasured physical or cognitive limitations that require the person to be accompanied most of the time. Globally, the two counterintuitive signs may be due to multicollinearity. For example, hearing and vision complaints are highly correlated, and spending less than 8 h per day alone is highly correlated with needing auxiliary instruments to perform the ADLs as well as living with someone else. High correlations between included variables affect the efficiency of the estimators, which may result in unexpected estimates. Also intriguingly, former and current smokers rate their health better than those who never smoked. Smoking status may also be capturing unobserved characteristics. For instance, people aged 55+ who still smoke possibly never had any serious health condition that would induce them to quit. Former smokers may have quit in time to avoid serious health damages. In the SHARE model, living with someone else has an estimated negative association with self-assessed health. The reasons for that may be the same ones mentioned above regarding the negative estimated coefficient associated with spending less than 8 h per day alone in the EPEPP model. For example, living with someone else is highly correlated with marital status, which may introduce significant multicollinearity in the model. Finally, in the SHARE model divorced individuals tend to have higher SAI scores than married individuals. Again, this finding may be due to multicollinearity or unobserved characteristics related to both health and selection into divorce (e.g., urban or rural area of residence, traditional values such as the idea that marriage is for life).

The MAB indicators that stand out in both the EPEPP and SHARE models are health complaints, difficulties performing the ADLs, felling depressed, feeling nervous, lacking energy, having someone to confide in, and exercising. This list includes indicators from all three domains of the MAB—biological, psychological, and social. Thus, a meaningful number of factors appear relevant in both models, providing external validity to our approach. It should be noted that lack of statistical significance of other MAB indicators may be attributable to the specific samples used or to lack of statistical power. It may also be the case that people simply do not consider some factors when asked to assess their health status. For instance, when self-evaluating their health status, people may be more likely to consider fear of falling, which is not measured here, than past falls, which is measured but not statistically significant.

Combining the two datasets allowed for improvements in statistical power, as the sample size increased substantially. It also implied two main drawbacks. First, several variables, including self-assessed health, had to be recoded. Still, our explorations suggest that this doesn't represent a significant problem. Second, we had to exclude health complaints. Health complaints appeared relevant in both the EPEPP and SHARE models. Excluding this indicator remains a drawback to be addressed in future work.

Difficulties performing the IADLs and living with someone else, as well as age and gender, were excluded from the final model based on statistical criteria. Conceptually and given our experience, there are some reasons why these variables may appear as not relevant for self-assessed health. The IADLs include tasks that some people do not have the ability to perform or are used to request help with, such as managing money and using transportation. Unlike difficulties in the ADLs, difficulties in the IADLs do not necessarily capture disability. Living with someone else may loose importance in our model because related variables, such as marital status and having someone to confide in, are included. Besides, one may argue that it is the need to live with someone else rather than living with someone else or not that is relevant for self-assessed health. Such need is determined by the individual's bad health and disability, which is captured by other variables in the model. Finally, age and gender may affect individuals' perception of their health status mainly due to external factors, e.g., social misconceptions such as the idea that older ages are necessarily associated with worse health. Once other biopsychosocial factors are taken into account, it seems plausible that age and gender should no longer play a role.

The individual SAI scores calculated based on Model 2 have the expected distributions according to most individual characteristics. A few distributions may appear intriguing because they are unadjusted for other characteristics. For example, men tend to have higher SAI scores than women. This may be partly explained by the male–female health-survival paradox—the phenomenon that women experience greater longevity but higher rates of disability and poor health than men at more advanced ages [e.g., Ref. (21)]. As seen above, once other characteristics are taken into account, there are no significant differences in self-assessed health due to gender. As discussed above, smoking status and marital status may be capturing both observed and unobserved characteristics, which may explain the higher SAI scores among current and former smokers, as well as among divorced individuals. Finally, SAI scores tend to be higher in the SHARE sample than in the EPEPP sample. This may be partly related to the different socioeconomic environments that people faced in 2005–2006 and 2011 (before and after the financial crisis).

The SAI in Practice

If the SAI is to be a useful tool for individuals to assess their aging status, in addition to an absolute value, it should have a relative component. The absolute value allows monitoring one's aging status over time, while the relative component allows individuals to position themselves with respect to their peers. Thus, to illustrate how a tool based on the SAI might look like in practice, we consider ten hypothetical individuals, characterized in **Table 3**. The individuals' characteristics are chosen to illustrate how the SAI changes as a result of changes in the various selected indicators. For each individual, we calculate his or her SAI score, and present it along with the distribution of the SAI among his or her peers (people aged ±2 years in the sample) in **Figure 1**.

Consider for example Mary, a 68-year-old overweight woman. She has no difficulties moving around indoors or performing the ADLs. She is not depressed or nervous, and does not lack energy. She has a perfect score in time awareness. She is married and has someone to confide in. She has 4 years of education and had a manual job prior to retirement. She engages in moderate physical activities but not in more vigorous ones and does not smoke. Mary has a SAI score of 0.61, which puts her in the middle quintile of the distribution of the SAI among her peers (**Figure 1A**).

Take a second example, Michael, who is just like Mary except he is not in good shape emotionally. He has a SAI score of 0.44,

TABLE 3 | Characteristics of the hypothetical individuals.

Panel (A)

	Mary	**James**	**Margaret**	**John**	**Michael**
Age	68	**78**	**78**	**78**	68
BMI	Overweight	Overweight	Overweight	Overweight	Overweight
Difficulties moving around indoors	No	**Yes**	**Yes**	**Yes**	No
Number of difficulties in the activities of daily living (ADLs)	Zero	**Five**	**Five**	**Five**	Zero
Depressed	No	No	No	No	**Yes**
Nervous	No	No	No	No	**Yes**
Lack of energy	No	No	No	No	**Yes**
Time awareness	Four	Four	Four	**Zero**	Four
Marital status	Married	Married	**Widowed**	**Widowed**	Married
Has someone to confide in	Yes	Yes	**No**	**No**	Yes
Years of education	Four	Four	Four	Four	Four
Type of job: manual work	Yes	Yes	Yes	Yes	Yes
Vigorous physical activities	No	No	No	No	No
Moderate physical activities	Yes	**No**	**No**	**No**	Yes
Smoking status	Non-smoker	Non-smoker	Non-smoker	Non-smoker	Non-smoker
Database	EPEPP	EPEPP	EPEPP	EPEPP	EPEPP
Selfie Aging Index (SAI) score	0.61	0.36	0.32	0.27	0.44
Quintile (compared to individuals within ±2 years of age)	3rd	1st	1st	1st	1st

Panel (B)

	Linda	**Charles**	**Susan**	**Elisabeth**	**William**
Age	**58**	**58**	**58**	68	**58**
BMI	Overweight	Overweight	**Normal weight**	Overweight	Overweight
Difficulties moving around indoors	No	No	No	No	No
Number of difficulties in the ADLs	Zero	Zero	Zero	Zero	Zero
Depressed	No	No	No	No	No
Nervous	No	No	No	No	No
Lack of energy	No	No	No	No	No
Time awareness	Four	Four	Four	Four	Four
Marital status	Married	Married	Married	Married	Married
Has someone to confide in	Yes	Yes	Yes	Yes	Yes
Years of education	**Twelve**	**Twelve**	**Twelve**	Four	Four
Type of job: manual work	**No**	**No**	**No**	Yes	Yes
Vigorous physical activities	No	No	**Yes**	No	No
Moderate physical activities	Yes	Yes	Yes	Yes	Yes
Smoking status	Non-smoker	**Smoker**	Non-smoker	Non-smoker	Non-smoker
Database	EPEPP	EPEPP	EPEPP	**SHARE**	EPEPP
SAI score	0.71	0.76	0.77	0.69	0.61
Quintile (compared to individuals within ±2 years of age)	5th	5th	5th	5th	3rd

The characteristics that differ from those of Mary are in bold.

which puts him in the bottom quintile of the distribution of the SAI among his peers (**Figure 1E**). Besides comparing individuals with different characteristics, the SAI can be used to infer what would happen if someone's characteristics changed. In this example, Michael's SAI score represents what we might expect of Mary's if her emotional status would deteriorate.

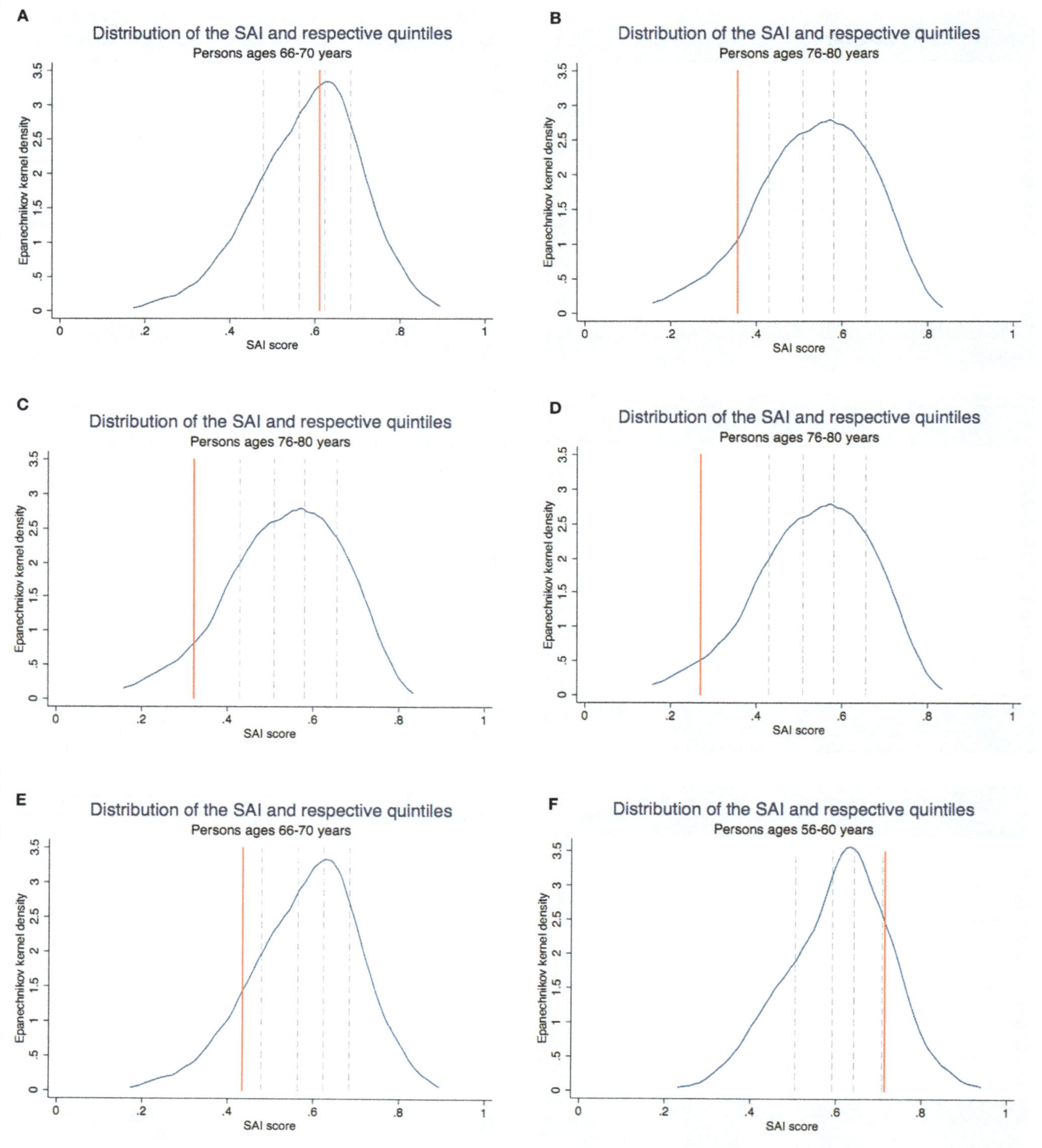

FIGURE 1 | Continued

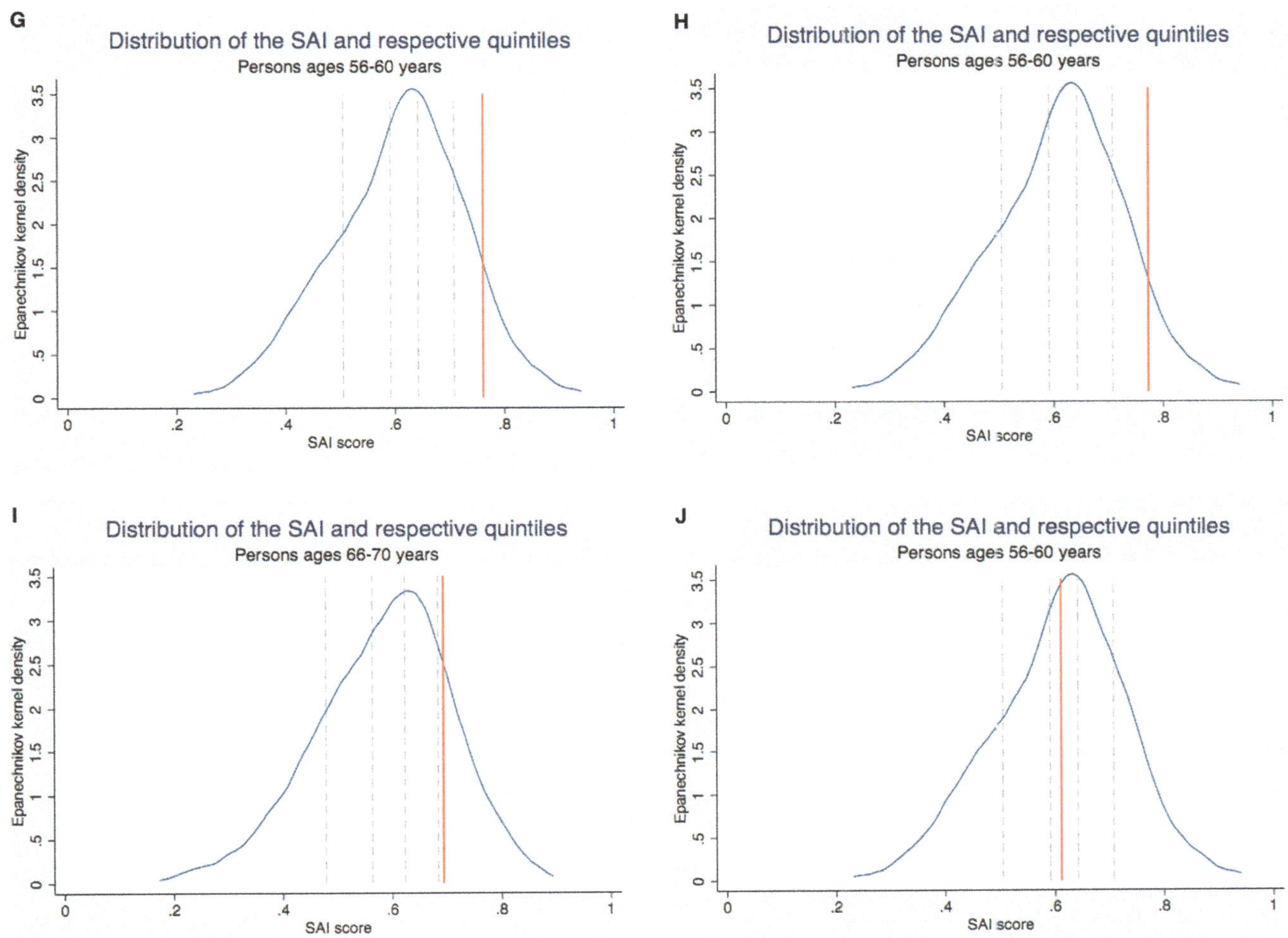

FIGURE 1 | Selfie Aging Index (SAI) scores of the hypothetical individuals. **(A)** Mary. **(B)** James. **(C)** Margaret. **(D)** John. **(E)** Michael. **(F)** Linda. **(G)** Charles. **(H)** Susan. **(I)** Elisabeth. **(J)** William.

As a final example, consider William. He has the same characteristics as Mary except he is 58 instead of 68. Given that age is not included in the SAI's calculation, William and Mary's scores are equal, but they compare themselves to different reference groups. Mary's peers are individuals aged 66–70 and William's are individuals aged 56–60. As the SAI distributions in the two age groups are very similar, in the end both William and Mary are in the middle quintile of the distributions of the SAI among their respective peers (**Figures 1A,J**).

CONCLUSION

Our results shed light on various factors that contribute significantly to healthy and active aging. Two examples are mental health and exercise, which deserve more attention from individuals themselves, health-care professionals, and public health policy.

This study provides several lines for future research. Other methods to construct multidimensional indices should be tested and results should be compared with the ones presented here. Our methodology can be applied to data from other countries, to compare healthy and active aging across countries. The effectiveness of the SAI as a tool to promote healthy and active aging at the individual and aggregate levels should be investigated.

This study develops the SAI to measure healthy and active aging at the individual level. It is designed thinking about its possible implementation as a tool for individuals to monitor their aging status. For this reason, it is completely based on self-assessed indicators. The goal is that the SAI allows each person to take a *selfie* of her aging status without requiring a health-care professional to operate the camera. We illustrate how the SAI may be implemented in practice and provide it with a relative component, whereby individuals can compare themselves to their peers. The SAI also has promising applications for health-care professionals. Though it does not replace the clinical assessment of health problems, it may motivate health-care professionals to adopt a more encompassing view of individuals' health and aging status. The SAI is useful to inform the design of public health policies targeting the most vulnerable groups. In conclusion, the SAI has the potential to put the individual at the center of the healthy and active aging discussion, contribute to patient empowerment and promote patient-centered care. It can become a useful instrument to monitor healthy and active aging for different actors, including individuals themselves, health-care professionals, and policy makers.

AUTHOR CONTRIBUTIONS

JG wrote the manuscript, and all remaining authors revised it critically.

ACKNOWLEDGMENTS

The authors appreciate the comments of participants at the annual encounter III Jornadas Científicas NOVAsaúde, the Ageing and Independent Living (AgIL) Workshop, and the Conferência Nacional de Economia da Saúde.

FUNDING

This study was funded by NOVAsaúde and partially supported by the Portuguese Foundation for Science and Technology through the project UID/MAT/00297/2013.

REFERENCES

1. Bousquet J, Kuh D, Bewick M, Standberg T, Farrell J, Pengelly R, et al. Operational definition of active and healthy ageing (AHA): a conceptual framework. *J Nutr Health Aging* (2015) 19(9):955–60. doi:10.1007/s12603-015-0589-6
2. UNECE/EC. *Active Ageing Index 2014: Analytical Report*. Report prepared by Asghar Zaidi of Center for Research on Ageing, University of Southampton and David Stanton, under contract with United Nations Economic Commission for Europe (Geneva), co-funded by European Commission's Directorate General for Employment, Social Affairs and Inclusion, Brussels (2015).
3. Zaidi A, Gasior K, Hofmarcher M, Lelkes O, Marin B, Rodrigues R, et al. *Active Ageing Index 2012 – Concept, Methodology and Final Results*. European Centre for Social Welfare Policy and Research, Vienna (2013). Available from: http://www.euro.centre.org/data/1453740620_84975.pdf
4. AARP. *Surveying the Ageing Landscape*. (2017). Available from: http://journal.aarpinternational.org/a/b/2014/03/surveying-the-aging-landscape
5. HelpAge. *Global AgeWatch Index 2015*. (2017). Available from: http://www.helpage.org/global-agewatch/
6. Barros PP, Almeida SV. How relevant is active ageing? Evidence from Portugal. In: Zaidi A, Harper S, Howse K, Lamura G, Perek-Bialas J, editors. *Building Evidence for Active Ageing Policies: Active Ageing Index and Its Potential*. Palgrave McMillan (2015).
7. Barslund M, von Werder M, Zaidi A. Inequality in active ageing: evidence from a new individual-level index for European countries. *Ageing Soc* (2017). doi:10.1017/S0144686X17001052
8. Bowling A. Enhancing later life: how older people perceive active ageing? *Aging Ment Health* (2008) 12(3):293–301. doi:10.1080/13607860802120979
9. Kusumastuti S, Derks MGM, Tellier S, di Nucci E, Lund R, Mortensen EL, et al. Successful ageing: a study of the literature using citation network analysis. *Maturitas* (2016) 93:4–12. doi:10.1016/j.maturitas.2016.04.010
10. Lara J, Godfrey A, Evans E, Heaven B, Brown LJE, Barron E, et al. Towards measurement of the Healthy Ageing Phenotype in life-style based intervention studies. *Maturitas* (2013) 76:189–99. doi:10.1016/j.maturitas.2013.07.007
11. Kuh D, Karunananthan S, Bergman H, Cooper R. A life-course approach to healthy ageing: maintaining physical capability. *Proc Nutr Soc* (2014) 73:237–48. doi:10.1017/S0029665113003923
12. Botelho MA. *Autonomia Funcional em Idosos: Caracterização multidimensional em idosos utentes de um centro de saúde urbano [Seniors' Functional Autonomy: Multidimensional Characterization of Elderly Users of an Urban Health Center]*. 1st ed. Porto, Portugal: Edições Bial (2000).
13. Fontes A, Botelho MA, Fernandes A. A biopsychosocial evaluation method and the International Classification of Functioning, Disability, and Health (ICF). *Educ Gerontol* (2014) 40(9):686–99. doi:10.1080/03601277.2011.559856
14. Lindeboom M, Kerkhofs M. Health and work of the elderly: subjective health measures, reporting errors and endogeneity in the relationship between health and work. *J Appl Econ* (2009) 24:1024–46. doi:10.1002/jae.1077
15. Sirven N, Debrand T. Social participation and healthy ageing: an international comparison using SHARE data. *Soc Sci Med* (2008) 67:2017–26. doi:10.1016/j.socscimed.2008.09.056
16. Steptoe A, Wright C, Kunz-Ebrecht SR, Iliffe S. Dispositional optimism and health behavior in community-dwelling older people: associations with healthy ageing. *Br J Health Psychol* (2006) 11:71–84. doi:10.1348/135910705X42850
17. Mota-Pinto A, Rodrigues V, Botelho A, Veríssimo MT, Morais A, Alves C. A sociodemographic study of ageing in the Portuguese population: the EPEPP study. *Arch Gerontol Geriatr* (2011) 52:304–8. doi:10.1016/j.archger.2010.04.019
18. Oliveira CR, Rosa MS, Mota-Pinto A, Botelho MA, Morais A, Veríssimo MT. *Estudo do Perfil do Envelhecimento da População Portuguesa [Study of the Ageing Profiles of the Portuguese Population]*. (2010). Available from: http://rihuc.huc.min-saude.pt/bitstream/10400.4/992/1/ACS%20EPEPP%20LIVRO.pdf
19. Rodrigues V, Mota-Pinto A, de Sousa B, Botelho MA, Alves C, de Oliveira CR. The aging profile of the Portuguese population: a principal component analysis. *J Community Health* (2014) 39(4):747–52. doi:10.1007/s10900-014-9821-2
20. Malter F, Börsch-Supan A. *SHARE Wave 4, Innovations and Methodology*. (2013). Available from: http://www.share-project.org/fileadmin/pdf_documentation/Method_FRB_FINAL.pdf
21. Alberts SC, Archie EA, Gesquiere LR, Altmann J, Vaupel JW, Christensen K. The male-female health-survival paradox: a comparative perspective on sex differences in ageing and mortality. In: Weinstein M, Lane MA, editors. *Sociality, Hierarchy, Health: Comparative Biodemography: A Collection of Papers*. Washington, DC: The National Academies Press, National Research Council (2014). p. 339–64. Committee on Population, Division of Behavioral and Social Sciences and Education.

4

Functional Capacity and Levels of Physical Activity in Aging: A 3-Year Follow-up

Maria Teresa Tomás[1], Alejandro Galán-Mercant[2], Elvis Alvarez Carnero[3] and Beatriz Fernandes[1]*

[1] Escola Superior de Tecnologia da Saúde de Lisboa (ESTeSL), Instituto Politécnico de Lisboa, Lisboa, Portugal,
[2] Health Science Department, Jaén University, Jaén, Spain, [3] Translational Research Institute for Metabolism and Diabetes, Florida Hospital, Orlando, FL, United States

Edited by:
Giuseppe Liotta,
Università degli Studi di Roma Tor Vergata, Italy

Reviewed by:
Liang-Yu Chen,
Taipei Veterans General Hospital, Taiwan
Ricardo Brandão Oliveira,
Rio de Janeiro State University, Brazil

***Correspondence:**
Maria Teresa Tomás
teresa.tomas@estesl.ipl.pt

Over the last decades, the world elderly population has increased exponentially and this tendency will continue during the coming years; from 2000 to 2050, people over 60 will double and those over 80 will quadruple. Loss of independence occurs as people age due to mobility restrictions, frailty, and decreased functional fitness and cognitive abilities. Evidence has shown that appropriate programs and policies contribute to keep older adults healthy and independent over time. The purpose of this chapter is to report the results of our 3-year follow-up study designed to characterize functional physical fitness in a sample of Portuguese community-dwelling older adults to propose a set of functional parameters that decline the most. We studied a group of 43 elderly people, aged 60 and over. Variables assessed on the participants were anthropometric measurements, functional capacity with the Senior Fitness Test battery (muscle strength, aerobic endurance, flexibility, agility, and dynamic balance), handgrip strength, levels of physical activity, and balance. Three years after the first assessment, a second assessment of the same variables was conducted. We analyzed what were the variables that, for this group, were related with a healthier aging and the relation with different physical activity levels. Our study showed that the distance covered in 6-min walk test and handgrip strength seem to explain a great amount of variability on functional variables that have changed on this period (68% of balance, lower and upper functional strength, respectively) and the active participants showed less decrements with aging in anthropometric and functional variables than those inactive or insufficiently active ($p < 0.05$). Greater importance should be given to prescription of exercise targeting older adults and, specifically, walking and manual activities should be given more attention as components of a community exercise program.

Keywords: predictors of disability, functional capacity, physical activity levels, aging, handgrip, 6 min walk test

INTRODUCTION

Aging is a gradual, life-long process and highly variable characterized by a progressive and cumulative generalized impairment of physiological functions (1), which may be explained at least by genetic factors, multiple morbidities, and non-genetic factors (specially nutrition, lifestyle, and physical activity) (1).

Nowadays, the increase in human life expectancy and the reduction in death rates has made the number of older adults to grow. Portugal is not an exception and, the rate of older people has risen until 148.7% in 2016 (2), which makes authorities and health care professionals be concerned with the retirement impact on levels of functional limitations (3).

According to Chen and colleagues, it is important to study disability as a process over time since it is very informative on the disability process of an aging population (4). So, a comprehensive follow-up of functional impairment rates and its relationship with disability over time may be the basic strategy to find out which factors contribute to a greater or lesser risk of disability and, thus, to promote strategies to a healthier aging process.

Body composition and cardiorespiratory fitness are the most studied health-related variables of physical fitness and function. Changes in body composition with a loss of muscle mass, bone mass, water content along with musculoskeletal and neuromotor function may predispose older adults to a functional decline with risk of disability increasingly high (5). In addition, changes in cardiorespiratory function with a decrement resulting as much as 50% by the age of 70 contribute also to a higher risk of disability (6). These previous findings have been partially confirmed in longitudinal studies focused on aging and disability, where independent associations of aging were found between lower mobility and mortality (7), and survival (8), dynapenia and abdominal obesity with disability worsening (9), cardiorespiratory fitness and muscle function (10), or cognitive/mental state or/and comorbidities and chronic diseases (11–13).

Although older adults are generally less active, physical activity and exercise training have beneficial effects on neuromuscular adaptations (muscle and myofiber hypertrophy with gains in strength and power (14)) in healthy older adults, depending on clinical status and the training modality exercise training, specially endurance training improves different aspects of muscle oxygenation (15). In fact endurance and resistance training programs have proved to be effective to the positive increment in aerobic capacity and thus also in functional capacity of participants as so in cognitive function and in the reduction of the risk for chronic diseases (16, 17). However, a great variability exists in functional responses to exercise and in levels of adherence and preferences (18). Particularly, changes in body composition with a loss of muscle mass, bone mass, and water content along with musculoskeletal and neuromotor function predisposed older adults to a functional decline with risk of disability increasingly high (5).

Despite this increment in research, it remains the need to identify the best predictors for functional capacity and what is the contribution of physical activity to maintain this capacity with aging.

It was our purpose to characterize longitudinally functional physical fitness in a sample of Portuguese community-dwelling older adults and find plausible associations between functional, and anthropometric variables, and differences across physical activity levels and cardiometabolic comorbidities in this population over a 3-year period.

MATERIALS AND METHODS

Population

Participants were recruited for this longitudinal study in day care centers and senior universities and were eligible if they were older than 60 years and independent in activities of daily living (ADL). Participants were excluded if they were unable to ambulate without assistance. Body composition, functional fitness, and physical activity assessments were carried out in all participations who met the inclusion criteria at beginning of the study (M1) and 3 years later (M2).

After an explanation of the study and after a signed informed consent, in accordance with the Declaration of Helsinki, participants performed a battery of tests to assess functional physical fitness. All study procedures were approved by the institutional review boards of the participating institutions.

Body Composition

Weight and height were measured using a digital balance with a stadiometer (SECA®). Body mass index (BMI) was calculated ($BMI = kg/m^2$). An anthropometric tape was used for measuring waist (WC) and hip circumferences (HP) as markers of regional adiposity. Waist circumference was measured at the smallest circumference above the umbilicus and below the xiphoidal process (19) and hip circumference was measured at the highest circumference of the buttocks in a level horizontal plane. Ratio waist–hip was found by dividing the waist circumference (cm) by hip circumference (cm) (20, 21).

Body Composition was assessed using anthropometric measurements (height, weight, waist, and hip circumference) and BMI and waist to hip ratio (WHR) were calculated.

Whole-body skeletal muscle mass (SMM) was estimated using the following Al-Gindan et al. (22) equations:

$$\begin{aligned} \text{SMM}(\text{kg})\text{in male} = 39.5 &+ (0.665\ \text{weight(kg)}) \\ &-(0.185\ \text{WC}(\text{cm})) - (0.418\ \text{HC}(\text{cm})) \\ &-(0.08\ \text{age (years)}), \\ &r^2 = 0.79;\ \text{SEE} = 2.7\,\text{kg}: \end{aligned} \quad (1)$$

and

$$\begin{aligned} \text{SMM}(\text{kg})\text{in females} = 2.89 &+ (0.255\ \text{weight(kg)}) \\ &-(0.175\ \text{HC(cm)}) - (0.038\ \text{age(years)}) \\ &+(0.118\ \text{Height}(\text{cm})); \\ &r^2 = 0.59;\ \text{SEE} = 2.1\text{kg} \end{aligned} \quad (2)$$

where WC, waist circumference, HC, Hip circumference.

Functional Fitness and Disability

The Senior Fitness Test battery was used to assess functional capacity. This battery consists of six items to assess lower limbs strength and flexibility, upper body strength and flexibility, agility and dynamic balance, and aerobic endurance. All the tests were performed according to guidelines and protocols for administration (6). Briefly, lower limbs strength was measured with the 30 s chair stand test. An arm curl test was utilized for upper body strength assessment, which consists of carrying out as many forearm curls as possible within 30 s with 2.27 kg (5 lb) and 3.63 kg (8 lb) dumbbells for women and men, respectively. The chair sit-and-reach and the back scratch tests were used to assess lower and upper body flexibility, respectively. The 8-foot up and go tests were used to assess mobility. To measure aerobic endurance we used the 6-min walk test (6MWT) (23), and estimated distance walked was calculated with a validated equation (24).

$$6\text{MWD}(\text{m}) = 218 + (5.14\ \text{Height}) - (5.32\ \text{Age}) - (1.80\ \text{Weight}) + (51.31\ \text{Sex}), \quad (3)$$

where $F = 0$; $M = 1$; $r^2 = 0.66$.

Isometric strength was assessed with a handgrip test using the American Society of Hand Therapists (ASHT) protocol. It was measured at both hands (in kg; JAMAR® dynamometer). ASHT recommends a sitting position with shoulder adducted, elbow flexed at 90° for arm and wrist in neutral position and wrist between 0° to 30° of dorsal flexion (25).

Balance was assessed with the Berg Balance Scale (BBS) (26) because it is easy to use, it takes ~15–20 min to complete and is appropriate for clinical and community settings. It consists on 14 items that the subject must complete safely. Each item is scored from 0 (unable to complete the task) to 4 (independent and safe performance). Maximum score is 56 points (26).

In addition, participants completed and *ad hoc* questionnaire about comorbidities or non-communicable diseases and musculoskeletal pain conditions.

Physical Activity

Levels of physical activity (LPA) were assessed and subjects were classified in sedentary/inactive, insufficiently active or active according the classification of physical behavior (19). An active participant was considered who perform 30 min of moderate activity at least 5 days a week and/or 20 min of vigorous activity 3 days per week or a combination of both.

Statistical Analysis

For all statistical analysis, the IBM SPSS 21.0 package for Macintosh was used (SPSS Inc., IBM Company, Chicago, IL, USA). The confidence level was established with a statistically significant p-value of less than 0.05. All variables were inspected and confirmed for a non-normal distribution prior to analysis (Kolmogorov–Smirnov normality test). Basic characteristics of the participants were obtained by analyzing frequencies (%), or calculating mean and SD (mean ± SD).

Differences of performance, body composition, and functional fitness between M1 and M2 were analyzed by Wilcoxon signed-rank test. In addition, differences by sex were carried out using a Mann–Whitney *U* test.

The association between comorbidities and functional variables at M1 and M2 were analyzed with Wilcoxon Signed Rank test or a Mann–Whitney *U* test, for comorbidities with significant impact on functional variables.

Linear regression models were performed for the clinical variables that had significant differences between two measures (differences in clinical variables were dependent variables and physical fitness and body composition as independent). Finally, a Kruskal–Wallis analysis was conducted to find differences in functional variables between physical inactive, insufficiently active and active.

RESULTS

Baseline (M1) and 3 years later (M2) characteristics of participants aged between 60 and 91 years, all Caucasian, are described in **Table 1**.

Fourteen percent had a normal BMI at M1 but this percentage was increased to 21% at M2. There were not underweight cases and the prevalence of obesity was 23.3% (BMI > 30.0).

Only six participants reported none disease or musculoskeletal issue. Eighty six percent reported one to four comorbidities and 58.1% present multibordity (2 or more chronic conditions): type II diabetes was present in 18.6% of all the participants, hypercholesterolemia in 32.6%, and hypertension in 74.4%. Musculoskeletal complaints were present in 74.4% of participants. Overall, 33.3% participants suffered one or more falls in the previous year (at M1). Almost all the anthropometrical and body composition characteristics changed over the 3-year follow-up period (**Table 1**). Males reduced their weight and BMI while females decreased SMM and had small although significant increment in WHR (**Table 1**).

Most our participants were sedentary or inactive (37.2%) or insufficiently active (39.5%) and only 23.3% were active at M1. These latter results were similar at M2: 39.5% were sedentary, 30.2% insufficiently active, and 30.2% were active.

Regarding physical fitness capacity, there were only a few components with significant alteration over time (**Table 2**). Males reduced flexibility with a small increase in upper limb strength (arm curl). Among females, we could observe a decrease in balance and muscle strength. No changes in functional aerobic capacity variables were verified in both sexes (**Table 2**). Although 58.3% of males and 48.4% of females presented values for the handgrip that were classified as poor (19) at M1, only 8.3% of males and 12.9% of females presented values on handgrip strength that could be classified as having sarcopenia at M2.

Balance assessed by BBS was significantly reduced only in women. Nevertheless, a change of 6 points in BBS score indicated with 95% of confidence that a genuine change in function has occurred (27) and this occurred for 18.6% of our sample (three males and five females).

Women reduced lower limbs (30 s chair stand test) strength at M2 but not mobility, although they took longer to complete the test, the decrement in mobility was not significant (8-foot-up-and-go test). BBS results informed that our participants have an increased risk of 43% of falling, 16% risk for suffering multiple falls, and 24% risk for suffering an injurious fall.

Table 3 shows the differences on functional variables between diabetic and non-diabetic groups, and participants with or without hypercholesterolemia at M1 and M2 (only for those

TABLE 1 | Variables of characterization of participants (12 males; 31 females; total $n = 43$) (mean ± SD) or n (%) for characterization of comorbidities.

	M1	M2	p
Age (years)			
M	73.50 ± 8.84	76.50 ± 8.85	**0.000**
F	73.94 ± 8.78	76.81 ± 8.68	**0.000**
T	73.81 ± 8.69	76.72 ± 8.62	**0.000**
Weight (kg)$^{\alpha, \beta}$			
M	83.76 ± 12.93	81.67 ± 12.37	**0.031**
F	65.42 ± 7.69	64.54 ± 7.98	NS
T	70.54 ± 12.47	69.31 ± 12.08	**0.009**
Height (m)$^{\alpha, \beta}$			
M	1.69 ± 0.08	1.69 ± 0.08	NS
F	1.53 ± 0.06	1.53 ± 0.06	NS
T	1.58 ± 0.09	1.57 ± 0.09	NS
BMI			
M	29.21 ± 4.05	28.59 ± 3.75	**0.028**
F	27.99 ± 3.36	27.69 ± 3.46	NS
T	28.34 ± 3.56	27.94 ± 3.52	**0.041**
WHR$^{\alpha, \beta}$			
M	0.96 ± 0.09	0.97 ± 0.10	NS
F	0.82 ± 0.06	0.85 ± 0.07	**0.04**
T	0.86 ± 0.09	0.88 ± 0.09	**0.003**
SMM$^{\alpha, \beta}$			
M	26.70 ± 6.51	24.51 ± 6.36	NS
F	16.31 ± 2.12	16.05 ± 1.95	**0.031**
T	19.21 ± 6.05	18.26 ± 5.18	**0.009**
Diabetes type II [*n* (%)]			
M	4 (33.3%)		
F	4 (12.9%)		
Hypercholesterolemia [*n* (%)]			
M	5 (41.7%)		
F	9 (29.0%)		
Hypertension [*n*(%)]			
M	11 (91.7%)		
F	21 (67.7%)		
Cardiopulmonary conditions [*n*(%)]			
M	8 (66.7%)		
F	11 (35.5%)		
Musculoskeletal complaints [*n* (%)]			
M	8 (66.7%)		
F	24 (77.4%)		
Number of comorbidities [*n* (%)]			
0	6 (14%)		
1	12 (27.9%)		
2	16 (37.2%)		
3	7 (16.3%)		
4	2 (4.7%)		

M, male; F, female; T, total; BMI, body mass index (weightheight^2); WHR, waist to hip ratio (circumference of the waist/circumference of the hip); SMM, skeletal muscle mass [according to equations in Al-Gindan et al. (22)]; M1, first moment of assessment; M2, second moment of assessment; $p < 0.05$ based on Wilcoxon signed-rank test for differences between M1 and M2, respectively, for males or females; α, β, $p < 0.05$ based on Mann–Whitney U test for differences between males and females on M1 and M2, respectively.
NS = Not Significant.

TABLE 2 | Values for functional fitness variables by gender (12 males; 31 females; total $n = 43$) (mean ± SD).

	M1	M2	P Wilcoxon
6MWT (m)α			
M	480.45 ± 98.38	479.67 ± 120.25	NS
F	394.21 ± 106.59	402.27 ± 117.13	NS
T	418.28 ± 110.37	424.38 ± 121.81	NS
% of ED-6MWT			
M	79.97 ± 11.99	81.51 ± 15.38	NS
F	78.91 ± 16.36	82.31 ± 19.01	NS
T	79.21 ± 15.14	82.08 ± 17.87	NS
Chair sit-and-reach test (cm)			
M	−4.13 ± 9.11	−9.58 ± 11.12	NS
F	−1.31 ± 9.42	−5.03 ± 9.68	NS
T	−2.09 ± 9.31	−6.30 ± 10.18	**0.015**
Back scratch test (cm)			
M	−14.00 ± 14.37	−18.83 ± 16.41	**0.041**
F	−10.15 ± 10.03	−13.47 ± 12.89	NS
T	−11.22 ± 11.36	−14.96 ± 13.96	**0.006**
30 s chair stand test			
M	13.33 ± 2.71	14.08 ± 4.29	NS
F	11.35 ± 3.68	12.80 ± 3.80	**0.008**
T	11.91 ± 3.52	13.19 ± 3.94	**0.008**
Arm curl test			
M	14.58 ± 2.78	17.17 ± 5.41	**0.029**
F	13.26 ± 4.19	14.71 ± 4.00	**0.015**
T	13.63 ± 3.86	15.40 ± 4.51	**0.001**
Right handgrip (kg)$^{\alpha, \beta}$			
M	38.58 ± 9.34	38.58 ± 9.98	NS
F	26.13 ± 7.09	25.74 ± 6.31	NS
T	29.60 ± 9.53	29.33 ± 9.41	NS
Left handgrip (kg)$^{\alpha, \beta}$			
M	37.08 ± 11.52	36.29 ± 10.78	NS
F	23.06 ± 5.73	23.35 ± 5.44	NS
T	26.98 ± 9.94	26.97 ± 9.28	NS
8-foot up-and-go test (s)			
M	6.66 ± 1.54	6.85 ± 2.25	NS
F	8.27 ± 2.89	8.47 ± 3.76	NS
T	7.83 ± 2.67	8.01 ± 3.45	NS
Berg scale			
M	54.33 ± 1.72	51.83 ± 4.47	NS
F	52.74 ± 3.54	49.87 ± 6.18	**0.000**
T	53.19 ± 3.20	50.42 ± 5.77	**0.000**

Legend: M, male; F, female; T, total; 6MWT, 6 min walk test; % of ED-6MWT, percentage of the estimated distance on 6MWT; $p < 0.05$ based on Wilcoxon signed-rank test for differences between M1 and M2, respectively, for males or females; α, β, $p < 0.05$ based on Mann–Whitney U test for differences between males and females on M1 and M2, respectively.
NS = Not Significant.

variables with significant differences at least in one time point). In summary, only type II diabetes and cholesterolemia conditions seemed to influence the performance in endurance capacity, Berg scale and flexibility (type diabetes), and strength (hypercholesterolemia). Longitudinal changes in endurance capacity (6MWT) were reduced in diabetic participants but not in non-diabetic ones (**Table 3**).

Anthropometrical and functional variables were statistically different across LPA and a better profile in functional capacity and anthropometry was showed for active when compared with inactive participants (**Table 4**). Distribution of comorbidities was similar among the physical activity level groups.

Finally, the linear regression models showed the best predictors of functional tests.

The first linear regression model to the dependent variable "Berg Balance Scale" was associated with 6MWT and "Right Handgrip" adjusted to weight was significant ($F = 27.076$; $p = 0.000$; $R^2 = 0.681$, and SEE = 3.400). The contribution of each predictor to the model was significant with a standardized Beta coefficient of 0.635 ($p = 0.000$) and 0.313 ($p = 0.039$), respectively. The whole model explained 68% of the variance.

The second linear regression model to the dependent variable "30 s chair stand test" was associated with 6MWT adjusted to weight ($F = 26.192$; $p = 0.000$; $R^2 = 0.567$, and SEE = 2.658). The contribution of the predictor to the model had standardized Beta coefficient of 0.779 ($p = 0.000$) with 57% of the variance explained by the model.

"Arm curl test" was correlated with 6MWT and "Left Handgrip" adjusted to weight (F = 12.190; $p = 0.000$; R2 = 0.484 and SEE = 3.362). The contribution of each predictor to the model was significant with a standardized Beta coefficient of 0.406 ($p = 0.009$) and 0.416 ($p = 0.024$), respectively (the model explained 48% of the variance).

Lower flexibility ("Chair Sit-and-Reach Test") was associated with upper flexibility ("Back Scratch Test") ($F = 9.111$; $p = 0.001$; $R^2 = 0.313$, and SEE = 8.646). The contribution of the predictor to the model was significant with a standardized Beta coefficient of 0.529 ($p = 0.000$) and the model explained 31% of the variance. Regarding, upper flexibility ("Back Scratch Test") was correlated with BBS ($F = 6.894$; $p = 0.003$; $R^2 = 0.256$, and SEE = 12.34) The contribution of the predictor to the model was significant with a standardized Beta coefficient of 0.500 ($p = 0.001$) and the model explained 26% of the variance.

Summarizing, physical function predictors, 6MWT and handgrip strength were the best predictors.

TABLE 3 | Values for functional fitness variables related with comorbidities (12 males; 31 females; Total $n = 43$) (mean ± SD).

	M1	M2	P Wilcoxon
Diabetes Mellitus			
6MWT (m)			
Non-diabetes ($n = 35$)	431.35 ± 113.04	442.118 ± 123.85	NS
Diabetes ($n = 8$)	361.09 ± 80.25	349.01 ± 81.07	NS
U Mann–Whitney	NS	**0.026**	
Back Scratch Test (cm)			
Non-Diabetes ($n = 35$)	−8.84 ± 10.26	−12.38 ± 13.05	**0.027**
Diabetes ($n = 8$)	−21.63 ± 10.51	−26.25 ± 12.82	NS
U Mann–Whitney	**0.006**	**0.005**	
Berg scale			
Non-Diabetes ($n = 35$)	53.54 ± 3.14	51.11 ± 5.91	**0.000**
Diabetes ($n = 8$)	51.63 ± 3.20	47.38 ± 4.14	NS
U Mann–Whitney	**0.033**	**0.022**	
Hypercholesterolemia			
Left handgrip (kg)			
Non-High Cholesterol ($n = 29$)	24.38 ± 6.09	24.22 ± 6.34	NS
High Cholesterol ($n = 14$)	32.36 ± 13.89	32.64 ± 11.28	NS
U Mann–Whitney	NS	**0.045**	

6MWT, 6 min' walk test; p < 0.05 based on Wilcoxon signed-rank test for differences between M1 and M2, respectively, for comorbidities; p < 0.05 based on Mann–Whitney test for differences between M1 and M2, respectively, for comorbidities.
NS = Not Significant.

Alternative or Additional

Finally, we could not find associations between changes in functional capacity tests and Berg scale or improvement in comorbidities.

DISCUSSION

To better understand the complex nature of physical function decline among older adults, we pursued two directions. First, we evaluated and identified the progression of physical function decline over a 3-year follow-up in a sample of people older than 60 years. Our results showed differences between gender in the anthropometric and functional variables after follow-up period, and these differences could be associated with changes in body composition across the aging process which is not a new finding. The level of functional fitness decreased with age, and the decrease was more important in females. On the other hand, this prospective longitudinal study showed the association between functional variables related to the balance, risk of falls, strength, physical fitness tests, and comorbidities. Our data bring knowledge to understand the variables that suffer the worst decrease with aging and may contribute to create more efficient strategies focused in these functional variables. In this scenario, the most important finding in this study is the relevance of 6MWT as predictor of other functional capacities and the influence of type II diabetes in 6MTW performance and age-related impairment.

The specific sexual phenotype of change for body weight was not new (BMI was reduced for male participants, but not for females); this adaptation followed the sarcopenic obesity paradigm since women did not lose weight in 3 years, but they increased waist and hip circumference (regional adiposity markers), and decreased whole-body skeletal muscle mass (SMM), which may increase the risk of hip fractures in the presence of a

TABLE 4 | Kruskal–Wallis analysis for differences in anthropometrical and functional variables between physical inactive, insufficiently active and active participants.

	Inactive ($n = 17$), mean ± SD	Insufficiently active ($n = 13$), mean ± SD	Active ($n = 12$), mean ± SD	*p*-Value
BMI (kg/m^2)	28.64 ± 3.53	27.92 ± 4.34	27.26 ± 2.79	NS
WHR	0.89 ± 0.11	0.88 ± 0.07	0.87 ± 0.10	NS
SMM (kg)	16.42 ± 4.00	19.47 ± 7.04	19.56 ± 4.08	**0.032**
6MWT (m)	334.12 ± 109.64	449.07 ± 86.63	525.50 ± 71.83	**0.000**
% of ED-6MWT (%)	72.32 ± 20.02	84.27 ± 13.53	93.54 ± 10.54	**0.006**
Chair sit-and-reach test (cm)	−9.65 ± 10.99	−5.65 ± 9.56	−2.57 ± 8.86	NS
Back scratch test (cm)	−22.23 ± 13.77	−8.76 ± 11.23	−11.65 ± 13.23	**0.011**
30 s chair stand test (repetitions)	10.88 ± 3.40	14.46 ± 3.47	14.92 ± 3.77	**0.009**
Arm curl test (repetitions)	12.65 ± 2.91	17.54 ± 5.12	16.85 ± 3.95	**0.004**
Right handgrip (kg)	23.29 ± 6.29	32.85 ± 9.90	33.69 ± 8.55	**0.003**
Left handgrip (kg)	21.12 ± 5.90	31.62 ± 10.92	29.96 ± 7.33	**0.001**
8-foot up-and-go test (s)	10.49 ± 3.96	6.59 ± 1.81	6.01 ± 1.27	**0.000**
Berg scale	46.29 ± 6.54	52.77 ± 3.46	53.46 ± 2.69	**0.001**

BMI, body mass index; WHR, waist to hip ratio; SMM, skeletal muscle mass; % of ED-6MWT, percentage of the estimated distance on 6MWT. p < 0.05; NS = Not Significant.

loss of balance. Previous studies (28, 29) concluded that greater abdominal obesity measured by WHR increased the risk of hip fracture considerably. The mechanism for an increased fracture risk with increasing WHR after adjusting for BMI might be mechanical instability and impaired balance induced by an increased body size in the abdominal region, leading to a fall (30). It has been suggested that carrying excess weight on the torso rather than on the hips increases the risk of falls that result in hip fracture, perhaps due to a higher center of gravity (28). This paradigm that explains a relationship between the increasing in the WHR and increment in the risk of falls was partially confirmed with our results of differences in the BBS variables, which suffered biggest significant changes (see **Table 2**). Other previous studies have investigated the relationship between obese and the risk of falls and fear of falls in older women (31–33). In general, results from our study are aligned with previous studies (34–37) and also with the study of Bird et al. (38) were balance decreased without loss of strength.

The influence of physical activity in functional capacity was confirmed in our group of age with a dose–response effect, so LPA were positively associated with performance in functional tests showing better results for those who are more active. Although only 30% of the participants accomplish physical activity guidelines (physical activity at least three times a week) the deleterious effect of PA on physical function impairment may not be related with a fixed quantity of PA, which may indicate that even low amounts of PA must promote significant benefits for physical function.

Our data highlighted that balance seems to be greatly explained by aerobic functional capacity (6MWT) and strength (handgrip). These results are in accordance with a previous study, which has shown that higher lower-limb function, balance, and mobility are associated with better walking ability and distance covered in the 6MWT by healthy older adults (39). Our study revealed that 6MWT and ha handgrip strength are also related with the BBS. Handgrip strength has been used as an outcome to measure muscle strength because it has been identified as strongly related with lower extremity muscle power, knee extension torque, and calf cross-sectional muscle area (40, 41) and could predict functional decline (42, 43). These findings reveal not only major relevance of cardiorespiratory fitness but also strength for preserving a good functional capacity. The main result from functional capacity were those related with comorbidities, although functional capacity were barely affected by group of comorbidities, so type II diabetes seemed to affect functional capacity (lower distance on 6MWT, lower flexibility, and lower balance than participants without diabetes type II). Furthermore participants with diabetes present a higher decrement on distance walked on 6MWT, which can potentiate the functional decline and risk of disability associated with aging. This topic should be object of more studies since this association may be a determinant of a frailty phenotype (44–46). In addition, we noticed that 39.5% at M1 and 35.7% of participants at M2 walked less than 400 m on 6MWT, which is a cut-off point to classify sarcopenia with limited mobility; on average, diabetic participants walked way below of this cut-off latter, representing their high susceptibility to be classified as sarcopenic obese and higher risk of frailty (47, 48). Regarding handgrip data, values split by hypercholesterolemia group were paradoxical since hypercholesterolemia group had higher values of strength, nevertheless the proportion of males and body weight values in the group of hypercholesterolemia were higher than in the group without hypercholesterolemia (35.7 vs 24.9%)., which may explain our results. Although the fact of having or not having multimorbidity [the presence of 2 or more chronic conditions (49)] may put older people in higher risk of frailty our results did not confirm this hypothesis.

Physical decline, including muscle weakness, balance dysfunction and mobility problems are related to functional decline, contributing to limit functional capacity while performing ADL and increasing the risk of falling (50, 51). Individualized intervention programs should address fall risks previously identified and they should include balance training, aerobic endurance, muscle strengthening, and flexibility (50).

Improvements in balance may rely in specific balance training programs (38) but also in other strategies. Our results may suggest that exercise prescription for older people should include also aerobic endurance and muscle training (50) as guidelines state, with recommendations to walk at least 30 min a day (52). Physical activity such as walking in different environments should be prescribed as an activity of daily living with benefits on physical capacity especially in balance and specially to those that do not meet the recommended 150 min per week of physical activity of moderate intensity and have or are at risk for chronic diseases (53), with special attention to groups of participants with comorbidities such as diabetes.

Strengths and Limitations

This was a longitudinal study that analyzed whether aging-related changes could be related with a lower decrement in functional variables such as muscle strength, flexibility, or mobility. However, the time interval was too short to found undeniable or high predictive value in variables of disability.

Although our study has a well-defined target population (day care centers and senior universities), participants were volunteers, and this could be a small bias which could be overcome by a larger sample. In addition, the small size of the sample is also a limitation that prevents a more accurate analysis of the results.

A higher time interval and a larger sample should be considered in future studies.

CONCLUSION

Results of this 3-year follow-up study confirmed the relevance of endurance and strength capacities, which may be improved across physical activity levels in combination with other body composition and physical function variables. The main relevance was the influence of type II diabetes 6MWT impairment in the second time point, which may confirm the deleterious consequences of the disease on cardiovascular capacity and sarcopenia; in addition, these results must provide construct validity of 6MWT. Finally, our results suggested that the loss of functional capacity must be more related with qualitative variables than morphological (for example, SMM) since we could not find any relationship between changes in body composition and physical function variables.

When prescribing exercise or programs for promoting health targeting this population greater attention should be given in walking activities and activities that use hands since these specific components seems to have a major impact in functional physical condition.

ETHICS STATEMENT

After an explanation of the study, participants signed an informed consent. All procedures were in accordance with the Declaration of Helsinki. All study procedures were approved by the institutional review boards of the participating institutions.

AUTHOR CONTRIBUTIONS

MTT, AG-M, EC, and BF have equally contributed to this manuscript, in designing the study. Data were collected by MTT, AG-M, and BF and were analyzed by all authors. Data interpretation and manuscript preparation were undertaken by MTT, AG-M, EC, and BF. All authors approved the final version of the paper.

ACKNOWLEDGMENTS

The authors wish to thank to Loures Municipality all the logistical support for the assessment of participants on two the moments.

FUNDING

This work was developed upon European Innovation Partnership for Active and Healthy Ageing (EIP-AHA) commitment without any financial support. A specific grant for supporting the publishing of knowledge was obtained from the institution of Portuguese authors (IPL/2016/SFQ2017_ESTeSL).

REFERENCES

1. Kirkwood TBL. Why and how are we living longer? *Exp Physiol* (2017) 102(9):1067–74. doi:10.1113/EP086205
2. PORDATA. *Retrato de Portugal, PORDATA*. 1a edição. Lisboa: Fundação Francisco Manuel dos Santos (2017).
3. van Zon SKR, Bültmann U, Reijneveld SA, de Leon CFM. Functional health decline before and after retirement: a longitudinal analysis of the health and retirement study. *Soc Sci Med* (2016) 170:26–34. doi:10.1016/j.socscimed.2016.10.002
4. Chen CM, Su YY, Mullan J, Huang MS, Chiu HC. Trajectories of disability and their relationship with health status and social service use. *Exp Aging Res* (2015) 41(3):240–58. doi:10.1080/0361073X.2015.1021641
5. Magyari P, Lite R, Kilpatrick MW, Schoffstall JE. *ACSM's Resources for the Exercise Physiologist – A Practical Guide for the Health Fitness Professional*. 2nd ed. American College of Sports Medicine, editor. Philadelphia: Wolters Kluwer Health (2018).
6. Rikli R, Jones CJ. *Senior Fitness Test Manual*. 2nd ed. Rikli R, Jones CJ, editors. Champaign, IL: Human Kinetics (2013).
7. Bergland A, Jørgensen L, Emaus N, Strand BH. Mobility as a predictor of all-cause mortality in older men and women: 11.8 year follow-up in the Tromsø study. *BMC Health Serv Res* (2017) 17(1):22. doi:10.1186/s12913-016-1950-0
8. Franzon K, Byberg L, Sjögren P, Zethelius B, Cederholm T, Kilander L. Predictors of independent aging and survival: a 16-year follow-up report in octogenarian men. *J Am Geriatr Soc* (2017) 65(9):1953–60. doi:10.1111/jgs.14971
9. Rossi AP, Fantin F, Caliari C, Zoico E, Mazzali G, Zanardo M, et al. Dynapenic abdominal obesity as predictor of mortality and disability worsening in older adults: a 10-year prospective study. *Clin Nutr* (2016) 35(1):199–204. doi:10.1016/j.clnu.2015.02.005
10. Distefano G, Goodpaster BH. Effects of exercise and aging on skeletal muscle. *Cold Spring Harb Perspect Med* (2017):a029785. doi:10.1101/cshperspect.a029785
11. Nagarkar A, Kashikar Y. Predictors of functional disability with focus on activities of daily living: a community based follow-up study in older adults in India. *Arch Gerontol Geriatr* (2017) 69:151–5. doi:10.1016/j.archger.2016.11.015
12. Veronese N, Stubbs B, Trevisan C, Bolzetta F, De Rui M, Solmi M, et al. What physical performance measures predict incident cognitive decline among intact older adults? A 4.4 year follow up study. *Exp Gerontol* (2016) 81:110–8. doi:10.1016/j.exger.2016.05.008
13. Onoda K, Ishihara M, Yamaguchi S. Decreased functional connectivity by aging is associated with cognitive decline. *J Cogn Neurosci* (2012) 24(11):2186–98. doi:10.1162/jocn_a_00269
14. Cartee GD, Hepple RT, Bamman MM, Zierath JR. Exercise promotes healthy aging of skeletal muscle. *Cell Metab* (2016) 23(6):1034–47. doi:10.1016/j.cmet.2016.05.007
15. Fiogbé E, de Vassimon-Barroso V, de Medeiros Takahashi AC. Exercise training in older adults, what effects on muscle oxygenation? A systematic review. *Arch Gerontol Geriatr* (2017) 71:89–98. doi:10.1016/j.archger.2017.03.001
16. Chodzko-Zajko WJ, Proctor DN, Fiatarone Singh MA, Minson CT, Nigg CR, Salem GJ, et al. Exercise and physical activity for older adults. *Med Sci Sports Exerc* (2009) 41(7):1510–30. doi:10.1249/MSS.0b013e3181a0c95c
17. de Asteasu MLS, Martínez-Velilla N, Zambom-Ferraresi F, Casas-Herrero Á, Izquierdo M. Role of physical exercise on cognitive function in healthy older adults: a systematic review of randomized clinical trials. *Ageing Res Rev* (2017) 37:117–34. doi:10.1016/j.arr.2017.05.007
18. Chmelo EA, Crotts CI, Newman JC, Brinkley TE, Lyles MF, Leng X, et al. Heterogeneity of physical function responses to exercise training in older adults. *J Am Geriatr Soc* (2015) 63(3):462–9. doi:10.1111/jgs.13322
19. American College of Sports Medicine. *ACSM's Health-Related Physical Fitness Assessment Manual*. 3rd ed. In: Kaminsky L, editor. Baltimore: Wolters Kluwer, Lippincott Williams & Wilkins (2010).
20. Heyward V. *Advanced Fitness Assessment & Exercise Prescription*. 3rd ed. Champaign: Human Kinetics (1997).
21. Haff GG, Dumke C. *Laboratory Manual for Exercise Physiology*. Champaign: Human Kinetics (2012).
22. Al-Gindan YY, Hankey C, Govan L, Gallagher D, Heymsfield SB, Lean ME. Derivation and validation of simple equations to predict total muscle mass from simple anthropometric and demographic data. *Am J Clin Nutr* (2014) 100(4):1041–51. doi:10.3945/ajcn.113.070466
23. ATS. ATS statement: guidelines for the six-minute walk test. *Am J Respir Crit Care Med* (2002) 166:111–7. doi:10 1164/ajrccm.166.1.at1102
24. Troosters T, Gosselink R, Decramer M. Six minute walking distance in healthy elderly subjects. *Eur Respir J* (1999) 14(2):270–4. doi:10.1034/j.1399-3003.1999.14b06.x
25. Rantanen T, Guralnik JM, Foley D, Masaki K, Leveille S, Curb JD, et al. Midlife hand grip strength as a predictor of old age disability. *JAMA* (1999) 281(6):558–60. doi:10.1001/jama.281.6.558
26. Berg KO, Wood-Dauphinee SL, Williams JI, Maki B. Measuring balance in the elderly: validation of an instrument. *Can J Public Health* (1992) 83 (Suppl 2):S7–11.
27. Donoghue D; Physiotherapy Research and Older People (PROP) Group, Stokes EK. How much change is true change? The minimum detectable change of the Berg Balance Scale in elderly people. *J Rehabil Med* (2009) 41(5):343–6. doi:10.2340/16501977-0337
28. Parker ED, Pereira MA, Virnig B, Folsom AR. The association of hip circumference with incident hip fracture in a cohort of postmenopausal women: the Iowa Women's Health Study. *Ann Epidemiol* (2008) 18(11):836–41. doi:10.1016/j.annepidem.2008.07.007
29. Søgaard AJ, Holvik K, Omsland TK, Tell GS, Dahl C, Schei B, et al. Abdominal obesity increases the risk of hip fracture. A population-based study of 43,000

women and men aged 60-79 years followed for 8 years. Cohort of Norway. *J Intern Med* (2015) 277(3):306–17. doi:10.1111/joim.12230
30. Corbeil P, Simoneau M, Rancourt D, Tremblay A, Teasdale N. Increased risk for falling associated with obesity: mathematical modeling of postural control. *IEEE Trans Neural Syst Rehabil Eng* (2001) 9(2):126–36. doi:10.1109/7333.928572
31. Rossi-Izquierdo M, Santos-Pérez S, Faraldo-García A, Vaamonde-Sánchez-Andrade I, Gayoso-Diz P, Del-Río-Valeiras M, et al. Impact of obesity in elderly patients with postural instability. *Aging Clin Exp Res* (2016) 28(3):423–8. doi:10.1007/s40520-015-0414-4
32. Dutil M, Handrigan GA, Corbeil P, Cantin V, Simoneau M, Teasdale N, et al. The impact of obesity on balance control in community-dwelling older women. *Age (Omaha)* (2013) 35(3):883–90. doi:10.1007/s11357-012-9386-x
33. Lim E. Sex differences in fear of falling among older adults with low grip strength. *Iran J Public Health* (2016) 45(5):569–77.
34. Milanovic Z, Jorgić B, Trajković N, Sporis G, Pantelić S, James N. Age-related decrease in physical activity and functional fitness among elderly men and women. *Clin Interv Aging* (2013) 8:549. doi:10.2147/CIA.S44112
35. Bassey EJ. Longitudinal changes in selected physical capabilities: muscle strength, flexibility and body size. *Age Ageing* (1998) 27(Suppl 3):12–6. doi:10.1093/ageing/27.suppl_3.12
36. Jenkins KR. Body-weight change and physical functioning among young old adults. *J Aging Health* (2004) 16(2):248–66. doi:10.1177/0898264303262626
37. Forrest KYZ, Zmuda JM, Cauley JA. Patterns and determinants of muscle strength change with aging in older men. *Aging Male* (2005) 8(3–4):151–6. doi:10.1080/13685530500137840
38. Bird M-L, Pittaway JK, Cuisick I, Rattray M, Ahuja KDK. Age-related changes in physical fall risk factors: results from a 3 year follow-up of community dwelling older adults in Tasmania, Australia. *Int J Environ Res Public Health* (2013) 10(11):5989–97. doi:10.3390/ijerph10115989
39. Caballer VB, Lisón JF, Rosado-Calatayud P, Amer-Cuenca JJ, Segura-Orti E. Factors associated with the 6-minute walk test in nursing home residents and community-dwelling older adults. *J Phys Ther Sci* (2015) 27(11):3571–8. doi:10.1589/jpts.27.3571
40. Lauretani F, Russo CR, Bandinelli S, Bartali B, Cavazzini C, Di Iorio A, et al. Age-associated changes in skeletal muscles and their effect on mobility: an operational diagnosis of sarcopenia. *J Appl Physiol* (2003) 95(5):1851–60. doi:10.1152/japplphysiol.00246.2003
41. Cruz-Jentoft AJ, Baeyens JP, Bauer JM, Boirie Y, Cederholm T, Landi F, et al. Sarcopenia: European consensus on definition and diagnosis: report of the European Working Group on Sarcopenia in Older People. *Age Ageing* (2010) 39(4):412–23. doi:10.1093/ageing/afq034
42. Olguín T, Bunout D, de la Maza MP, Barrera G, Hirsch S. Admission handgrip strength predicts functional decline in hospitalized patients. *Clin Nutr ESPEN* (2017) 17:28–32. doi:10.1016/j.clnesp.2016.12.001
43. Owusu C, Margevicius S, Schluchter M, Koroukian SM, Berger NA. Short physical performance battery, usual gait speed, grip strength and vulnerable elders survey each predict functional decline among older women with breast cancer. *J Geriatr Oncol* (2017) 8(5):356–62. doi:10.1016/j.jgo.2017.07.004
44. Marengoni A, Angleman S, Melis R, Mangialasche F, Karp A, Garmen A, et al. Aging with multimorbidity: a systematic review of the literature. *Ageing Res Rev* (2011) 10(4):430–9. doi:10.1016/j.arr.2011.03.003
45. Guaraldi G, Silva AR, Stentarelli C. Multimorbidity and functional status assessment. *Curr Opin HIV AIDS* (2014) 9(4):386–97. doi:10.1097/COH.0000000000000079
46. Portz JD, Kutner JS, Blatchford PJ, Ritchie CS. High symptom burden and low functional status in the setting of multimorbidity. *J Am Geriatr Soc* (2017) 65(10):2285–9. doi:10.1111/jgs.15045
47. Hubbard RE, Lang IA, Llewellyn DJ, Rockwood K. Frailty, body mass index, and abdominal obesity in older people. *J Gerontol A Biol Sci Med Sci* (2010) 65(4):377–81. doi:10.1093/gerona/glp186
48. Toosizadeh N, Wendel C, Hsu C-H, Zamrini E, Mohler J. Frailty assessment in older adults using upper-extremity function: index development. *BMC Geriatr* (2017) 17(1):117. doi:10.1186/s12877-017-0509-1
49. Barnett K, Mercer SW, Norbury M, Watt G, Wyke S, Guthrie B. Epidemiology of multimorbidity and implications for health care, research, and medical education: a cross-sectional study. *Lancet* (2012) 380(9836):37–43. doi:10.1016/S0140-6736(12)60240-2
50. Rose DJ. Preventing falls among older adults: no "one size suits all" intervention strategy. *J Rehabil Res Dev* (2008) 45(8):1153–66. doi:10.1682/JRRD.2008.03.0041
51. Rubenstein LZ, Josephson KR. The epidemiology of falls and syncope. *Clin Geriatr Med* (2002) 18(2):141–58. doi:10.1016/S0749-0690(02)00002-2
52. WHO. *Global Recommendations on Physical Activity for Health.* Geneva: World Health Organization (2010). 60 p.
53. Sallis R, Franklin B, Joy L, Ross R, Sabgir D, Stone J. Strategies for promoting physical activity in clinical practice. *Prog Cardiovasc Dis* (2015) 57(4):375–86. doi:10.1016/j.pcad.2014.10.003

5

Cholesterol Removal from Adult Skeletal Muscle Impairs Excitation–contraction Coupling and Aging Reduces Caveolin-3 and Alters the Expression of other Triadic Proteins

Genaro Barrientos[1†], *Paola Llanos*[2†], *Jorge Hidalgo*[1], *Pura Bolaños*[3], *Carlo Caputo*[3], *Alexander Riquelme*[4], *Gina Sánchez*[4,5,6], *Andrew F. G. Quest*[6,7,8] *and Cecilia Hidalgo*[1,4,6*]

[1] Physiology and Biophysics Program, Institute of Biomedical Sciences, School of Medicine, University of Chile, Santiago, Chile, [2] Institute for Research in Dental Sciences, Faculty of Dentistry, University of Chile, Santiago, Chile, [3] Centre of Biophysics and Biochemistry, Venezuelan Institute for Scientific Research, Caracas, Venezuela, [4] Biomedical Neuroscience Institute, School of Medicine, University of Chile, Santiago, Chile, [5] Pathophysiology Program, Institute of Biomedical Sciences, School of Medicine, University of Chile, Santiago, Chile, [6] Center for Molecular Studies of the Cell, School of Medicine, University of Chile, Santiago, Chile, [7] Laboratory of Cell Communication, Program in Cell and Molecular Biology, Institute of Biomedical Sciences, School of Medicine, University of Chile, Santiago, Chile, [8] Advanced Center for Chronic Diseases and Network for Metabolic Stress Signaling, University of Chile, Santiago, Chile

Edited by:
Brian McDonagh,
University of Liverpool, UK

Reviewed by:
Nazareno Paolocci,
Johns Hopkins University, USA
John James Mackrill,
University College Cork, Ireland

***Correspondence:**
Cecilia Hidalgo,
Facultad de Medicina, Center for Molecular Studies of the Cell and Physiology and Biophysics Program, Biomedical Neuroscience Institute, Instituto de Ciencias Biomédicas, Universidad de Chile, Independencia 1027, Santiago 8380453, Chile
chidalgo@med.uchile.cl

† These authors have contributed equally to this work.

Cholesterol and caveolin are integral membrane components that modulate the function/location of many cellular proteins. Skeletal muscle fibers, which have unusually high cholesterol levels in transverse tubules, express the caveolin-3 isoform but its association with transverse tubules remains contentious. Cholesterol removal impairs excitation–contraction (E–C) coupling in amphibian and mammalian fetal skeletal muscle fibers. Here, we show that treating single muscle fibers from adult mice with the cholesterol removing agent methyl-β-cyclodextrin decreased fiber cholesterol by 26%, altered the location pattern of caveolin-3 and of the voltage dependent calcium channel Cav1.1, and suppressed or reduced electrically evoked Ca^{2+} transients without affecting membrane integrity or causing sarcoplasmic reticulum (SR) calcium depletion. We found that transverse tubules from adult muscle and triad fractions that contain ~10% attached transverse tubules, but not SR membranes, contained caveolin-3 and Cav1.1; both proteins partitioned into detergent-resistant membrane fractions highly enriched in cholesterol. Aging entails significant deterioration of skeletal muscle function. We found that triad fractions from aged rats had similar cholesterol and RyR1 protein levels compared to triads from young rats, but had lower caveolin-3 and glyceraldehyde 3-phosphate dehydrogenase and increased Na^+/K^+-ATPase protein levels. Both triad fractions had comparable NADPH oxidase (NOX) activity and protein content of NOX2 subunits ($p47^{phox}$ and $gp91^{phox}$), implying that NOX activity does not increase during aging. These findings show that partial cholesterol removal impairs E–C coupling and alters caveolin-3 and Cav1.1 location pattern, and that aging reduces caveolin-3 protein content and modifies the expression of other triadic proteins. We discuss the possible implications of these findings for skeletal muscle function in young and aged animals.

Keywords: transverse tubules, Ca^{2+} transients, RyR1, Cav1.1, GAPDH, NADPH oxidase, Na^+/K^+-ATPase

Introduction

In skeletal muscle, action potentials propagate into the fiber interior through the transverse tubule (T-tubule) system, an intracellular membrane network composed of narrow tubules around 40–85 nm in diameter that originate from deep invaginations of the surface plasma membrane (Melzer et al., 1995; Jayasinghe and Launikonis, 2013). The T-tubule network contains Cav1.1 voltage-dependent Ca^{2+} channels (Anderson et al., 1994)—also known as dihydropyridine receptors (DHPR)—which play a crucial role in skeletal muscle excitation–contraction (E–C) coupling. Skeletal muscle T-tubules form arrangements called triads with the two adjacent terminal cisternae of the sarcoplasmic reticulum (SR) (Franzini-Armstrong, 1972). At the triads, the T-tubule Cav1.1 channels physically interact with the type-1 ryanodine receptor (RyR1), Ca^{2+} release channels present in junctional SR (Marks et al., 1989; Zalk et al., 2007). Muscle depolarization triggers voltage-dependent Cav1.1 conformational changes (Rios et al., 1993; Minarovic and Meszaros, 1998) that elicit RyR1-mediated Ca^{2+} release (Anderson and Meissner, 1995; Fill and Copello, 2002); the ensuing increase in myoplasmic Ca^{2+} concentration ($[Ca^{2+}]$) triggers muscle contraction.

Reports regarding T-tubule lipid composition from vertebrate muscles have revealed some unusual features, characterized by high cholesterol and sphingolipid contents (Lau et al., 1979; Rosemblatt et al., 1981; Hidalgo et al., 1986), which endow T-tubule membranes with an unusually rigid lipid environment similar to that present in thermophilic bacteria (Hidalgo, 1985). The high cholesterol and sphingolipid levels of T-tubule membranes, which are significantly higher than those present in plasma membranes, are comparable to those reported in lipids rafts and caveolae (Smart et al., 1999). Previous studies indicate that treatment of cultured C2C12 muscle cells with the cholesterol-binding drug Amphotericin B considerably reduces the tubular elements connected to the surface (Carozzi et al., 2000). Similarly, treatment of fetal skeletal muscle cells from mice with the cholesterol-lowering agent MβCD decreases surface-connected tubular elements and disorganizes the T-tubule system (Pouvreau et al., 2004). Previous reports indicate that cholesterol removal impairs E–C coupling in amphibian (Launikonis and Stephenson, 2001) and skeletal muscles from fetal mice (Pouvreau et al., 2004). To test the hypothesis that T-tubule cholesterol content is important for E–C coupling in adult muscle, the first aim of the present work was to examine in single skeletal muscle fibers from adult mice the effects of partial cholesterol removal with MβCD on electrically evoked Ca^{2+} transients.

Caveolins are a particular class of membrane proteins that associate directly with cholesterol in lipid rafts and constitute structural components of caveolae. The scaffolding domain of caveolin participates in protein-protein interactions and the regulation of signal transduction events (Williams and Lisanti, 2004). Striated muscle tissue expresses mainly the caveolin-3 protein isoform (Song et al., 1996); yet, few studies have addressed the role of caveolin-3 in striated muscle function. In cardiac muscle cells, caveolin-3 associates with Cav1.2 (L-type) Ca^{2+} channels (Balijepalli et al., 2006). The expression levels of caveolin-3 in skeletal muscle modulate Ca^{2+} currents through Cav1.1 L-type calcium channels and caveolin-3 mutations reduce Cav1.1 currents without altering Cav1.1 expression levels (Weiss et al., 2008), suggesting a role for caveolin-3 in the E–C coupling process. Additionally, recent studies reported direct interaction of caveolin-3 with skeletal muscle RyR1 (Whiteley et al., 2012) and suggested inhibition of mechano-sensitive cation channels by caveolin-3 (Huang et al., 2013). The precise location of caveolin-3 in skeletal muscle fibers remains contentious. Previous studies reported that caveolin-3 is present in the sarcolemma (skeletal muscle surface plasma membrane) associated with the dystrophin complex (Song et al., 1996), and that during muscle differentiation caveolin-3 associates with developing T-tubules but is absent from mature T-tubules (Parton et al., 1997). A later study in soleus muscle from adult rats, however, reported that while caveolin-3 occurs at the highest density on the plasma membrane, it is also present in T-tubules (Ralston and Ploug, 1999). Caveolin-3 knockout mice present T-tubule system abnormalities (Galbiati et al., 2001), consistent with a T-tubule location, and also exhibit muscle degeneration (Hagiwara et al., 2000). A more recent study reported the presence of caveolin-3 in isolated SR vesicles (Li et al., 2006), albeit the low cholesterol content of these membranes (Lau et al., 1979; Rosemblatt et al., 1981) makes this location unlikely. Hence, to test the hypothesis that in adult muscle fibers caveolin-3 is present in the T-tubules, the second aim of this work was to study caveolin-3 location in adult mammalian skeletal muscle.

Aging entails significant deterioration of skeletal muscle function (Miller et al., 2014). Among other changes, a decreased intracellular Ca^{2+} peak associates with the reduction in muscle force observed during aging (Booth et al., 1994; Wang et al., 2000). Age-related changes in T-tubule protein and lipid composition might contribute to the observed defects in skeletal muscle function. In fact, previous work suggested that aged rats have uncoupled Cav1.1-RyR1 channels (Renganathan et al., 1997) and display a 60% reduction in Cav1.1 protein levels (O'connell et al., 2008). No information is available, however, on changes in T-tubule cholesterol and caveolin-3 levels during aging. Therefore, to test the hypothesis that aging brings about

Abbreviations: Cav1.1, Voltage-dependent Ca^{2+} channels; Ca^{2+}, Calcium; DHPR, Dihydropyridine receptor; DRM, Detergent resistant membranes; E-C coupling, excitation–contraction coupling; FDB, Flexor digitorium brevis; GAPDH, Glyceraldehyde 3-phosphate dehydrogenase; HRS, Heavy sarcoplasmic reticulum; LSR, Light reticulum; MβCD, Methyl-β-cyclodextrin; NOX, NADPH-oxidase; RyR1, Type-1 ryanodine receptor; SR, Sarcoplasmic reticulum; T-tubules, Transverse tubules.

changes in transverse tubule components, which might contribute to aged-related defective skeletal muscle function, the third aim of the present study was to investigate if aging modifies T-tubule cholesterol levels and to compare, in addition, the levels of key triadic proteins including caveolin-3 in young and aged rats. For this purpose, we used triad-enriched membrane fractions obtained from adult skeletal muscle that contain ~10% attached T-tubules (Hidalgo et al., 1993), and which after isolation maintain the morphological features found in intact muscle (Wagenknecht et al., 2002). In particular, we investigated if caveolin-3 levels change in aged animals since alterations in the levels of this scaffolding protein may result in ion channel dysregulation, among other effects.

Our results show that partial cholesterol extraction from isolated single skeletal fibers impaired E–C coupling and altered Cav1.1 and caveolin-3 distribution. We also found caveolin-3 in T-tubules and T-tubule-containing triad fractions but not in SR membranes, and in cholesterol-enriched detergent-resistant membrane (DRM) fractions from T-tubules or triads. We observed significantly decreased caveolin-3 and glyceraldehyde 3-phosphate dehydrogenase (GAPDH) and increased Na^+/K^+-ATPase levels in triads from aged rats, but we did not detect changes in cholesterol and RyR1 protein levels. We discuss the possible implications of these findings for skeletal muscle E–C coupling in young and aged animals.

Materials and Methods

Animals

Male New Zealand white rabbits (6-month-old), Balb/C mice (8-week-old) and Sprague Dawley rats (3 or 24 months-old) were obtained from the Animal Facility at the Faculty of Medicine, Universidad de Chile. Room temperature was kept constant at 21°C, and light was maintained on a 12:12 h light-dark cycle. Mice were sacrificed by quick cervical dislocation. Rabbits and rats were euthanized by intraperitoneal overdose of sodium pentobarbital (100 mg/kg). All experiments were carried out following the guidelines provided by National Institutes of Health (USA) and the regulations for the Care and Use of Animals for Scientific Purposes; the Bioethics Committee of the Faculty of Medicine, Universidad de Chile approved all animal procedures performed in this work.

Materials

All reagents used were of analytical grade. Protease inhibitors (leupeptin, pepstatin A, benzamidine, and phenylmethylsulfonyl fluoride) were from Sigma-Aldrich (St. Louis, MO), MagFluo-4 AM and Fluo-4 AM were from Invitrogen (Carlsbad, CA), and Matrigel was from BD Biosciences (San Jose, CA). Paraformaldehyde was from Electron Microscopy Science (Hatfield, PA), Dulbecco's modified Eagle's medium supplemented with 10% fetal bovine serum was from Invitrogen (Carlsbad, CA) and was supplemented with 0.1 mg/ml penicillin–streptomycin from Sigma-Aldrich (St. Louis, MO). The BCA protein assay kit was from Pierce Biotechnology, Inc. (Rockford, IL), commercial BSA was from Sigma-Aldrich (St. Louis, MO) and Dako anti-fading reagent was from Dako (Denmark). Horseradish peroxidase-conjugated anti-IgG (anti-mouse or anti-rabbit) were from Santa Cruz Biotechnology, Inc. (Santa Cruz, CA). Antibodies against the $\alpha 1s$ subunit of Cav1.1 were from Affinity BioReagents (Golden, CO; mouse monoclonal) or from Santa Cruz Biotechnology, Inc. (Santa Cruz, CA; rabbit polyclonal). Alexa Fluor-488 anti-mouse and Alexa Fluor-633 anti-rabbit antibodies were from Invitrogen (Carlsbad, CA). Caveolin-3 antibodies were from BD Biosciences (San Jose, CA) or Santa Cruz Biotechnology (Santa Cruz, CA), $gp91^{phox}$ and $p47^{phox}$ antibodies were from Santa Cruz Biotechnology (Santa Cruz, CA), GAPDH antibody was from Sigma-Aldrich (St. Louis, MO), RyR1 (34C) and Na^+/K^+-ATPase (α6F) antibodies were from Developmental Studies Hybridoma Bank http://dshb.biology.uiowa.edu/. The Amplex Red Cholesterol Assay kit was from Invitrogen (Carlsbad, CA), the total cholesterol assay kit was from Labtest (Sao Paulo, Brazil) and the ECL kit was from Thermo Fisher Scientific Inc. (Rockford, IL).

Fiber Isolation from Adult Skeletal Muscle

Flexor digitorum brevis (FDB) muscles were dissected from 8 week-old mice and single intact myofibers were isolated enzymatically as described (Carroll et al., 1995; Barrientos et al., 2009). Isolated fibers were plated on Matrigel-coated coverslips and maintained in Dulbecco's modified Eagle's medium supplemented with 10% fetal bovine serum and 0.1 mg/ml penicillin–streptomycin. Fibers were kept overnight in an incubator under 5% CO_2, and experiments were conducted within 12–24 h of plating.

Immunofluorescence

Dissociated single fibers from adult mice FDB muscles were plated on 35 mm coverslips coated with Matrigel. After washing with PBS, fibers were fixed by incubation for 10 min at room temperature with PBS supplemented with 4% paraformaldehyde. Next, fibers were rinsed with PBS, permeabilized with 0.1% TritonX-100 in PBS, rinsed with PBS and blocked for 1 h with PBS-1% BSA at room temperature. Fibers were incubated overnight with polyclonal rabbit antibodies against caveolin-3 (1:100, Santa Cruz Biotechnology; Santa Cruz, CA,) and Cav1.1 (1:100). Fibers were washed and incubated 1 h with Alexa Fluor-488 anti-mouse and Alexa Fluor-633 anti-rabbit antibodies. Samples treated with Dako anti-fading reagent were stored at 4°C until use.

Fluorescence Recording and Field Stimulation

All records were collected from single fibers bathed in mammalian Ringer solution (mM: 145 NaCl, 2.5 KCl, 1.0 $MgSO_4$, 2.5 $CaCl_2$, 10 glucose, 10 Hepes/Tris, pH 7.4). Fibers were incubated for 40 min at room temperature with 10 μM MagFluo-4 AM in mammalian Ringer solution containing 0.01% pluronic acid. Alternatively, fibers were loaded at room temperature for 40 min in mammalian Ringer plus 0.01% pluronic acid with the higher affinity Ca^{2+} dye Fluo-4 AM (10 μM). Fibers adhering spontaneously to the glass bottom of the experimental chamber were selected for fluorescence recording. The experimental chamber was mounted on the stage of an inverted Nikon Diaphot

TMD microscope equipped for epifluorescence. Fibers were illuminated with a xenon lamp (100 W) only during recording to avoid dye photobleaching. The characteristic wavelengths of filter combinations (excitation/dichroic/barrier) were (nm) 450–490/510/520. Light signals were collected from a spot of approximately 12 μm diameter, with a photomultiplier connected to a Nikon P1 amplifier. This procedure allowed recording from several fibers within the microscope field (Calderon et al., 2011).

Field stimulation leading to intracellular Ca^{2+} transients was elicited by applying supra-threshold rectangular current pulses (0.2–0.4 ms duration) through two platinum plate electrodes placed on either side along the experimental chamber. The amplifier output was connected to an Axon Instruments TL1 DMA interface. Data were acquired and analyzed using the Axon Instruments pCLAMP 6 software. Fluorescence values are expressed as $\Delta F/F_{rest}[(F - F_{rest})/F_{rest}]$, where F_{rest} correspond to the basal fluorescence recorded before stimulation (Capote et al., 2005).

Membrane Fractions

Triad-enriched fractions (hereafter referred to as triads) containing on average 10% attached T-tubules were isolated from rabbit or rat muscle as described previously (Hidalgo et al., 1993). T-tubule membranes, heavy sarcoplasmic reticulum (HRS) and light reticulum (LSR) from skeletal muscle were isolated as previously described (Rosemblatt et al., 1981), with some modifications. Briefly, 100 g of back muscles from rabbit or 15 g from the back and hind limb skeletal muscles from male rats were homogenized in four volumes of buffer A (mM: 100 KCl. 20 MOPS-Tris, pH 7.0). The suspension was centrifuged at 10,000 × g and the sediment was homogenized in buffer A, adjusted to 0.6 M KCl by solid salt addition and centrifuged for 1 h at 100,000 × g. The pellets were resuspended in buffer A containing a combination of protease inhibitors (1 μg/ml leupeptin, 1 μg/ml pepstatin, 0.4 mM benzamidine 1 mM phenylmethanesulfonylfluoride), and sedimented at 100,000 × g. The pellets were resuspended in sucrose buffer (buffer B; mM: 300 sucrose, 20 MOPS-Tris, pH 7.0, plus 1 μg/ml leupeptin, 1 μg/ml pepstatin, 0.4 mM benzamidine) and centrifuged at 100,000 × g. The resulting pellets were resuspended in buffer B, loaded on a discontinuous sucrose gradient (45, 35, 27.5, and 25% w/v) and centrifuged at 100,000 × g overnight. T-tubules were collected from the 25/27.5% interface. The HSR and LSR fractions were collected from the 35/45 and the 27.5/35% interfaces, respectively. Fractions were resuspended in buffer B, centrifuged for 30 min at 100,000 × g and the pellets were resuspended in a minimum volume of buffer B, frozen in liquid N_2 and stored at −80°C until use.

Junctional T-tubule fractions were prepared from triads as described (Horgan and Kuypers, 1987). Briefly, the triad fraction was loaded on top of an ion-free sucrose gradient (1.4–0.74 M) and centrifuged 16 h at 100,000 × g. This treatment separates the junctional T-tubule membranes from the triads and yields a light fraction containing junctional T-tubules. This fraction was collected, diluted in 20 mM MOPS/Tris, pH 7.2 supplemented with 1 μg/ml leupeptin, 1 μg/ml pepstatin, 0.4 mM benzamidine, and centrifuged for 1 h at 100,000 × g. The pellet, resuspended in a small volume of buffer B containing 1 μg/ml leupeptin, 1 μg/ml pepstatin, was stored at −80°C until use.

Detergent-resistant Membrane (DRM) Fractions

DRM fractions were prepared from triads and T-tubule membranes as described (Brown and Waneck, 1992; Sargiacomo et al., 1993) with minor modifications. Briefly, membrane fractions were resuspended and mixed in 2 ml (final volume) of Mes buffer saline (MBS, in mM: 150 NaCl, 25 Mes/NaOH, pH 6.5) containing 1% Triton X-100 and protease inhibitors (1 μg/ml leupeptin, 1 μg/ml pepstatin, 1 mM phenylmethanesulfonylfluoride, 0.4 mM benzamidine) and incubated for 15 min at 4°C. The suspensions, adjusted to 40% (w/v) sucrose by adding 2 ml of ice-cold 80% sucrose (w/v) in MBS, were placed at the bottom of an ultracentrifuge tube: two equal volume layers of 30 and 5% sucrose were added on top, and the gradients were centrifuged at 100,000 × g for 20 h. The light opalescent band confined to the 5–30% interface was collected, diluted three times with MBS and centrifuged at 100,000 × g for 1 h. The fractions thus obtained were resuspended in buffer B, frozen in liquid nitrogen and stored at −80°C until use.

SDS/PAGE and Western Blot Analysis

Membrane preparations were heat-denatured in SDS-containing sample buffer with reducing agents and loaded onto Tris-glycine 4–12% acrylamide gradient SDS-containing gels. Following electrophoresis at 100 V, proteins were transferred to nitrocellulose membranes at 100 V for 1 h. Membranes, blocked with 5% nonfat dry milk in Tris-saline buffer (mM: 140 NaCl, 20 Tris-HCl, pH 7.6) plus 0.2% Tween 20 were probed with specific antibodies directed against T-tubule or SR proteins. Horseradish peroxidase-conjugated anti-mouse or anti-rabbit IgG were used as secondary antibodies. Immunoblots were developed using an ECL kit and automated image capture was performed with the ChemiDoc system (Bio-Rad, Hercules, CA). All blot quantifications involved measuring band intensities; the amount of protein loaded in each lane was checked by Coomassie blue staining.

Other Procedures

NOX activity was determined as described previously (Sanchez et al., 2008). Protein concentration was determined by the BCA protein assay using commercial BSA as a standard. Cholesterol content was determined using the colorimetric total cholesterol kit or the fluorescence Amplex Red Cholesterol Assay kit, as detailed in the text. Electron microscopy (EM) analysis of DRM fractions was performed as described (Badizadegan et al., 2000).

Statistical Analysis

To detect significant differences between two groups, statistical analysis of data, presented as Mean ± SE, was determined with the Student's *t*-test (two-tailed); a value of $p < 0.05$ was considered statistically significant.

Results

Membrane Cholesterol Reduction Impairs Skeletal Muscle E–C Coupling

To study whether decreasing the high T-tubule cholesterol levels affects the E–C coupling process, we measured electrically induced Ca^{2+} transients in FDB fibers from adult mice before and after addition of the cholesterol-lowering agent MβCD. The representative experiment illustrated in **Figure 1A** shows Ca^{2+} transients recorded in fibers loaded with the low-affinity Ca^{2+} probe MagFluo-4 before or 5, 20, and 25 min after perfusion with 1% MβCD, which abolished Ca^{2+} transients after 25 min. This treatment impaired Ca^{2+} transients in all fibers tested, isolated from six different animals. Of note, MβCD abolished Ca^{2+} transients in 26 of the 30 fibers tested and in the remaining 4 fibers it significantly reduced Ca^{2+} transient amplitude by 51.3 ± 27.6 (%).

To assay whether MβCD treatment modified resting myoplasmic free [Ca^{2+}], which did not display apparent changes in fibers loaded with the low affinity Ca^{2+} probe MagFluo-4 (**Figure 1A**), we loaded fibers with Fluo-4, a high affinity fluorescent Ca^{2+} probe, and determined Ca^{2+} transients elicited by electrical field stimulation. The representative experiment illustrated in **Figure 1B** shows that initial stimulation at 20 Hz elicited significant Ca^{2+} transients in two fibers recorded in parallel. After perfusion with 1% MβCD, both fibers displayed for about 8 min Ca^{2+} transients of similar magnitudes in response to stimulation at 0.1 Hz, after which time the response declined abruptly and vanished within 2 min (**Figure 1B**). The same results were obtained in 26 fibers from five different mice treated with MβCD. In contrast, and in agreement with previous findings (Barrientos et al., 2009), control fibers (18 fibers from 5 mice) loaded with Fluo-4 AM in mammalian Ringer solution containing 0.01% pluronic acid, responded with Ca^{2+} transients of equal magnitude for at least 30 min when stimulated at 0.1 Hz (not shown).

Perfusion with 1% MβCD produced an increase in resting fluorescence coincident with the decline in Ca^{2+} transient amplitude, as evidenced from the parallel records from two fibers illustrated in **Figure 1B**; the Fluo-4 fluorescence increase reached a plateau 9–11 min after MβCD addition. Average fluorescence values recorded 20 min after MβCD addition showed a small but significant baseline fluorescence increase in MβCD-treated fibers ($n = 25$) relative to the controls ($n = 17$) (**Figure 1C**). This increase was observed at levels far from probe saturation, as indicated by the considerably higher fluorescence increase produced by the initial stimulation at 20 Hz. From this higher value and the K_d (345 μM) for Fluo-4, we estimate that the net increase in resting [Ca^{2+}] was < 100 nM. Perfusion with 10 mM caffeine after MβCD removal, when resting [Ca^{2+}] reached a plateau, produced a transient and significant increase in fluorescence (**Figure 1B**). The caffeine-stimulated fluorescence increase was observed in a large fraction (23/26) of MβCD-treated fibers and in all (18/18) control fibers.

These combined results indicate that perfusion with 1% MβCD, which decreases cholesterol levels by 26% in FDB fibers from adult muscle (**Table 1**), abolishes electrically evoked Ca^{2+} transients without significantly perturbing the membrane permeability barrier, as indicated by the lack of massive increase in myoplasmic [Ca^{2+}]. Additionally, the stimulatory effects of caffeine strongly suggest that the lack of response to electrical stimulation in MβCD-treated fibers is not due to SR depletion and presumably reflects impaired E–C coupling.

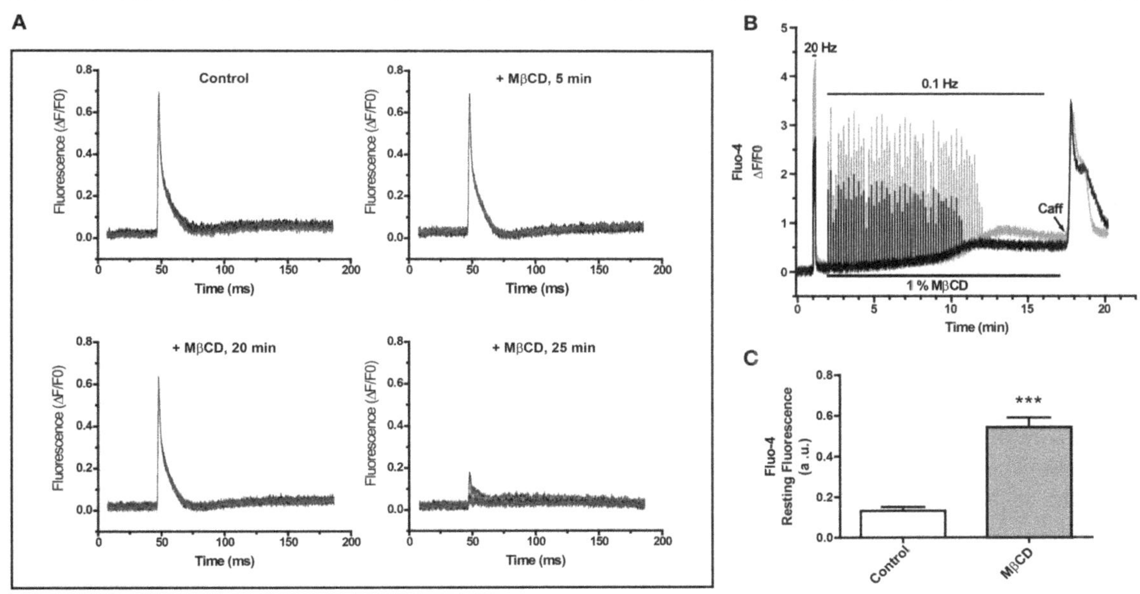

FIGURE 1 | Perfusion of single fibers from adult skeletal muscle with MβCD abolishes calcium transients and increases resting calcium levels. (A) FDB fibers were loaded with the low affinity Ca^{2+} sensor Mag-Fluo-4 and Ca^{2+} transients were elicited by electrical field stimulation. Fluorescence was evaluated before and after the addition of 1% MβCD. Each panel shows 10 transients, collected at 10 s intervals at the times indicated in the figure. **(B)** Ca^{2+} transients were elicited by electric field stimulation of FDB fibers loaded with Fluo-4, a high affinity Ca^{2+} probe. The traces show the fluorescence of two fibers and their responses to field stimulation at 20 or 0.1 Hz. The continuous line at the top represents the period of electric field stimulation, the lower continuous line indicates the period of perfusion with MβCD. The arrowhead indicates addition of 10 mM caffeine. **(C)** Average Fluo-4 resting fluorescence collected 20 min after initiation fluorescence recording in control ($n = 17$) or MβCD-treated ($n = 25$) fibers.

TABLE 1 | Cholesterol content in mice skeletal fibers and membrane fractions.

Assayed sample	Cholesterol (μg/mg protein)
SKELETAL FDB FIBERS	
A. Control	17.6 ± 1.2 (4)
B. MβCD-treated	13.1 ± 1.4 (4)
MEMBRANE FRACTIONS	
C. T-tubules (rabbit)	271.6 ± 14.8 (3)
D. DRM from T-tubules (rabbit)	1233.0 ± 69.55 (4)
Ratio D/C	4.5
E. Triads (rabbit)	41.5 ± 2.3 (4)
F. DRM from Triads (rabbit)	184.3 ± 4.9 (4)
Ratio F/E	4.4
G. Plasma membrane (Ortegren et al., 2004)	143
H. Caveolae (Ortegren et al., 2004)	400.5 ± 21
Ratio H/G	2.8

Total cholesterol content was measured, with the exception of the DRM fractions, with a commercial colorimetric kit; cholesterol content of DRM fractions was determined with the Amplex Red kit (for details see Materials and Methods). FDB cholesterol content was measured in sonicated whole fiber homogenates. Data represent Mean ± SE; the number of different preparation assayed is given in parenthesis.

Caveolin-3 Associates with T-tubule and Triad Membranes and is Absent from SR Fractions

Previous reports suggest a role for caveolin-3 in skeletal muscle E–C coupling (Weiss et al., 2008; Whiteley et al., 2012), which, as reported here, is sensitive to cholesterol removal from adult fibers. The caveolin proteins bind directly to cholesterol (Murata et al., 1995) and their presence in membranes correlates directly with membrane cholesterol levels (Toselli et al., 2005); however, the location of caveolin-3 in T-tubule membranes remains debatable. Accordingly, we tested here the location of caveolin-3 by immunohistochemistry of adult fibers from mice and by Western blot analysis of membrane fractions isolated from rabbit or rat skeletal muscle.

As illustrated in **Figure 2A**, caveolin-3 co-localizes with Cav1.1 in FDB fibers from adult mice skeletal muscle. Treatment of with 1% MβCD, which reduced cholesterol content by 26% (**Table 1**), produced a significant change in the distribution of both Cav1.1 (**Figure 2B**) and caveolin-3 (**Figure 2C**). After MβCD treatment, both proteins exhibited a decrease in the characteristic banding pattern displayed by control fibers, suggesting that partial reduction of fiber cholesterol content alters the typical array of Cav1.1 in the T-tubule membrane (**Figure 2B**) and reduces the association of caveolin-3 with T-tubules (**Figure 2C**). Similar results were obtained in 3–9 fiber preparations from each mouse, out of a total of four mice.

The representative Western blot illustrated in **Figure 3A** shows that caveolin-3 is present in T-tubules (lanes 1–2) and triads (lanes 5–6) isolated from rabbit skeletal muscle, but is absent from the LSR (lane 3) and HSR (lane 4) fractions, which are highly enriched in Ca^{2+}-ATPase and RyR1/calsequestrin, respectively (not shown). We obtained similar results in 3 independent preparations. The separate blots shown in **Figure 3B** confirm that T-tubule and triad fractions contain Cav1.1. These findings show unambiguously that caveolin-3 is present in T-tubules and T-tubule-containing triads but is absent from SR membranes. To further assay the specific association of caveolin-3 with T-tubule membranes, we dissociated triads isolated from rabbit muscle to generate a light fraction enriched in junctional T-tubule membranes (Horgan and Kuypers, 1987). The representative whole gel (stained with Coomassie blue) illustrated in **Figure 3C** (left) shows that the protein profile of T-tubules isolated from whole rabbit skeletal muscle (lane 1) is very similar to that of the junctional T-tubule fraction obtained from dissociated triads (lane 2). The respective Western blots shown at right in **Figure 3C** also indicate that both T-tubule fractions contain comparable caveolin-3 and Cav1.1 protein levels. Similar results were obtained in two different preparations. We also found caveolin-3 in triads from rat (**Figure 3D**, lane 2) that at equal protein loads migrated slightly faster but displayed similar band density as the caveolin-3 band present in triads from rabbit skeletal muscle (**Figure 3D**, lane 1). Junctional T-tubules isolated from rat triads also contained significant levels of caveolin-3 (data not shown).

Detergent Resistant Membranes (DRM) from Skeletal Muscle Contain High Cholesterol Levels, Caveolin-3 and Cav1.1

Incubation of T-tubules or triads with 1% Triton [X-100] (for details, see Experimental Procedures) yielded a light DRM fraction at the 5/30% sucrose interface. This fraction was visible to the naked eye, as illustrated in **Figure 4A** for the DRM fraction isolated from rabbit T-tubules; the representative electron micrograph of the DRM isolated from triads (rabbit) illustrated in **Figure 4B** revealed the presence of unilamellar vesicles (arrowheads) associated with electron-dense material.

DRM fractions isolated from triads migrated at a higher sucrose density (25–28% sucrose, w/v) than DRM fractions from T-tubules (16–18% sucrose, w/v). Both fractions had higher cholesterol contents than the corresponding initial fractions, albeit DRM fractions from triads had lower cholesterol levels than DRM fractions from T-tubules (**Table 1**). For comparison, the isolated caveolae and plasma membrane cholesterol levels (400 and 143 μg/mg protein, respectively) reported in the literature (Ortegren et al., 2004) yield a caveolae/plasma membrane cholesterol ratio of 2.8. Our results yield almost two-fold higher values for the ratios between the cholesterol contents of DRM from T-tubules or triads relative to the original membranes (**Table 1**). Immunoblot analysis (**Figure 4C**) revealed a significant enrichment in caveolin-3 in DRM fractions from triads (rabbit, lane 1; rat, lane 2) when compared to the original triad fractions (rat, lane 4; rabbit, lane 5) or to the junctional T-tubule membranes from rabbit (lane 3). As illustrated in **Figure 4D**, DRM fractions from triads (lanes 1–2) or T-tubules (lanes 3–4) also contained significant levels of the Cav1.1 protein.

To further test the association of caveolin-3 with cholesterol, we treated T-tubules or triads from rabbit with increasing concentrations of MβCD, centrifuged the fractions at 100,000 × g for 5 min and determined cholesterol and caveolin-3 protein contents in the resulting pellets and supernatants, respectively. As illustrated in **Figure 4E**, treatment with MβCD produced a

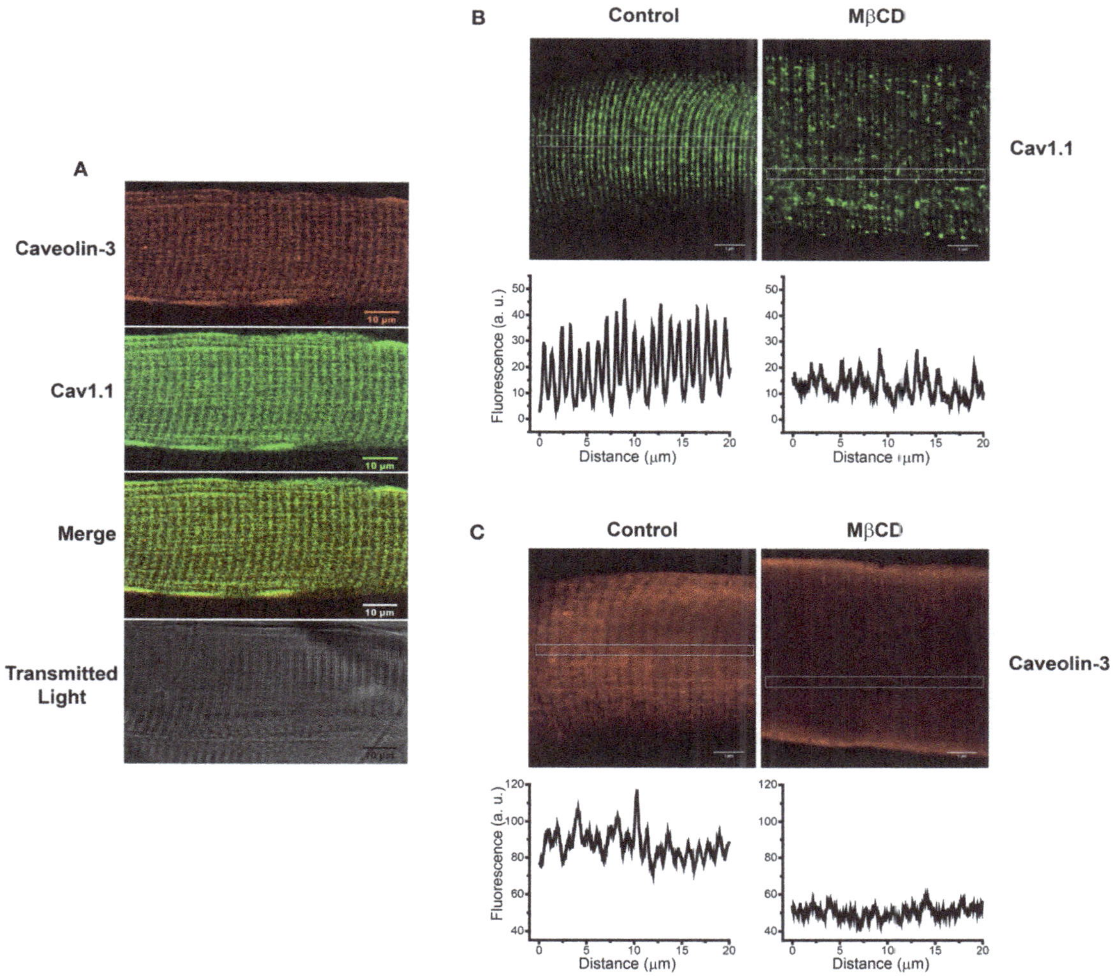

FIGURE 2 | Caveolin-3 is associated to T-tubules membranes in intact FDB fibers from adult skeletal muscle; treatment with MβCD alters the distribution of Cav1.1 and caveolin-3. (A) Immunohistochemistry of a single FDB fiber isolated from skeletal muscle of adult mice. The top panel shows caveolin-3 in red, the central panel shows Cav1.1 in green, the panel with the merged image shows the superposition of both fluorescence signals, and the lower panel shows the transmitted light image. **(B)** Distribution of Cav1.1 (green) in control (left panel) and fibers treated with 1% MβCD (right panel). The graphs under each image illustrate the horizontal fluorescence profiles collected from the rectangular region of interest (ROI) indicated in the images. **(C)** Distribution of caveolin-3 (red) in control (left panel) and MβCD-treated fibers (right panel). The graphs under each image illustrate the horizontal fluorescence profiles collected from the rectangular ROI indicated in each image. Scale bar: 5 μm.

concentration-dependent decrease in the cholesterol content of pellets from T-tubules (open circles) and triads (open squares). Analysis of caveolin-3 content in the respective supernatants of MβCD-treated fractions (**Figure 4F**) revealed that the soluble fractions from T-tubules contained caveolin-3 (lanes 1–4) whereas, the soluble fractions from triads lacked this protein (lanes 5–8).

Triads from Aged Rats Contain Decreased Protein Levels of Caveolin-3 and GAPDH

The representative Western blot illustrated in **Figure 5A** shows that triads from aged rats (24-month-old) contain significantly lower caveolin-3 protein contents than triads from young (3-month-old) rats. Likewise, triads from aged rats contain lower GAPDH levels (**Figure 5B**). Results from 6 aged and 6 young rats indicate both reductions are statistically significant (**Figures 5A,B**).

Triads from Aged Rats Contain Increased Na^+/K^+-ATPase α1 Subunit Protein Levels

The representative Western blot illustrated in **Figure 5C** indicates that triads from aged rats contain significant higher Na^+/K^+-ATPase α1 subunit levels than triads from young rats. Results from 6 aged and 6 young rats indicate that these differences are statistically significant (**Figure 5C**).

Triad RyR1 Protein Levels and Cholesterol Content Do Not Change with Age

Triads from young or aged rats contained comparable RyR1 protein levels, as shown in the representative Western blot

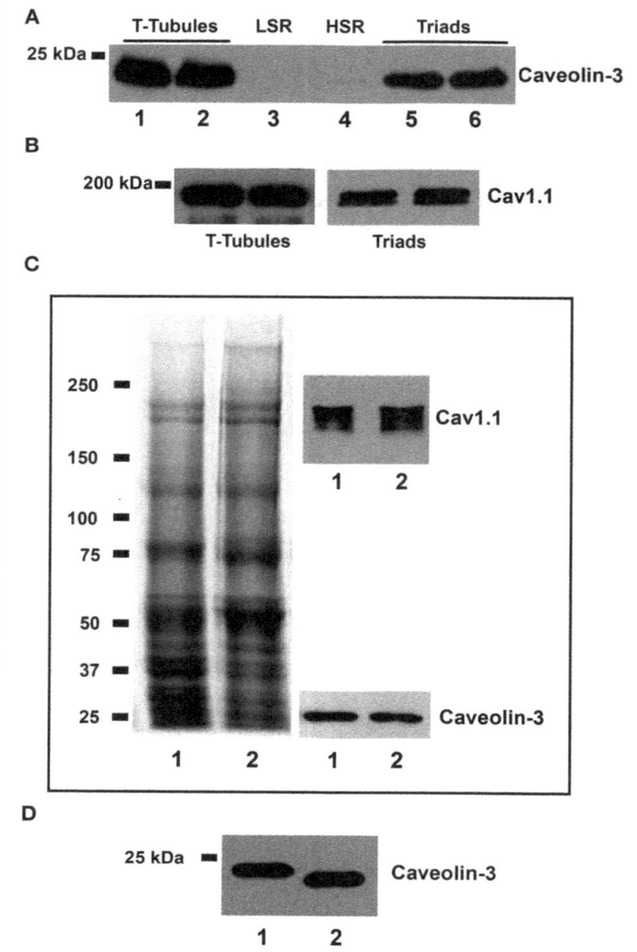

FIGURE 3 | Caveolin-3 is associated to T-tubules and triad fractions from adult skeletal muscle. (A) The representative upper blot shows membrane fractions from rabbit skeletal muscle, resolved by SDS/PAGE, transferred and tested with caveolin-3 or Cav1.1 antibodies. Each lane was loaded with 20 μg of protein. T-tubules, lanes 1 and 2; LSR, lane 3; HSR, lane 4; triads, lanes 5 and 6. **(B)** Separate blot showing that T-tubule and triad fractions contain Cav1.1. **(C)** The left panel shows a Coomassie blue stained gel; lane 1: T-tubules (20 μg), lane 2: junctional T-tubules (20 μg). The right panel shows the corresponding Western blots for caveolin-3 and Cav1.1, in the same samples loaded on the left panel. **(D)** Western blot of triad fractions; each lane was loaded with 20 μg of protein. Lane 1: triads from rabbit; lane 2: triads from rat.

illustrated in **Figure 5D** and by the average results from 6 young and 6 aged animals summarized in the graph shown in **Figure 5D**. We obtained inconclusive results regarding Cav1.1 protein levels. Triad fractions from four aged rats displayed similar Cav1.1 protein contents as young rats, but triads from two aged rats had significantly higher Cav1.1 protein levels. All six triad fractions assayed had comparable RyR1 and cholesterol contents (see below), presumably ruling out significant differences in T-tubule content among these fractions.

Triads from aged rats contain on average 51.3 ± 2.6 μg cholesterol/mg protein ($n = 6$; Mean ± SE); these values are not significantly different from the levels determined in triads from young rats: 53.2 ± 3.5 μg cholesterol/mg protein ($n = 6$; Mean ± SE).

Determination of NOX Subunits (gp91^{phox} and p47^{phox}) Protein Contents and NOX Activity in Young and Aged Rats

As illustrated by the representative Western blot and the graph illustrated in **Figure 6A**, gp91^{phox} protein levels did not change with age. The same observation applies to p47^{phox} protein levels (**Figure 6B**); in this case, we observed a tendency toward a decrease with age, which was not statistically significant. In concordance with the lack of change of both gp91^{phox} and p47^{phox} protein levels, we found similar NOX activities in triads from young and aged rats (**Figure 6C**).

To summarize, the above results show that aging decreased caveolin-3 and GAPDH protein levels, increased the levels of the Na^+/K^+-ATPase protein, but did not modify either RyR1, gp91^{phox} and p47^{phox} protein levels or NOX activity.

Discussion

In this work, we addressed three related aspects. First, we tested the effects of the cholesterol-lowering agent MβCD on Ca^{2+} transients elicited by electrical field stimulation of skeletal fibers from adult mice, and found that MβCD reduced Ca^{2+} transients without disrupting fiber membrane integrity or emptying the SR of its Ca^{2+} content. Second, using several experimental strategies we determined unambiguously that caveolin-3, a cholesterol-associated protein, is present in T-tubules but not in HSR and LSR vesicles. Additionally, we found that treatment with MβCD altered the distribution of both Cav1.1 and caveolin-3 in FDB fibers from adult mice. Third, we found decreased caveolin-3 and GAPDH and increased Na^+/K^+-ATPase α1 subunit protein contents in triad fractions from aged rats, with no apparent age-related changes in cholesterol levels or RyR1, gp91^{phox} and p47phox protein contents. We subsequently discuss the possible implications of these findings for skeletal muscle function in young and aged animals.

Treatment with MβCD Suppresses Depolarization-induced Ca^{2+} Transients

As reported previously, single skeletal muscle fibers from fetal mice treated with MβCD display defective E–C coupling but retain normal voltage dependence and exhibit similar action potentials as control fibers (Pouvreau et al., 2004). Our results in FDB fibers from adult mice indicate that MβCD partially removed cholesterol from these fibers, in agreement with our previous report (Llanos et al., 2015), suppressed Ca^{2+} transients in most fibers or significantly reduced their amplitude, and altered the distribution of both caveolin-3 and Cav1.1. Our determinations of Fluo-4 fluorescence suggest that MβCD treatment induced a moderate increase (≤2-fold) in myoplasmic resting [Ca^{2+}] and preserved caffeine-induced Ca^{2+} release. Altogether, results from previous studies combined with the

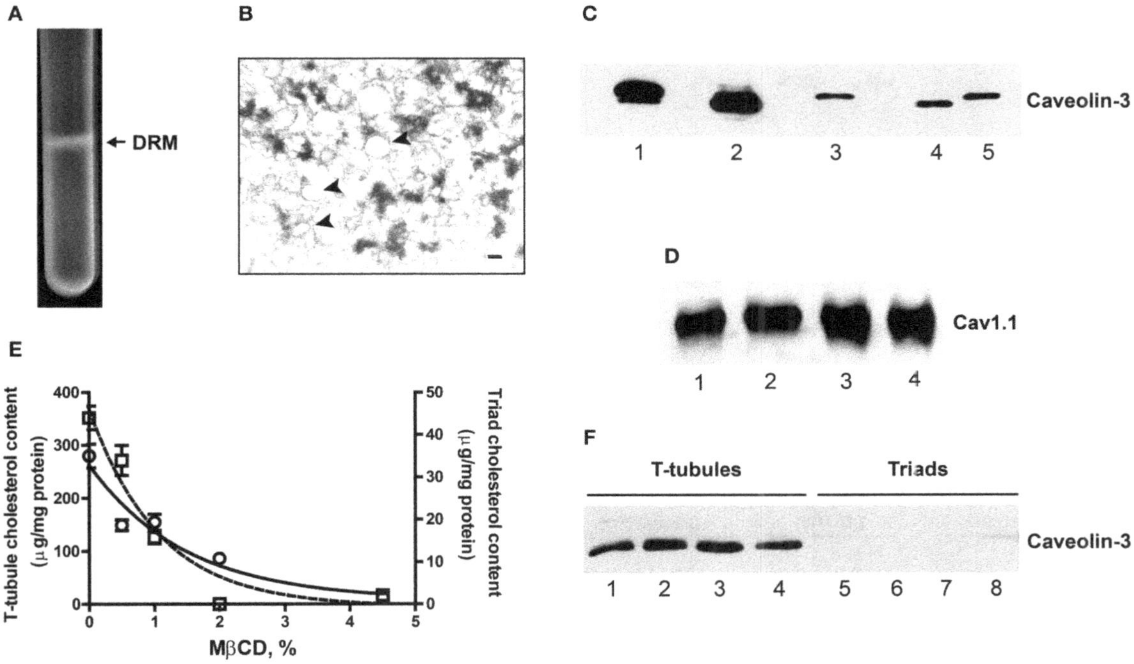

FIGURE 4 | DRM fractions from triads are enriched in caveolin-3 and contain Cav1.1. (A) Photograph of a centrifuge tube after 16 h of centrifugation of a sucrose gradient loaded with Triton X-100-treated triads, showing the appearance of an opalescent band containing the DRM fraction (for details, see the Experimental Procedures Section). **(B)** Representative EM photograph of a DRM fraction from triads. Unilamellar vesicles appear associated to electron dense material (arrows). Magnification: 150,000×; calibration bar, 20 nm. **(C)** Representative Western blot revealed with caveolin-3 antibodies. Lanes 1 and 2: 15 μg DRM isolated from triads from rabbit or rat, respectively. Lane 3: 15 μg of junctional T-tubules from triads from rabbit. Lanes 4 and 5: 20 μg, triads from rat or rabbit, respectively. Spaces between thes lanes correspond to empty lanes. **(D)** Western blot revealed with Cav1.1 antibodies. Lanes 1 and 2: 13 μg, DRM from triads from rabbit. Lanes 3 and 4: 6 μg, DRM from T-tubules from rabbit. **(E)** T-tubule and triads fractions from rabbit were treated with increasing MβCD concentrations, pelleted at 100,000 × g and the membrane cholesterol and soluble caveolin-3 were evaluated (for details, see Experimental Procedures Section). The graph shows the cholesterol content of MβCD-treated T-tubules (left y-axis) or triads (right y-axis). **(F)** Western blot showing caveolin-3 protein content in the supernatants of MβCD-treated T-tubules (lanes 1–4) or triads (lanes 5–8). Similar results were obtained in two different experiments.

present findings suggest that partial cholesterol removal affects T-tubule components, such as Cav1.1, which participate directly in the E–C coupling process. In fact, we found that MβCD treatment caused significant disarray in the regular pattern of Cav1.1 distribution. This alteration may underlie the selective and marked reduction in Cav1.1-mediated currents produced by MβCD, since a previous study indicates that membrane cholesterol removal from skeletal fibers from fetal mice specifically targets Cav1.1 channel function since T-type Ca^{2+} currents remain unaltered (Pouvreau et al., 2004). Of note, statin treatment to inhibit cholesterol synthesis (Istvan and Deisenhofer, 2001) produces T-tubule structural abnormalities in human patients (Voigt et al., 2013). A decrease in T-tubule cholesterol content may contribute to the skeletal muscle dysfunction described in patients undergoing statin therapy; in fact, as many as 25% of statin users who exercise may experience defective skeletal muscle function (Dirks and Jones, 2006). There is no information, however, regarding T-tubule cholesterol levels in these subjects. In addition, cholesterol removal may affect caveolin-3 distribution and function, in particular its role in E–C coupling, as discussed below.

Association of Caveolin-3 with T-tubules and DRM Fractions

Previous studies associated caveolin-3 with the T-tubule system only during development (Parton et al., 1997), and reported that in adult skeletal muscle caveolin-3 was exclusively present in association with the sarcolemmal membrane (Parton et al., 1997). Moreover, other studies described caveolin-3 in association with the SR membrane (Li et al., 2006). Our results in three different mammalian species—mice, rabbit and rat—show conclusively that in adult mammalian skeletal muscle this protein is associated to T-tubule and not to SR membranes, suggesting an evolutionary conserved role for caveolin-3 in T-tubule system development and preservation of structural integrity in adult muscle.

Here, we show that DRM fractions from either T-tubules or triads are highly enriched in cholesterol and caveolin-3 with respect to the original membrane fractions, and also contain Cav1.1. Our results complement previous studies showing the presence of both caveolin-3 and Cav1.2 in DRM obtained from cardiac tissue (Balijepalli et al., 2006). EM images of DRM obtained from triads revealed the presence of membrane-associated electron dense material, suggesting that in addition to

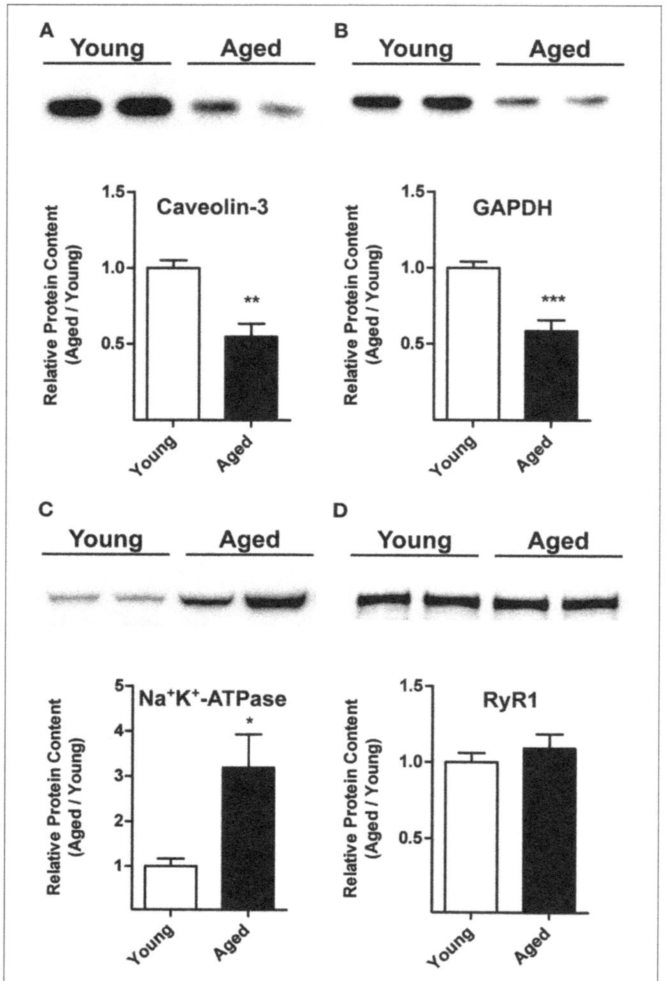

FIGURE 5 | Caveolin-3, GAPDH, Na^+/K^+-ATPase, and RyR1 protein contents in triads from young or aged rats. (A,B) The top panels illustrate representative Western blots. Each lane was loaded with 10 μg of protein assayed for caveolin-3 and GAPDH, respectively. **(C)** The top panel illustrates a representative Western blot for Na^+/K^+-ATPase; each lane was loaded with 30 μg of protein. **(D)** The top panel illustrates a representative Western blot for RyR1; each lane was loaded with 5 μg of protein. Each lane in the blots illustrated in **(A–D)** corresponds to triad fractions from different rats. The lower graphs in **(A–D)** present values (Mean ± SE) collected from triad fractions from 6 young and 6 aged rats. $^*p < 0.05$; $^{**}p < 0.01$; $^{***}p < 0.001$.

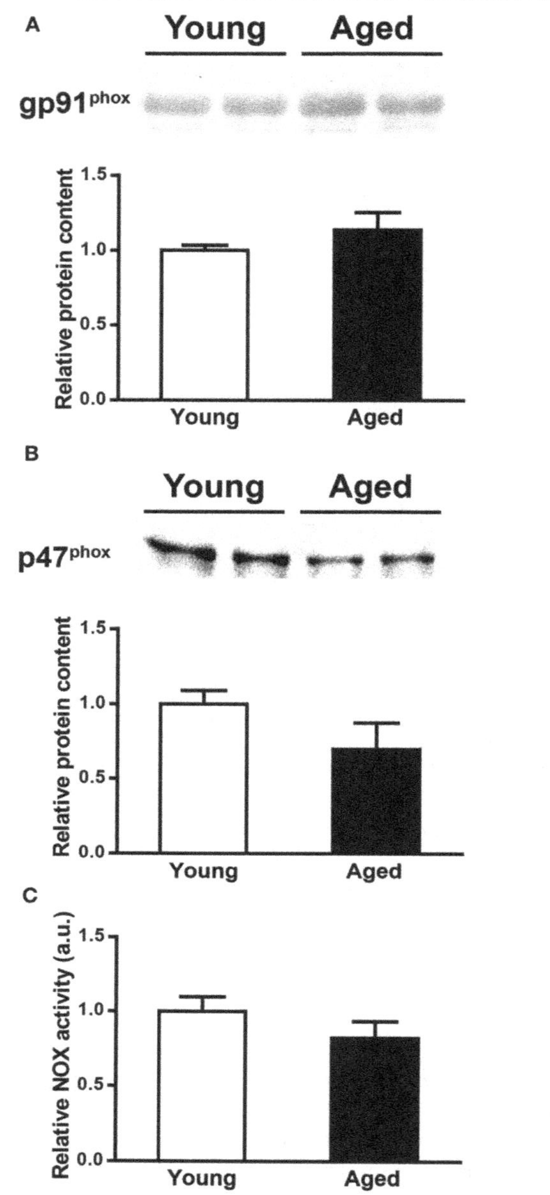

FIGURE 6 | gp91^{phox} and p47^{phox} protein levels and NOX activity in triads from young or aged rats. (A) The top panel illustrates a representative Western blot for gp91^{phox}; each lane was loaded with 40 μg of protein of triad fraction from different rats. **(B)** The top panel illustrates a representative Western blot for p47^{phox}; each lane was loaded with 15 μg of protein of triad fraction from different rats. The lower graphs in **(A,B)** summarize values (Mean ± SE) collected from triad fractions from 6 young and 6 aged rats. **(C)** NOX activity of triad fractions from young or aged rats; values (Mean ± SE) correspond to 6 young and 6 aged rats.

caveolin-3 and Cav1.1, other proteins of the E–C coupling complex remain associated with DRM fractions. In fact, we found that DRM fractions from triads migrated at higher sucrose densities than DRM from T-tubules, indicating higher protein to lipid ratios in the former fractions. Our results also reveal that cholesterol extraction from T-tubules and triads with MβCD produced concurrent caveolin-3 extraction to the supernatants only in isolated T-tubules. Previous work showed that caveolin-3 interacts both with Cav1.1 (Couchoux et al., 2011) and RyR1 (Whiteley et al., 2012); the persistence of this T-tubule/SR protein complex in triads may explain why removing cholesterol did not extract caveolin-3 from these fractions.

Caveolin-3 and Skeletal Muscle Function

The levels of caveolin-3 are critical for the correct functioning of skeletal muscle, because changes in the expression of this protein produce pathological phenomena (Galbiati et al., 2000; Hagiwara et al., 2000). Caveolin-3 reduction in skeletal muscle myotubes from mice induces the opening of non-selective mechano-sensitive ion channels while caveolin-3 overexpression produces a small decrease in mechano-sensitive currents, suggesting that normal caveolin-3 expression contributes to protection of the sarcolemma from mechanical damage (Huang et al., 2013). Skeletal muscle also expresses caveolin-1 (Kawabe et al., 2001; Li et al., 2006); however, caveolin-1 does not restore completely the function of caveolin-3, since caveolin-3 knockout mice present T-tubule system abnormalities (Galbiati et al., 2001) and exhibit muscle degeneration (Hagiwara et al., 2000). Interestingly, mice null for caveolin-3 and caveolin-1 develop severe heart disease (Park et al., 2002), while caveolin-3 over expression induces a Duchenne-like phenotype in mice (Aravamudan et al., 2003). Furthermore, mice null for caveolin-3 and caveolin-1 display insulin resistance, glucose intolerance and decreased insulin-induced glucose uptake; re-expression of these proteins reverses these conditions (Capozza et al., 2005). The insulin receptor is unstable in caveolin-3 null mice; insulin binding induces its degradation suggesting that caveolin-3 stabilizes the insulin receptor (Capozza et al., 2005). Of note, caveolin-3 reduction in cardiac muscle cells produces severe alterations in cardiac function, characterized by considerable tissue degeneration, fibrosis, decreased cardiac function, and decreased activity of nitric oxide synthase (Aravamudan et al., 2003). Altogether, these reports suggest that alterations in caveolin-3 levels induce pathological conditions in skeletal and cardiac muscle.

Recent studies reported that caveolin-3 interacts with Cav1.1 (Couchoux et al., 2011) and RyR1 (Whiteley et al., 2012), suggesting that the two Ca^{2+} channels directly involved in E–C coupling establish functional links with caveolin-3. Cholesterol removal, which affects the distribution of both caveolin-3 and Cav1.1, may affect these functional connections giving rise to the defective E–C coupling responses reported in amphibian (Launikonis and Stephenson, 2001), fetal (Pouvreau et al., 2004) and adult rat skeletal muscle, where we found that partial cholesterol extraction inhibited Ca^{2+} transients. These effects are similar to the reported effects of aging on E–C coupling (Booth et al., 1994; Wang et al., 2000). Early studies indicated that rat skeletal muscle from 12-month-old rats had higher caveolin content than muscle from 3-month-old rats; however, whether this increase reflects augmented expression of caveolin-3, caveolin-1, or both was not evaluated (Munoz et al., 1996). Other early studies suggested that aging produces uncoupling between Cav1.1 and RyR1, with the consequent muscle weakness (Renganathan et al., 1997). Our results indicate that triad fractions from skeletal muscle of 24-month-old rats had 2-fold lower caveolin-3 protein levels than triads from young rats. As described above, caveolin-3 interacts with Cav1.1 and RyR1, forming a supra-molecular complex. Reduction in caveolin-3 protein levels during aging is likely to remodel or alter the integrity of this complex, causing E–C uncoupling. A decrease in caveolin-3 levels may also modify T-tubule architecture and T-tubule related signal transduction pathways, such as insulin-dependent glucose uptake.

Caveolin-3 binds directly to cholesterol (Murata et al., 1995) and sphingolipids (Haberkant et al., 2008). We found that DRM fraction from T-tubules or triads contained both caveolin-3 and Cav1.1; the possible association of these two proteins in cholesterol-enriched membrane regions supports the proposed role of caveolin-3 in regulating Cav1.1 function (Weiss et al., 2008). While we did not detect significant differences in cholesterol content between triads from young or aged rats, a marked reduction in caveolin-3 protein content during aging may affect the local cholesterol distribution in T-tubule membranes, altering the function of the caveolin-3-containing RyR1/Cav1.1 supramolecular complex, and hence E–C coupling. Accordingly, it would be of interest to investigate in future studies if restoring caveolin-3 levels in the skeletal muscle of aged animals improves their defective E–C coupling.

Changes in Other Triadic Proteins during Aging

RyR1 and Cav1.1

Our results in triads from skeletal muscle of 24-month-old rats confirm that RyR1 protein content does not change with rodent age (Russ et al., 2011). Previous reports suggest a drastic reduction of Cav1.1 and no significant change of RyR1 protein levels in total fractions from skeletal muscles of 30-month-old rats (O'connell et al., 2008). We obtained inconclusive results regarding changes in Cav1.1 protein levels with age, but we did not observe an age-related Cav1.1 reduction.

Na^+/K^+-ATPase

In rat skeletal muscle, aging causes muscle type-specific alterations in Na^+/K^+-ATPase activity and increases the expression of the enzyme α1 and β1-subunits, measured in total muscle homogenates (Sun et al., 1999). Immunohistochemistry analysis showed increased expression of the α1-subunit in white but not in red gastrocnemius muscle, which displays mainly a sarcolemmal pattern (Zhang et al., 2006). Increased expression of the Na^+/K^+-ATPase enzyme during aging, which we confirmed in triad fractions from aged muscle, may be relevant for muscle function during aging. Reduction of caveolin-3 content activates non-selective mechano-sensitive ion channels in skeletal muscle (Huang et al., 2013), whereas in cardiac muscle caveolin-3 regulates Kv1.5 potassium currents by modulating the number of functional channels in the membrane (Folco et al., 2004). Accordingly, decreased T-tubule caveolin-3 levels may result in increased Na^+ and K^+ fluxes via non-selective ion channels during aging, which if not compensated by active ion transport by the Na^+/K^+-ATPase would result in decreased excitability of skeletal muscle fibers, thereby contributing to contractile fatigue (Welle, 2002). Therefore, the increased Na^+/K^+-ATPase protein levels displayed by triads from aged rat muscle may reflect an adaptation mechanism to compensate for the increment of ionic T-tubule membrane permeability induced by the low caveolin-3 levels observed in aged muscle.

GAPDH

In addition to decreased caveolin-3 content, triads from aged rats displayed significant reductions in GAPDH protein content. Our results agree with previous reports showing that aged skeletal muscles display decreased levels of GAPDH mRNA

(Touchberry et al., 2006) and protein (Vigelso et al., 2015). In skeletal muscle, GAPDH binds to RyR1, Cav1.1 and the T-tubule membrane (Brandt et al., 1990), forming a complex that may functionally couple glycolysis with SERCA-mediated Ca^{2+} transport into the SR (Xu et al., 1995). SR-associated glycolytic enzymes may produce ATP locally, resulting in modifications of myoplasmic Ca^{2+} signals, either via SERCA-mediated Ca^{2+} uptake into the SR and/or via RyR1-mediated Ca^{2+} release, because ATP is a well-characterized physiological RyR agonist (Fill and Copello, 2002; Bull et al., 2007). The higher Na^{+}/K^{+}-ATPase levels displayed by triads from aged rats, combined with their reduced GAPDH content, suggest that aged muscle has a reduced capacity to generate ATP locally at the triads, which may result in inhibition of SR Ca^{2+} uptake and reduced RyR1 activity. We propose that these combined factors contribute to disrupt normal Ca^{2+} signaling, thereby reducing muscle contractility in aged skeletal muscle. Future studies should address this proposal.

NOX

Skeletal muscle activity increases ROS production (Reid et al., 1992; Borzone et al., 1994). In several tissues, the diverse NOX isoforms contribute to ROS generation (Bedard and Krause, 2007). Skeletal muscle expresses NOX4 mRNA as well as the mRNA for the gp91^{phox} subunit of the NOX2 isoform (Cheng et al., 2001; Shiose et al., 2001), in addition to expressing proteins of the NOX2 complex (Javeshghani et al., 2002), but the role of NOX in activity-dependent ROS production in skeletal muscle remains inconclusive. For instance, NOX-mediated ROS production in diaphragm muscle does not contribute to the ROS increase produced by heat stress (Zuo et al., 2003). Nonetheless, skeletal muscle T-tubules express several NOX2 subunits and NOX2-generated ROS stimulate SR Ca^{2+} release, presumably as a result of NOX2-induced RyR1 redox modifications (Hidalgo et al., 2006). Recent studies using the ROS-sensitive probe rhoGFP indicate that contraction and stretching of skeletal muscle both activate NOX (Pal et al., 2013). We found that triads from young or aged rats contained similar p47^{phox} and gp91^{phox} protein levels and comparable NOX activities. Our results strongly suggest that NOX-generated ROS do not contribute to the increased resting ROS levels of aged muscle; however, we cannot rule out differential effects of exercise on NOX-dependent ROS production as a function of age. It has been proposed that mitochondrial and NOX are possible ROS sources in aged skeletal muscle (Bejma and Ji, 1999). Our results support a predominant mitochondrial origin for the reported increase in resting ROS production in skeletal muscle (Vasilaki et al., 2006; Umanskaya et al., 2014), which results in increased RyR1 oxidation (Andersson et al., 2011).

Concluding Remarks

In this work, we show that partial cholesterol extraction from single skeletal fibers isolated from mice adult skeletal muscle eliminated or significantly reduced electrically evoked Ca^{2+} transients, without affecting membrane permeability or causing SR calcium depletion. We propose that partial cholesterol removal impairs E–C coupling by modifying the interactions of the cholesterol-associated protein caveolin-3 with RyR1 and Cav1.1. In support of this proposal, we found caveolin-3 associated with the cholesterol-rich T-tubule membranes, but not with SR membranes; moreover, caveolin-3 is present together with Cav1.1 in cholesterol-enriched DRM fractions from T-tubules or triads. In addition, we observed significantly decreased caveolin-3 and GAPDH and increased Na^{+}/K^{+}-ATPase levels in triads from aged rats, but we did not detect changes in cholesterol or RyR1 protein levels. These findings suggest that age-related changes in triadic proteins, and in particular the decrease in caveolin-3 protein content, are likely to alter T-tubule related signal transduction pathways and to produce defective E–C coupling of aged skeletal muscle. Our results contribute to the field of muscle physiology by suggesting that cholesterol and caveolin-3 are important for the normal E–C coupling process, and that alterations in their levels contribute to the defective function of aged skeletal muscle.

Author Contributions

GB and PL performed experiments, analyzed data, and contributed to manuscript writing. PB, CC and AR performed experiments and analyzed data. GS performed experiments, analyzed data and critically reviewed the manuscript. JH analyzed data, contributed to the discussion of results and critically reviewed the manuscript. AQ and CH supervised the study, analyzed data and provided funding. CH wrote the manuscript and is the guarantor of this work and, as such, had full access to all the data in the study and takes responsibility for the integrity of the data and the accuracy of the data analysis.

Acknowledgments

This work was financed by FONDECYT (grants 1090071, 1140545, 1130250), FONDECYT-FONDAP (15130011), Millennium Science Initiative (BNI-P-09-015F), and CONICYT-Research Ring (ACT-1111). The funding agencies had no role in study design, data collection and analysis, decision to publish, or preparation of the manuscript. We thank L. Montecinos, M. Silva, F. Mieres, and S. Guzman for their skilled technical assistance.

References

Andersson, D. C., Betzenhauser, M. J., Reiken, S., Meli, A. C., Umanskaya, A., Xie, W., et al. (2011). Ryanodine receptor oxidation causes intracellular calcium leak and muscle weakness in aging. *Cell Metab.* 14, 196–207. doi: 10.1016/j.cmet.2011.05.014

Anderson, K., Cohn, A. H., and Meissner, G. (1994). High-affinity [3H]PN200-110 and [3H]ryanodine binding to rabbit and frog skeletal muscle. *Am. J. Physiol.* 266, C462–C466.

Anderson, K., and Meissner, G. (1995). T-tubule depolarization-induced SR Ca2+ release is controlled by dihydropyridine receptor- and Ca(2+)-dependent mechanisms in cell homogenates from rabbit skeletal muscle. *J. Gen. Physiol.* 105, 363–383. doi: 10.1085/jgp.105.3.363

Aravamudan, B., Volonte, D., Ramani, R., Gursoy, E., Lisanti, M. P., London, B., et al. (2003). Transgenic overexpression of caveolin-3 in the heart induces a cardiomyopathic phenotype. *Hum. Mol. Genet.* 12, 2777–2788. doi: 10.1093/hmg/ddg313

Badizadegan, K., Dickinson, B. L., Wheeler, H. E., Blumberg, R. S., Holmes, R. K., and Lencer, W. I. (2000). Heterogeneity of detergent-insoluble membranes from human intestine containing caveolin-1 and ganglioside G(M1). *Am. J. Physiol. Gastrointest. Liver Physiol.* 278, G895–G904. doi: 10.1016/S0016-5085(00)84524-2

Balijepalli, R. C., Foell, J. D., Hall, D. D., Hell, J. W., and Kamp, T. J. (2006). Localization of cardiac L-type Ca(2+) channels to a caveolar macromolecular signaling complex is required for beta(2)-adrenergic regulation. *Proc. Natl. Acad. Sci. U.S.A.* 103, 7500–7505. doi: 10.1073/pnas.0503465103

Barrientos, G., Bose, D. D., Feng, W., Padilla, I., and Pessah, I. N. (2009). The Na+/Ca2+ exchange inhibitor 2-(2-(4-(4-nitrobenzyloxy)phenyl)ethyl)isothiourea methanesulfonate (KB-R7943) also blocks ryanodine receptors type 1 (RyR1) and type 2 (RyR2) channels. *Mol. Pharmacol.* 76, 560–568. doi: 10.1124/mol.109.057265

Bedard, K., and Krause, K. H. (2007). The NOX family of ROS-generating NADPH oxidases: physiology and pathophysiology. *Physiol. Rev.* 87, 245–313. doi: 10.1152/physrev.00044.2005

Bejma, J., and Ji, L. L. (1999). Aging and acute exercise enhance free radical generation in rat skeletal muscle. *J. Appl. Physiol.* 87, 465–470.

Booth, F. W., Weeden, S. H., and Tseng, B. S. (1994). Effect of aging on human skeletal muscle and motor function. *Med. Sci. Sports Exerc.* 26, 556–560. doi: 10.1249/00005768-199405000-00006

Borzone, G., Zhao, B., Merola, A. J., Berliner, L., and Clanton, T. L. (1994). Detection of free radicals by electron spin resonance in rat diaphragm after resistive loading. *J. Appl. Physiol.* 77, 812–818.

Brandt, N. R., Caswell, A. H., Wen, S. R., and Talvenheimo, J. A. (1990). Molecular interactions of the junctional foot protein and dihydropyridine receptor in skeletal muscle triads. *J. Membr. Biol.* 113, 237–251. doi: 10.1007/BF01870075

Brown, D., and Waneck, G. L. (1992). Glycosyl-phosphatidylinositol-anchored membrane proteins. *J. Am. Soc. Nephrol.* 3, 895–906.

Bull, R., Finkelstein, J. P., Humeres, A., Behrens, M. I., and Hidalgo, C. (2007). Effects of ATP, Mg2+, and redox agents on the Ca2+ dependence of RyR channels from rat brain cortex. *Am. J. Physiol. Cell Physiol.* 293, C162–C171. doi: 10.1152/ajpcell.00518.2006

Calderon, J. C., Bolanos, P., and Caputo, C. (2011). Kinetic changes in tetanic Ca(2)(+) transients in enzymatically dissociated muscle fibres under repetitive stimulation. *J. Physiol.* 589, 5269–5283. doi: 10.1113/jphysiol.2011.213314

Capote, J., Bolanos, P., Schuhmeier, R. P., Melzer, W., and Caputo, C. (2005). Calcium transients in developing mouse skeletal muscle fibres. *J. Physiol.* 564, 451–464. doi: 10.1113/jphysiol.2004.081034

Capozza, F., Combs, T. P., Cohen, A. W., Cho, Y. R., Park, S. Y., Schubert, W., et al. (2005). Caveolin-3 knockout mice show increased adiposity and whole body insulin resistance, with ligand-induced insulin receptor instability in skeletal muscle. *Am. J. Physiol. Cell Physiol.* 288, C1317–C1331. doi: 10.1152/ajpcell.00489.2004

Carozzi, A. J., Ikonen, E., Lindsay, M. R., and Parton, R. G. (2000). Role of cholesterol in developing T-tubules: analogous mechanisms for T-tubule and caveolae biogenesis. *Traffic* 1, 326–341. doi: 10.1034/j.1600-0854.2000.010406.x

Carroll, S. L., Klein, M. G., and Schneider, M. F. (1995). Calcium transients in intact rat skeletal muscle fibers in agarose gel. *Am. J. Physiol.* 269, C28–C34.

Cheng, G., Cao, Z., Xu, X., Van Meir, E. G., and Lambeth, J. D. (2001). Homologs of gp91phox: cloning and tissue expression of Nox3, Nox4, and Nox5. *Gene* 269, 131–140. doi: 10.1016/S0378-1119(01)00449-8

Couchoux, H., Bichraoui, H., Chouabe, C., Altafaj, X., Bonvallet, R., Allard, B., et al. (2011). Caveolin-3 is a direct molecular partner of the Cav1.1 subunit of the skeletal muscle L-type calcium channel. *Int. J. Biochem. Cell Biol.* 43, 713–720. doi: 10.1016/j.biocel.2011.01.011

Dirks, A. J., and Jones, K. M. (2006). Statin-induced apoptosis and skeletal myopathy. *Am. J. Physiol. Cell Physiol.* 291, C1208–C1212. doi: 10.1152/ajpcell.00226.2006

Fill, M., and Copello, J. A. (2002). Ryanodine receptor calcium release channels. *Physiol. Rev.* 82, 893–922. doi: 10.1152/physrev.00013.2002

Folco, E. J., Liu, G. X., and Koren, G. (2004). Caveolin-3 and SAP97 form a scaffolding protein complex that regulates the voltage-gated potassium channel Kv1.5. *Am. J. Physiol. Heart Circ. Physiol.* 287, H681–H690. doi: 10.1152/ajpheart.00152.2004

Franzini-Armstrong, C. (1972). Studies of the triad. 3. Structure of the junction in fast twitch fibers. *Tissue Cell* 4, 469–478. doi: 10.1016/S0040-8166(72)80023-5

Galbiati, F., Engelman, J. A., Volonte, D., Zhang, X. L., Minetti, C., Li, M., et al. (2001). Caveolin-3 null mice show a loss of caveolae, changes in the microdomain distribution of the dystrophin-glycoprotein complex, and t-tubule abnormalities. *J Biol. Chem.* 276, 21425–21433. doi: 10.1074/jbc.M100828200

Galbiati, F., Volonte, D., Chu, J. B., Li, M., Fine, S. W., Fu, M., et al. (2000). Transgenic overexpression of caveolin-3 in skeletal muscle fibers induces a Duchenne-like muscular dystrophy phenotype. *Proc. Natl. Acad. Sci. U.S.A.* 97, 9689–9694. doi: 10.1073/pnas.160249097

Haberkant, P., Schmitt, O., Contreras, F. X., Thiele, C., Hanada, K., Sprong, H., et al. (2008). Protein-sphingolipid interactions within cellular membranes. *J. Lipid Res.* 49, 251–262. doi: 10.1194/jlr.D700023-JLR200

Hagiwara, Y., Sasaoka, T., Araishi, K., Imamura, M., Yorifuji, H., Nonaka, I., et al. (2000). Caveolin-3 deficiency causes muscle degeneration in mice. *Hum. Mol. Genet.* 9, 3047–3054. doi: 10.1093/hmg/9.20.3047

Hidalgo, C. (1985). Lipid phase of transverse tubule membranes from skeletal muscle. An electron paramagnetic resonance study. *Biophys. J.* 47, 757–764. doi: 10.1016/S0006-3495(85)83978-3

Hidalgo, C., Jorquera, J., Tapia, V., and Donoso, P. (1993). Triads and transverse tubules isolated from skeletal muscle contain high levels of inositol 1,4,5-trisphosphate. *J. Biol. Chem.* 268, 15111–15117.

Hidalgo, C., Parra, C., Riquelme, G., and Jaimovich, E. (1986). Transverse tubules from frog skeletal muscle. Purification and properties of vesicles sealed with the inside-out orientation. *Biochim. Biophys. Acta* 855, 79–88. doi: 10.1016/0005-2736(86)90191-4

Hidalgo, C., Sanchez, G., Barrientos, G., and Racena-Parks, P. (2006). A transverse tubule NADPH oxidase activity stimulates calcium release from isolated triads via ryanodine receptor type 1 s -glutathionylation. *J. Biol. Chem.* 281, 26473–26482. doi: 10.1074/jbc.M600451200

Horgan, D. J., and Kuypers, R. (1987). Isolation of transverse tubules by fractionation of sarcoplasmic reticulum preparations in ion-free sucrose density gradients. *Arch. Biochem. Biophys.* 253, 377–387. doi: 10.1016/0003-9861(87)90191-3

Huang, H., Bae, C., Sachs, F., and Suchyna, T. M. (2013). Caveolae regulation of mechanosensitive channel function in myotubes. *PLoS ONE* 8:e72894. doi: 10.1371/journal.pone.0072894

Istvan, E. S., and Deisenhofer, J. (2001). Structural mechanism for statin inhibition of HMG-CoA reductase. *Science* 292, 1160–1164. doi: 10.1126/science.1059344

Javeshghani, D., Magder, S. A., Barreiro, E., Quinn, M. T., and Hussain, S. N. (2002). Molecular characterization of a superoxide-generating NAD(P)H oxidase in the ventilatory muscles. *Am. J. Respir. Crit. Care Med.* 165, 412–418. doi: 10.1164/ajrccm.165.3.2103028

Jayasinghe, I. D., and Launikonis, B. S. (2013). Three-dimensional reconstruction and analysis of the tubular system of vertebrate skeletal muscle. *J. Cell Sci.* 126, 4048–4058. doi: 10.1242/jcs.131565

Kawabe, J. I., Grant, B. S., Yamamoto, M., Schwencke, C., Okumura, S., and Ishikawa, Y. (2001). Changes in caveolin subtype protein expression in aging rat organs. *Mol. Cell. Endocrinol.* 176, 91–95. doi: 10.1016/S0303-7207(01)00472-5

Lau, Y. H., Caswell, A. H., Brunschwig, J. P., Baerwald, R., and Garcia, M. (1979). Lipid analysis and freeze-fracture studies on isolated transverse tubules and sarcoplasmic reticulum subfractions of skeletal muscle. *J. Biol. Chem.* 254, 540–546.

Launikonis, B. S., and Stephenson, D. G. (2001). Effects of membrane cholesterol manipulation on excitation-contraction coupling in skeletal muscle of the toad. *J. Physiol.* 534, 71–85. doi: 10.1111/j.1469-7793.2001.00071.x

Li, C., Duan, W., Yang, F., and Zhang, X. (2006). Caveolin-3-anchored microdomains at the rabbit sarcoplasmic reticulum membranes. *Biochem. Biophys. Res. Commun.* 344, 1135–1140. doi: 10.1016/j.bbrc.2006.04.024

Llanos, P., Contreras-Ferrat, A., Georgiev, T., Osorio-Fuentealba, C., Espinosa, A., Hidalgo, J., et al. (2015). The cholesterol-lowering agent methyl-beta-cyclodextrin promotes glucose uptake via GLUT4 in adult muscle fibers and reduces insulin resistance in obese mice. *Am. J. Physiol. Endocrinol. Metab.* 308, E294–E305. doi: 10.1152/ajpendo.00189.2014

Marks, A. R., Tempst, P., Hwang, K. S., Taubman, M. B., Inui, M., Chadwick, C., et al. (1989). Molecular cloning and characterization of the ryanodine receptor/junctional channel complex cDNA from skeletal muscle sarcoplasmic reticulum. *Proc. Natl. Acad. Sci. U.S.A.* 86, 8683–8687. doi: 10.1073/pnas.86.22.8683

Melzer, W., Herrmann-Frank, A., and Luttgau, H. C. (1995). The role of Ca2+ ions in excitation-contraction coupling of skeletal muscle fibres. *Biochim. Biophys. Acta* 1241, 59–116. doi: 10.1016/0304-4157(94)00014-5

Miller, M. S., Callahan, D. M., and Toth, M. J. (2014). Skeletal muscle myofilament adaptations to aging, disease, and disuse and their effects on whole muscle performance in older adult humans. *Front. Physiol.* 5:369. doi: 10.3389/fphys.2014.00369

Minarovic, I., and Meszaros, L. G. (1998). Fluorescent probing with felodipine of the dihydropyridine receptor and its interaction with the ryanodine receptor calcium release channel. *Biochem. Biophys. Res. Commun.* 244, 519–524. doi: 10.1006/bbrc.1998.8233

Munoz, P., Mora, S., Sevilla, L., Kaliman, P., Tomas, E., Guma, A., et al. (1996). Expression and insulin-regulated distribution of caveolin in skeletal muscle. Caveolin does not colocalize with GLUT4 in intracellular membranes. *J. Biol. Chem.* 271, 8133–8139. doi: 10.1074/jbc.271.14.8133

Murata, M., Peranen, J., Schreiner, R., Wieland, F., Kurzchalia, T. V., and Simons, K. (1995). VIP21/caveolin is a cholesterol-binding protein. *Proc. Natl. Acad. Sci. U.S.A.* 92, 10339–10343. doi: 10.1073/pnas.92.22.10339

O'connell, K., Gannon, J., Doran, P., and Ohlendieck, K. (2008). Reduced expression of sarcalumenin and related Ca2+ -regulatory proteins in aged rat skeletal muscle. *Exp. Gerontol.* 43, 958–961. doi: 10.1016/j.exger.2008.07.006

Ortegren, U., Karlsson, M., Blazic, N., Blomqvist, M., Nystrom, F. H., Gustavsson, J., et al. (2004). Lipids and glycosphingolipids in caveolae and surrounding plasma membrane of primary rat adipocytes. *Eur. J. Biochem.* 271, 2028–2036. doi: 10.1111/j.1432-1033.2004.04117.x

Pal, R., Basu Thakur, P., Li, S., Minard, C., and Rodney, G. G. (2013). Real-time imaging of NADPH oxidase activity in living cells using a novel fluorescent protein reporter. *PLoS ONE* 8:e63989. doi: 10.1371/journal.pone.0063989

Park, D. S., Woodman, S. E., Schubert, W., Cohen, A. W., Frank, P. G., Chandra, M., et al. (2002). Caveolin-1/3 double-knockout mice are viable, but lack both muscle and non-muscle caveolae, and develop a severe cardiomyopathic phenotype. *Am. J. Pathol.* 160, 2207–2217. doi: 10.1016/S0002-9440(10)61168-6

Parton, R. G., Way, M., Zorzi, N., and Stang, E. (1997). Caveolin-3 associates with developing T-tubules during muscle differentiation. *J. Cell Biol.* 136, 137–154. doi: 10.1083/jcb.136.1.137

Pouvreau, S., Berthier, C., Blaineau, S., Amsellem, J., Coronado, R., and Strube, C. (2004). Membrane cholesterol modulates dihydropyridine receptor function in mice fetal skeletal muscle cells. *J. Physiol.* 555, 365–381. doi: 10.1113/jphysiol.2003.055285

Ralston, E., and Ploug, T. (1999). Caveolin-3 is associated with the T-tubules of mature skeletal muscle fibers. *Exp. Cell Res.* 246, 510–515. doi: 10.1006/excr.1998.4305

Reid, M. B., Shoji, T., Moody, M. R., and Entman, M. L. (1992). Reactive oxygen in skeletal muscle. II. Extracellular release of free radicals. *J. Appl. Physiol.* 73, 1805–1809.

Renganathan, M., Messi, M. L., and Delbono, O. (1997). Dihydropyridine receptor-ryanodine receptor uncoupling in aged skeletal muscle. *J. Membr. Biol.* 157, 247–253. doi: 10.1007/s002329900233

Rios, E., Karhanek, M., Ma, J., and Gonzalez, A. (1993). An allosteric model of the molecular interactions of excitation-contraction coupling in skeletal muscle. *J. Gen. Physiol.* 102, 449–481. doi: 10.1085/jgp.102.3.449

Rosemblatt, M., Hidalgo, C., Vergara, C., and Ikemoto, N. (1981). Immunological and biochemical properties of transverse tubule membranes isolated from rabbit skeletal muscle. *J. Biol. Chem.* 256, 8140–8148.

Russ, D. W., Grandy, J. S., Toma, K., and Ward, C. W. (2011). Ageing, but not yet senescent, rats exhibit reduced muscle quality and sarcoplasmic reticulum function. *Acta Physiol.* 201, 391–403. doi: 10.1111/j.1748-1716.2010.02191.x

Sanchez, G., Escobar, M., Pedrozo, Z., Macho, P., Domenech, R., Hartel, S., et al. (2008). Exercise and tachycardia increase NADPH oxidase and ryanodine receptor-2 activity: possible role in cardioprotection. *Cardiovasc. Res.* 77, 380–386. doi: 10.1093/cvr/cvm011

Sargiacomo, M., Sudol, M., Tang, Z., and Lisanti, M. P. (1993). Signal transducing molecules and glycosyl-phosphatidylinositol-linked proteins form a caveolin-rich insoluble complex in MDCK cells. *J. Cell Biol.* 122, 789–807. doi: 10.1083/jcb.122.4.789

Shiose, A., Kuroda, J., Tsuruya, K., Hirai, M., Hirakata, H., Naito, S., et al. (2001). A novel superoxide-producing NAD(P)H oxidase in kidney. *J. Biol. Chem.* 276, 1417–1423. doi: 10.1074/jbc.M007597200

Smart, E. J., Graf, G. A., Mcniven, M. A., Sessa, W. C., Engelman, J. A., Scherer, P. E., et al. (1999). Caveolins, liquid-ordered domains, and signal transduction. *Mol. Cell. Biol.* 19, 7289–7304.

Song, K. S., Scherer, P. E., Tang, Z., Okamoto, T., Li, S., Chafel, M., et al. (1996). Expression of caveolin-3 in skeletal, cardiac, and smooth muscle cells. Caveolin-3 is a component of the sarcolemma and co-fractionates with dystrophin and dystrophin-associated glycoproteins. *J. Biol. Chem.* 271, 15160–15165. doi: 10.1074/jbc.271.25.15160

Sun, X., Nagarajan, M., Beesley, P. W., and Ng, Y. C. (1999). Age-associated differential expression of Na(+)-K(+)-ATPase subunit isoforms in skeletal muscles of F-344/BN rats. *J. Appl. Physiol.* 87, 1132–1140.

Toselli, M., Biella, G., Taglietti, V., Cazzaniga, E., and Parenti, M. (2005). Caveolin-1 expression and membrane cholesterol content modulate N-type calcium channel activity in NG108-15 cells. *Biophys. J.* 89, 2443–2457. doi: 10.1529/biophysj.105.065623

Touchberry, C. D., Wacker, M. J., Richmond, S. R., Whitman, S. A., and Godard, M. P. (2006). Age-related changes in relative expression of real-time PCR housekeeping genes in human skeletal muscle. *J. Biomol. Tech.* 17, 157–162.

Umanskaya, A., Santulli, G., Xie, W., Andersson, D. C., Reiken, S. R., and Marks, A. R. (2014). Genetically enhancing mitochondrial antioxidant activity improves muscle function in aging. *Proc. Natl. Acad. Sci. U.S.A.* 111, 15250–15255. doi: 10.1073/pnas.1412754111

Vasilaki, A., Mansouri, A., Van Remmen, H., Van Der Meulen, J. H., Larkin, L., Richardson, A. G., et al. (2006). Free radical generation by skeletal muscle of adult and old mice: effect of contractile activity. *Aging Cell* 5, 109–117. doi: 10.1111/j.1474-9726.2006.00198.x

Vigelso, A., Dybboe, R., Hansen, C. N., Dela, F., Helge, J. W., and Guadalupe-Grau, A. (2015). GAPDH and beta-actin protein decreases with aging making Stain-Free technology a superior loading control in Western Blotting of human skeletal muscle. *J. Appl. Physiol.* 118, 386–394. doi: 10.1152/japplphysiol.00840.2014

Voigt, T., Sebald, H. J., Schoenauer, R., Levano, S., Girard, T., Hoppeler, H. H., et al. (2013). Annexin A1 is a biomarker of T-tubular repair in skeletal muscle of nonmyopathic patients undergoing statin therapy. *FASEB J.* 27, 2156–2164. doi: 10.1096/fj.12-219345

Wagenknecht, T., Hsieh, C. E., Rath, B. K., Fleischer, S., and Marko, M. (2002). Electron tomography of frozen-hydrated isolated triad junctions. *Biophys. J.* 83, 2491–2501. doi: 10.1016/S0006-3495(02)75260-0

Wang, Z. M., Messi, M. L., and Delbono, O. (2000). L-Type Ca(2+) channel charge movement and intracellular Ca(2+) in skeletal muscle fibers from aging mice. *Biophys. J.* 78, 1947–1954. doi: 10.1016/S0006-3495(00)76742-7

Weiss, N., Couchoux, H., Legrand, C., Berthier, C., Allard, B., and Jacquemond, V. (2008). Expression of the muscular dystrophy-associated caveolin-3(P104L) mutant in adult mouse skeletal muscle specifically alters the Ca(2+) channel function of the dihydropyridine receptor. *Pflugers Arch.* 457, 361–375. doi: 10.1007/s00424-008-0528-z

Welle, S. (2002). Cellular and molecular basis of age-related sarcopenia. *Can. J. Appl. Physiol.* 27, 19–41. doi: 10.1139/h02-002

Whiteley, G., Collins, R. F., and Kitmitto, A. (2012). Characterization of the molecular architecture of human caveolin-3 and interaction with the skeletal muscle ryanodine receptor. *J. Biol. Chem.* 287, 40302–40316. doi: 10.1074/jbc.M112.377085

Williams, T. M., and Lisanti, M. P. (2004). The Caveolin genes: from cell biology to medicine. *Ann. Med.* 36, 584–595. doi: 10.1080/07853890410018899

Xu, K. Y., Zweier, J. L., and Becker, L. C. (1995). Functional coupling between glycolysis and sarcoplasmic reticulum Ca2+ transport. *Circ. Res.* 77, 88–97. doi: 10.1161/01.RES.77.1.88

Zalk, R., Lehnart, S. E., and Marks, A. R. (2007). Modulation of the ryanodine receptor and intracellular calcium. *Annu. Rev. Biochem.* 76, 367–385. doi: 10.1146/annurev.biochem.76.053105.094237

Zhang, L., Morris, K. J., and Ng, Y. C. (2006). Fiber type-specific immunostaining of the Na+,K+-ATPase subunit isoforms in skeletal muscle: age-associated differential changes. *Biochim. Biophys. Acta* 1762, 783–793. doi: 10.1016/j.bbadis.2006.08.006

Zuo, L., Pasniciuc, S., Wright, V. P., Merola, A. J., and Clanton, T. L. (2003). Sources for superoxide release: lessons from blockade of electron transport, NADPH oxidase, and anion channels in diaphragm. *Antioxid. Redox Signal.* 5, 667–675. doi: 10.1089/152308603770310347

6

Potential Molecular Mechanisms Underlying Muscle Fatigue Mediated by Reactive Oxygen and Nitrogen Species

*Edward P. Debold**

Department of Kinesiology, University of Massachusetts, Amherst, MA, USA

Edited by:
Brian McDonagh,
University of Liverpool, UK

Reviewed by:
Leonardo F. Ferreira,
University of Florida, USA
D. George Stephenson,
La Trobe University, Australia
James Nathan Cobley,
Abertay University, UK

****Correspondence:***
Edward P. Debold,
Department of Kinesiology, University of Massachusetts, 158 Totman Bldg., 30 Eastman Lane, Amherst, MA 01003, USA
edebold@kin.umass.edu

Intense contractile activity causes a dramatic decline in the force and velocity generating capacity of skeletal muscle within a few minutes, a phenomenon that characterizes fatigue. Much of the research effort has focused on how elevated levels of the metabolites of ATP hydrolysis might inhibit the function of the contractile proteins. However, there is now growing evidence that elevated levels of reactive oxygen and nitrogen species (ROS/RNS), which also accumulate in the myoplasm during fatigue, also play a causative role in this type of fatigue. The most compelling evidence comes from observations demonstrating that pre-treatment of intact muscle with a ROS scavenger can significantly attenuate the development of fatigue. A clear advantage of this line of inquiry is that the molecular targets and protein modifications of some of the ROS scavengers are well-characterized enabling researchers to begin to identify potential regions and even specific amino acid residues modified during fatigue. Combining this knowledge with assessments of contractile properties from the whole muscle level down to the dynamic motions within specific contractile proteins enable the linking of the structural modifications to the functional impacts, using advanced chemical and biophysical techniques. Based on this approach at least two areas are beginning emerge as potentially important sites, the regulatory protein troponin and the actin binding region of myosin. This review highlights some of these recent efforts which have the potential to offer uniquely precise information on the underlying molecular basis of fatigue. This work may also have implications beyond muscle fatigue as ROS/RNS mediated protein modifications are also thought to play a role in the loss of muscle function with aging and in some acute pathologies like cardiac arrest and ischemia.

Keywords: muscle, fatigue, reactive oxygen species, myosin, troponin, tropomyosin

Introduction

Intense exercise can be sustained for only a few minutes before the force and motion generating capacity of skeletal muscle is severely compromised; a phenomenon which defines fatigue (Westerblad et al., 1991; Fitts, 1994; Allen, 2009). Understanding the mechanisms through which this occurs is important to our basic understanding of muscle but also for the development of therapies to improve the physical function of the elderly and chronically ill, so debilitated by fatigue. The extent and rate of fatigue from intense exercise is dependent on numerous factors including the intensity of contraction as well as the rate and duration of stimulation (Fitts, 1994). In humans there are many potential sites of failure and many transient intracellular biochemical changes, including the accumulation of metabolites of ATP hydrolysis (Fitts, 1994). The role of accumulating metabolites has been particularly well-studied, detailed in other reviews (Westerblad et al., 1991; Fitts, 1994, 1996; Cooke, 2007; Enoka and Duchateau, 2007; Allen et al., 2008; Allen, 2009; Debold, 2012). Although less well-studied, there is growing evidence that elevated levels of reactive oxygen and nitrogen species (ROS/RNS) accumulate during intense contractile activity and play a causative role in the fatigue process (Westerblad and Allen, 2011).

Some of the most compelling evidence comes from the observation that pre-treatment with exogenous ROS scavengers attenuates the rate and extent of fatigue in intact muscle (see **Figure 1**). While this is most pronounced in isolated muscle preparations (Shindoh et al., 1990; Moopanar and Allen, 2005, 2006) where the *ex vivo* nature of the preparations might augment the level of ROS (Halliwell, 2014), it has also been observed in exercising humans (Reid et al., 1994; Medved et al., 2004; Ferreira et al., 2011; Slattery et al., 2014). The preventative effect of ROS scavengers is most obvious in humans when fatigue is induced with low stimulation frequencies (Reid et al., 1994), but it is also dependent on the variant of ROS scavenger (Hernández et al., 2012). Thus, there is evidence that ROS/RNS scavengers can delay fatigue and that the accumulation of ROS is linked to the onset and extent of fatigue, which provide compelling support for a causative role. The molecular mechanisms underlying these effects remain unclear but in the last 5–10 years several research groups have made significant advances that have identified specific contractile proteins modified by ROS/RNS and their impact on molecular function (Callahan et al., 2001; Moopanar and Allen, 2005, 2006; Prochniewicz et al., 2008; Dutka et al., 2011; Klein et al., 2011; Mollica et al., 2012; Moen et al., 2014b; Cheng et al., 2015). This review focuses on these recent efforts that highlight the potential molecular mechanism of ROS/RNS mediated fatigue.

What are ROS/RNS and How Do They Affect Muscle Function?

ROS/RNS are chemically reactive molecules making them capable of transiently or permanently damaging cell membranes

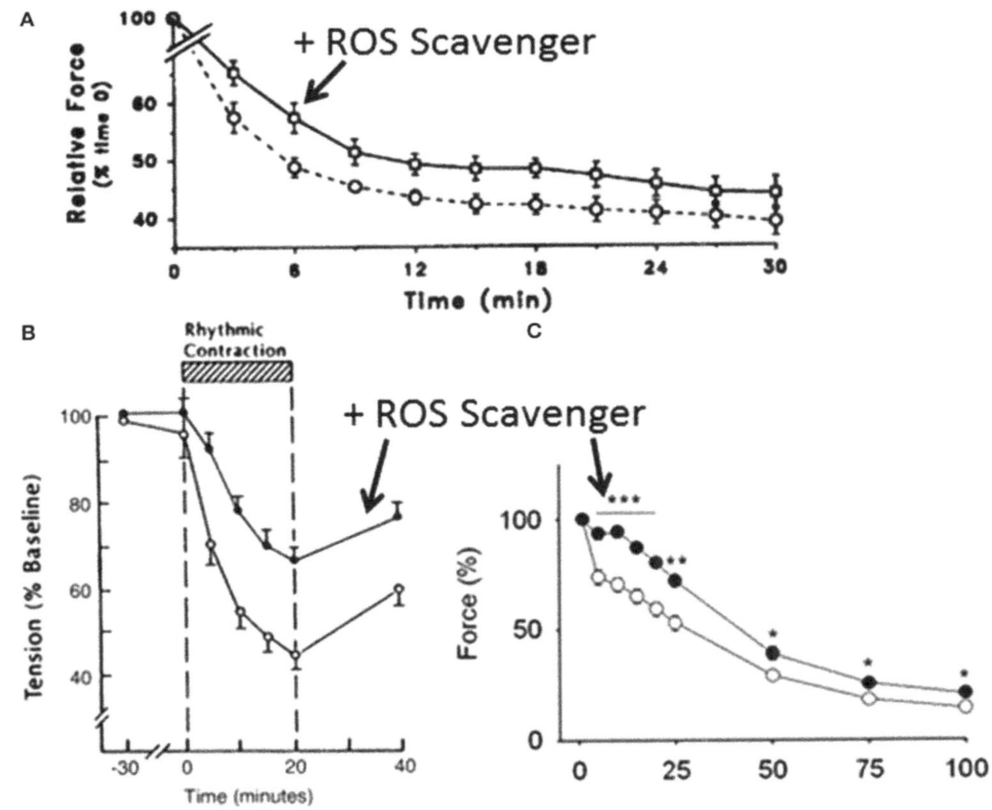

FIGURE 1 | Effect of reactive oxygen species scavengers on fatigue. (A) Effect of pretreatment with ROS scavenger, *N*-acetylcysteine (circles) vs. control (squares) on the fatigue profile of the tibialis anterior muscle in humans stimulated at 10 Hz with a surface electrode. The drop in force was significant under both conditions but the force was greater with *N*-acetylcysteine treatment. Reprinted from Reid et al. (1994) with rights and permission from American Society for Clinical Investigation. **(B)** Effect of the *N*-acetylcysteine on the development of diaphragm fatigue in an anesthetized intact rabbit preparation. Reprinted from Shindoh et al. (1990) with permission. **(C)** Effect of *N*-acetylcysteine on the development of fatigue in isolated mouse extensor digitorum longus muscle. Reprinted from Katz et al. (2014) with permission. *, ** and *** indicate significantly different from corresponding control value (open circles) at $p < 0.05$, $p < 0.01$, and $p < 0.001$ respectively.

and proteins (Moen et al., 2014b). The most important species of ROS/RNS for muscle contraction appear to be hydrogen peroxide (H_2O_2), superoxide ($O_2^{-\cdot}$) as well as nitric oxide which is a precursor to the RNS peroxynitrite ($ONOO^-$), and involved in the S-Nitrosylation of proteins (Reid, 2001a). ROS were originally thought to be primarily generated in the mitochondria as a by-product of oxidative phosphorylation, however more recent findings suggest that the amount generated in the mitochondria is likely quite low, with an upper estimate of ~0.15% (St-Pierre et al., 2002). Instead newer measurements suggest that the primary source of ROS in the cytosol is generated by membrane bound NADPH oxidases (Sakellariou et al., 2011, 2013). For a detailed description of ROS/RNS generating reactions the reader is directed to several excellent reviews (Reid, 2001b; Allen et al., 2008; Powers et al., 2011). Regardless of the source, free radicals are continually produced in muscle cells. At rest, low levels are generated and thought to play an important role in maintaining normal muscle function (Reid, 2001b). In fact, when levels of ROS are low, as might occur at rest or even in the early stages of fatigue, they appear to enhance not inhibit force production (Reid, 2001b) and may even help to delay the onset of fatigue (Mollica et al., 2012). However, as contraction intensifies and/or becomes prolonged, ROS/RNS become elevated and are thought to inhibit proper function of muscle proteins (Reid, 2001a). Consistent with this idea, at higher concentrations, certain ROS inhibit contractile function in isolated muscle fibers (Andrade et al., 1998). When excessively elevated, the reactive nature of ROS/RNS mean that they can induce structural modifications to contractile proteins at cysteine and methionine residues, including for example the formation of disulfide bridges between neighboring cysteine residues either within or between proteins. These modifications may be benign or could depress the function of key contractile proteins. Therefore, goal of much of the recent research in this area has focused on linking loss of contractile protein function to a specific structural alteration; recent advances in biochemical and biophysical techniques are making this a tractable problem.

Skeletal muscle fatigue from intense contractile activity could result from the failure anywhere along the muscle activation pathway, from the firing of neurons in the motor cortex to the generation of force and motion by an actomyosin cross-bridge. A wealth of evidence suggests that this type of fatigue is primarily due to a failure that is distal to the central nervous system (Merton, 1954; Cady et al., 1989; Westerblad et al., 1991). Thus, it is thought that the mechanisms that underlie the role for ROS/RNS in fatigue are also mediated distal to the neuromuscular junction (Westerblad and Allen, 2011). Based on the idea that fatigue originates peripherally there are four key sites at which ROS/RNS mediated fatigue could potentially develop (Westerblad and Allen, 2011): (1) compromised ability to depolarize the sarcolemma; (2) reduction in the amount of Ca^{++} released from the sarcoplasmic reticulum (SR); (3) a decrease in the Ca^{++}-sensitivity of the thin filament; and (4) a direct effect on myosin's ability to bind to and translocate an actin filament.

Do ROS Contribute to Fatigue by Affecting Membrane Excitability and/or Ca^{++} Release from the SR?

A decrease in membrane excitability is one potential mechanism, and based on observations in intact fibers this is believed to occur during fatigue (Juel, 1988), with the effect most pronounced deep within the t-tubules (Balog et al., 1994). Presumably this results from the inability to restore the Na^+/K^+ balance with repeated contractions (Juel, 1988) due to ROS modifications of the Na^+/K^+ pump acting to inhibit its function (McKenna et al., 2006). Interestingly, pretreatment of humans with *N*-acetylcysteine (NAC) (a thiol containing compound (Ferreira and Reid, 2008) that spurs the resynthesize glutathione, a major endogenous antioxidant) increased time to fatigue at 92% of VO_2 peak by ~25% (McKenna et al., 2006). Subsequent biochemical analysis of muscle biopsies revealed that NAC attenuated the decline Na^+/K^+ pump activity, suggesting that this type of fatigue may involve ROS/RNS modification of proteins responsible for maintaining membrane excitability.

However, a distinctly different conclusion was reached by authors using intact fibers that were exposed to elevated levels of exogenous H_2O_2. These findings consistently show that elevated H_2O_2 decreases isometric force but not the intracellular $[Ca^{++}]$ (Andrade et al., 1998, 2001), suggesting that the signal to the SR to release Ca^{++} and thus membrane excitability is not compromised by ROS in these preparations. Part of the discrepancy in the findings may be due to different stimulation rates employed since the experiments on isolated preparations typically show little or no effect on intracellular Ca^{++}-levels with fatigue typically stimulate the muscle at 40 Hz or greater, a rate at which ROS scavengers have little effect on fatigue (Ferreira and Reid, 2008). Another issue may be the timing of the exposure to the oxidants as it has been shown that different regions of the contractile proteins are accessible based on the level of Ca^{++}-activation (Gross and Lehman, 2013). Or the discrepancy may be related to the use of exogenous H_2O_2, which has been hypothesized to exert different effects than those generated endogenously (Forman, 2007).

If membrane excitability were compromised by fatigue it should translate into a weaker signal activating the voltage sensitive receptors of the t-tubules (DHPR) and in turn less release of Ca^{++} by the ryanodine receptors (RyR), causing less activation of the thin filament and thus less cross-bridge formation and force generation (Balog and Fitts, 1996). Support for this notion comes from observations in mechanically skinned fibers in which fatigue, accelerated by higher temperatures, was mitigated by the superoxide scavenger Tiron (van der Poel and Stephenson, 2007). Consistent with this observation studies utilizing vesicles with RYR channels have demonstrated that this channel can be oxidized and that this can affect its ability to release Ca^{++} by increasing their sensitivity to Ca^{++}-induced-Ca^{++}-release (CICR) (Marengo et al., 1998). Likewise, exposure of skinned muscle fibers to H_2O_2 can also increase CICR. Furthermore, NO has been shown to exert regulatory effects on the RYR channels in skeletal muscle (Sun et al., 2001, 2003).

Despite these modifications, exposure of isolated intact muscle preparations to exogenous ROS have generally demonstrated insignificant effects on Ca^{++} released from the SR in response to an action potential (Lamb and Posterino, 2003; Posterino et al., 2003), even at higher temperatures(Place et al., 2009). This suggests that Ca^{++} release is not susceptible to ROS when activated via the nerve whereas it is when stimulated artificially in skinned fibers. Further support for this notion comes from observations showing that the ROS scavenger, Tiron, significantly attenuates the development of fatigue in intact fibers without altering the intracellular [Ca^{++}] (Moopanar and Allen, 2005). Therefore, despite the findings in skinned muscle fibers most current evidence in intact preparations suggests that ROS/RNS mediated fatigue is not due to a loss of membrane excitability or an inability to release Ca^{++} but rather to an effect downstream of Ca^{++} release (Westerblad and Allen, 2011).

Does ROS Contribute to Fatigue by Decreasing Myofilament Ca^{++}-Sensitivity?

During normal muscle activation Ca^{++} release from the SR is followed by a series of complex molecular events that ultimately lead to tropomyosin moving over the surface of actin to reveal the myosin binding sites (Gordon et al., 2000). During fatigue disruption of any one of these steps would disrupt thin filament activation leading a decrease in Ca^{++}-sensitivity. These steps include the binding of Ca^{++} to the calcium binding subunit of troponin (TnC), which triggers the c-terminal domain of the inhibitory subunit of Tn (TnI) to retract from its binding site on actin (Takeda et al., 2003), that allows tropomyosin (Tm) to move further into the groove in actin making the myosin binding sites more accessible (Gordon et al., 2000). In the most widely accepted model of thin filament activation Tm is believed be in a dynamic equilibrium among three positions on actin (Galinska-Rakoczy et al., 2008) with the filament only fully activated when a myosin molecule is strongly bound to actin (McKillop and Geeves, 1993). This is required because the strong-binding of myosin moves Tm a further distance away from the myosin binding sites allowing for neighboring myosins to strongly bind to the filament (Galinska-Rakoczy et al., 2008). Therefore, ROS/RNS could elicit fatigue by either altering Tn's ability to bind Ca^{++} and communicate this signal to its other subunits and Tm, and/or by disrupting myosin's ability to strongly bind to actin. This effect may be particularly relevant because in the latter stages of fatigue, through mechanisms independent of ROS, Ca^{++} release from the SR is compromised (Lee et al., 1991) resulting in a lower intracellular level of Ca^{++} with any given level of stimulation.

Some of the earliest efforts, in chemically skinned cardiac muscle fibers, found that exposure to elevated levels of superoxide had a large effect on maximal force but did not reduce Ca^{++}-sensitivity (MacFarlane and Miller, 1992). Similarly, exposure of rabbit diaphragm fibers to superoxide reduced maximal force but did not change the concentration of Ca^{++} required to reach half maximal force (pCa_{50}) (Darnley et al., 2001). Skinned single skeletal muscle fibers to respond similarly to elevated ROS, seeing a decrease in maximal isometric force with no change in Ca^{++}-sensitivity (van der Poel and Stephenson, 2002). Although this study was focused on determining the effects of elevated temperatures on contractile function, the findings are relevant to the role of ROS in muscle fatigue because they indicated that the depression in function at higher temperatures was due to elevated levels of superoxide. Consistent with this idea, the depression in maximal isometric force could be reversed by the disulphide reducing agent dithiotheritol (DTT) (van der Poel and Stephenson, 2002), which is similar to what is seen with fatigue (Moopanar and Allen, 2005). Collectively these findings suggest that ROS have a pronounced, depressive effect on maximal isometric force and little impact on Ca^{++}-sensitivity. Thus, these findings point toward ROS potentially having a direct effect on actomyosin and not the regulatory proteins troponin and tropomyosin.

However, these findings stand in stark contrast to the results from intact muscle preparations which have consistently observed that ROS decreases Ca^{++}-sensitivity while exerting minimal effects on maximal isometric force (Andrade et al., 1998, 2001; Moopanar and Allen, 2005, 2006). For example, elevated levels of H_2O_2 produced a pronounced rightward shift in the force-calcium relation in intact muscle fibers without affecting the intracellular Ca^{++} concentration (**Figure 2**), suggesting that the H_2O_2 decreased the Ca^{++}-sensitivity of the myofilaments (Andrade et al., 1998). This work was confirmed and extended in a more recent where intact muscle was fatigued in the presence of DTT (Moopanar and Allen, 2006). In this study living mouse fast muscle fibers were stimulated to fatigue while simultaneously measuring isometric force and intracellular levels of Ca^{++}, enabling the ability to directly determine the

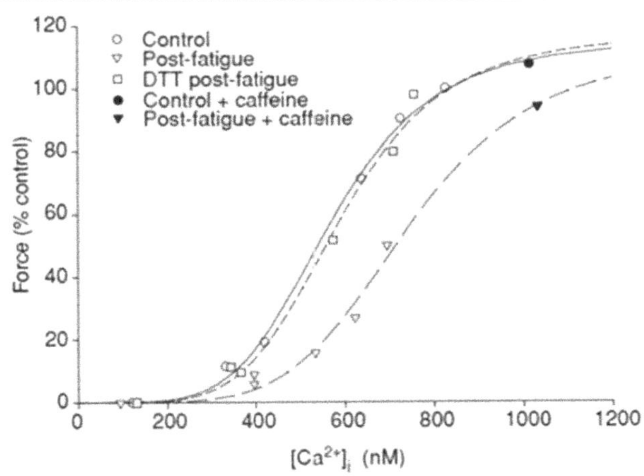

FIGURE 2 | ROS mediated fatigue and Ca^{++}-sensitivity. Force-calcium relation plotted during fatigue of intact mouse flexor brevis muscle fibers stimulated at 100 Hz, at 37°C. Force expressed relative to rested value under control conditions. Fatigue under control conditions produced a strong rightward shift in the relation and depressed maximal force. Maximal force but not Ca^{++}-sensitivity was restored with caffeine. Treatment with dithiothreitol (DTT) restored Ca^{++}-sensitivity. Reprinted from Moopanar and Allen (2006) with permission from John Wiley and Sons publishing company.

force-calcium relationship in an intact fiber during fatigue. Consistent with prior experiments in intact muscle, Ca^{++} release was compromised by fatigue but this was not reversed by DTT, indicating no role for ROS. Ca^{++}-sensitivity however was depressed and was fully reversed by DTT. While subsequent findings suggested that iron leeching off the stimulating electrode in these experiments likely drove the ROS concentration higher than originally reported (Reardon and Allen, 2009a,b) it remains clear that elevated levels of ROS mediated the depressive effects on force. Therefore, these findings suggest that elevated levels of ROS decrease the Ca^{++}-sensitivity of the myofilaments and that this may be the primary mechanism through which ROS induces fatigue in intact muscle.

It is not clear why the results from skinned muscle fibers differ so strongly from those using intact muscle fibers. While it can be argued that intact fibers, which can be exposed to a fatiguing protocol, represent the more physiologically relevant findings, a careful delineation of the differences between these findings may provide key insights into the mechanisms underlying ROS induced muscle fatigue. Along this line of thought, a recent report focused on prolonged low-frequency force depression observed that both the SR Ca^{++}-release and myofilament sensitivity can be altered by fatiguing stimulation in intact fibers (Cheng et al., 2015). To explain these findings they suggested a model where the mechanism of ROS mediated fatigue is dependent on the stimulation protocol, with one type of protocol superoxide is generated in the mitochondria and owing to its proximity and possible physical connections to the SR (Boncompagni et al., 2009) directly affects the DHP and RyR channels, and as a result reduces Ca^{++} release, but has no effect on Ca^{++}-sensitivity. In contrast, other types of fatigue protocols, and exposures to exogenous ROS/RNS, result in a more broad cytosolic elevation of ROS (e.g., exogenous H_2O_2 exposure) that modifies the thick and thin filaments of the sarcomere, leading to a decrease in Ca^{++}-sensitivity.

Since DTT targets disulphide linkages the findings of Moopanar and Allen (2006) suggest that these types of modifications are driving the ROS mediated fatigue, but it is unclear which of the contractile proteins involved determining the Ca^{++}-sensitivity are modified by the ROS. However, related work in diaphragm muscle fatigued under hypoxic conditions may offer insight (de Paula Brotto et al., 2001). In response to fatiguing stimulation there was evidence of TnI and TnC degradation, both of which are integral to proper thin filament activation. The loss in force during fatigue was attributed to the cleavage of these subunits of Tn which the authors speculated resulted from ROS modification that targeted them for proteolysis (de Paula Brotto et al., 2001). The authors also speculated that although hypoxia might generate a greater and more diverse pool of ROS that the same ROS might also appear during physiological fatigue because muscle is thought to become hypoxic to some extent during fatigue even under normoxic conditions (Babcock et al., 1995).

Alternatively fatigue may not lead to cleavage of TnI but rather might induce post-translational modifications of Tn/Tm. In support of this notion a recent study focused on identifying the mechanisms of the increased Ca^{++}-sensitivity following a treatment that oxidizes cysteine residues (disulphide 2,2′-dithiodipyridine or DTDP) found that the effects could be attributed to the addition of a glutathione to a specific cysteine residue (Cys133) in TnI (Mollica et al., 2012). This residue is in a crucial mobile region of TnI that switches between being bound to actin (low Ca^{++}) and bound to a hydrophobic patch on the N-lobe of TnC (High Ca^{++}) (Takeda et al., 2003). Therefore, this modification likely would lead to this region more readily associating with TnC and therefore could explain the increased Ca^{++}-sensitivity under the conditions tested. This effect appears to increase with exercise and thus the authors suggested it may help delay the onset of, rather than contribute to, fatigue. Thus, this effect is the opposite of the depressive effects described above but highlights that the regulatory proteins can be post-translationally modified in response to exercise. It would be interesting to determine if the modification is lost as fatigue becomes more severe or if other alterations that lead to depressed Ca^{++}-sensitivity appear in the same crucial region of TnI.

Yet another possible explanation for these observations would be the oxidation-induced dissociation of TnC from the troponin complex and thus the thin filament. This notion is supported by evidence showing that oxidation of the Cys 98 residue of the D/E helix of TnC reduces its affinity for the thin filament and the effect is readily reversed by exposure to DTT (Pinto et al., 2011). It will be informative to understand the mechanisms underlying this event in more detail and how it might impact fatigue in future work.

Overall these data demonstrate strong evidence that the ROS/RNS mediated fatigue could involve alterations in the structure and function of the muscle regulatory proteins that is consistent with the observed decrease in Ca^{++} sensitivity.

Is Myosin's Function Affected by ROS/RNS During Fatigue?

The skinned fibers studies demonstrating that elevated levels of ROS/RNS decrease maximal isometric force but not Ca^{++}sensitivity suggest that under these conditions ROS/RNS may act by modifying myosin and/or actin. Such targets and modifications have yet to be thoroughly investigated but some recent work focused on understanding the broad effects of oxidative stress on muscle have highlighted that myosin may have redox sensitive residues in the actomyosin interface (Prochniewicz et al., 2008; Klein et al., 2011; Moen et al., 2014a,b) that affect its function. Consistent with others, this group has shown that non-physiological concentrations of H_2O_2 (5–50 mM) can reduce the maximal isometric force, maximal ATPase rate and Ca^{++} -sensitivity of chemically skinned skeletal muscle fibers (Prochniewicz et al., 2008). Electron paramagnetic resonance labeling experiments revealed that the treatment increases the fraction of myosin heads in the strongly bound state in relaxed conditions (i.e., low Ca^{++}). With more heads in a strongly bound state at rest, less heads will be able to go through the weak-to-strong force generating transition upon activation, and thus this may explain the decrease in maximal isometric force in the muscle fibers in response to H_2O_2. Further, analysis using mass spectrometry showed the addition of multiple oxygen atoms on both myosin's heavy and light chains, which occurred exclusively at methionine residues. This provides a link between the loss of force generation with a modification to a specific residue on myosin. In a follow up study, using myosin expressed in *Dictyostelium Discoideum* (*Dicty*), the authors demonstrated that most of H_2O_2's effects on myosin function can be attributed to oxidation at a single methionine residue (M394) in the actin-binding interface (Klein et al., 2011). This hypothesis is further supported by more recent work demonstrating that the depressive effects of oxidation at this site can be completely reversed by exposure to methionine sulfoxide reductase targeting the M394 site (Moen et al., 2014a). Interestingly in human skeletal muscle myosin this residue is a Cys not a Met, but the effects of oxidation at this residue when it is changed to a Cys in the *Dicty* construct are nearly identical to those when M394 is oxidized (Moen et al., 2014a). Thus, this is an interesting line of experiments and highlights that myosin can be modified by ROS species which are elevated during fatigue, and that the functional differences are attributable to the modification at a single residue in the actomyosin interface. It will be important to determine if the modification also happens in human skeletal muscle during fatigue and to demonstrate that it contributes to the depressive effects seen during fatigue. This would be particularly exciting because presumably it could be readily reversed.

Acknowledgments

EPD is funded by the American Heart Association (GIA#14GRNT20450002).

References

Allen, D. G. (2009). Fatigue in working muscles. *J. Appl. Physiol.* 106, 358–359. doi: 10.1152/japplphysiol.91599.2008

Allen, D. G., Lamb, G. D., and Westerblad, H. (2008). Skeletal muscle fatigue: cellular mechanisms. *Physiol. Rev.* 88, 287–332. doi: 10.1152/physrev.00015.2007

Andrade, F. H., Reid, M. B., Allen, D. G., and Westerblad, H. (1998). Effect of hydrogen peroxide and dithiothreitol on contractile function of single skeletal muscle fibres from the mouse. *J. Physiol.* 509(Pt 2), 565–575. doi: 10.1111/j.1469-7793.1998.565bn.x

Andrade, F. H., Reid, M. B., and Westerblad, H. (2001). Contractile response of skeletal muscle to low peroxide concentrations: myofibrillar calcium sensitivity as a likely target for redox-modulation. *FASEB J.* 15, 309–311. doi: 10.1096/fj.00-0507fje

Babcock, M. A., Johnson, B. D., Pegelow, D. F., Suman, O. E., Griffin, D., and Dempsey, J. A. (1995). Hypoxic effects on exercise-induced diaphragmatic fatigue in normal healthy humans. *J. Appl. Physiol. (1985)* 78, 82–92.

Balog, E. M., and Fitts, R. H. (1996). Effects of fatiguing stimulation on intracellular Na+ and K+ in frog skeletal muscle. *J. Appl. Physiol. (1985)* 81, 679–685.

Balog, E. M., Thompson, L. V., and Fitts, R. H. (1994). Role of sarcolemma action potentials and excitability in muscle fatigue. *J. Appl. Physiol. (1985)* 76, 2157–2162.

Boncompagni, S., Rossi, A. E., Micaroni, M., Hamilton, S. L., Dirksen, R. T., Franzini-Armstrong, C., et al. (2009). Characterization and temporal development of cores in a mouse model of malignant hyperthermia. *Proc. Natl. Acad. Sci. U.S.A.* 106, 21996–22001. doi: 10.1073/pnas.0911496106

Cady, E. B., Jones, D. A., Lynn, J., and Newham, D. J. (1989). Changes in force and intracellular metabolites during fatigue of human skeletal muscle. *J. Physiol.* 418, 311–325. doi: 10.1113/jphysiol.1989.sp017842

Callahan, L. A., She, Z. W., and Nosek, T. M. (2001). Superoxide, hydroxyl radical, and hydrogen peroxide effects on single-diaphragm fiber contractile apparatus. *J. Appl. Physiol. (1985)* 90, 45–54.

Cheng, A. J., Bruton, J. D., Lanner, J. T., and Westerblad, H. (2015). Antioxidant treatments do not improve force recovery after fatiguing stimulation of mouse skeletal muscle fibres. *J. Physiol.* 593, 457–472. doi: 10.1113/jphysiol.2014.279398

Cooke, R. (2007). Modulation of the actomyosin interaction during fatigue of skeletal muscle. *Muscle Nerve* 36, 756–777. doi: 10.1002/mus.20891

Darnley, G. M., Duke, A. M., Steele, D. S., and MacFarlane, N. G. (2001). Effects of reactive oxygen species on aspects of excitation-contraction coupling in chemically skinned rabbit diaphragm muscle fibres. *Exp. Physiol.* 86, 161–168. doi: 10.1113/eph8602109

Debold, E. P. (2012). Recent insights into the molecular basis of muscular fatigue. *Med. Sci. Sports Exerc.* 44, 1440–1452. doi: 10.1249/mss.0b013e31824cfd26

de Paula Brotto, M., van Leyen, S. A., Brotto, L. S., Jin, J. P., Nosek, C. M., and Nosek, T. M. (2001). Hypoxia/fatigue-induced degradation of troponin I and troponin C: new insights into physiologic muscle fatigue. *Pflugers Arch.* 442, 738–744. doi: 10.1007/s004240100587

Dutka, T. L., Mollica, J. P., and Lamb, G. D. (2011). Differential effects of peroxynitrite on contractile protein properties in fast- and slow-twitch skeletal muscle fibers of rat. *J. Appl. Physiol. (1985)* 110, 705–716. doi: 10.1152/japplphysiol.00739.2010

Enoka, R. M., and Duchateau, J. (2007). Muscle fatigue: what, why and how it influences muscle function. *J. Physiol.* 586, 11–23. doi: 10.1113/jphysiol.2007.139477

Ferreira, L. F., Campbell, K. S., and Reid, M. B. (2011). Effectiveness of sulfur-containing antioxidants in delaying skeletal muscle fatigue. *Med. Sci. Sports Exerc.* 43, 1025–1031. doi: 10.1249/MSS.0b013e3182019a78

Ferreira, L. F., and Reid, M. B. (2008). Muscle-derived ROS and thiol regulation in muscle fatigue. *J. Appl. Physiol. (1985)* 104, 853–860. doi: 10.1152/japplphysiol.00953.2007

Fitts, R. H. (1994). Cellular mechanisms of muscle fatigue. *Physiol. Rev.* 74, 49–94.

Fitts, R. H. (1996). Muscle fatigue: the cellular aspects. *Am. J. Sports Med.* 24, S9–S13.

Forman, H. J. (2007). Use and abuse of exogenous H2O2 in studies of signal transduction. *Free Radic. Biol. Med.* 42, 926–932. doi: 10.1016/j.freeradbiomed.2007.01.011

Galinska-Rakoczy, A., Engel, P., Xu, C., Jung, H., Craig, R., Tobacman, L. S., et al. (2008). Structural basis for the regulation of muscle contraction by troponin and tropomyosin. *J. Mol. Biol.* 379, 929–935. doi: 10.1016/j.jmb.2008.04.062

Gordon, A. M., Homsher, E., and Regnier, M. (2000). Regulation of contraction in striated muscle. *Physiol. Rev.* 80, 853–924.

Gross, S. M., and Lehman, S. L. (2013). Accessibility of myofilament cysteines and effects on ATPase depend on the activation state during exposure to oxidants. *PLoS ONE* 8:e69110. doi: 10.1371/journal.pone.0069110

Halliwell, B. (2014).Cell culture, oxidative stress, and antioxidants: avoiding pitfalls. *Biomed. J.* 37, 99–105. doi: 10.4103/2319-4170.128725

Hernández, A., Cheng, A., and Westerblad, H. (2012). Antioxidants and skeletal muscle performance: "common knowledge" vs. experimental evidence. *Front. Physiol.* 3:46. doi: 10.3389/fphys.2012.00046

Juel, C. (1988). Muscle action potential propagation velocity changes during activity. *Muscle Nerve* 11, 714–719. doi: 10.1002/mus.880110707

Katz, A., Hernández, A., Caballero, D. M., Briceno, J. F., Amezquita, L. V., Kosterina, N., et al. (2014). Effects of N-acetylcysteine on isolated mouse skeletal muscle: contractile properties, temperature dependence, and metabolism. *Pflugers Arch.* 466, 577–585. doi: 10.1007/s00424-013-1331-z

Klein, J. C., Moen, R. J., Smith, E. A., Titus, M. A., and Thomas, D. D. (2011). Structural and functional impact of site-directed methionine oxidation in myosin. *Biochemistry* 50, 10318–10327. doi: 10.1021/bi201279u

Lamb, G. D., and Posterino, G. S. (2003). Effects of oxidation and reduction on contractile function in skeletal muscle fibres of the rat. *J. Physiol.* 546, 149–163. doi: 10.1113/jphysiol.2002.027896

Lee, J. A., Westerblad, H., and Allen, D. G. (1991). Changes in tetanic and resting [Ca2+]i during fatigue and recovery of single muscle fibres from *Xenopus laevis*. *J. Physiol.* 433, 307–326. doi: 10.1113/jphysiol.1991.sp018427

MacFarlane, N. G., and Miller, D. J. (1992). Depression of peak force without altering calcium sensitivity by the superoxide anion in chemically skinned cardiac muscle of rat. *Circ. Res.* 70, 1217–1224. doi: 10.1161/01.RES.70.6.1217

Marengo, J. J., Hidalgo, C., and Bull, R. (1998). Sulfhydryl oxidation modifies the calcium dependence of ryanodine-sensitive calcium channels of excitable cells. *Biophys. J.* 74, 1263–1277. doi: 10.1016/S0006-3495(98)77840-3

McKenna, M. J., Medved, I., Goodman, C. A., Brown, M. J., Bjorksten, A. R., Murphy, K. T., et al. (2006). N-acetylcysteine attenuates the decline in muscle Na+,K+-pump activity and delays fatigue during prolonged exercise in humans. *J. Physiol.* 576, 279–288. doi: 10.1113/jphysiol.2006.115352

McKillop, D. F., and Geeves, M. A. (1993). Regulation of the interaction between actin and myosin subfragment 1: evidence for three states of the thin filament. *Biophys. J.* 65, 693–701. doi: 10.1016/S0006-3495(93)81110-X

Medved, I., Brown, M. J., Bjorksten, A. R., Murphy, K. T., Petersen, A. C., Sostaric, S., et al. (2004). N-acetylcysteine enhances muscle cysteine and glutathione availability and attenuates fatigue during prolonged exercise in endurance-trained individuals. *J. Appl. Physiol (1985)* 97, 1477–1485. doi: 10.1152/japplphysiol.00371.2004

Merton, P. A. (1954). Voluntary strength and fatigue. *J. Physiol.* 123, 553–564. doi: 10.1113/jphysiol.1954.sp005070

Moen, R. J., Cornea, S., Oseid, D. E., Binder, B. P., Klein, J. C., and Thomas, D. D. (2014a). Redox-sensitive residue in the actin-binding interface of myosin. *Biochem. Biophys. Res. Commun.* 453, 345–349. doi: 10.1016/j.bbrc.2014.09.072

Moen, R. J., Klein, J. C., and Thomas, D. D. (2014b). Electron paramagnetic resonance resolves effects of oxidative stress on muscle proteins. *Exerc. Sport Sci. Rev.* 42, 30–36. doi: 10.1249/JES.0000000000000004

Mollica, J. P., Dutka, T. L., Merry, T. L., Lamboley, C. R., McConell, G. K., McKenna, M. J., et al. (2012). S-glutathionylation of troponin I (fast) increases contractile apparatus Ca2+ sensitivity in fast-twitch muscle fibres of rats and humans. *J. Physiol.* 590, 1443–1463. doi: 10.1113/jphysiol.2011.224535

Moopanar, T. R., and Allen, D. G. (2005). Reactive oxygen species reduce myofibrillar Ca2+ sensitivity in fatiguing mouse skeletal muscle at 37 degrees C. *J. Physiol.* 564, 189–199. doi: 10.1113/jphysiol.2005.083519

Moopanar, T. R., and Allen, D. G. (2006). The activity-induced reduction of myofibrillar Ca2+ sensitivity in mouse skeletal muscle is reversed by dithiothreitol. *J. Physiol.* 571, 191–200. doi: 10.1113/jphysiol.2005.101105

Pinto, J. R., de Sousa, V. P., and Sorenson, M. M. (2011). Redox state of troponin C cysteine in the D/E helix alters the C-domain affinity for the thin filament of vertebrate striated muscle. *Biochim. Biophys. Acta* 1810, 391–397. doi: 10.1016/j.bbagen.2010.11.008

Place, N., Yamada, T., Zhang, S. J., Westerblad, H., and Bruton, J. D. (2009). High temperature does not alter fatigability in intact mouse skeletal muscle fibres. *J. Physiol.* 587, 4717–4724. doi: 10.1113/jphysiol.2009.176883

Posterino, G. S., Cellini, M. A., and Lamb, G. D. (2003). Effects of oxidation and cytosolic redox conditions on excitation-contraction coupling in rat skeletal muscle. *J. Physiol.* 547, 807–823. doi: 10.1113/jphysiol.2002.035204

Powers, S. K., Nelson, W. B., and Hudson, M. B. (2011). Exercise-induced oxidative stress in humans: cause and consequences. *Free Radic. Biol. Med.* 51, 942–950. doi: 10.1016/j.freeradbiomed.2010.12.009

Prochniewicz, E., Spakowicz, D., and Thomas, D. D. (2008). Changes in actin structural transitions associated with oxidative inhibition of muscle contraction. *Biochemistry* 47, 11811–11817. doi: 10.1021/bi801080x

Reardon, T. F., and Allen, D. G. (2009a). Iron injections in mice increase skeletal muscle iron content, induce oxidative stress and reduce exercise performance. *Exp. Physiol.* 94, 720–730. doi: 10.1113/expphysiol.2008.046045

Reardon, T. F., and Allen, D. G. (2009b). Time to fatigue is increased in mouse muscle at 37 degrees C; the role of iron and reactive oxygen species. *J. Physiol.* 587, 4705–4716. doi: 10.1113/jphysiol.2009.173005

Reid, M. B. (2001a). Invited Review: redox modulation of skeletal muscle contraction: what we know and what we don't. *J. Appl. Physiol. (1985)* 90, 724–731.

Reid, M. B. (2001b). Nitric oxide, reactive oxygen species, and skeletal muscle contraction. *Med. Sci. Sports Exerc.* 33, 371–376. doi: 10.1097/00005768-200103000-00006

Reid, M. B., Stokic, D. S., Koch, S. M., Khawli, F. A., and Leis, A. A. (1994). N-acetylcysteine inhibits muscle fatigue in humans. *J. Clin. Invest.* 94, 2468–2474. doi: 10.1172/JCI117615

Sakellariou, G. K., Pye, D., Vasilaki, A., Zibrik, L., Palomero, J., Kabayo, T., et al. (2011). Role of superoxide-nitric oxide interactions in the accelerated age-related loss of muscle mass in mice lacking Cu,Zn superoxide dismutase. *Aging Cell* 10, 749–760. doi: 10.1111/j.1474-9726.2011.00709.x

Sakellariou, G. K., Vasilaki, A., Palomero, J., Kayani, A., Zibrik, L., McArdle, A., et al. (2013). Studies of mitochondrial and nonmitochondrial sources implicate nicotinamide adenine dinucleotide phosphate oxidase(s) in the increased skeletal muscle superoxide generation that occurs during contractile activity. *Antioxid. Redox. Signal.* 18, 603–621. doi: 10.1089/ars.2012.4623

Shindoh, C., DiMarco, A., Thomas, A., Manubay, P., and Supinski, G. (1990). Effect of N-acetylcysteine on diaphragm fatigue. *J. Appl. Physiol. (1985)* 68, 2107–2113.

Slattery, K. M., Dascombe, B., Wallace, L. K., Bentley, D. J., and Coutts, A. J. (2014). Effect of N-acetylcysteine on cycling performance after intensified training. *Med. Sci. Sports Exerc.* 46, 1114–1123. doi: 10.1249/MSS.0000000000000222

St-Pierre, J., Buckingham, J. A., Roebuck, S. J., and Brand, M. D. (2002). Topology of superoxide production from different sites in the mitochondrial electron transport chain. *J. Biol. Chem.* 277, 44784–44790. doi: 10.1074/jbc.M207217200

Sun, J., Xin, C., Eu, J. P., Stamler, J. S., and Meissner, G. (2001). Cysteine-3635 is responsible for skeletal muscle ryanodine receptor modulation by NO. *Proc. Natl. Acad. Sci.U.S.A.* 98, 11158–11162. doi: 10.1073/pnas.201289098

Sun, J., Xu, L., Eu, J. P., Stamler, J. S., and Meissner, G. (2003). Nitric oxide, NOC-12, and S-nitrosoglutathione modulate the skeletal muscle calcium release channel/ryanodine receptor by different mechanisms. An allosteric function for O2 in S-nitrosylation of the channel. *J. Biol. Chem.* 278, 8184–8189. doi: 10.1074/jbc.M211940200

Takeda, S., Yamashita, A., Maeda, K., and Maéda, Y. (2003). Structure of the core domain of human cardiac troponin in the $Ca^{(2+)}$-saturated form. *Nature* 424, 35–41. doi: 10.1038/nature01780

van der Poel, C., and Stephenson, D. G. (2002). Reversible changes in $Ca^{(2+)}$-activation properties of rat skeletal muscle exposed to elevated physiological temperatures. *J. Physiol.* 544, 765–776. doi: 10.1113/jphysiol.2002.024968

van der Poel, C., and Stephenson, D. G. (2007). Effects of elevated physiological temperatures on sarcoplasmic reticulum function in mechanically skinned muscle fibers of the rat. *Am. J. Physiol. Cell Physiol.* 293, C133–C141. doi: 10.1152/ajpcell.00052.2007

Westerblad, H., and Allen, D. G. (2011). Emerging roles of ROS/RNS in muscle function and fatigue. *Antioxid. Redox. Signal.* 15, 2487–2499. doi: 10.1089/ars.2011.3909

Westerblad, H., Lee, J. A., Lannergren, J., and Allen, D. G. (1991). Cellular mechanisms of fatigue in skeletal muscle. *Am. J. Physiol.* 261, C195–C209.

7

Health and Lifestyles Factors Associated with Osteoarthritis among Older Adults in Portugal

Natália Duarte[1]*, Ana Maria Rodrigues[2,3], Jaime Da Cunha Branco[4], Helena Canhão[5], Susan L. Hughes[6] and Constança Paúl[1]

[1] Research Unit on Ageing, Instituto de Ciências Biomédicas Abel Salazar (ICBAS), Centro de Investigação em Tecnologias e Serviços de Saúde (CINTESIS), University of Porto, Porto, Portugal, [2] EpiReumaPt Study Group—Sociedade Portuguesa de Reumatologia, Lisboa, Portugal, [3] EpiDoc Unit—Unidade de Epidemiologia em Doenças Crónicas (CEDOC, NMS/UNL), Unidade de Investigação em Reumatologia, Instituto de Medicina Molecular, Faculdade de Medicina da Universidade de Lisboa, Lisboa, Portugal, [4] EpiReumaPt Study Group—Centro de Estudos de Doenças Crónicas (CEDOC) da NOVA Medical School, Universidade Nova de Lisboa (NMS/UNL), Centro Hospitalar Lisboa Ocidental (CHLO-EPE), Sociedade Portuguesa de Reumatologia, Lisbon, Portugal, [5] EpiReumaPt Study Group—Centro de Estudos de Doenças Crónicas (CEDOC), EpiDoC Unit, NOVA Medical School, Universidade Nova de Lisboa (NMS/UNL), Escola Nacional de Saúde Publica, Universidade Nova de Lisboa, Sociedade Portuguesa de Reumatologia, Serviço de Reumatologia do Hospital de Santa Maria, Centro Hospitalar Lisboa Norte (CHLN-EPE), Lisboa, Portugal, [6] Community Health Sciences, School of Public Health, Center for Research on Health and Aging, University of Illinois at Chicago, Chicago, IL, United States

Edited by:
Xenofon Baraliakos, Rheumazentrum Ruhrgebiet, Germany

Reviewed by:
Rainer Klocke, Dudley Group NHS Foundation Trust, United Kingdom
Cristina Pamfil, Iuliu Haţieganu University of Medicine and Pharmacy, Romania

***Correspondence:**
Natália Duarte
nduarte@unifai.eu,
nataliascduarte@gmail.com

Objective: This study aimed to identify independent associations of sociodemographic, functionality, physical activity, physical and mental health, and osteoarthritis (OA), among older adults.

Methods: A sample of 1,645 older adults (50+ years) observed by rheumatologists, from EpiReumaPt, a population-based study was analyzed. A structured interview included sociodemographic data, chronic non-communicable disease, and physical activity. Functional ability was assessed by the Health Assessment Questionnaire Disability Index; depression and anxiety were assessed by Hospital Anxiety and Depression Scale. OA (knee OA and/or hip OA and/or hand OA) was defined after medical evaluation by rheumatologists according to expert opinion combined with the fulfillment of the American College of Rheumatology classification criteria.

Results: 1,059 participants (64.9%) met the OA classification criteria. Statistically significant differences were found between persons with and without OA in all sociodemographic variables, non-communicable diseases, functional status, physical activity, depression, and anxiety. In the unadjusted logistic regression models, all variables were associated with OA. The final adjusted model explained 32% of the variance. Those who are female with higher age, have more than five comorbidities, and lower levels of function and physical activity were more likely to meet the criteria for a diagnosis of OA.

Discussion: We have analyzed data from a population-based study and found that a diagnosis of OA was independently associated with age, female gender, higher number of comorbidities, physical disability, and low levels of physical activity. These results reinforce the usefulness of the development of a multidimensional assessment to design and test effective interventions for this population.

Keywords: predictors, rheumatic disease, aging, disability, comorbidity, women

INTRODUCTION

Osteoarthritis (OA) is the most prevalent rheumatic disease in the general population (1), and its prevalence is known to increase gradually with age (2). The World Health Organization (WHO) Scientific Group on Rheumatic Diseases estimates that 10% of the world's population 60 years or older has significant clinical problems that can be attributed to OA (3).

Osteoarthritis is a major contributor to functional impairment and loss of independence in older persons causing difficulties in maintaining their activities of daily living (4). Data from the *Global Burden of Disease Project* identify the common causes of years of healthy life lost due to disability in people older than 60 years and identify OA as one of the 10 most relevant causes of disability in this population (5).

Because of the high prevalence of this disease and its impact on independence and quality of life among patients, researchers have been studying factors associated with OA prevalence. Sociodemographic variables, such as age and gender, have been the most studied factors, but studies have also analyzed the association of OA with comorbidities [e.g., Ref. (6, 7)], psychological factors (8, 9), and physical activity (10, 11).

Currently, few studies have compared people with and without OA, furthermore, most studies have analyzed associated factors separately and the comparative contribution of each variable is unknown.

The objectives of this study are (1) to compare people with and without OA with respect to sociodemographic characteristics, functionality, physical activity, non-communicable chronic diseases, and presence of anxiety and depression symptoms; and (2) to identify independent associations between sociodemographic characteristics, functionality, physical activity, physical health and psychological symptoms, and OA.

MATERIALS AND METHODS

Sample

Data from EpiReumaPt project, which is a national, cross-sectional, and population-based study, were used (12). This study population comprised adults (≥18 years old) living in the community, in the Portugal mainland and islands (Azores and Madeira). Exclusion criteria were resident of an institution, and inability to speak Portuguese or to complete the assessment protocol. Participants were selected through a process of multi-stage random sampling. The sample was stratified by region and population size.

EpiReumaPt involved a three-stage approach. The first stage included the selection of potential participant household/families using a random selection process. In each household, the adult with the most recent birthday was recruited and completed a structured interview (sociodemographic, socioeconomic, anxiety and depression symptoms, lifestyle habits, chronic non-communicable diseases, health resources utilization data), and a screening for rheumatic diseases. In the second stage, all participants who screened positive for at least one rheumatic disease plus 20% of participants with no rheumatic symptoms were invited to be assessed by a rheumatologist. In the last phase, a team of three experienced rheumatologists revised all the clinical, laboratory, and imaging data and confirmed the diagnoses using validated criteria (12). Details of the EpiReumaPt methodology have been published previously (12–14).

In this study, the sample consisted of adults 50+ years old who participated in the second phase of EpiReumaPt study and were evaluated by a rheumatologist to confirm the presence or absence of OA (knee OA and/or hip OA and/or hand OA). OA was defined by rheumatologists according to expert opinion combined with the fulfillment of the American College of Rheumatology classification criteria for knee OA, hip OA, and hand OA, as described earlier (15–17).

Sociodemographic data, physical function, anxiety and depression symptoms, lifestyle (e.g., physical activity), and chronic non-communicable diseases were collected during the first stage of the EpiReumaPt project.

Measurements

Sociodemographic data included age, gender, marital status, education, and work status. Marital status was categorized in three categories: without partner (single and divorced people), married, and widower. Work status was categorized as employed full time, part-time, not currently employed (domestic employed, unemployed, and students), and retired.

Number of current chronic non-communicable diseases was assessed using a comprehensive list which included the following 14 diseases: high blood pressure, high cholesterol, heart disease, diabetes mellitus, chronic lung disease, problems in the digestive tract, renal colic, neurological disease, allergies, mental or psychiatric illness, cancer, thyroid and parathyroid problems, hypogonadism, hyperuricemia, and other rheumatic diseases (OA was excluded from this list).

The Health Assessment Questionnaire Disability Index [HAQ-DI; (18)] was used to assess level of functional ability. HAQ-DI measures difficulties with the performance of 20 daily activities retrospectively over the preceding week with four possible responses: no difficulty (0 points), some difficulty (1 point), much difficulty (2 points), and unable to do (3 points). The 20 activities are classified into 8 categories with 2 or 3 activities each: dressing and grooming, arising eating, walking, personal hygiene, reaching, gripping, and usual activities (i.e., shopping, doing chores, getting in and out of a car) (18, 19). The score for each category is the single response within the category with the highest score (greater difficulty). The total score is computed as the mean of the eight category scores. As in previous studies, we did not correct HAQ-DI scores for use of assistive devices (19, 20).

To assess physical activity, participants were asked about the amount of time (minutes) per week they dedicated to physical activity. Answers were categorized as <150 or ≥150 min, based on the physical activity recommendations of the WHO (21) for older adults.

Depression and anxiety were assessed by Hospital Anxiety and Depression Scale [HADS; (22, 23)]. The HADS is a short instrument with two subscales that both have seven items that assess presence of clinical anxiety and depression. The scale has a maximum score of 21 for both anxiety and depression subscales. People with scores between 0 and 7 are considered normal, scores between 8 and 10 are borderline, and a score ≥11 indicates a mood disorder. In data analysis, anxiety and depression were considered as dichotomous variables (i.e., a participant with a score ≥11 on either subscale was considered depressed or anxious).

Ethical Issue

EpiReumaPt was approved by the National Committee for Data Protection and by NOVA Medical School Ethics Committee. All participants provided informed consent, and the study was performed according to the principles established by the Declaration of Helsinki.

Statistical Analysis

Participants (N = 1,645) were divided in two groups: group 1 (n = 1,059) consisted of participants meeting the OA diagnostic criteria; and group 2 (n = 586) consisted of participants without OA diagnosis or others rheumatic diseases. There were no missing data except for physical activity (n = 485).

Descriptive analysis was used to describe the main characteristics of the sample, using frequencies (absolute and relative) or means and SDs, depending on the type of the variable. The comparison of groups defined by the presence/absence of OA (group 1: with OA and group 2: without OA) was performed using independent samples t-test for continuous variables and Chi-square test for categorical variables. Univariate logistic regression models, with presence of OA as the outcome, were performed to identify a set of factors that could predict OA presence, including sociodemographic characteristics, comorbidities, functional status, physical activity, depression, and anxiety. The final multivariable model with backward elimination included variables with p-values <0.05. Odds ratios (ORs) and 95% confidence intervals were used to assess the results. All statistical analyses were performed using Statistical Package for the Social Sciences (SPSS, version 24, IBM), and α = 0.05 was used to determine significance level.

RESULTS

Characteristics of the Sample

The sample comprised 1,645 participants. The mean age of the sample was 65.3 years (SD = 9.3) and 63.2% (n = 1,040) were women. Most of the participants were married (n = 1097, 66.7%) and had 4 years of education (n = 847, 54.5%). Regarding work status, the majority were retired (n = 1050, 63.8%). With respect to number of self-reported chronic non-communicable diseases, most participants reported 0–2 (n = 720, 43.8%) and 3–4 (n = 540, 32.8%) chronic diseases. Hypertension (n = 857, 52.1%) and high cholesterol (n = 805, 48.9%) were the most frequently reported diseases. Among rheumatic diseases, osteoporosis was the most frequently self-reported disease (n = 190, 11.6%). With respect to functional status, the mean score of HAQ-DI for the total sample was 0.55 (SD = 0.65) out of 3, indicating low levels of limitations. The majority of the sample met the ≥150 min of physical exercises per week (n = 306; 63.1%). Depressive symptoms were found in 10.6% (n = 174) and anxiety was found in 13.8% (n = 227) of the total sample.

Sample consisted of 1,059 adults with OA diagnosis (64.4%) and 586 without OA diagnosis (35.6%). Among people with OA, 12.5% (n = 132) were classified as having hip OA, 44.7% (n = 473) hand OA, and 68.6% knee OA (n = 726). Among persons with an OA diagnosis, 36.6% (n = 388) reported the presence of other rheumatic diseases. In this sample, the additional rheumatic diseases most commonly reported were osteoporosis (n = 190, 11.6%) and rheumatoid arthritis (n = 91, 5.5%).

Statistically significant differences were found between groups (with and without OA) in all sociodemographic variables (i.e., age, gender, marital status, education, and work status), non-communicable diseases, functional status, physical activity, depression, and anxiety (**Table 1**). Participants with OA were older (mean = 67.1, SD = 9.1) than participants without OA (mean = 62.1, SD = 8.9). The proportion of women with OA (n = 774, 73.1%) was higher than among persons without OA (n = 266; 45.4%). More participants with OA were

TABLE 1 | Sociodemographic and health description of the sample and comparison of groups [with and without osteoarthritis (OA) diagnosis].

	Total (n = 1,645)	With OA (n = 1,059)	Without OA (n = 586)	p
	n (%)	n (%)	n (%)	
Age (years)[a]	65.3 (9.3)	67.1 (9.1)	62.1 (8.9)	<0.001
Gender				
Male	605 (36.8)	285 (26.9)	320 (54.6)	<0.001
Female	1,040 (63.2)	774 (73.1)	266 (45.4)	
Marital status				
Without partner	214 (13.0)	124 (11.7)	90 (15.4)	<0.001
Married	1,097 (66.7)	666 (63.5)	425 (72.5)	
Widower	334 (20.3)	263 (24.8)	71 (12.1)	
Education				
0–3 years	242 (14.7)	194 (18.3)	48 (8.2)	<0.001
4 years	847 (54.5)	580 (54.8)	267 (45.6)	
5–9 years	274 (16.7)	140 (13.2)	134 (22.9)	
10+ years	282 (17.1)	145 (13.7)	137 (23.4)	
Work status				
Full time employed	295 (17.9)	119 (11.2)	176 (30.0)	<0.001
Partial time employed	52 (3.2)	33 (3.1)	19 (3.2)	
Without labor activity	248 (15.1)	158 (14.9)	90 (15.4)	
Retired	1,050 (63.8)	749 (70.9)	301 (51.4)	
Non-communicable diseases				
0–2	720 (43.8)	355 (33.5)	365 (62.3)	<0.001
3–4	540 (32.8)	367 (34.7)	173 (29.5)	
5 or +	385 (23.4)	337 (31.8)	48 (8.2)	
Physical disability[a] **(HAQ)**	0.55 (0.65)	0.70 (0.67)	0.28 (0.53)	<0.001
Physical activity per week (n = 485)				
<150 min	179 (36.9)	115 (43.2)	64 (29.2)	0.001
≥150 min	306 (63.1)	151 (56.8)	155 (70.8)	
Depressive symptoms				
Present	174 (10.6)	143 (13.5)	31 (5.3)	<0.001
Non-present	1,471 (89.4)	916 (86.5)	555 (94.7)	
Anxiety symptoms				
Present	227 (13.8)	172 (16.2)	55 (9.4)	<0.001
Non-present	1,418 (86.2)	887 (83.8)	531 (90.6)	

[a]*Mean (SD).*

married (n = 666, 63.5%), in comparison to persons without OA (n = 425, 72.5%). Widowers were the second most common category represented, 263 (24.8%) in participants with OA compared to 71 (12.1%) in those without OA. Regarding work status, the majority of participants in both groups were retired (persons with OA: n = 749, 70.7%; persons without OA: n = 301, 51.4%). Among participants with OA, the second most frequent category was "without labor activity" (n = 158, 14.9%), whereas for persons without OA, the second most common category was "full time employed" (n = 176, 30.0%). Most persons with OA reported presence 3–4 non-communicable diseases (n = 367, 34.7%), compared to 0–2 non-communicable diseases (n = 365, 62.3%) among persons without OA. Individuals with OA were significantly less active (56.8% met the recommendation of ≥150 min of physical activity per week) than those without OA (70.8% met the recommendation of ≥150 min of physical activity per week). With respect to functional status, participants with OA showed significantly higher levels of functional limitations (mean = 0.70, SD = 0.67) than persons without OA (mean = 0.28, SD = 0.58). Percentage of depressive symptoms was also higher among individuals with OA (n = 143, 13.5%) compared to participants without OA (n = 93; 8.7%). Similar results were found for anxiety, persons with OA showed a higher percentage of anxiety symptoms (n = 172, 13.8%) than people without OA (n = 55, 9.4%).

Multivariate Predictors of OA

Using OA as the outcome, unadjusted logistic regression models found that all of the variables shown in **Table 1** were associated with presence of this chronic disease (**Table 2**). The final adjusted model contains only significant variables, and the non-significant variables were excluded, one by one, from the model. The variables were removed in the following sequence: marital status ($p = 0.387$), work status ($p = 0.216$), depression ($p = 0.512$), and anxiety ($p = 0.066$). In the final adjusted model, age, gender, number of comorbidities, physical disability, and physical activity remained statistically significant and the model explained 32% of the variance. People who were older (OR = 1.048, $p < 0.001$) and female (OR = 3.192, $p < 0.001$) were more likely to have OA. People with more than five comorbidities were more likely to report OA than people with 0–2 comorbidities (OR = 4.484, $p < 0.001$). Functional disability was also associated with OA. Specifically, persons with higher levels functional disability were more likely to report OA than those with lower levels of disability

TABLE 2 | Associations of potential explanatory variables with osteoarthritis (OA).

			Unadjusted			Adjusted		
	N	**Cases of OA**	**Odds ratio (OR)**	**95% confidence intervals (CI 95%)**	***p***	**OR**	**CI 95%**	***p***
Age	1,645	67.1 (9.1)	1.063	1.051–1.076	<0.001	1.048	1.021–1.076	<0.001
Gender					<0.001			<0.001
Male	605	285 (26.9%)	1	–	–	1	–	–
Female	1,040	774 (73.1%)	3.269	2.643–4.038	<0.001	3.192	2.040–4.994	<0.001
Marital status					<0.001	–	–	–
Without partner	214	124 (11.7%)	1	–	–			
Married	1,097	672 (63.5%)	1.148	0.852–1.545	0.364			
Widower	334	263 (24.8%)	2.689	1.844–3.921	<0.001			
Education					<0.001			0.037
≥10 years	282	145 (13.7%)	1	–	–	1	–	–
5–9 years	274	140 (13.2%)	0.975	0.708–1.377	0.939	0.583	0.321–1.059	0.076
4 years	847	580 (54.8%)	2.052	1.559–2.702	<0.001	1.182	0.715–1.956	0.515
0–3 years	242	194 (18.3%)	3.819	2.578–5.656	<0.001	0.503	0.192–1.313	0.160
Work status					<0.001	–	–	–
Full time employed	295	119 (11.2%)	1	–	–			
Partial time employed	52	33 (3.1%)	2.569	1.395–4.730	0.002			
Without labor activity	248	158 (14.9%)	2.596	1.833–3.677	<0.001			
Retired	1,050	749 (70.9%)	3.814	2.814–4.813	<0.001			
Comorbidities					<0.001			<0.001
0–2	720	355 (33.5%)	1	–	–	1	–	–
3–4	540	367 (34.7%)	2.181	1.729–2.752	<0.001	2.850	1.801–4.511	<0.001
5 or more	385	337 (31.8%)	7.219	5.160–10.099	<0.001	4.484	2.348–8.561	<0.001
Physical disability (HAQ)	1,645	0.70 (0.67)[a]	3.871	3.081–4.865	<0.001	1.926	1.186–3.126	<0.001
Physical activity per week					0.002			0.027
≥150 min	306	151 (56.8%)	1	–	–	1	–	–
<150 min	179	115 (43.2%)	1.844	1.263–2.694	0.002	1.630	1.056–2.516	0.027
Depression					<0.001	–	–	–
No	1,471	916 (86.5%)	1	–	–			
Yes	174	143 (13.5%)	2.795	1.869–4.179	<0.001			
Anxiety					<0.001	–	–	–
No	1,418	887 (83.8%)	1	–	–			
Yes	227	143 (16.2%)	1.872	1.357–2.584	<0.001			

[a]*Mean (SD).*

(OR = 1.926, $p < 0.001$). Physical activity was also associated with OA persons; people with lower levels of physical activity were more likely to report OA than those with higher levels of physical activity (OR = 1.630, $p = 0.027$).

DISCUSSION

The results from this study showed a positive association between older age, female gender, comorbidities (higher number of non-communicable diseases), disability, physical activity level, and presence of OA; findings that are consistent with previous results reported in the literature on OA. According to *A National Public Health Agenda for Osteoarthritis* (24), OA prevalence increases substantially at age 45. Also, the *World Health Organization World Report on Ageing and Health* (25) showed a higher rate of knee and hip OA in people above 65 years and in females. Women reported higher percentage of OA than men; these results highlight the importance of considering gender differences among people with OA. We developed an exploratory analysis of this same sample, and the results showed that women had lower levels of education, more non-communicable diseases, higher levels of disability, and depressive and anxiety symptoms than men. These results indicate that interventions that seek to improve function among persons with OA should consider the profile of the largely female population of persons with OA to maximize adherence to and impact of interventions in this population.

Other sociodemographic variables tested: marital status, and work status, lost their significance in the adjusted model, probably because people with OA and with low levels of education are mostly women (n = 554, 52.3%) and had higher levels of physical activity (n = 73, 15.1%), furthermore, retired people was the oldest group (mean age = 70.9, SD = 7.4) and had the highest level of disability (mean = 0.77, SD = 0.69). Prior studies have analyzed the impact of sociodemographic characteristics in OA, for example, Cleveland et al. (26) explored the relationship between functional status/disability and sociodemographic status in people with OA and found that persons with lower education, non-homeowners, or lower income were more likely to have increased disability.

Persons with OA seem to have a higher number of others non-communicable diseases. This result is consistent with a systematic review on multimorbidity which showed that depression, hypertension, diabetes, arthritis, asthma, and OA were prone to be comorbid with other conditions (7).

We found a positive relationship between physical disability and OA. The mean disability score, in this study among persons with OA, was 0.70, higher than the mean score that was reported for a general population (0.49) (19), but very similar to the mean reported in a population with OA (0.80) (19). The same authors have stated referred that HAQ-DI scores of 0–1 are generally considered to represent mild to moderate difficulty functioning. According to the WHO (27), among people with OA, 80% had mobility disability and 25% were unable to perform activities of daily living independently. On the one hand, OA appears to have a high impact in disability; on the other hand, low levels of functioning promote sedentary behavior which is a risk factor for OA as well as for weight gain, general de-conditioning, and possibly the onset of other chronic conditions.

Our results showed that 56.8% of people with OA met the physical activity recommendations. This percentage is lower than the level of physical activity performed by people without OA, suggesting that the presence of OA can be a barrier to physical activity participation. The *National Food, Nutrition and Physical Activity Survey* Report (28) found low levels of physical activity in the general Portuguese population. In this national report, only 36% of young adults (15–21 years), 27% of adults, and 22% of older adults (65–84 years) met the actual recommendations for physical activity. This issue is particularly important for adults with OA, because this group is physically inactive and at risk of disability due to joint limitations (4). Several studies confirm the importance of physical activity for arthritis and have shown that increased physical activity is associated with improved disability in people with arthritis and in OA symptomatology relief (4, 25, 29). International organizations recognize regular physical activity as one of the most important non-pharmacological therapies for OA (30–32).

One study that explored the physical activity levels in knee OA patients concluded that only 41% of patients reported sufficient levels of physical activity (33). Badley and Ansari (10) concluded that physical inactivity accounted for an estimated 21% of disability attributed to arthritis and randomized clinical trials demonstrated that structured physical activity can reduce the risk of developing disability in people with OA (34).

In this study, symptoms of depressive and anxiety symptoms were higher in people with OA than in people without OA. However, in the adjusted model, these two variables ceased to be significant. According to Eurostats (35), in 2014, 7.1% of the population of EU-28 reported having chronic depression. Portugal with 11.9% was top ranked in the share of total population reporting chronic depression. Stubbs et al. (9) concluded that in Europe there is a prevalence of 19.9% of depressive symptoms in people with OA, lower than the prevalence found in studies conducted in USA (23.1%). Few studies have analyzed the symptoms of anxiety among OA patients, as most of the studies focused in the rheumatic disease in general [e.g., Ref. (36)].

Despite the results, study of psychological morbidity continued among people with OA remains important because it can affect the diagnosis and the adherence to treatment (36–38). Depressive symptoms appear to act as a potential barrier to physical activity and social participation for people with OA (9).

This study has some limitations, namely, the cross-sectional nature of the data; and the missing information about the time of duration of OA and pain, which could help us to understand the relationship between specific variables like physical activity and disability. Physical activity was assessed in a reduced number of participants which could limit the interpretation of the results. Those without a physical activity assessment could be more inactive than those who filled all the evaluation. The prevalence of OA is overestimated in this sample when compared with the Portuguese population (50+ years). This aspect is related to the general objectives of EpiReumaPt that focus on people with rheumatic diseases and with the criteria for sample selection in this study. The amount of variance in OA explained by the model was low (32%), which limits the interpretation of the results. The variance explained could be improved by the inclusion of other biological variables, such as body mass index and muscle strength. Other limitations of the EpiReumaPt initiative were reported by Branco et al. (12). The main strengths of the study are first the large national population-based sample and second, the fact that the OA diagnosis was made by rheumatologists who are experts in performing these evaluations. A final strength of the dataset and design is that it enabled a systematize comparison of the characteristics of person with and without OA using a large number of sociodemographic, disease, and functional status variables.

In this paper, we have analyzed older adults (+50) from a population-based study and found that a diagnosis of OA was independently associated with age, female gender, higher number of comorbidities, physical disability, and low levels of physical activity. These results reinforce the need to of the develop multidimensional assessments to design and evaluate effective interventions for this population.

ETHICS STATEMENT

EpiReumaPt was approved by the National Committee for Data Protection and by NOVA Medical School Ethics Committee. All participants provided informed consent, and the study was performed according to the principles established by the Declaration of Helsinki.

AUTHOR CONTRIBUTIONS

ND contributed to the conception, design, analysis, and interpretation of data for the work. She agreed to be accountable for all aspects of the work in ensuring that questions related to the accuracy or integrity of any part of the work are appropriately investigated and resolved. AR, JB, HC, and SH revised the work critically for important intellectual content and approved the final version to be published. CP contributed to the design, analysis, and interpretation of the data for the work; revised the work critically for important intellectual content; and approved the final version to be published.

ACKNOWLEDGMENTS

The EpiReumaPt Study Group would like to acknowledge the invaluable help of Henrique de Barros, MD PhD; João Eurico da Fonseca, MD PhD; José António Pereira da Silva, MD PhD; Francisco George, MD; Rui André, MD; Luís Maurício, MD; Faculdade de Medicina da Universidade de Coimbra, Faculdade de Medicina da Universidade de Lisboa, Faculdade de Medicina da Universidade do Porto, Liga Portuguesa Contra as Doenças Reumáticas, Associações de Doentes com Doença Reumática, Administrações Regionais de Saúde (Norte, Centro, Lisboa e Vale do Tejo, Alentejo e Algarve), Governo Regional da Madeira, Governo Regional dos Açores, Associação Nacional de Freguesias, Associação Nacional dos Municípios Portugueses, Câmara Municipal de Lisboa.

FUNDING

EpiReumaPt was endorsed by the Alto *Patrocínio da Presidência da República* and was supported by a Grant from Directorate-General of Health. The project was also sponsored by Fundação Calouste Gulbenkian, Fundação Champalimaud, Fundação AstraZeneca, Abbvie, Merck Sharp & Dohme, Pfizer, Roche, Servier, Bial, D3A Medical Systems, Happybrands, *Centro de Medicina Laboratorial Germano de Sousa, Clínica Médica da Praia da Vitória, CAL-Clínica, Galp Energia, Açoreana Seguros*, and individual support of rheumatologists. The work was supported by a doctoral fellowship of the Portuguese Foundation for Science and Technology (Reference: SFRH/BD/111533/2015).

REFERENCES

1. Van der Pas S, Castell MV, Cooper C, Denkinger M, Dennison EM, Edwards MH, et al. European project on osteoarthritis: design of a six-cohort study on the personal and societal burden of osteoarthritis in an older European population. *BMC Musculoskelet Disord* (2013) 14:1–11. doi:10.1186/1471-2474-14-138
2. Martin JA, Buckwalter JA. Aging, articular cartilage chondrocyte senescence and osteoarthritis. *Biogerontology* (2002) 3(5):257–64. doi:10.1023/A:1020185404126
3. Woolf AD, Pfleger B. Burden of major musculoskeletal conditions. *Bull World Health Organ* (2003) 81(9):646–56.
4. Song J, Gilbert AL, Chang RW, Pellegrini CA, Ehrlich-Jones LS, Lee J. Do inactive older adults who increase physical activity experience less disability evidence from the osteoarthritis initiative. *Optom Vis Sci* (2017) 94(1):26–32. doi:10.1097/RHU.0000000000000473
5. World Health Organization. *Global Health Estimates 2013: Deaths by Cause, Age, Sex and Regional Grouping 2000–2012*. Geneva: World Health Organization (2013).
6. Louati K. An overview of osteoarthritis in 2016. *Rev Infirm* (2017) 223:16–8. doi:10.1016/j.revinf.2016.06.002
7. Xu X, Mishra GD, Jones M. Evidence on multimorbidity from definition to intervention: an overview of systematic reviews. *Ageing Res Rev* (2017) 37:53–68. doi:10.1016/j.arr.2017.05.003
8. Ramprasad KS, Veeranna HD, Adarsha HM. Prevalence of mood variances in patients with osteoarthritis of knee. *Scholars J Appl Med Sci* (2014) 2(3C):1095–7.
9. Stubbs B, Aluko Y, Myint PK, Smith TO. Prevalence of depressive symptoms and anxiety in osteoarthritis: a systematic review and meta-analysis. *Age Ageing* (2016) 45(2):228–35. doi:10.1093/ageing/afw001
10. Badley EM, Ansari H. Arthritis and arthritis-attributable activity limitations in the United States and Canada: a cross-border comparison. *Arthritis Care Res (Hoboken)* (2010) 62:308–15. doi:10.1002/acr.20100
11. Hutton I, Gambie G, McLean G, Butcher H, Gow P, Dalbeth N. What is associated with being active in arthritis? Analysis from the obstacles to action study. *Int Med J* (2010) 40:512–20. doi:10.1111/j.1445-5994.2009.01989.x
12. Branco J, Rodrigues AM, Gouveia N, Eusébio M, Ramiro S, Machado PM, et al. Prevalence of rheumatic and musculoskeletal disease and their impact on health-related quality of life, physical function and mental health in Portugal: results from EpiReumaPt – a national health survey. *RMD Open* (2016) 2(1):e000166. doi:10.1136/rmdopen-2015-000166
13. Gouveia N, Rodrigues AM, Ramiro S, Machado P, Costas LP, Mourão AF, et al. EpiReumaPt: how to perform a national population based study – a practical guide. *Acta Reumatol Port* (2015) 40:128–36.
14. Rodrigues AM, Gouveia N, da Costa LP, Eusébio M, Ramiro S, Machado P, et al. EpiReumaPt – the study of Rheumatic and musculoskeletal disease in Portugal: a detailed view of the methodology. *Acta Reumatol Ogica Port* (2015) 40(2):110–24.

15. Altman R, Alarcon G, Appelrouth D, Bloch D, Borenstein D, Brandt K, et al. The American-College-of-Rheumatology criteria for the classification and reporting of osteoarthritis of the Hip. *Arthritis Rheum* (1991) 34(5):505–14. doi:10.1002/art.1780340502
16. Altman R, Alarcon G, Appelrouth D, Bloch D, Borenstein D, Brandt K, et al. The American-College-of-Rheumatology criteria for the classification and reporting of osteoarthritis of the hand. *Arthritis Rheum* (1990) 33(11):1601–10. doi:10.1002/art.1780331101
17. Altman R, Asch E, Bloch D, Bole G, Borenstein D, Brandt K, et al. Development of criteria for the classification and reporting of osteoarthritis – classification of osteoarthritis of the knee. *Arthritis Rheum* (1986) 29(8):1039–49. doi:10.1002/art.1780290816
18. Fries JF, Spitz P, Kraines RG, Holman HR. Measurement of patient outcomes in arthritis. *Arthritis Rheum* (1980) 23:137–45. doi:10.1002/art.1780230202
19. Bruce B, Fries JF. The Stanford Health Assessment Questionnaire: dimensions and practical applications. *Health Qual Life Outcomes* (2003) 1:20. doi:10.1186/1477-7525-1-20
20. Cuperus N, Vlieland TPMV, Mahler EAM, Kersten CC, Hoogeboom TJ, Ende CHM. The clinical burden of generalized osteoarthritis represented by self-reported health-related quality of life and activity limitations: a cross-sectional study. *Rheumatol Int* (2015) 35:871–7. doi:10.1007/s00296-014-3149-1
21. World Health Organization. *Global Recommendations on Physical Activity for Health*. Switzerland: World Health Organization (2010).
22. Pais-Ribeiro J, Silva I, Ferreira T, Martins A, Meneses R, Baltar M. Validation study of a Portuguese version of the hospital anxiety and depression scale. *Psychol Health Med* (2007) 12(2):225–35; quiz 235–227. doi:10.1080/13548500500524088
23. Zigmond AS, Snaith RP. The hospital anxiety and depression scale. *Acta Psychiatr Scand* (1983) 67(6):361–70. doi:10.1111/j.1600-0447.1983.tb09716.x
24. Centers for Disease Control and Prevention and Arthritis Foundation. *The National Public Health Agenda for Osteoarthritis*. (2010). Available from: www.cdc.gov/arthritis/docs/OAAgenda.pdf
25. Briggs AM, Cross MJ, Hoy DG, Sanchez-Riera L, Blyth FM, Woolf AD, et al. Musculoskeletal health conditions represent a global threat to healthy aging: a report for the 2015 World Health Organization world report on ageing and health. *Gerontologist* (2016) 56(S2):S243–55. doi:10.1093/geront/gnw002
26. Cleveland RJ, Renner JB, Jordan JM, Callahan LF. Progression of disability is associated with socioeconomic measures in the Johnston country osteoarthritis project. *Osteoarthritis Cartilage* (2014) 22:S57–489. doi:10.1016/j.joca.2014.02.412
27. World Health Organization. *Burden of the Musculoskeletal Conditions at the Start of the New Millennium; Report of a WHO Scientific Group*. Geneva: World Health Organization (2003). Technical Report Series, no 919.
28. Lopes C, Torres D, Oliveira A, Severo M, Alancão V, Guiomar S, et al. *The National Food, Nutrition and Physical Activity Survey*. (2017). Available from: https://ian-af.up.pt/sites/default/files/IAN-AF_%20Relatório%20Resultados_v1.5_0.pdf
29. Zhang W, Nuki G, Moskowitz RW, Abramson S, Altman RD, Arden NK, et al. OARSI recommendations for the management of hip and knee osteoarthritis. *Osteoarthritis Cartilage* (2010) 18(4):476–99. doi:10.1016/j.joca.2010.01.013
30. Hochberg MC, Altman RD, April KT, Benkhalti M, Guyatt G, McGowan J, et al. American College of Rheumatology. American College of Rheumatology 2012 recommendations for the use of nonpharmacologic and pharmacologic therapies in osteoarthritis of the hand, hip, and knee. *Arthritis Care Res* (2012) 64:465–74. doi:10.1002/acr.21596
31. McAlindon TE, Bannuru RR, Sullivan MC, Arden NK, Berenbaum F, Bierma-Zeinstra SM, et al. OARSI guidelines for the non-surgical management of knee osteoarthritis. *Osteoarthritis Cartilage* (2014) 22:363–88. doi:10.1016/j.joca.2014.01.003
32. Fernandes L, Hagen KB, Bijlsma JW, Andreassen O, Christensen P, Conaghan PG, et al. EULAR recommendations for the non-pharmacological core management of hip and knee osteoarthritis. *Ann Rheum Dis* (2013) 72:1125–35. doi:10.1136/annrheumdis-2012-202745
33. Wallis JA, Webster KE, Levinger P, Taylor NF. What proportion of people with hip and knee osteoarthritis meet physical activity guidelines? A systematic review and meta-analysis. *Osteoarthritis Cartilage* (2013) 21(11):1648–59. doi:10.1016/j.joca.2013.08.003
34. Penninx BW, Messier SP, Rejeski WJ, Wlliamsor JD, DiBari M, Cavazzini C, et al. Physical exercise and prevention of disability in activities of daily living in older persons with osteoarthritis. *Arch Intern Med* (2001) 161(19):2309–16. doi:10.1001/archinte.161.19.2309
35. Eurostats. *Mental Health and Related Issues Statistics*. (2017). Available from: http://ec.europa.eu/eurostat/statistics-explained/index.php/Mental_health_and_related_issues_statistics#Publications
36. Murphy LB, Sacks JJ, Brady TJ, Hootman JM, Chapman DP. Anxiety and depression among US adults with arthritis: prevalence and correlates. *Arthritis Care Res* (2012) 64(7):968–76. doi:10.1002/acr.21685
37. Yohannes AM, Baldwin RC. Medical co-morbidities in late-life depression. *Psychiatric Times* (2008) 25:52–5.
38. Yohannes AM, Caton S. Management of depression in older people with osteoarthritis: a systematic review. *Aging Ment Health* (2010) 14(4):637–51. doi:10.1080/13607860903483094

8

The Quadruple Helix-Based Innovation Model of Reference Sites for Active and Healthy Ageing in Europe: The Ageing@Coimbra Case Study

João O. Malva[1,2], Alda Amado[1,3], Alexandra Rodrigues[1,4], Anabela Mota-Pinto[1,5,6], Ana F. Cardoso[1,7], Ana M. Teixeira[1,8], Ana Todo-Bom[1,6,9], António Devesa[1,10], António F. Ambrósio[1,2], António L. Cunha[1,11], Bárbara Gomes[1,2,12], Carina Dantas[1,13], Cidalina Abreu[1,7], Isabel Santana[1,9,14], Jean Bousquet[15], João Apóstolo[1,7], Lúcia Santos[1,16], Lúcio Meneses de Almeida[1,17], Maddalena Illario[18], Rafaela Veríssimo[19], Vitor Rodrigues[1,5] and Manuel T. Veríssimo[1,2,9]*

[1] Ageing@Coimbra, EIP on AHA Reference Site, Coimbra, Portugal, [2] Faculty of Medicine, Coimbra Institute for Clinical and Biomedical Research (iCBR), and CNC.IBILI, University of Coimbra, Coimbra, Portugal, [3] Instituto de Segurança Social, Centro Distrital de Coimbra, Coimbra, Portugal, [4] Comissão de Coordenação e Desenvolvimento Regional do Centro, Coimbra, Portugal, [5] Centre of Investigation in Environment, Genetics and Oncobiology (CIMAGO), Faculty of Medicine, University of Coimbra, Coimbra, Portugal, [6] Faculty of Medicine, General Pathology Institute, University of Coimbra, Coimbra, Portugal, [7] Centre for Evidence Based Practice, Health Sciences Research Unit: Nursing (UICISA: E), Nursing School of Coimbra, Coimbra, Portugal, [8] Research Center for Sport and Physical Activity, Faculty of Sport Sciences and Physical Education, University of Coimbra, Coimbra, Portugal, [9] University of Coimbra Hospital, CHUC, Coimbra, Portugal, [10] Municipality of Coimbra, Coimbra, Portugal, [11] Pedro Nunes Institute, Laboratory of Automatics and Systems, Coimbra, Portugal, [12] King's College London, Cicely Saunders Institute of Palliative Care, Policy and Rehabilitation, London, United Kingdom, [13] Caritas Coimbra, Coimbra, Portugal, [14] Center for Neuroscience and Cell Biology (CNC), University of Coimbra, Coimbra, Portugal, [15] Contre les Maladies Chroniques pour un Vleilissement Active (MACVIA) en France en EIP on AHA Reference Site, Montpellier, France, [16] Portuguese Pharmaceutical Society – Center Region Branch, Coimbra, Portugal, [17] Regional Health Authority, ARS Centro, Coimbra, Portugal, [18] Division for Health Innovation, Campania Region and Federico II University Hospital Naples (R&D and DISMET), Naples, Italy, [19] Centro Hospitalar de Gaia/Espinho, Gaia, Portugal

Edited by:
Helena Canhao, Unidade EpiDoC, Epidemiologia de doenças crônicas, Portugal

Reviewed by:
Mario Ulises Pérez-Zepeda, Instituto Nacional de Geriatría, Mexico
Jose Luiz Telles, Escola Nacional de Saúde Pública, Brazil

***Correspondence:**
João O. Malva
jomalva@fmed.uc.pt

Challenges posed by demographic changes and population aging are key priorities for the Horizon 2020 Program of the European Commission. Aligned with the vision of the European Innovation Partnership on Active and Healthy Ageing (EIP on AHA), the development, exchange, and large-scale adoption of innovative good practices is a key element of the responses required to ensure all European citizens remain as active and healthy as possible as they age. Urged by the need of developing scalable disruptive innovation across Europe, the European Commission and the EIP on AHA created the Reference Sites; local coalition of partners that develop good practices to support AHA. Ageing@Coimbra is an example of how this can be achieved at a regional level. The consortium comprises over 70 institutions that develop innovative practices to support AHA in Portugal. Ageing@Coimbra partners support a regional network of stakeholders that build a holistic ecosystem in health and social care, taking into consideration the specificities of the territories, living environments and cultural resources (2,243,934 inhabitants, 530,423 aged 65 or plus live in the Centre Region of Portugal). Good practices in reducing the burden of brain diseases that affect cognition and memory impairment in older people and tackling social isolation in urban and rural areas are among the top priorities of Ageing@Coimbra. Profiting from the collaborative work of academia, business companies, civil society, and authorities, the quadruple helix of Ageing@Coimbra supports: early diagnosis of frailty and disease; care and cure; and active, assisted, and independent living. This paper describes, as a Community Case Study, the creation of a Reference Site of the EIP on AHA, Ageing@Coimbra, and its impact in Portugal. This Reference Site can motivate other regions to develop innovative formulas to federate stakeholders and networks, building consortia at regional level. This growing movement, across Europe, is inspired by the quadruple helix concept and by the replication of innovative good practices; creating new Reference Sites for the benefit of Citizens.

Keywords: ageing (aging), European commission, innovation, active and healthy aging, reference sites

INTRODUCTION

Europe faces the global challenge of population aging with strong impact in the quality of life of individuals and families, society cohesion, health, and economic resources of citizens and member states. The percentage of people aged 65 or over in the population is expected to grow from 18.4% in 2013 to 28.4% in 2060 for the average of European countries (1). The growth will be particularly evident in the oldest old (aged 80 or over), who will increase from 5.1% in 2013 to 11.8% in 2060. European projections of old-age dependency ratios (people aged 65 or over versus people aged 15–64) reveal that the current ratio of 1 person aged 65 or over per 4 working-age people will rise to a ratio of 1 person aged 65 or over to 2 working-age people in 2060 (1). This poses huge challenges for sustaining retirement and care in later life.

Portugal stands in a particular challenging position in the overall EU28 scenario. The Portuguese population is aging rapidly with an Ageing Index (people aged 65 or over per 100 people aged less than 15) of 143.9 in 2015 compared to 27 in 1960.[1] The percentage of people aged 80 years or over was 5.4% in 2013 and it is expected to grow to 16.1% in 2060, reaching the highest value of all EU28 countries (1).

Within Portugal, the population living in the Centre Region is particularly old due to the increase in life expectancy, migration of young adults and decrease in birth rate. Within the Centre Region, some areas are already facing the demographic scenarios expected for the European landscape in 2060, e.g., municipalities with Ageing Index above 700.[2]

Taking together, the demographic landscape of Europe, with a particularly and striking case in Portugal, urges the need of defining new strategies and implementing actions to deliver innovative and disruptive solutions. These solutions are expected to have impact at the individual, family, labor, societal, and economic dimensions to support individual health and well-being, at all ages, and deliver solutions to support health and social care sustainability. As we will elaborate bellow, the EIP on AHA movement, and the particular case of Ageing@Coimbra (as a Community Case Study), may be inspiring for the required change management processes, delivering solutions for the challenges of aging and opening new opportunities for economic growth.

BACKGROUND AND RATIONALE

The European Innovation Partnership on Active and Healthy Ageing

The EIP on AHA[3] is a coalition of European partners promoted by the European Commission to develop, implement, and replicate at large-scale innovative good practices to support AHA of European citizens.

The EIP on AHA grew from recognition that the quality of life of older people is strongly affected by life style habits across the life cycle in all ages. Many older people suffer from multiple chronic conditions that demand continuous support by medical and social care providers and limit functional independence. Ultimately, poor health in later life strongly impacts on health and economic resources, human suffering, human dignity of individuals, and families (2).

The EIP on AHA fosters collaborative work of European partners to support three main strategic pillars of AHA: (1) prevention, screening, and early diagnosis; (2) care and cure; (3) independent living and active aging. EIP on AHA partners are organized in six action groups: A1, adherence to prescription and medical plans; A2, personalized health management and prevention of falls; A3, lifespan health promotion and prevention of age-related frailty and disease; B3, replicating and tutoring integrated care for chronic diseases; C2, development of interoperable independent living solutions; D4, innovation for age-friendly buildings, cities and environments.

The main goal is to achieve a triple win for Europe: (1) Health and quality of life of European citizens; (2) Sustainable and efficient care systems; and (3) Growth and expansion of EU industry.

EIP on AHA is a wide interdisciplinary and transdisciplinary network that seeks innovative collaborative models, removing silos and developing citizen-centered processes. EIP on AHA

[1] http://www.pordata.pt/ (Accessed: April 24, 2018).

[2] https://www.ine.pt/ (Accessed: April 24, 2018).

[3] https://ec.europa.eu/eip/ageing/home_en (Accessed: April 24, 2018).

partners joint academia, health, and social care providers, citizens and patient associations and several other stakeholder groups with innovators, entrepreneurs, and business partners. The aim is to deliver knowledge and user-based competence into innovative good practices, products, and services. Only disruptive innovation and knowledge-based added value will deliver efficient meaningful large-scale interventions to face the societal challenges, opening, at the same time, new opportunities for entrepreneurs, business activity, and job creation (3, 4).

The Reference Sites Collaborative Network

Reference Sites have been defined by the EIP on AHA as "inspirational ecosystems, delivering creative and workable solutions that improve the lives and health of older people."[4] Reference Sites effort is to foster and create innovative solutions and scale-up and replicate these solutions across Europe.

Reference Sites include regions, cities, integrated hospitals, or care organizations that focus on innovative and holistic approaches to support AHA. Reference Sites show diverse levels of impact and maturity toward the goal standard of regional ecosystems aligning actors across the quadruple helix: academia, authorities, business, and civil society. The impact of the activities of Reference Sites provides evidence of innovative components, and indicators are measurable in line with the Monitoring and Assessment Framework of the EIP on AHA (MAFEIP), under the dimensions "Quality of life," "Sustainability of health-care systems," and "Economic growth and jobs."[5]

The first call for Reference Sites by the European Commission resulted in the award of 32 Reference Sites in 2013. The second call led to a total of 74 Reference Sites in 2016. Recently (November, 2017), the Reference Sites launched a non-profit association based in Brussels to promote synergies and collaborative work (e.g., twinning activities)—the Reference Site Collaborative Network (5).

METHODS

The Ageing@Coimbra—Creation of a Bottom-Up Innovative Quadruple Helix-Based Consortium

The Ageing@Coimbra Consortium[6] was formally created in January 2013 as a response of the Centre Region of Portugal to the first call for Reference Sites to develop and implement innovative good practices to support AHA.

Ageing@Coimbra is an informal network of 5 founder and 65 associated partners that build a "quadruple helix", aligning: (1) public institutions (e.g., municipalities, health and social care authorities), (2) academia (e.g., universities and research institutions), (3) industry partners (e.g., business companies, business incubators, and clusters), and (4) civil society organizations (e.g., third age universities, cultural, and civic organizations). The consortium was founded under a leadership initiative of the University of Coimbra, the Municipality of Coimbra, the Regional Health Authority, the University of Coimbra Hospital, and the Pedro Nunes Institute (technology transfer, business incubator and business accelerator affiliated with the University of Coimbra). The Administrative Authority of the Centre Region of Portugal ("Comissão de Coordenação e Desenvolvimento Regional do Centro," CCDRC) has been a major supporter and driver for the success of Ageing@Coimbra, actively engaging in the implementation of activities, international visibility and ownership of responsibility to include AHA in the key priorities of the Smart Specialization Strategy (RIS3) of the Center Region of Portugal. In 2017, CCDRC launched a regional competition to award three cases of good practices in three clusters: Knowledge, Health, and Life.

Ageing@Coimbra was the first EIP on AHA Reference Site in Portugal. The innovative formula and lean governance structure created an inclusive partnership with agility, rapid implementation, and growth potential. Concordantly, other regions in Portugal (e.g., Porto metropolitan area, Algarve) and regions in other European countries (e.g., Asturias in Spain, Lodz in Poland) embraced Ageing@Coimbra example to replicate the model and launched new reference sites in 2016, or they will do so in a future call expected for 2019. The same example has replication potential in other countries in Europe and globally (e.g., Northeast Brazil).

RESULTS

The Ageing@Coimbra, Consortium—Reference Site in Portugal

As an active member of EIP on AHA Action Groups, Ageing@Coimbra participates in the collaborative activities and delivers success cases of projects and good practices.

A1 Action Group: Adherence to Medical Plans

Multimorbidity and the related prescription of multiple drugs are becoming common problems among older people, frequently associated with poor health outcomes, being inadequate and/or poor adherence to medical plans one of the relevant factors that compromise the success of treatments (6). Therefore, in agreement with the overall goals and triple win defined by the EIP on AHA, the A1 Action Group aims to contribute to the improvement of adherence to medical plans and medication at European level. Ageing@Coimbra has been actively involved in this Action Group and, since 2015, is coordinating the work and activities of one of the four strategic objectives agreed for this group's renovated Action Plan, related to the reinforcement of the multidisciplinary and integrated approach to improve adherence to prescription and to tackle inappropriate polypharmacy.

The collaborative work of Ageing@Coimbra in the A1 Action Group resulted in the successful development of the third Health Program Project SIMPATHY (Stimulating Innovative Management of Polypharmacy and Adherence in the Elderly), a project coordinated by the Scottish Government (Grant Agreement 663082)[7] (6–8) (**Figure 1**).

[4]https://ec.europa.eu/eip/ageing/reference-sites_en (Accessed: April 24, 2018).
[5]http://mafeip.eu/ (Accessed: April 24, 2018).
[6]www.ageingcoimbra.pt/en/ (Accessed: April 24, 2018).

[7]www.simpathy.eu (Accessed: April 24, 2018).

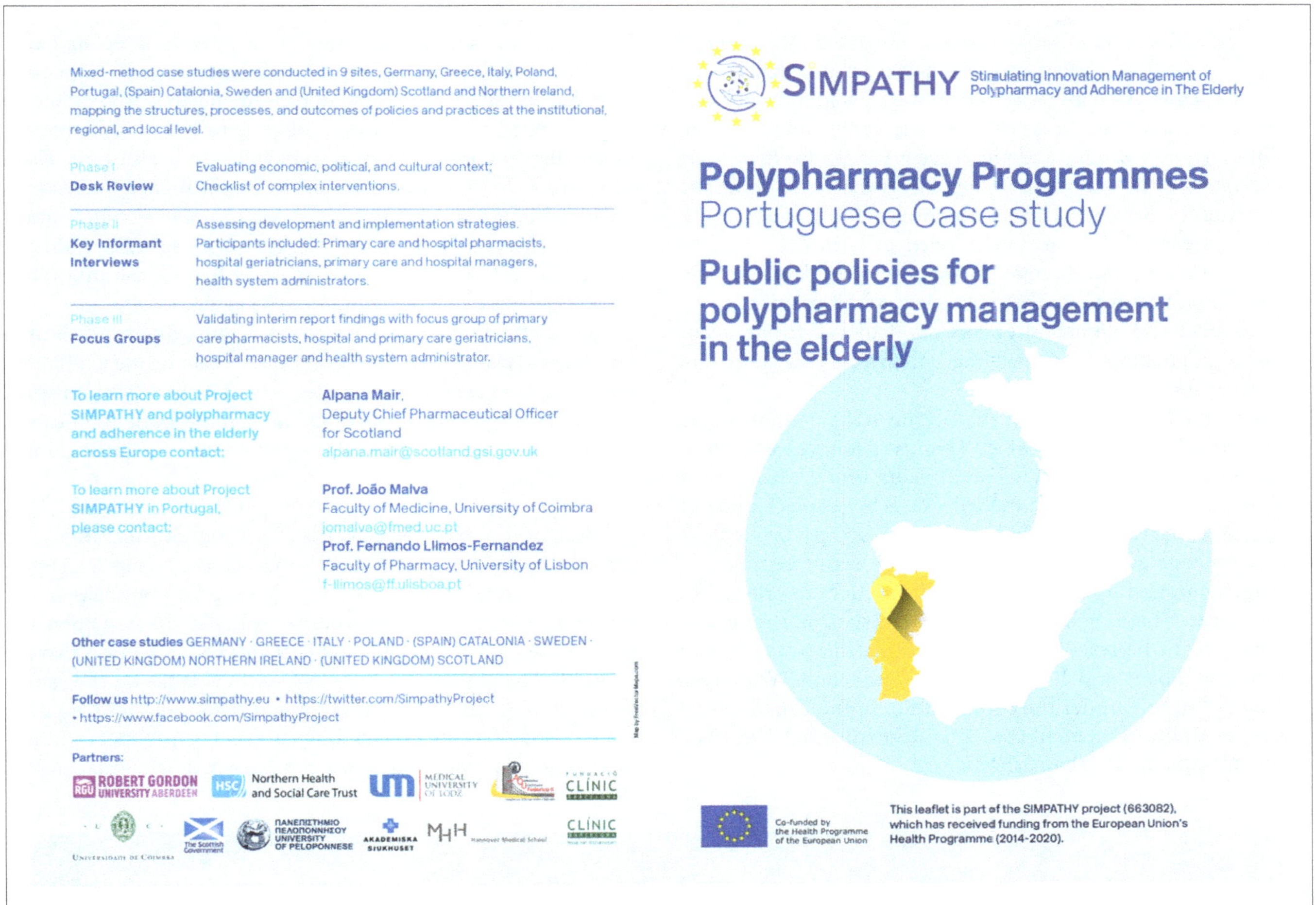

FIGURE 1 | Flyer of SIMPATHY case study in Portugal. SIMPATHY in Portugal recognized the lack of policy guidelines for polypharmacy management across the country.

A2 Action Group: Personalized Health Management and Prevention of Falls

The relevance of the topic addressed in the A2 Action Group is supported by the Joint Declaration of the European Stakeholders Alliance for Active Ageing through Falls Prevention[8] "*falls are a major indicator of increasing frailty and loss of independence and mobility in older people.*" The main objective of the A2 Action Group has been to deliver EU wide evidence-based, validated and operational programs for the prevention, early identification, and minimization of risk and management of falls in order to reduce falls and the personal, system, and societal consequences of fall-related injuries. In order to reach relevant joint achievements and goals four different areas of collaborative work are being developed: (1) implementation of an integrated and person-centered service pathway for fall prevention and management; (2) data collection for evidence-based interventions on falls; (3) awareness, information, and education, to support the training of the workforce; (4) Governance: innovation, sustainability, and scaling-up, including models for exploitation, business analysis, and strategies for falls prevention technologies take up.

The collaborative work of Ageing@Coimbra in the A2 group resulted in joint activities and collaborative work in the Prevention of Falls Network for Dissemination (ProFouND), an EC funded initiative dedicated to the dissemination and implementation of best practices in falls prevention across Europe.[9]

Also, within the scope of the A2 action group, the Project "Good practices to develop physical activity programs at work—FitWork" was developed within the framework of the ERASMUS + SPORT program aimed at developing good practices to implement physical activity programs at work attending to specific risks of workplaces (muscular–skeletal disorders and sedentary workplaces). The project is coordinated by Instituto de Biomecánica de Valencia and more information can be found at.[10]

A3 Action Group: Lifespan Health Promotion and Prevention of Age-Related Frailty and Disease

Reflecting a growing awareness of the need for better care and sustainable and effective health services, the A3 Action Group aims to contribute to AHA with a life-course approach, implementing the shift from reactive disease management to anticipatory care of

[8]http://www.eunaapa.org/wp-content/uploads/2015/09/Joint-Declaration_Sept-2015.pdf (Accessed: April 24, 2018).

[9]http://profound.eu.com (Accessed: April 24, 2018).

[10]www.fitwork.eu (Accessed: April 24, 2018).

functional decline through community-based prevention, early diagnosis, and screening programs, and integrated care management systems. This patient-centered approach involving social and health-care systems is based on innovative solutions that support interactions in the areas of nutrition, frailty and functional decline, cognitive decline and physical activity. It also fosters the development of networks strengthening education and training of the health workforce, citizens empowerment through health and ICT literacy, and advancing knowledge on the determinants of frailty and chronic diseases to support early detection and sustainable interventions. The joint effort of A3 partners is the improvement and alignment of services delivered to the needs of older populations and enabling caregivers' education and empowerment.

To ensure the scalability of the EIP on AHA commitments on frailty, the FOCUS project (*Frailty Management Optimization through EIPAHA Commitments and Utilization of Stakeholders' Input*) was launched (9). This project aims at a critical reduction of frailty burden in Europe by deploying knowledge and tools on frailty diagnosis/screening and management, and by supporting good practices developed in this context. The FOCUS Consortium consists of a multidisciplinary team representing Centre-North (the Netherlands) and South (Spain and Italy), East (Poland), and West (UK, Portugal) Europe, under the coordination of the University of Valencia (Grant Agreement 664367). More information can be found at http://focus-aha.eu/home.

B3 Action Group: Integrated Care

The B3 Action Group main goal is to provide integrated care to older people with chronic conditions through a people-centered approach, foreseeing improvements in quality of life by implementing integrated care programs to reduce unnecessary hospitalization and improve the efficiency of health care. These programs are multidisciplinary, well-coordinated, accessible, anchored in the community and home care settings, and stimulate the interplay between health and social systems, industry, academia, and health-care users in order to establish innovative responses to the challenges imposed by aging.

Within the scope of the B3 Action Group, Ageing@Coimbra and Porto4Health References Sites collaborate as the key Portuguese partners of MACVIA-Fr Reference Site in a Twinning project on the large-scale deployment of a Smartphone Application (App) to monitor and control the symptoms of allergic rhinitis (5, 10) (**Figure 2**).

C2 Action Group: Independent Living Solutions

The objective of the C2 Action Group is to develop interoperable independent living solutions, including guidelines for business models. This should boost the deployment of open and personalized solutions for active and independent living that are supported by global standards and new evidence on the return of investment. The C2 Action Group provides essential input to the creation of a new market for cost-effective products and services that help older people live a more active and independent

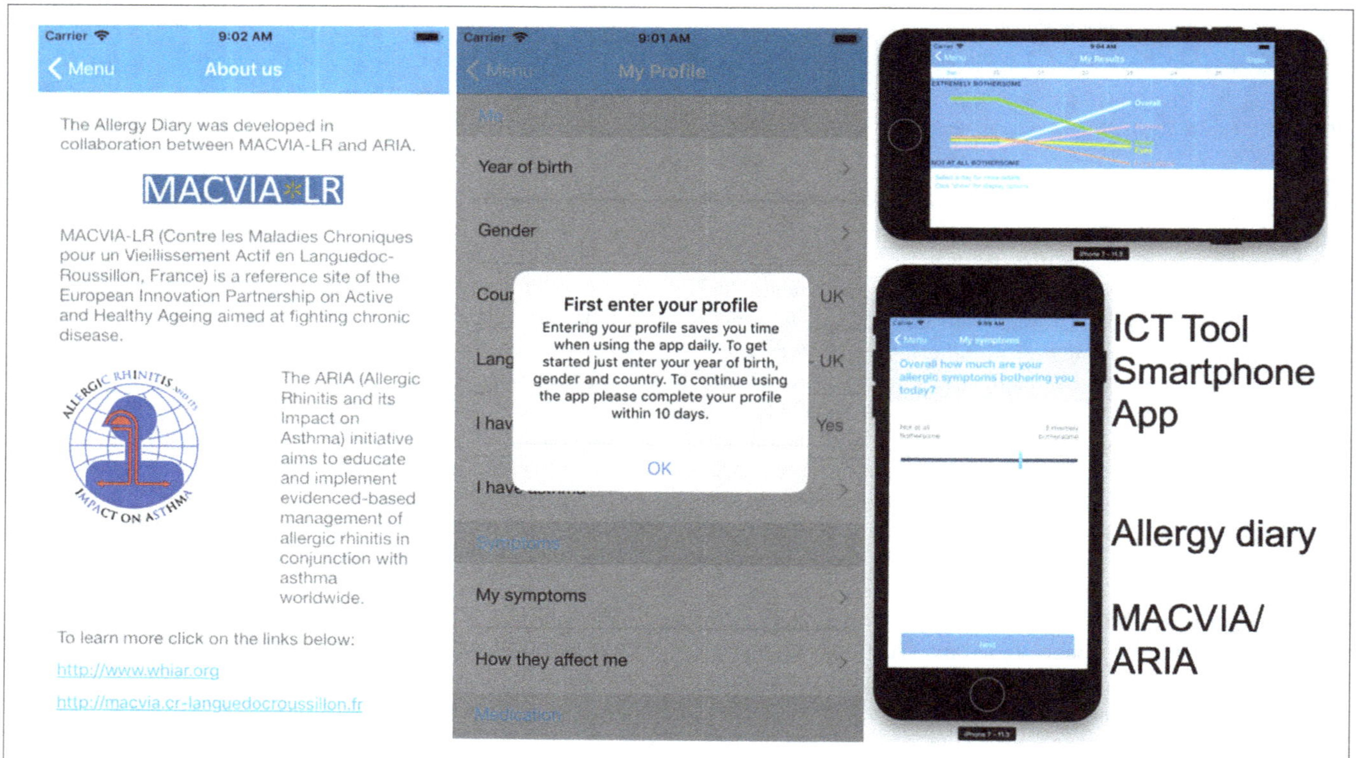

FIGURE 2 | MACVIA/ARIA allergy diary Smartphone Application (App) developed by the MACVIA-Fr Reference Site, adopted and replicated across EU and non-EU countries; 15931 users—AT 655; AU 196; BE 164; BR 2039; CA 34; CH 905; CZ 5; DE 814; DK 151; ES 736; FI 456; FR 1029; GB 962; GR 240; IT 1970; LT 394; MX 905; NL 603; PL 968; PT 2264; SE 174; TR 260 (November 22, 2017).

life. This reinforces ongoing research and innovation activities in Europe (and elsewhere), supported through public–private partnerships.

Within the scope of the C2 Action Group, in 2017, the AAL Forum, the biggest European event in the field of Technologies for AHA was organized in Coimbra, by the Pedro Nunes Institute, in partnership with the Portuguese Foundation for Science and Technology and some of the Ageing@Coimbra core partners. The theme of the Forum was "Bridging the gaps between technology solutions and aging well. What can YOU do?" Interoperable solutions were discussed as crucial to assure the value of the digital solutions, for example contributing for the integration between social and health care.

An inspirational fresh addition to this year's AAL Forum exhibition hall was the attendance of over 120 end-users above the age of 65, all eager to give their honest opinion on what they saw. Exhibitors had approximately 7 min to present and sell their AAL solution to the guests, which turned out to be more of a challenge than the majority of exhibitors expected (**Figure 3**). After visiting each of the exhibition stands, the group of over 65's had the hard job of picking their three favorite stands.

For the first time in the AAL Forum, the jury responsible for awarding the Exhibition Prize was constituted only by end-users above the age of 65. This activity was supported by Ageing@Coimbra and the Administrative Authority of the Centre Region of Portugal.

Another example of the collaborative work of Ageing@Coimbra members within the scope of C2 Action Group is well represented by the project GrowMeUp, funded under the H2020 call PHC-19-2014 "Advancing active and healthy aging with ICT: service robotics within assisted living environments"; coordinated by the University of Coimbra and including the active partnership with Caritas Coimbra as an end-user organization (Grant Agreement 643647).[11]

[11] www.growmeup.eu (Accessed: April 24, 2018).

D4 Action Group: Age-Friendly Environments

The D4 Action Group has its main roots on the concept of Age-Friendly Environments, as envisaged by the World Health Organization[12] (WHO), referring to physical and social environments as key determinants for health, well-being and the participation of people as they age. In that sense, the main objective of the D4 Action Group is to contribute to a more inclusive society and communities across Europe by empowering older persons through scaled up inclusive solutions.[13] Caritas Coimbra is main coordinator of the domain 8 of this action group—connect and leverage local and regional age-friendly environments—which fosters wide participation of different stakeholders across Europe, supporting networking, transfer of experience and the upscale of good practices.

Caritas Coimbra is also a founder member and Vice-President of the European Covenant on Demographic Change, an organization that aims to gather local, regional, and national authorities as well as other stakeholders in order to cooperate and implement evidence-based solutions to support AHA.[14] The Covenant comprises more than 150 members—local and regional authorities, industries, research centers/universities, civil society organizations—to link up, benefit from each other's experience and work together to promote initiatives on age-friendly environments across the EU.

The collaborative work of Ageing@Coimbra in D4 group includes the leadership of the University of Coimbra in the H2020 project Euro-Healthy (Shaping European Policies to Promote Health Equity) with a key goal to deliver a Population Health Index and a Web Geographic Information System (Web-GIS) addressing health inequity across the EU (Grant Agreement 643398) (11).[15]

[12] http://www.who.int/ageing/projects/age-friendly-environments/en/ (Accessed: April 24, 2018).

[13] https://ec.europa.eu/eip/ageing/action-groups-eip-aha/d4-age-friendly-environments_en (Accessed: April 24, 2018).

[14] www.agefriendlyeurope.org (Accessed: April 24, 2018).

[15] www.euro-healthy.eu (Accessed: April 24, 2018).

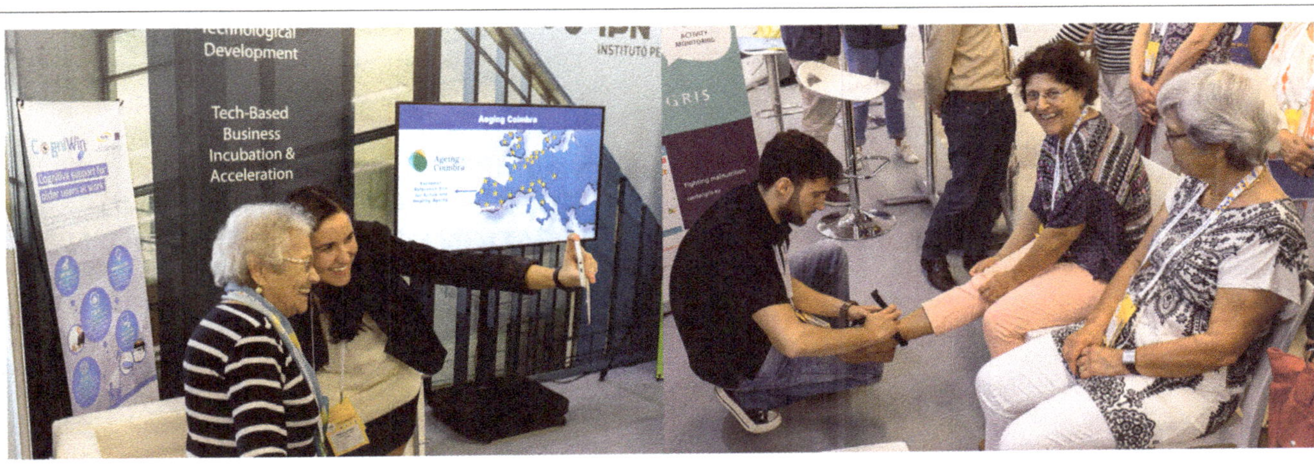

FIGURE 3 | Older citizens (identified through Third Age Universities and Social Care Providers) experience and evaluate technologies at the AAL Forum 2017 (Coimbra, October 2–4, 2017). Over 120 old citizens tested, evaluated, and provided recommendations for technology developers. The identified participants and the AAL Forum organization expressed written agreement for the inclusion of these photos in the present publication.

AGEING@COIMBRA INNOVATION CLUSTERS ON BRAIN AGEING AND ON SOCIAL ISOLATION

Ageing@Coimbra Provides an Integrated Pipeline in Biomarkers for Neurodegenerative Diseases

The area of biomarkers for neurodegenerative diseases, particularly concerning Alzheimer's disease, profits from the solid basis of neuroscience research provided by CNC.IBILI. Fundamental research is transferred from bench to bedside by means of knowledge-based genetics, biochemical, imaging, and neuropsychology biomarkers of cognitive dysfunction.

Genetics and biochemical biomarkers currently used to identify risk factors and biomarkers of Alzheimer's disease include APP, tau, amyloid beta 1-42, genotyping for PSEN1, PSEN2, APP, ApoE (12).

The Faculty of Psychology of the University of Coimbra provides neuropsychology tests to screen for functional and memory competence of older adults including Adults and Older Adults Functional Assessment Inventory (IAIFA), World Health Organization Quality of Life-OLD module, Geriatric Depression Scale (GDS-15), cognitive performance (MOCA, ACE-R).

The early diagnosis pipeline is complemented with robust brain imaging tools to ensure high quality diagnosis of putative neurodegenerative conditions. The Applied Nuclear Sciences Institute (ICNAS) pipeline launches innovative cyclotron-based synthesis methods of radiotracers including PET/FDG, PET/PiB, PET/PK11195, and other radiotracers upgrading the diagnosis tools.

This integrated approach, aligning technologies and professionals/resources for a better public service results in relevant assets for Ageing@Coimbra stakeholders, creating the most valuable and reliable integrated health service in Alzheimer's diseases in Portugal; with recognized impact in the Health Cluster Portugal, the Joint Program in Neurodegenerative Diseases, and the EIT Health Knowledge Innovation Community (KIC).

The diagnostics pipeline for early detection of Alzheimer's disease contributes to better health-care management and also to liaise with patient associations (e.g., Alzheimer's disease; Alzheimer Portugal) for better social care and support to patients and care providers.

Social Isolation—Mobile Units, Continuous Integrated Care, and Healthy Food

The territory of the Center Region of Portugal offers peculiar conditions as a regional living laboratory. In the region, about 23% of residents are aged 65 or over living in diverse environments, urban versus rural, highly dense versus low-density territories. In inland areas, especially in the mountain area, low-density territories also create geographic barriers to mobility especially of frail people contributing to social isolation. On the other hand, social isolation is also a burden of older persons living alone in urban areas of the Centre Region of Portugal.

These particular conditions create a local need to develop integrated care and personalized solutions to support older people living in socially challenging conditions.

The majority of municipalities in the Region have been equipped with health mobile units to deliver primary care and social care support to frail older people living in rural isolated areas. The added value of these services is well recognized by users and professionals, showing increase demand in terms of individual requests by the citizens and attracted interest by other municipalities.

Portugal launched in 2016 a new coordination structure of the National Network for Integrated Care Units. This network provided complementary health and social care support to populations, being socially isolated frail older people the main beneficiaries. The regional network includes 3 main units for palliative care, 9 units for convalescence care, and more than 62 integrated home care teams. Ageing@Coimbra links with integrated home care teams in close collaboration with the regional health authority, the national insurance office, and municipalities.

The social support to isolated frail older people in the region is a key priority for local players, including municipalities. Several important actions support intergeneration activities to tackle social isolation, ICT literacy, polypharmacy, and adherence to therapy strategies, assisted living programs, innovative strategies to engage older citizens with meaningful activities, and an humanitarian approach in health care—both in rural and urban areas.

The regional health authority launched a program ("pão.come") to reduce the content of salt in the daily food of Portuguese citizens, in particular the amount of salt in bakery. Traditionally, Portuguese citizens use excess salt in food, specially in bakery. This fact has been associated with high-prevalence of cerebrovascular diseases (13). Interestingly, the population of the Centre Region faces a major change in the profile of cerebrovascular diseases. The number of fatalities and permanent impairment conditions has been reduced significantly. Two major driving forces can account for the success of the "pão.come" program: (1) effective reduction of salt in bread that contributes to reduce the global numbers of stroke and cerebrovascular conditions; (2) the implementation of special priority channels (green way) in hospitals for people suffering from stroke and acute cerebrovascular diseases.

A schematic representation of the innovation clusters of Ageing@Coimbra (promoting healthy brain; social isolation) is depicted in **Figure 4**.

FUNDAMENTAL AND APPLIED RESEARCH IN AGEING, CARE AND INNOVATION IN GERIATRIC MEDICINE

Fundamental and Applied Research

Research on the mechanisms of aging-related diseases is a solid and established research area at the University of Coimbra and at the Center for Neuroscience and Cell Biology of Coimbra. Research in this area delivers high-impact and highly cited publications, international collaborations, advanced training of Ph.D., and postdoctoral students as well as entrepreneurship training and new spin off companies. Highlighting the priority of aging research, in 2016, a new ERA Chair group (H2020 Widespread, Grant Agreement 669088) was appointed by the

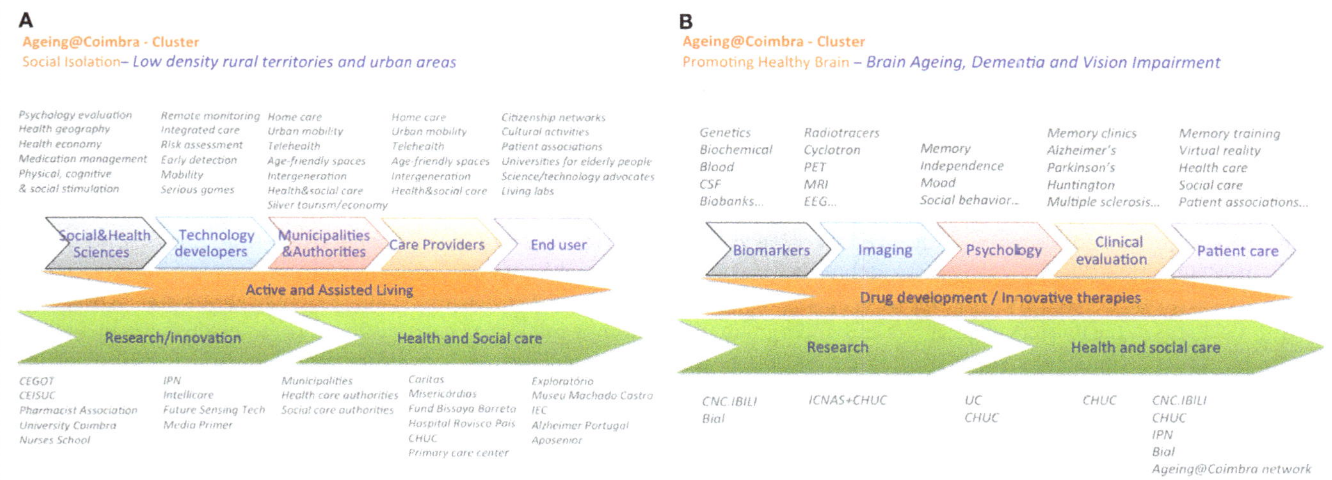

FIGURE 4 | Innovation cluster of Ageing@Coimbra on **(A)** "Social isolation: Low-density territories and urban areas," **(B)** "Promoting Healthy Brain: Brain aging, dementia, and vision impairment." The innovation pipeline represents the integration of stakeholder's activities from fundamental research into clinical or end-user applications.

Faculty of Medicine of the University of Coimbra to develop a research program, advanced teaching and translational research in cardiovascular aging (14).[16]

EIT Health

In 2015, three founder members of Ageing@Coimbra, the University of Coimbra, University of Coimbra Hospital and Pedro Nunes Institute, were accepted, as Associated Partners, in the new KIC in Active Living and Healthy Ageing from EIT Health. Together with the pharmaceutical company BIAL, they formed a cluster of Innostars, a legal entity member of EIT Health.

EIT Health is a powerful consortium of more than 140 members from academia and industry partners that develop collaborative market-driven projects to tackle societal challenges: (1) promote healthy living; (2) support active aging; (3) improve health care. Projects deliver better training of students, executives, and citizens (Campus); transform innovative ideas into products and services (Innovation Projects); and create and catapult business creation (Accelerator).[17]

Geriatric Medicine

The University of Coimbra Hospital offers a well-established multidisciplinary geriatric assessment service. The knowledge gathered by the clinical team supported the creation of a new clinical service entirely dedicated to AHA, including daily clinical care, a hospital residence, outpatient consultations and community health-care services. The key pillars of the new unit enclose clinical care of geriatric patients, training of new health-care professionals and research on aging and geriatrics.

The clinical unit on AHA establishes strong links with other hospital specialty services for prevalent and multimorbid conditions, including Neurodegenerative and Psychiatric Diseases, Pneumology and Respiratory Diseases, Immunology, Cardiovascular Diseases, Diabetes, Cancer, Musculoskeletal Diseases, among others.

Geriatric Medicine profits from the institutional collaboration of the University of Coimbra Hospital and the Rehabilitation Hospital Rovisco Pais and other local Hospital units in the region. Dedicated patient-centered rehabilitation services profiting from holistic approaches and multidisciplinary care are key success factors to prevent and treat geriatric frailty, particularly ortogeriatric frailty. Long-term care and palliative care multidisciplinary services in the region offer support to patients and families affected by long-term functional dependence and end-of life care for older patients and their families, including a hospital palliative care team offering support across clinical services at the University of Coimbra Hospital and two inpatient palliative care units, at the Portuguese Cancer Institute—Coimbra and Cantanhede Hospital (the latter also offering home care support). Reinforcing this strategic area, the Calouste Gulbenkian Foundation supports a "Professorship in Palliative Care" at the Faculty of Medicine of the University of Coimbra to strengthen research and education in Palliative Care in the Centre Region.

Health Literacy and Professional Training

The training of formal caregivers (working in institutions for older people), or informal caregivers (providing non-remunerated care for older people) is extremely important, especially when taking into account the growing older population that depends on care for chronic and degenerative diseases.

The University of Coimbra, together with Ageing@Coimbra, knowing the demand for specialized caregivers' training and the need to reach an audience with time limitations and geographically dispersed, concluded that a distance learning modality (e-learning course) was among the most appropriate responses. The Distance Learning Course, "Active and Healthy Ageing,"

[16]http://erachair.uc-biotech.pt/team/ (Accessed: April 24, 2018).
[17]www.eithealth.eu/home (Accessed: April 24, 2018).

which is a method of active learning providing training in the basic care areas of older people, was created by a team of lecturers of the Faculty of Medicine.[18]

Health literacy in aging is also a priority topic in postgraduate training. The Faculty of Medicine offers a masters degree in geriatrics and gerontology, where medical doctors can learn and upgrade their knowledge in age and age-related chronic diseases. Geriatrics in Coimbra is supported by advanced teaching, clinical health care and professional training. Advanced teaching at the Faculty of Medicine of the University of Coimbra includes the Ph.D. program in health sciences, the Ph.D. program in aging and chronic diseases, the masters in geriatrics and undergraduate training in geriatrics under the scope of the masters course in medicine. Postgraduate training of health-care professionals also includes the annual course on Ageing and Geriatrics (in 2017, we celebrate its 16th Edition).

Nursing School of Coimbra promotes the implementation of the comprehensive geriatric assessment at a national level. The activities include cultural adaptation and validation of tools for use in the field of geriatrics and participation in the development of national and international web platforms to support National and European strategy to intervene on older adults' frailty and to involve stakeholders in this process. The measurable impact of work of Nursing School of Coimbra is also observable in prevention of cognitive decline in advanced age by promoting the implementation of cognitive stimulation-based practice in different health-care contexts and by enabling multidisciplinary teams to implement autonomously this practice in different regions of Portugal. In addition, Nursing School of Coimbra is also training health professionals at a national level by enabling them to achieve critical reasoning, questioning of the ongoing practices and seeking and evaluating information to support Evidence-Based Practice. Nursing School of Coimbra is also offering postgraduate programs in Geriatric Health and Ageing, Health, and Citizenship.

Social Participation

Ageing@Coimbra profits from the engagement of several institutional partners that promote the social inclusion and participation of seniors in meaningful social activities and long-life learning. These institutions include Third Age Universities, Citizenship Associations, Science Centers, Museums, among others. Together, these institutions mobilize thousands of older citizens and their families in a number of activities involving the society: including heart and cardiovascular diseases awareness; Diabetes; Brain Awareness Week; International Day of the Older Person; European Scientists Night; among others.

GOOD PRACTICES AGEING@COIMBRA, 2017

In 2017, the Regional Authority of Centre Region, in a partnership with Ageing@Coimbra, launched a call to award good practices supporting AHA and age-friendly territories in the 100 Municipalities of the Region. This initiative contributes to (1) identify innovative good practices; (2) publicly recognize individual and institutional stakeholders; (3) disseminate knowledge to support adoption and scaling-up in other territories. The call awarded, in 2017, three categories: (1) Life+ ("Vida+"), to support healthy life styles; (2) Health+ ("Saúde+"), supporting innovative health care for older people; and (3) knowledge+ (Conhecimento+), to support research and technology applied to AHA.

We received 128 valid applications from diverse thematic and geographic origins, including 74 applications for the category "Life," 38 for "Health," and 16 applications for "Knowledge," from a total of 118 institutions. These institutions included 34 municipalities, 12 social care providers, and several citizenship associations and universities, from a total of 49 municipalities (**Figure 5**).

"Life" projects include programs for physical activity, with or without assessment of health parameters, multidimensional evaluation (clinics, social and gerontology), intergenerational dialog, therapy by arts, creation, and development of informatics platforms. The winner "Novas Primaveras," submitted by the Arts and Music Association of Pousos village, describes a program focused on therapy for older people through arts. This good practice was launched in 2004 and involves (currently) 12,711 direct and 84 indirect users from 30 Institutions, engaging users in music, dancing, theater, poetry, and other artistic expressions.

"Health" projects enclosed areas related with new mobile health units to support home care, implementation of new methodologies of health care (primary, non-formal, long-term, dementia), prevention of frailty in older people, screening and diagnosis of disease, physical and cognitive stimulation and rehabilitation,

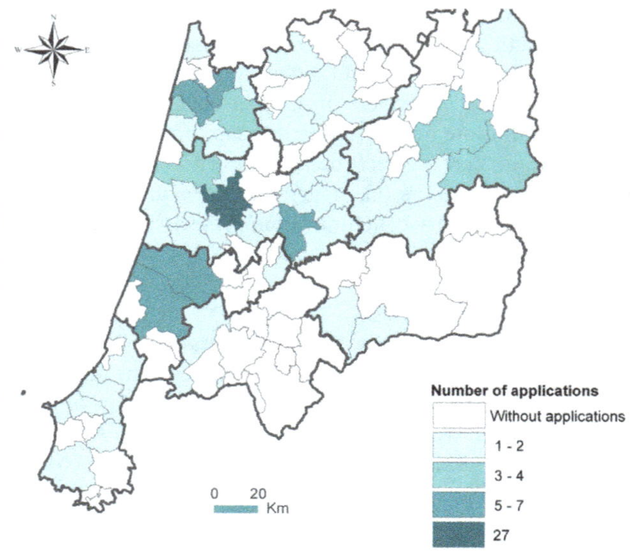

FIGURE 5 | Number of applications for the award of good practices on AHA ("Boas Práticas de Envelhecimento Ativo e Saudável da Região Centro"). The contest involved stakeholders from 49 of the 100 municipalities of Centro Region, that submitted 1 or more application, per municipality, of the total of 128 good practices (blue color scale for number of application per municipality).

[18] http://www.ed.uc.pt/educ/curso?id=127 (Accessed: April 24, 2018).

monitoring of chronic diseases using ICT's, support of patients in hospital and care residence settings (arts, comedy), health literacy, and health promotion. The winner good practice described specialized care for dementia patients ("Cuidados especializados para demência") submitted by the network of care providers "União das Misericórdias Portuguesas—Unidade de Cuidados Continuados Bento XVI (Fátima)". This dementia care residence is a pilot unit established in 2013, including environmental, professional, therapeutics competences, recognized as a reference model for the care of patients with cognitive impairment and dementia. It includes 20 beds for mid-term care and rehabilitation (up to 90 days) and 30 beds for long-term care and maintenance (up to 180 days).

"Knowledge" projects include: research and application of programs and new models; application of ICT solutions; collaborative models using telehealth and teleassistance; intergenerational approaches; infrastructures; equipment and access to knowledge; multimorbidity research and care; AHA and longevity, databases and population profiling. The winner was a project submitted by the Faculty of Medicine of the University of Coimbra and the Center for Neuroscience and Cell Biology: "NoMicro Technologies." This project describes the development of a technology to support healing of chronic wounds and prevention of infection by pathogens. NoMicro Technologies is currently in a phase of preclinical proof of concept.

In conclusion, the number and quality of the applications received in the call exceeded the best expectations of the organizing committee, reflecting the growing involvement and awareness of stakeholders of the Centre Region to support AHA of citizens.

DISCUSSION

Standing on the big societal challenges created by the impact of population aging in individual's health, but also for efficiency and sustainability of the health and social care systems, the movement created by EIP on AHA addresses the individual's and societal hurdles, under a positive perspective of stimulating the economic growth and job creation.

The collaborative work developed by EIP on AHA partners, under the scope of the six active action groups or under the scope of the quadruple helix-based Reference Sites, has delivered an impressive number of ground-transforming good practices, innovation schemes, and change management process, with big societal impact and economic potential.[19]

EIP on AHA Reference Sites like Ageing@Coimbra have shown to be instrumental bodies for helping the European Commission in the implementation of policies, including the "Blueprint for Digital Transformation on Health and Care in an Ageing Society"[20] and "Boosting Innovation on Active and Healthy Ageing in the Digital Single Market."[21] The goal of the blueprint is to reach out in 2018 more than 50 European Regions that will invest in the implementation and/or deployment of large-scale digital solutions for health and care. EIP on AHA is one of the key champions pre-identified by the European Commission that contributed to the Blueprint and committed to deliver results. The Digital Single Market Strategy unites regions, industry, and users around a shared vision on how digital innovation can transform health and care in Europe and will create the background for the impact expected for the Blueprint policy implementation. The Reference Sites are seen as key elements and stakeholders of this transformation. Accordingly, the close interaction of EIP on AHA and Reference Sites with national/regional authorities and international organizations, including WHO, foster the impact of activities leveraged from regional to European and global dimensions (5).

The impact of Reference Sites in the European landscape is also revealed by the collaborative work under the twinning collaborative scheme, involving delivery of good practices by innovator regions/actor and adoption by twin Reference Sites. The example of the twinning project lead by MACVIA and adopted/replicated by Ageing@Coimbra, and many other Reference Sites is a good example of a successful twinning project with impact in the society (see text footnote 20).

The challenges imposed to societies by population aging and demographic changes are of paramount complexity. Innovative formulas to deliver practices and services and organization models, like those embedded in EIP on AHA Reference Sites and Ageing@Coimbra, might prove to be key elements of the change management schemes needed to deliver quality of life to citizens and sustainability of health and care systems, starting from pilot twinning schemes to large scale-up replication across Europe and Globally.

CONCLUSION

In conclusion, the innovative and successful example of Ageing@Coimbra as a Reference Site of EIP on AHA supports the adoption of bottom-up, inclusive, and holistic approaches to create regional networks and partnerships with the aim of supporting the creation and replication of good practices for Active and Healthy Ageing. This methodology has proven to be successful in Coimbra/Centro de Portugal and other regions of Portugal, as well as in other European countries. Other examples of innovative regions embracing this model may follow and reinforce the change management objectives pursued by the EIP on AHA and the European Commission. However, important hurdles related with poor commitment of partners, oversimplification of processes in lean management structures are also difficulties that need to be constantly monitored and overcome.

Ageing@Coimbra is a growing consortium, consolidating its unique position as an aging network in the Centre Region of Portugal, with strong collaborations with other Reference Sites and international networks. Ageing@Coimbra will support the replication of good practices emerging from its stakeholder members and will twin with other European partners to foster the adoption of innovative practices and technologies for the benefit of Centre Region and European citizens.

[19] http://www.scale-aha.eu/fileadmin/scaleaha/documents/scaleaha_d5.4_final-studyreport.pdf (Accessed: April 24, 2018).

[20] https://ec.europa.eu/digital-single-market/en/blueprint-digital-transformation-health-and-care-ageing-society (Accessed: April 24, 2018).

[21] https://ec.europa.eu/digital-single-market/en/node/84742 (Accessed: April 24, 2018).

AUTHOR CONTRIBUTIONS

JM: concept design, writing the text, editing figures, and manuscript correction. AA: concept design, manuscript correction. AR: concept design, writing the text, editing figures, and manuscript correction. AM-P: writing the text and manuscript correction. AFC: concept design; writing the text; and manuscript correction. AT: concept design; writing the text; and manuscript correction. AT-B: editing figures and manuscript correction. AD: concept design and manuscript correction. AFA: manuscript correction. ALC: concept design; writing the text; and manuscript correction. CD: concept design; writing the text; editing figures; and manuscript correction. BG: writing the text and manuscript correction. CA: concept design; writing the text; and manuscript correction. IS: manuscript correction. JB: editing figures and manuscript correction. JA: concept design; writing the text; and manuscript correction. LS: concept design; writing the text; and manuscript correction. LA: concept design and manuscript correction. MI: writing the text; manuscript correction. RV: manuscript correction. VR: concept design and manuscript correction. MV: concept design; writing the text; editing figures; and manuscript correction.

FUNDING

The authors acknowledge the collaboration of Dr. Armando Pereira and Dr. Inês Costa as staff members of the research management office of the Faculty of Medicine of the University of Coimbra (GGI, FMUC). The following funding sources supported projects involving Ageing@Coimbra members: Portuguese Foundation for Science and Technology (FCT-Portugal), Pest UID/NEU/04539/2013, COMPETE-FEDER POCI-01-0145-FEDER-007440; 3rd Health Program of the European Commission; Horizon 2020 (H2020) of the European Commission; Portugal 2020 (EU); Calouste Gulbenkian Foundation.

REFERENCES

1. European Commission. *Directorate-General for Economical and Financial Affairs Ageing Report*. European Commission (2015).
2. World Health Organization. *World Report on Ageing and Health*. World Health Organization (2015).
3. Lagiewka K. European innovation partnership on active and healthy ageing: triggers of setting the headline target of 2 additional healthy life years at birth at EU average by 2020. *Arch Public Health* (2012) 70(1):23. doi:10.1186/0778-7367-70-23
4. Bousquet J, Michel J-P, Strandberg T, Crooks G, Iakovidis I, Iglesia M. The European innovation partnership on active and healthy ageing: the European geriatric medicine introduces the EIP on AHA column. *Eur Ger Med* (2014) 5(6):361–2. doi:10.1016/j.eurger.2014.09.010
5. Bousquet J, Agache I, Aliberti MR, Angles R, Annesi-Maesano I, Anto JM, et al. Transfer of innovation on allergic rhinitis and asthma multimorbidity in the elderly (MACVIA-ARIA)-EIP on AHA twinning reference site (GARD research demonstration project). *Allergy* (2017) 73(1):77–92. doi:10.1111/all.13218
6. Mair M, Fernandez-Llimos F, Alonso A, Harrison C, Hurding S, Kempen T, et al. *Polypharmacy Management by 2030: A Patient Safety Challenge*. 2nd ed. SIMPATHY Consortium (2017).
7. Stewart D, Mair A, Wilson M, Kardas P, Lewek P, Alonso A, et al. Guidance to manage inappropriate polypharmacy in older people: systematic review and future developments. *Expert Opin Drug Saf* (2017) 16(2):203–13. doi:10.1080/14740338.2017
8. Stewart D, Gibson-Smith K, MacLure K, Mair A, Alonso A, Codina C, et al. A modified Delphi study to determine the level of consensus across the European union on the structures, processes and desired outcomes to the management of polypharmacy in older people. *PLoS One* (2017) 12(11):e018348. doi:10.1371/journal.pone.0188348
9. Cano A, Kurpas D, Bujnowska-Fedak M, Santana S, Holland C, Marcucci M, et al. FOCUS: frailty management optimisation through EIPAHA commitments and utilisation of stakeholders' input – an innovative European project in elderly care. *Fam Med Prim Care Rev* (2016) 18:373–6. doi:10.5114/fmpcr/63234
10. Caimmi D, Baiz N, Tanno LK, Demoly P, Arnavielhe S, Murray R, et al. Validation of the MASK-rhinitis visual analogue scale on smartphone screens to assess allergic rhinitis control. *Clin Exp Allergy* (2017) 47(12):1526–33. doi:10.1111/cea.13025
11. Santana P, Costa C, Freitas A, Stefanik I, Quintal C, Bana e Costa CA, et al. *Atlas of Population Health in European Union Regions*. Coimbra: University of Coimbra Press (2017).
12. van Waalwijk van Doorn LJ, Gispert JD, Kuiperij HB, Claassen JA, Arighi A, Baldeiras I, et al. Improved cerebrospinal fluid-based discrimination between Alzheimer's disease patients and controls after correction for ventricular volumes. *J Alzheimers Dis* (2017) 56(2):543–55. doi:10.3233/JAD-160668
13. Bibbins-Domingo K, Chertow GM, Coxson PG, Moran A, Lightwood JM, Pletcher MJ, et al. Projected effect of dietary salt reductions on future cardiovascular disease. *N Engl J Med* (2010) 362:590–9. doi:10.1056/NEJMoa0907355
14. Aday S, Zoldan J, Besnier M, Carreto L, Saif J, Fernandes R, et al. Synthetic microparticles conjugated with VEGF165 improve the survival of endothelial progenitor cells via microRNA-17 inhibition. *Nat Commun* (2017) 8(1):747. doi:10.1038/s41467-017-00746-7

9

Genetic Pathways of Aging and their Relevance in the Dog as a Natural Model of Human Aging

Sára Sándor and Enikő Kubinyi*

Department of Ethology, Eötvös Loránd University, Budapest, Hungary

Edited by:
Alexey Moskalev,
Komi Scientific Center (RAS),
Russia

Reviewed by:
Andrzej Bartke,
Southern Illinois University
United States
George A. Garinis,
Foundation for Research and
Technology Hellas, Greece

***Correspondence:**
Sára Sándor
sandorsara@gmail.com

Aging research has experienced a burst of scientific efforts in the last decades as the growing ratio of elderly people has begun to pose an increased burden on the healthcare and pension systems of developed countries. Although many breakthroughs have been reported in understanding the cellular mechanisms of aging, the intrinsic and extrinsic factors that contribute to senescence on higher biological levels are still barely understood. The dog, *Canis familiaris*, has already served as a valuable model of human physiology and disease. The possible role the dog could play in aging research is still an open question, although utilization of dogs may hold great promises as they naturally develop age-related cognitive decline, with behavioral and histological characteristics very similar to those of humans. In this regard, family dogs may possess unmatched potentials as models for investigations on the complex interactions between environmental, behavioral, and genetic factors that determine the course of aging. In this review, we summarize the known genetic pathways in aging and their relevance in dogs, putting emphasis on the yet barely described nature of certain aging pathways in canines. Reasons for highlighting the dog as a future aging and gerontology model are also discussed, ranging from its unique evolutionary path shared with humans, its social skills, and the fact that family dogs live together with their owners, and are being exposed to the same environmental effects.

Keywords: hallmarks of aging, animal aging models, family dogs, aging genetics, dementia research

INTRODUCTION

Dogs (*Canis familiaris*) are special in the animal kingdom in many aspects. Being the oldest domesticated species, they accompany humans for approximately 15,000–100,000 years (estimates depend on the different approaches used to study their origin; see Vila, 1997; Larson et al., 2012; Thalmann et al., 2013; Frantz et al., 2016; Botigué et al., 2017). Consequently, they have adapted to the special social environment of human communities in a way unmatched by any other species and thus earned their rightful title as man's best friend. They have also gained diverse functionality throughout the millennia, which resulted in a phenotypic variability unrivalled by any other species. Recently, the species has also been promoted to be a model of human physiology and disease. The sequencing of the dog genome (Lindblad-Toh et al., 2005) and the development of high-resolution genotyping arrays to support genome wide association studies (GWAS) (Hayward et al., 2016) were important steps to open up new perspectives of genetic investigations in dogs. Recently, a growing number of full genome sequences from various dog breeds have also been added to the genetic toolkit of canine researchers (Dreger et al., 2016a; Dreger et al., 2016b; Kim et al., 2018). The importance of these improvements is clearly visible through the expanding list of reported disease associated polymorphisms in dogs. Examples like the famous case of the narcolepsy causing mutation in the canine *Hypocretin Receptor 2* gene (Lin et al., 1999), which turned the focus of researchers to its human homolog's role in narcolepsy, have demonstrated how canine genetics can benefit humans.

Genetic analyses have also helped to shed light on the origin and evolution of dogs and on the divergence of breeds (vonHoldt et al., 2010; Axelsson et al., 2013; Skoglund et al., 2015; Frantz et al., 2016; Freedman et al., 2016; Wang et al., 2016) and have revealed numerous genetic variants responsible for their phenotypic variability. For example, several genes have been shown to affect the body size variability of dogs (Sutter et al., 2007; Hoopes et al., 2012; Rimbault et al., 2013; Plassais et al., 2017), which is unmatched by any other mammalian species. Importantly, dogs also show marked differences in their expected lifespan in connection with body mass. On average, giant sized breeds (above 50 kg) have an expected lifespan of 6–8 years, while small sized breeds (below 10 kg) can live up to 14–16 years (Jimenez, 2016).

This wide range of expected lifespans, together with other aspects, has made dogs promising as model organisms for aging research (Gilmore and Greer, 2015; Creevy et al., 2016; Kaeberlein et al., 2016; Mazzatenta et al., 2017; Hoffman et al., 2018). In this regard, family dogs living as animal companions with their owners could be even more relevant than laboratory dogs (Kaeberlein, 2016). Although laboratory dogs had been traditionally used for a wide range of investigations, including aging research (Cotman and Head, 2008), they have some major limitations. For example, they experience a less complex nutritional and environmental history during their life course than family dogs do, which could lead to major deviances in their base level behavioral parameters. Also, they usually represent only a few breeds. These aspects clearly reduce the power of laboratory dogs to correspond with highly variable natural populations, especially when we consider the range of different aging phenotypes. Actually, describing and characterizing human aging phenotypes is a main goal of researchers, as such variability leads to fundamental differences in individual courses of aging. Living a long life with poor health can negatively affect the welfare of both the elderly and their surroundings. Age-related dementia can especially make a major impact in this regard, rendering patients unable to live an independent life. Therefore, lifespan and healthspan are considered partly independent attributes of human aging, leading to the distinction between healthy aging and pathological aging. Furthermore, in respect to cognitive decline, which can hinder welfare even if no other diseases are present, some authors suggested to discriminate successful aging as a subtype of healthy aging, which is characterized by maintained ability to live an autonomous life until death (Rowe and Kahn, 1987; Rowe and Kahn, 2015). In this regard, family dogs clearly surpass laboratory dogs as models, because they are more abundant, are more variable, and are much more likely to reach an old age and to encounter various aging courses. Although the detailed phenotypic categorization of aging in dogs will require further efforts, definitions for frailty, for example, have already been proposed in the species (Hua et al., 2016).

Nevertheless, it still remains a question how exactly dogs, especially family dogs, can fit in the puzzle of aging genetics among many already well-established experimental models. Despite the huge progress in understanding the genetic basis of morphological variability of dogs, still very little is known about the functional relevance of canine homologs of conserved longevity genes. Currently, this may stand as an obstacle in the way of effectively utilizing dogs as aging models. As family dogs can provide unique insights into many aspects of human aging, the current lack of detailed information about the canine genetic pathways of aging should be overcome by future research approaches. In this review, we provide an overview of the evolutionary conserved biological mechanisms that contribute to aging, following the classification system proposed by López-Otín et al., 2013, and we summarize current knowledge about these pathways in dogs. We also briefly discuss the benefits and limitations of family dogs in aging research and propose possible future directions for canine aging genetic studies.

DOGS AS MODEL ANIMALS IN AGING RESEARCH

A plethora of different species has been involved in aging studies to unravel the genetic factors behind this complex biological process. Due to their short lifespan and easy handling under laboratory conditions, the yeast (*Saccharomyces cerevisiae*), the nematode worm *Caenorhabditis elegans*, the fruit fly (*Drosophila melanogaster*), and rodents (mice: *Mus musculus* and rats: *Rattus norvegicus*) all became important contributors to the discovery of longevity affecting genes. Recently, the turquoise killifish (*Nothobranchius furzeri*) has also been added to this palette (Hu and Brunet, 2018). The applicability of various genetic approaches (e.g., induced mutagenesis, RNA interference, gene trapping) in these organisms allowed researchers to specifically target genes for further investigations or to efficiently search for phenotype–genotype associations in mutants.

As most of the revealed pathways turned out to be highly conserved, findings made on model organisms seemed translatable to humans in most cases. However, human aging has characteristics, like the occurrence of age-related dementia, which do not have counterparts in many model organisms. Although this limitation has been overcome by different techniques to induce neurodegenerative processes in the central nervous system (CNS) of model animals, the findings of such studies may not be easily implemented in humans (Jucker, 2010; Puzzo et al., 2015; De Felice and Munoz, 2016). In addition, the interaction between genetic factors and environmental conditions can also vary in humans, meaning that certain variants can have beneficial effects in one context and adverse effects in another (Ukraintseva et al., 2016).

Therefore, studies on human populations are inevitable to understand human aging in its full complexity. Apparently, in this case the genetic toolkit is reduced to associative approaches.

With the advent of the genomic era, this has become less of a problem, and several genome wide association studies (GWAS) have actually reported lifespan affecting loci in humans (Deelen et al., 2011; Nebel et al., 2011; Sebastiani et al., 2012; Sebastiani and Perls, 2012; Beekman et al., 2013). However, longitudinal studies and testing the effects of anti-aging interventions are still more challenging in humans than in short-lived animals.

When all of these considerations are taken into account, the dog may rise as an excellent midline solution for the limitations of simple organisms and for the challenges human studies hold (Waters, 2011). Here are some examples, why:

1. Family dogs, on average, age about six to seven times faster than humans. The mean lifespan of companion dogs (purebred and crossbred together) from Europe and Japan were shown to be 12 and 13.7 years, respectively (O'Neill et al., 2013; Inoue et al., 2018), while the mean lifespan of European humans is 77.2, according to a UN report (Anon, 2019) and is around 83 years for Japanese people (Tokudome et al., 2016). Therefore, follow-up studies are much easier in the case of dogs, and have already been performed by several research groups to measure immunological, neuropathological, and metabolomic changes related to canine aging (Su et al., 2005; Greeley et al., 2006; Cotman and Head, 2008).
2. The fact that the mean lifespan of dogs can range from 5.5 to 14.5 years (Michell, 1999; O'Neill et al., 2013; Jimenez, 2016), depending on body size and breed, suggests that dogs, sharing their lives with humans, gained considerable advantages from this alliance by doubling their mean expected lifespan compared to wild wolves (Mech, 2006). This artificially enhances the proportion of individuals with age-related pathologies, which often show strong correspondences with human diseases, and thus can provide opportunities for translational studies.
3. Dogs are prone to develop human-like neurodegenerative disorders and are susceptible to age-related cognitive abnormalities. Almost one third of 11–12-year-old dogs and 70% of 15–16-year-old dogs were reported to show cognitive disturbances with symptoms corresponding to human senile dementia: spatial disorientation, social behavior disorders (e.g., problems with recognizing family members), repetitive (stereotype) behavior, apathy, increased irritability, sleep–wake cycle disruption, incontinence, and reduced ability to accomplish tasks (Neilson et al., 2001). Together, these symptoms constitute a typical, age-related, progressive pathological decline in dogs' mental abilities, which is usually referred to as "Canine Cognitive Dysfunction Syndrome" (CCD) (Cummings et al., 1996; Landsberg et al., 2012). To this day, a vast amount of literature has accumulated about CCD (Szabó et al., 2016; Chapagain et al., 2018), yet there is weak knowledge about the genetic factors influencing it. Importantly, cognitive decline in dogs was associated with β-amyloid accumulation in the prefrontal cortex, noradrenergic neuron loss in the locus coeruleus (Insua et al., 2010), and, lately, with the formation of tau tangles (Schmidt et al., 2015; Smolek et al., 2016), which can all be seen in humans in early stages of neurodegenerative diseases.
4. Dogs also correspond very well to humans in several metabolic and physiological features, some of which are consequences of domestication (Axelsson et al., 2013). These features have already been thoroughly described in laboratory dogs, as traditional test animals of the pharmacological industry. Therefore, the intestinal absorption profiles of many drugs and supplements are actually known to be very similar in dogs and humans (Roudebush et al., 2005).
5. Several studies from the last two decades (for a review on the history of dog behavioral research, see Feuerbacher and Wynne, 2011) have supported the notion that dogs possess cognitive abilities that are similar to human social skills in communication and learning (Topál et al., 2009; Bensky et al., 2013; Miklósi, 2014). Also, they have a prolonged postnatal period with high sensitivity for human contact and usually live in a close proximity with people, which makes them able to easily interpret many human actions (Miklósi and Kubinyi, 2016). Therefore, dogs can participate in special experimental protocols, which would not be possible with less trainable and sociable species.
6. Dogs share more ancestral genomic sequence with humans than rodents do (Lindblad-Toh et al., 2005), and linkage disequilibrium regions can be extensive within dog breeds, making it easier to pinpoint phenotype–marker associations, which can be later narrowed down by interbreed investigations. This provides particular prospects for GWAS (Boyko, 2011; Vaysse et al., 2011; Schoenebeck and Ostrander, 2014; Hayward et al., 2016).
7. Family dogs are plentiful and easily available at very little cost, so large datasets can be collected *via* the help of dog owners and veterinarians under citizen science approaches (Hecht and Rice, 2015; Stewart et al., 2015).

These points suggest that family dogs can become valuable models to study complex human traits like aging. However, researchers have to face some obstacles and limitations as well, which have to be addressed properly.

1. One of these limitations is the still deficient knowledge about the exact functions that conserved genetic pathways play in canine aging. On the one hand, this may seem to be a minor question, as all fundamental cellular senescence mechanisms were reported to be conserved. On the other hand, divergences may occur in each species regarding some of these mechanisms, as for example, both the telomere biology of flies and the somatic telomerase expression of mice were reported to show marked differences from humans (Kipling and Cooke, 1990; Levis et al., 1993; Prowse and Greidert, 1995). Furthermore, the genes and their functions linked to human age-related neurodegeneration may be fundamentally different from their homologs found in model organisms, or even missing from other species (Bitar and Barry, 2017). Consequently, in an ideal setting, each genetic pathway should be evaluated in each species intended for

translational studies before further efforts are put into costly and time-consuming investigations.

2. The variable living environment of family dogs has been discussed as a potential advantage over laboratory dogs; however, it also brings serious challenges to optimal study design. Integrative and cooperative approaches based on large datasets could help to overcome this limitation. Large-scale retrospective studies, which were based on veterinary databases, have already led to important findings regarding the differences in life expectancies between various breeds (Proschowsky et al., 2003; O'Neill et al., 2013; Inoue et al., 2018), or between lean and obese dogs (Salt et al., 2018). In this regard, citizen science approaches can have promising prospects in family dog research (Hecht and Rice, 2015; Stewart et al., 2015), as it was already indicated by a few examples (Hecht and Rice, 2015; Stewart et al., 2015; Ilska et al., 2017). Also, if studies need to involve pathological, histological, and molecular data about dogs that suffered from CCD, citizen science approaches must be expanded to involve a wider range of professionals, including veterinarians. Such interdisciplinary studies may become especially important in cases where family dogs are used as preclinical models to test the anti-aging effects of drugs (Kaeberlein et al., 2016).
3. Until now few studies involved family dogs in cellular and molecular level investigations, as this may require invasive methods or even the sacrifice of animals. Apparently, such approaches are not applicable in the case of family dogs, which, however, represent the valuable genetic and behavioral variability of the species. These issues were encountered by researchers, who aimed to study brains of non-laboratory dogs, and found it difficult to collect both behavioral and molecular data (which required medically advised euthanasia of the animals) from the same individuals within the time-frame of the study (Ghi et al., 2009). In this regard, the establishment and long-term maintenance of databanks and biobanks that collect behavioral, lifestyle, medical data, and biological materials from family dogs, by providing the opportunity for owners to donate their dogs' bodies for research purposes under appropriate ethical considerations, would be advantageous for canine genomics and aging research.
4. Similarly to invasive methods, genetic manipulations may seem less applicable in dogs than in experimental model organisms. Nevertheless, some groups have already applied targeted genetic manipulations in laboratory dogs to create better models of certain medical conditions (Zou et al., 2015). More importantly, therapeutic applications of gene editing have recently been applied on pet dogs suffering from Duchenne muscular atrophy, with promising results (Amoasii et al., 2018). Hence, it is likely that this line of canine genetics and medical research will continue to unfold its potentials.
5. Currently, methods, by which cognitive aging can be effectively assessed in dogs, are limited. Effective phenotypical categorization of canine age-related pathologies, including CCD, will be crucial for studies, which intend to assess the effects of anti-aging interventions on dogs.

THE HALLMARKS OF AGING IN DOGS

Most aging-related genes are components of essential metabolic and signaling pathways (**Figure 1**), like the ones regulating autophagic activity. Other genes make contribution to cellular processes that affect genomic integrity, either in a protective role (DNA repair mechanisms) or in a destructive manner (oxidative stress, transposons). Some genes may affect aging in a somewhat programmed manner, either through epigenetic modulations or by the altered maintenance of telomeres. Because of this large number of involved genetic—and environmental—factors, establishment of a conceptual framework that can systematically comprise all of them would be a first step to provide better insight into the aging process in its entirety. In this regard, recently nine main factors have been designated as fundamental hallmarks that contribute to the aging of animals, with a main focus on mammals (López-Otín et al., 2013). Each hallmark had to meet three criteria: they must affect longevity and healthspan either in a negative or positive manner and have to show age-related changes in measurable parameters. Thus, the following phenomena were defined as main contributors to mammalian aging (**Figure 1**): 1) genomic instability; 2) telomere attrition; 3) epigenetic alterations; 4) disruption of proteostasis; 5) deregulation of nutrient sensing; 6) mitochondrial dysfunction; 7) cellular senescence; 8) stem cell exhaustion; and 9) altered intercellular communication. Although some of these could not perfectly fit all of the criteria, they still make an effective framework to work with. Providing a systematic overview of the genetic pathways involved in the aging of dogs is also of high relevance, as it can help defining directions in canine aging research to support the progression of the species into an effective translational model. For example, in the case of the *apolipoprotein E* (*APOE*) gene, which has polymorphisms strongly associated with average lifespan and Alzheimer's risk in humans (Nebel et al., 2011; Broer et al., 2015), the translational relevance of the canine homolog is debatable, because *APOE*'s sequence was reported to have low conservation between the two species (Sarasa et al., 2010). Nevertheless, the function of the expressed protein may still be conserved. As *APOE* variants are major risk factors of human dementia, clarifying this question would be an important step to ensure clinical translatability of canine CCD research. In general, exploring more details about genetic pathways and gene variants involved in canine aging and age-related pathologies should be a major consideration of researchers who utilize dogs in aging research.

Genomic Instability

As organisms age, various forms of damage may accumulate in their genomes, leading to mutations, chromosomal rearrangements, and aneuploidy (Faggioli et al., 2012; Forsberg et al., 2012; Moskalev et al., 2013). Increased mutational burden in somatic cells eventually hinders cellular function and leads to terminal cellular senescence or apoptosis. In cases when cells escape death/senescence inducing processes, malignant transformations can occur as a consequence of genomic damage.

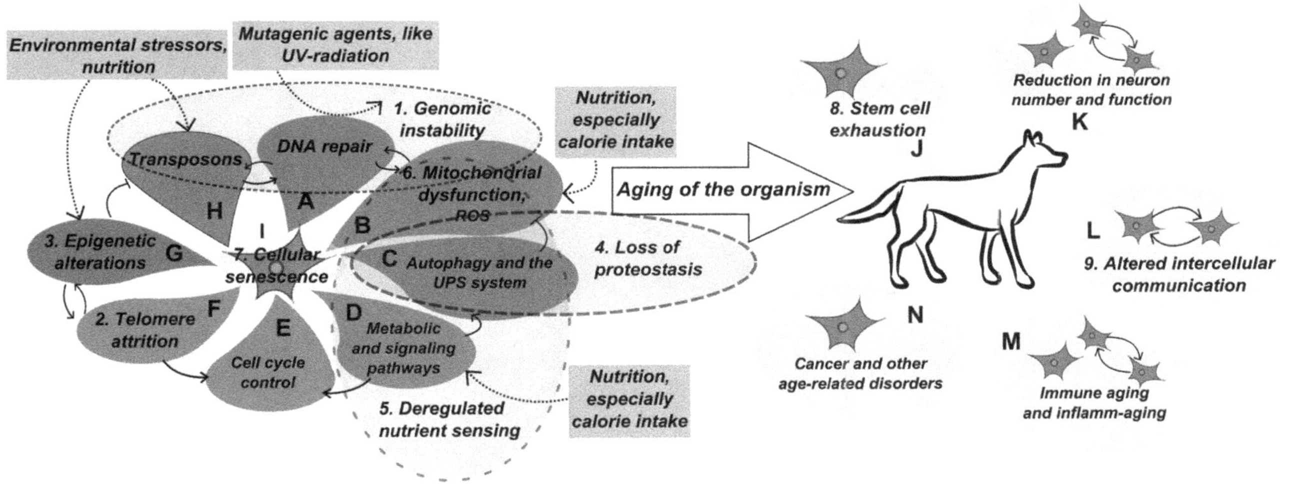

FIGURE 1 | Main mechanisms of aging.The figure depicts the mechanism that underlie cellular aging and, consequently, aging of a multicellular organism. The main mechanisms defined as hallmarks of aging by López-Otín et al. in 2013 are numbered according to their order in the main text. **(A)** The DNA repair machinery provides the first line of defence against mutagenic agents and also interacts with mobile DNA elements through repairing double strand breaks induced by transposons. Impaired function of this machinery can be a main contributor to *Genomic instability* (1). **(B)** Reactive oxygen species produced by mitochondrial respiration represent an inner source for DNA lesions, thus interact with the DNA repair machinery: proper functionality of DNA repair enzymes is required to protect cells from oxidative damage, however elevation in the level of oxidative stress may overburden the repair machinery. Age-related *Mitochondrial dysfunction* (6) can lead to increased oxidative and apoptotic burden. In addition, increased oxidative stress can also affect proteostasis. **(C)** Macroautophagy is a protective mechanism against malfunctioning mitochondria that might cause oxidative stress, while together with other clearance mechanisms it also functions to remove misfolded proteins and protein aggregates. It also functions as a mechanism for programmed cell death (indicated with dashed line between autophagy and cell cycle control). Together with the ubiquitin-proteasome system (not indicated separately on the figure) its malfunction may lead to *Loss of proteostasis* (4) in cells. **(D)** The activity of the autophagy machinery is strictly regulated by different signalling pathways, many of which function in metabolite sensing and cell growth control. Dysruption in these signaling pathways is summarized as *Deregeulated nutrient sensing* (5) by López-Otín et al (2013). **(E)** Cell cycle control is a main determinant of *Cellular senescence* (7). Also, on a multicellular level, dysregulation of cell cycle control may decrease lifespan by initiating tumour formation. **(F)** In many species telomeres function as a measuring mechanisms to limit the number of potential cell cycles. When telomere length reaches a critical shortness, it will activate cell cycle control mechanisms to render the cell into a senescent state. The telomerase enzyme was also shown to interact with global genomic chromatin maintenance. In general, *Telomere attrition* (2) is a main hallmark of aging in most mammalian species. **(G)** Epigenetic regulation involves two main mechanisms, the methylation of CpG islands and modification of the chromatin structure through histone proteins. Chromatin structure at telomeres is important for telomere maintenance and the repression of retroelements by CpG methylation may prevent DNA damage caused by transposon mobilisation. *Epigenetic alterations* (3) are also linked to aging in both humans and model organisms. **(H)** Derepression of mobile DNA elements, primarily of retroelements in mammalian genomes, may result in an increased frequency of double strand breaks and insertion mutagenesis leading to increased *Genomic instability* (1). **(I)** Altogether, the molecular mechanisms of aging eventually result in *Cellular senescence* (7). **(J)** Cellular senescence will lead to reduced function of tissues in a multicellular organism. *Depletion of tissue renewing stem cells* (8) is also a main hallmark of organismal aging and is a result of cellular senescence and increased activation / differentiation of dormant stem cells in certain tissues. **(K)** Loss of stem cells and cellular senescene will lead to functional decline in the central nervous system. **(L)** *Altered intercellular communication* (9) is also considered a main hallmark of aging in multicellular organisms, as coordinated activity of cells is essential for proper tissue functionality. **(M)** The immune system can be affected considerably by altered intercellular communication, and this could also lead to increased inflammation in the body, called inflamm-aging. The elevated levels of inflammation may also result from the increasing number of senescent / apoptotic cells. **(N)** Together with intracellular changes, mainly loss of genomic integrity, disrupted proteostasis and signalling pathways, the imbalanced function of the immune system will contribute to the occurrence of age-related diseases.

Therefore, various protective mechanisms have evolved to prevent or correct DNA damage. Genomic instability arises when the occurrence of deleterious events exceeds the capacity of the DNA damage response system. DNA damaging agents can originate from various extrinsic or intrinsic sources. Intrinsic factors involve oxidative damage, telomere attrition, and transposon insertions.

The DNA Repair Machinery

The DNA repair machinery involves divergent pathways, each aimed to correct certain forms of DNA damage (**Figure 2**). These protective mechanisms have been in the focus of cancer and aging research for a long time (Zimmermann, 1971; Lombard et al., 2005; Cho and Suh, 2014). Defects in DNA repair genes, like the *Bloom syndrome RecQ like helicase* (*BLM*) and the *Werner syndrome RecQ like helicase* (*WRN*), can lead to severe illnesses, called progeria syndromes in humans, which are characterized by premature aging and other symptoms, including cognitive disabilities and a higher rate of tumorigenesis (Ellis et al., 1995; Yu et al., 1996; Martin, 2005; Arora et al., 2014). Mutations in other DNA repair genes were also reported to increase cancer risk (Jeggo et al., 2016) and thus lead to a reduction in expected lifespan. More importantly, polymorphisms in several genes of the DNA damage response machinery have been actually linked to longevity in humans (Cho and Suh, 2014). Intriguingly, no canine progeria syndrome has been documented in scientific literature. On the other hand, several studies that investigated various forms of canine cancer revealed alterations in the DNA

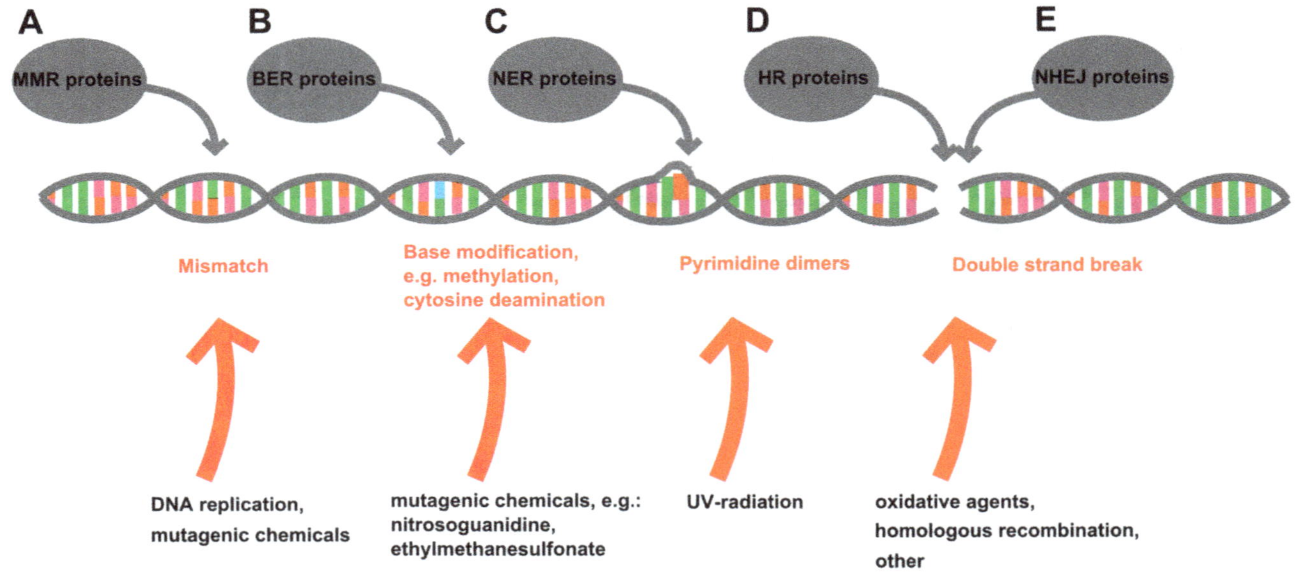

FIGURE 2 | The protective roles of the DNA repair machinery. The DNA repair machinery counteracts the effects of variable DNA damaging processes. In healthy cells, the repair machinery can balance these deleterious effects (represented by red arrows); however, in the case of increased mutagenic burden (e.g., exposure to UV radiation), or when members of the repair machinery are not functioning properly, the balance can be lost and a growing number of DNA lesions may cause the cells to die or turn malignant. **(A)** The function of the Mismatch Repair system (MMR) is coupled to DNA replication where mismatching base pairs can be formed spontaneously and are being identified and repaired by MMR proteins. **(B)** The Base Excision Repair (BER) system can detect damaged/chemically modified bases in the DNA helix, and remove them, resulting in an apurinated site, which will induce endonucleases to cut back the DNA strand. The single strand break is repaired by a DNA polymerase based on the sequence of the complementary strand, and the newly synthesized sequence is ligated to the original DNA strand by a ligase enzyme. **(C)** Mutations that disrupt the normal topology of the DNA double helix, like the UV-light induced formation of pyrimidine dimers, are corrected by the nucleotide excision repair (NER) system. This machinery recognizes aberrant DNA structure caused by chemically modified nucleotides and removes these nucleotides resulting in a single strand break, which will be filled in by DNA polymerase and ligase enzymes. **(D, E)** The most destructive form of DNA damage is double strand break (DSB), which could trigger an immediate apoptotic response if it fails to be repaired. Two distinct mechanisms are used by cells to repair DSB: one is homologous recombination (HR) and the other is non-homologous end joining (NHEJ). HR is a fundamental process also linked to meiosis in eukaryotic cells, and it provides a possibility to recover the damaged DNA strand in full length, by using a homologous DNA helix (e.g., the sister chromatid) as template. In contrast, NHEJ may link ends of double stranded DNA together randomly, which could lead to loss of sequences around the breakpoint. All types of DNA repair are indispensable for normal cellular and organismal function.

repair machinery, which corresponded to findings in human cancers. For example, a reduced DNA damage response capacity was observed in lymphomas of Golden retriever dogs (Thamm et al., 2013), and a lower expression of the *ATM serine/threonine kinase* (*ATM*) gene was found in canine mammary tumors (Raposo-Ferreira et al., 2016). Genetic variations in the *breast cancer 1* (*BRCA1*) and *tumor protein p53* (*TP53*) genes and the *MTAP-CDKN2A* locus were also linked to various forms of cancer in dogs (Kirpensteijn et al., 2008; Rivera et al., 2009; Shearin et al., 2012). While these findings clearly promote the dog as a natural model of human cancers, it is still unclear how exactly variations in DNA repair capacity contribute to the expected lifespan of dogs. A more detailed discussion of DNA repair in dogs can be found in the review of Grosse et al. (2014).

Nuclear Architecture

Genomic instability may also rise from altered nuclear architecture. Good examples are the Hutchinson-Gilford and the Néstor-Guillermo progeria syndromes, which were linked to mutations in *lamin* genes responsible for formation of the nuclear lamina (De Sandre-Giovannoli et al., 2003; Eriksson et al., 2003; Cabanillas et al., 2011). In addition, both the accumulation of progerin, which is an aberrant form of lamin A, and the reduced expression of lamin B1 were linked to aging (Freund et al., 2012; Golubtsova et al., 2016; Hilton et al., 2017), and lamins were also shown to regulate DNA damage response (Gonzalez-Suarez et al., 2009). Thus, the canine homologs of *lamins* could be promising targets in aging research. So far, a few studies have investigated them, mainly in regard to their possible role in hereditary diseases, like dilated cardiomyopathy of Doberman pinschers and Newfoundland dogs (Wiersma et al., 2007; Meurs et al., 2008) and elbow dysplasia in Bernese Mountain Dogs (Pfahler and Distl, 2012); however, only in the latter case an association was reported between disease occurrence and the *lamin B1* gene.

Oxidative Damage

Oxidative damage in cells mainly results from chemical interactions between cellular constituents and reactive oxygen species (ROS), which chemically act as free radicals, characterized by a high oxidative activity. These agents target macromolecules, such as DNA, lipids (Rubbo et al., 1994), and proteins (Stadtman and Levine, 2006), and thus may make a huge impact on cellular function. The sources of ROS are many: mitochondrial respiration (Liu et al., 2002; Murphy, 2009), ionizing radiation (Riley, 1994), and the activity of specific enzymes, such as the NADPH oxidase (Babior, 2004) and dual oxidase (DUOX) (Edens et al., 2001), are the main examples.

The amount of oxidative DNA lesions has been well documented to increase with age in different species. For example, in rats, Fraga et al. (1990) reported the age-related accumulation of 8-hydroxy-2-deoxyguanosine, which is a typical product of DNA oxidation. Furthermore, several studies confirmed that aged dogs show elevated levels of oxidative damage in their brains, indicated by the accumulation of carbonyl groups (Head et al., 2002; Skoumalova et al., 2003), lipofuscin (Rofina et al., 2004), 4-hydroxynonenal (Papaioannou et al., 2001; Rofina et al., 2004; Hwang et al., 2008), and malondialdehyde (Head et al., 2002) in neural tissue. In addition, as the reduced expression of antioxidant enzymes may also contribute to the increased oxidative burden in cells (Kiatipattanasakul et al., 1996), their role in neural aging and neurodegeneration should also be considered. In humans, for example, a mutation in superoxide dismutase 1 (SOD1), which is a main antioxidant enzyme in cells, has been linked to amyotrophic lateral sclerosis (ALS) (Orrell, 2000). Importantly, a mutation in the canine homolog of *SOD1* was also linked to an ALS like neurodegenerative process, called degenerative myelopathy (DM) (Awano et al., 2009).

Surprisingly, ROS have also been indicated as important and evolutionary conserved signaling molecules, which function in pathways that respond to availability of nutrients, changes in environmental oxygen levels, and exercise (Schieber and Chandel, 2014; Merry and Ristow, 2016). Hydrogen peroxide (H_2O_2), for example, plays an important role as signal transducer in the MAPK and Nf-Kβ pathways (Allen and Tresini, 2000) and also serves as activator of peroxiredoxins (Wood et al., 2003), which are crucial for maintaining redox balance of cells. Nitric oxide (NO) has long been indicated to play various physiological roles, with emphasis on the immune and cardiovascular systems (Lundberg et al., 2008). Thus, maintaining optimal levels of oxidative stress in cells could actually be more important for healthy aging than maximizing the neutralization of ROS by antioxidants. In accordance with this, some studies reported controversial effects of oxidative stress in aging and metabolic parameters. For example, it was demonstrated by Ristow et al. (2009) in a human study that supplementation with high doses of extrinsic antioxidants ameliorated the beneficial effects of exercise in volunteers. Furthermore, elevated levels of ROS were reported to either increase lifespan in yeast and worms (Doonan et al., 2008; Van Raamsdonk and Hekimi, 2009; Mesquita et al., 2010) while having no effect on mortality in mice (Van Remmen et al., 2003; Zhang et al., 2009) Also, the lifespan extension of worms promoted by reduced glucose availability was found to be accompanied by elevated levels of ROS in cells (Schulz et al., 2007). Such findings led to the reconsideration of the role oxidative stress plays in cellular senescence and resulted in a more refined view (López-Otín et al., 2013; Shadel and Horvath, 2015). In this regard, it is a question yet to be addressed, how lifelong antioxidant supplementation, often provided by high-quality commercial foods, may affect the healthspan of dogs.

Transposable Elements

The mobilization of endogenous transposable elements, called transposons, has recently gained attention as an intrinsic contributor to cellular senescence (Gorbunova et al., 2014). Transposons are present in the genomes of all organisms, from bacteria to mammals, and possess the ability to change their

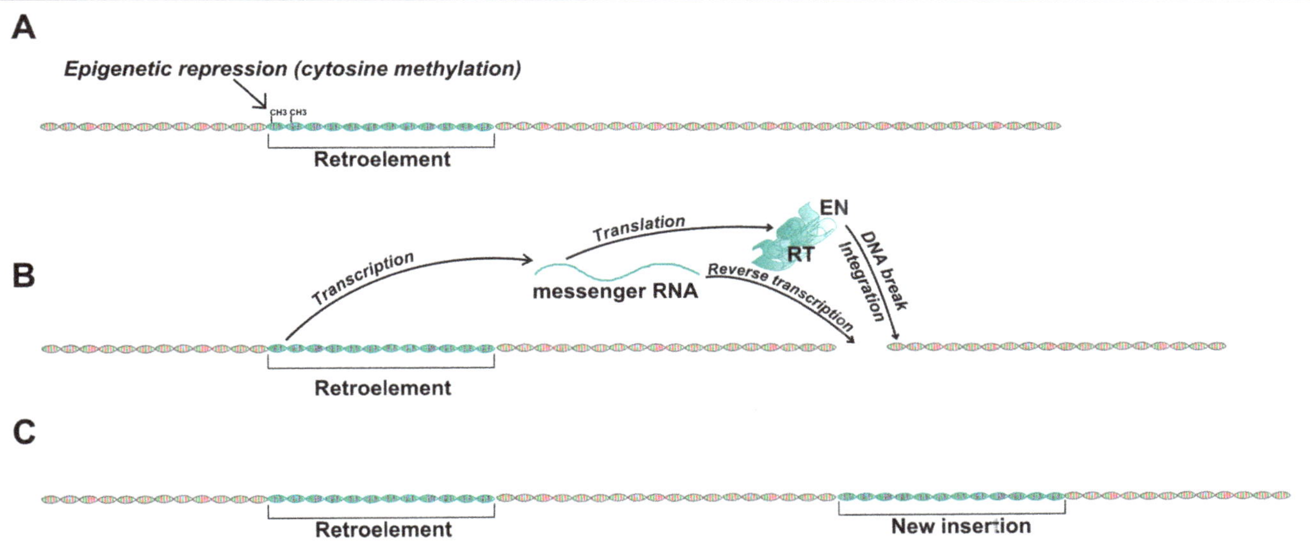

FIGURE 3 | Mobilization of retroelements in the genome. This picture shows the basic mechanism of retrotransposon mobilization. **(A)** Normally, activity of functional retroelements, like LINE-1, is repressed in somatic cells by methylation of CpG islands in their promoter regions. **(B)** Demethylation of the transposon promoter may result in transcriptional activation. The transcribed mRNA encodes the proteins necessary for retrotransposition, the Integrase (Int) and Reverse Transcriptase (RT), and also serves as template for reverse transcription. The reverse transcribed transposon DNA will be integrated into the genome by the Int protein, which first induces a double strand break. **(C)** The retroelement has copied itself into a new genomic region.

position in or between chromosomes. They can be categorized into two groups. Retrotransposons move by a replicative "copy and paste" mechanism, increasing in numbers in their host genome (**Figure 3**), while DNA transposons mainly follow a "cut and paste" mechanism, leaving only a short footprint behind (Wicker et al., 2007; Mandal and Kazazian, 2008). Since the human genome project revealed that around 55% of the human genome is composed of remains of transposable elements, mainly of retrotransposons, an increased attention has been paid to their role in genome evolution (Kazazian, 2004), especially in the formation of gene regulatory networks (Sundaram et al., 2014). While all DNA transposons have lost their mobility in the course of human evolution (Pace and Feschotte, 2007), several retroelements found in our genome are still active and can cause insertional mutations (Hancks and Kazazian, 2016). Human retroelements can be categorized into three groups: the *LTR* (*Long Terminal Repeat*) elements, the *LINE* (*Long Interspersed Nuclear Element*) transposons, and the *SINE* (*Short Interspersed Nuclear Element*) transposons (Mandal and Kazazian, 2008). Similar types of retroelements can be found in the dog genome; however, transposon-derived sequences make up only 34% of it (Lindblad-Toh et al., 2005). Importantly, active *LINE* and *SINE* elements are present in both species.

Active retroelements have been found responsible for several hereditary diseases in dogs by causing insertional mutations. For example, a *LINE-1* (*L1*) insertion in the gene of Factor IX was shown to segregate with mild hemophilia in German Wirehaired Pointers (Brooks et al., 2003), while a similar insertion in the *dystrophin* gene leads to Duchenne-like muscular dystrophy in Pembroke Welsh Corgi dogs (Smith et al., 2011). *SINE* elements were also shown to cause several inherited diseases, like recessive centronuclear myopathy in Labrador Retrievers (Tiret et al., 2005) and early canine retinal degeneration, which was linked to the *serine/threonine kinase 38 like* (*STK38L*) gene in Norwegian Elkhound–Beagle outcrosses by linkage mapping (Goldstein et al., 2010). A form of progressive retinal atrophy (PRA) in Tibetan Spaniels and Tibetan Terriers was also associated with a *SINE* insertion, but in the *family with sequence similarity 161 member A* (*FAM161A*) gene (Downs et al., 2014). Bandera's neonatal ataxia in Coton de Tulear dogs was shown to be caused by the disruption of the *glutamate metabotropic receptor 1* (*GRM1*) gene by recent retrotransposon mobilization, as the insertion was not found in other breeds (Zeng et al., 2011). Interestingly, several examples of non-disease causing insertional mutations are known, which alter morphology (Parker et al., 2009; Marchant et al., 2017) or coat color (Clark et al., 2006; Dreger and Schmutz, 2011) and thus have become selection criteria in many breeds. Beyond these examples, where the integration event can be revealed by a phenotypic effect or disease, the mobilization of retroelements seems common in dogs, as analyses of individual dog genomes showed that approximately half of annotated dog genes contain a SINEC_Cf type insertion in their introns (Wang and Kirkness, 2005). This high activity of retrotransposons in the lineage of domestic dogs can be explained by intense selection pressures that resulted from domestication, breeding strategies, and changing environment (Capy et al., 2000; Chénais et al., 2012). This hypothesis was actually supported by the findings of Koch et al. (2016), who compared the methylation patterns of wolf and dog genomes and found that almost half of the sites potentially relevant in domestication contained a *LINE* or *SINE* insertion.

Beyond the germ-line mutations discussed so far, a vast body of evidence indicates that retroelements can mobilize in somatic cells (Collier and Largaespada, 2007; Hunter et al., 2015) although this is strictly controlled by specific non-coding small RNAs and epigenetic regulation, including hypermethylation and transcriptional repression (Levin and Moran, 2011; Pizarro and Cristofari, 2016). As the general hypomethylation of the genome has long been documented to be an attribute of aging (Wilson and Jones, 1983; Singhal et al., 1987), more and more researchers have suggested a main role for somatic transposon mobilization in cellular senescence (Murray, 1990; Sturm et al., 2015; Pal and Tyler, 2016). Importantly, this hypothesis was also supported by experimental findings. For example, the artificial downregulation of the yeast *Ty1* element resulted in lower levels of age-related chromosome rearrangements in aged cells (Maxwell et al., 2011). Also, many of the 118 *L1* subfamilies of mice showed an elevated expression with age (De Cecco et al., 2013). In humans the hypomethylation of *LINE-1* and *Alu* (a *SINE* element abundant in the human genome) elements has been linked to cancer susceptibility (Zhu et al., 2011; Luo et al., 2014).

Because the activation of transposable elements can be induced by various environmental stressors as well (Hunter et al., 2015), including heavy metal toxicity (Morales et al., 2015), certain genotoxic agents (Stribinskis and Ramos, 2006), and even nutrition (Waterland and Jirtle, 2003), they represent another possible intracellular interface between the living environment/lifestyle and aging. In this regard, family dogs, which share their environment with their owners, can be valuable models to study how retrotransposons may contribute to aging and mortality under various circumstances. The age-related activity of retroelements has not yet been specifically assessed in dogs. However, in a study that investigated the elevated blood levels of *SINE* sequences in dogs with mammary tumors, it was shown that tumor-affected dogs above 10 years of age had higher levels of circulating *SINE* elements than younger dogs with tumors (Gelaleti et al., 2014).

Telomere Attrition and Aging

In most eukaryotic cells, shortening of the protective sequences at chromosome ends (**Figure 4A**), called telomeres, occurs with each DNA replication. Therefore, telomere shortening has been proposed as a key mechanism of cellular senescence and it also suggested the existence of an aging program in cells (Shampay and Blackburn, 1988; Harley et al., 1990; Hastie et al., 1990). This so called replicative aging limits the number of cell cycles a cell can go through before reaching its Hayflick limit and entering a senescent state (Hayflick, 1976). Furthermore, a recent study supported the conserved role of this aging program on the level of whole organisms by reporting clear correlations between the rate of telomere shortening and the lifespan of different mammalian and

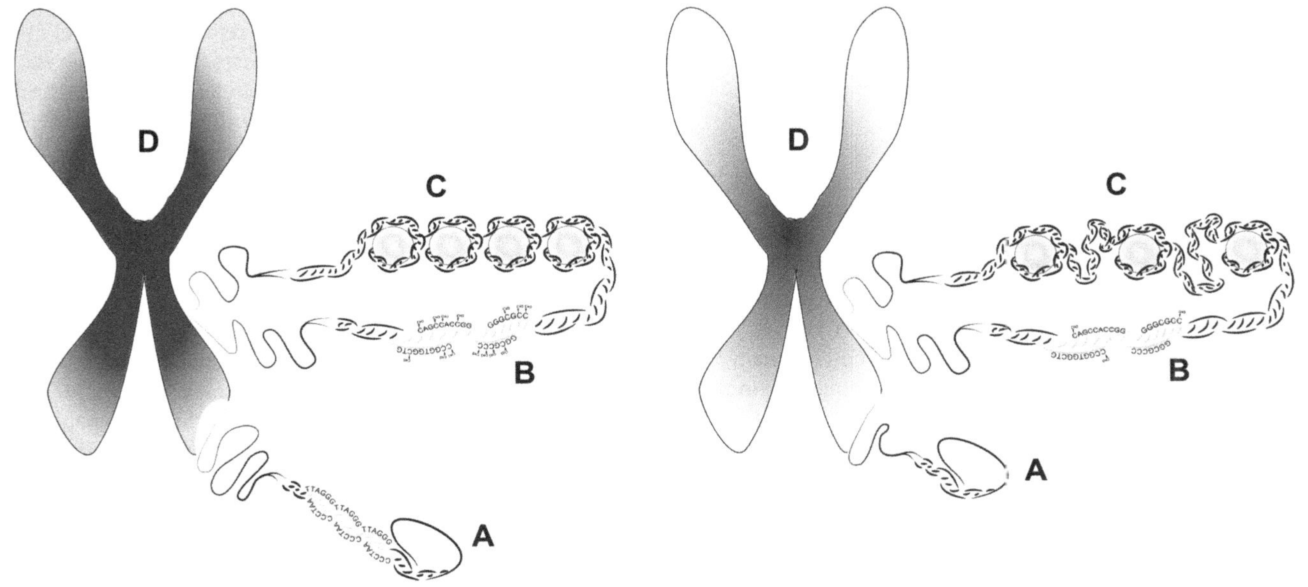

FIGURE 4 | The role of telomeres and epigenetics in chromosomal integrity and aging. The figure illustrates how shortening of telomeres and changes in the epigenetic pattern affect the overall structure of chromosomes. **(A)** Chromosome ends are protected by repetitive sequences called telomeres in most eukaryotic organisms. This telomere sequence, consisting of TTAGGG repeats, shortens with each DNA replication, which eventually triggers cellular senescence. **(B)** Chromatin changes occur on the first level of DNA packaging, when the DNA double strand is coiled up on nucleosomes. Tight coiling on nucleosomes results in a heterochromatic state, when the DNA double helix is not accessible to many proteins, including the transcription machinery. In contrast, reduction in the number of nucleosomes leads to a less coiled and less dense state rendering the DNA more open to transcription. **(C)** DNA methylation at CpG islands cause chemical changes directly in the DNA double helix. Cytosine methylation is usually linked to silencing of transcription. Methylation also interacts with chromatin structure: increased CpG methylation is usually linked to heterochromatic state. **(D)** Changes in chromosomal structure during aging is characterized by a decrease of heterochromatic regions (symbolized by darker color) and an increase of euchromatic regions (symbolized by lighter colors).

bird species (Whittemore et al., 2019). Importantly, telomere shortening is a characteristic only of somatic cells, while in germ line cells, telomere sequences are constantly restored by telomerase enzymes. The limited proliferative potential of somatic cells may seem disadvantageous for an individual, yet it may increase fitness by limiting the growth of malignant cells. In line with this, recent studies have suggested a trade-off between telomere length and cancer occurrence (Zhang et al., 2015; Stone et al., 2016). On the other hand, loss of telomeres can result in end-to-end chromosomal fusions, which might also lead to tumorigenesis (Hastie et al., 1990). These findings indicated that fine-tuning of telomere dynamics in somatic cells might be crucial for healthy aging, at the cost of reducing the maximal lifespan. In fact, polymorphisms in genes associated with telomerase function were shown to be linked with expected lifespan and disease predisposition in human populations (Atzmon et al., 2010; Soerensen et al., 2012b; Codd et al., 2013). Telomere dynamics may also play an influential role in neurodegeneration, as patients with Alzheimer's showed shorter average telomere length than healthy controls (Forero et al., 2016). Therefore, understanding the links between telomeres and age-related changes on the cellular level, which can lead to pathological processes, is a main goal in aging research. However, in some animals, including common laboratory models, telomerase biology does not entirely correspond to that described in humans. The laboratory mouse, for instance, was shown to exhibit a high variability of telomere length and telomerase expression in adult tissues (Kipling and Cooke, 1990; Prowse and Greidert, 1995; Greenberg et al., 1998; Martín-Rivera et al., 1998), indicating a lesser role of constant telomere attrition as a programmed aging inducer. More importantly, *D. melanogaster* was shown to possess a fundamentally different telomere structure than found in other animals, as chromosome ends of fruit flies are capped by transposon derived sequences (Levis et al., 1993). These facts clearly limit the applicability of these species as models of human telomere function (Wright and Shay, 2000; Smogorzewska and De Lange, 2002). Nevertheless, longevity of mice was still shown to be positively affected by gene therapy induced telomerase expression (de Jesus et al., 2012).

Contrary to mice, dogs were reported to have low or no telomerase expression in normal somatic tissues, a pattern similar to that in humans (Nasir et al., 2001). It was also reported by Yazawa et al. (1999) Yazawa et al. (2001). Furthermore, tumors in dogs often showed high levels of telomerase expression, similarly to human malignancies (Vonderheide et al., 1999; Lamb et al., 2015). Although very little is known about the molecular mechanisms regulating telomere maintenance and cell cycle arrest in dogs, such findings indicate that dogs may also share basic telomere biology with humans. Importantly, telomere length was shown to be variable across different dog breeds and was in correlation with expected lifespan (Fick et al., 2012). Also, telomere length in individual dogs was found to decrease with age (Nasir et al., 2001), similarly as described in humans (Harley et al., 1990; Hastie et al., 1990; Lindsey et al., 1991).

Epigenetic Alterations

Epigenetics refers to mechanisms that modulate gene expression by determining how the transcription apparatus can access different sections of the genomic DNA. The condensation procedure, which literally packs the DNA double helix into a dense structure, called chromatin, is one of the main mechanisms to provide epigenetic regulatory potentials (**Figure 4C**). The structure of chromatin is determined by histone proteins, which constitute the basic building blocks for DNA condensation, the nucleosomes. The more densely packed heterochromatic state renders the DNA inaccessible for RNA polymerases and thus inhibits gene expression, while genes positioned in euchromatic sites are open to transcription. However, not all of these genes can be transcribed, even if appropriate activating factors are present, as another epigenetic mechanism, the methylation of cytosines at specific GC-rich sites (called CpG islands), may block transcription (**Figure 4B**). This process has an important role in cellular differentiation and probably also acts as genomic "memory," storing information about the fate of individual cells (Bird, 2002; Halley-Stott and Gurdon, 2013). Abnormal somatic alterations in DNA methylation have been linked to various diseases, including schizophrenia (Hannon et al., 2015; Wockner et al., 2015). Furthermore, changes in chromatin structure and methylation pattern are often found in cancer (Daniel and Tollefsbol, 2015), where the disruption of cellular identity and concurrent dedifferentiation is a common phenomenon.

Interestingly, the genomic methylation pattern is erased and rewritten during spermato- and oogenesis and after fertilization in mammals (Geiman and Muegge, 2009; Seisenberger et al., 2012; Smith et al., 2012). The exact role these mechanisms play in aging, however, is still unknown.

In general, systemic changes in the ratio of heterochromatic and euchromatic regions (**Figure 4D**) and a global hypomethylation of the genome have been shown to accompany aging (Gentilini et al., 2013; Pal and Tyler, 2016). When focusing on specific genomic regions, however, both hypomethylation and hypermethylation should be taken into account (Maegawa et al., 2010). Actually, senescence-related changes in the DNA methylation profile may include both the activation of pro-aging genes and the repression of anti-aging genes, as in the case of *WRN* and *LMNA* (Fraga and Esteller, 2007). The remodeling of chromatin structure, induced by methylation and acetylation of certain histone protein residues, also shows complex age-related patterns (Fraga and Esteller, 2007; Han and Brunet, 2012). Importantly, both chromatin dynamics and DNA methylation were shown to interact with other age-related genetic pathways, like telomere-length control (Blasco, 2007). In turn, the telomerase enzyme was found to affect chromatin structure and DNA repair mechanisms (Masutomi et al., 2005). In addition, the epigenetic pattern is regulated by many factors other than developmental status, like stress, exercise, and diet (Daniel and Tollefsbol, 2015), which therefore can also affect aging through altering the expression of certain genes.

Although age associated changes in chromatin structure and DNA methylation patterns have been reported in several model animals, there can be major differences between species. For example, epigenetic regulation in *C. elegans* seems to be limited to chromatin remodeling by histone modifications, as m5C DNA methylation pattern does not exist in this organism (Bird, 2002), limiting its utilization as a model to study epigenetic changes in aging. Nevertheless, the histone demethylase UTX-1 was shown to regulate aging in worms (Jin et al., 2011).

In dogs, an increasing body of evidence has suggested epigenetic regulation behind species and breed-specific traits (Koch et al., 2016; Banlaki et al., 2017; Cimarelli et al., 2017). Importantly, a recent study demonstrated that changes in methylation status in DNA regions, which were homologous to regions with known age-sensitive methylation patterns in humans, were in strong correlation with chronological age in dogs and wolves (Thompson et al., 2017). This finding supported the applicability of the dog as a model of age-related epigenetic changes, while it also provided a molecular approach to determine the biological age of individual canines.

Regulation of Epigenetic Pattern

The regulation and maintenance of the epigenetic pattern are coordinated by various enzymes, which act downstream of metabolic and signaling pathways. Altered functions of these enzymes were shown to have a major impact on health and aging. Most importantly, *sirtuin* genes were among the first shown to affect longevity in yeast (Kaeberlein et al., 1999), *C. elegans* (Tissenbaum and Guarente, 2001), *Drosophila* (Rogina and Helfand, 2004), and mice (Calvanese et al., 2009). Sirtuins exert various enzymatic functions, including histone deacetylation, and thus play a key role in the maintenance of chromatin structure (Longo and Kennedy, 2006; Fraga and Esteller, 2007). They also interact with many signaling and metabolic pathways, and regulate oxidative metabolism, stress response, autophagy, and the maintenance of telomeres (Jia et al., 2012; Kim et al., 2012). In mammals, seven *sirtuins* are known with divergent functions (Guarente, 2011) and at least three of them—*SIRT1*, *SIRT3*, and *SIRT6*—have been implicated to modulate aging. Importantly, polymorphisms in *sirtuin* genes have been actually linked to human longevity (Kim et al., 2012; Albani et al., 2014).

Sirtuins and other histone-modifying enzymes, together with DNA methyltransferases, have been barely studied in dogs so far. However, as the sequence and function of *sirtuin* genes show a highly conserved nature (Greiss and Gartner, 2009; Gaur et al., 2017), they are likely to play similar roles in the aging of dogs as in other species. In fact, altered expression of *sirtuin* genes, mainly that of *SIRT1*, have been implicated in canine tumors (Marfe et al., 2012), similarly as in humans (Brooks and Gu, 2009). Several sirtuin-targeting drugs have been proposed as promising pharmacological interventions to fight disease and aging (Dai et al., 2018); therefore, they are likely to be utilized in the future as anti-aging therapeutics and may be applied in dogs as well. In this regard, some compounds that interact with histone-regulating enzymes have already been tested in dogs for various reasons. For example, the histone deacetylase inhibitors AR-42 and panobiostat showed promising results in dog cell line models of prostate cancer and B-cell lymphoma, respectively (Elshafae et al., 2017; Dias et al., 2018). More importantly, resveratrol, which has sirtuin-activating effect (Gertz et al., 2012), was reported to positively affect the immune function of healthy pet dogs (Mathew et al., 2018) and it also effectively inhibited the growth of canine hemangiosarcoma *in vitro* (Alderete et al., 2017). Actually, resveratrol is one of the most comprehensively studied naturally occurring compounds with suggested beneficial effects on health and aging. It was shown to activate SIRT1 and improve mitochondrial function in mice (Lagouge et al., 2006) and to reverse age-related cognitive decline in learning and memory in rats (Gocmez et al., 2016). However, its longevity benefits are still dubious. For example, it only increased the relative survival of mice when the animals received a high calorie diet (Baur et al., 2006). Longitudinal follow-up studies on family dogs may help to clarify this question, as these animals represent a naturally variable population regarding diet and genetic background.

Age-Related Changes in Gene Expression

Alterations in the epigenetic pattern, together with the availability of transcription factors and activation of signaling pathways, can influence the whole expressed mRNA content (the transcriptome) in cells. Not surprisingly, altered gene expression patterns were shown to correlate with aging in mice, humans, and dogs (Lee et al., 1999; Lee et al., 2000; Lu et al., 2004; Zahn et al., 2007; Swanson et al., 2009). Comparisons between species-specific expression profiles have already been implicated as powerful tools to identify evolutionary conserved regulatory pathways (de Magalhães et al., 2009). In this regard, further gene expression data from dogs, especially from individuals with CCD, may also help researchers to pinpoint the shared molecular pathways of human and canine neurodegeneration.

The expression of some microRNAs (miRNAs), which are small non-coding RNAs with important regulatory functions, was also shown to correlate with aging in humans and mice (Somel et al., 2010; Drummond et al., 2011; Inukai et al., 2012; Zhang et al., 2012). Furthermore, age-associated miRNAs—named as gero-miRNAs—were identified in various organisms and were shown to target mRNAs associated with longevity pathways (Gonskikh and Polacek, 2017). Thus, characterization of gero-miRNAs would be a crucial step in dog aging research to further support the role of the dog as a translational model of human aging. Efforts have already been made to provide a detailed annotation of canine miRNAs (Penso-Dolfin et al., 2016), including the establishment of a miRNA tissue atlas in Beagle dogs (Koenig et al., 2016).

Disruption of Proteostasis

Proteins represent the key functional components of cells. The totality of all protein types expressed simultaneously in a cell is called the proteome. Proteome integrity is indispensable for the optimal functionality of cells; therefore, several mechanisms have evolved to maintain its homeostasis—called proteostasis. Impairments in proteostasis can lead to cellular senescence and even severe diseases, called proteinopathies, which mainly affect the CNS and are caused by the excessive accumulation and aggregation of misfolded proteins (Pievani et al., 2014). Loss of proteostasis is hypothesized to be a general attribute of aging cells across different taxa (Koga et al., 2011). For example, it was reported to be an early sign of aging in worms (Ben-Zvi et al., 2009) and to be a characteristic change during both premature and normal aging in mice (Wilson et al., 2015).

Proteostasis is maintained by the orchestrated function of mechanisms, which provide protein quality control, support the folding of synthesized proteins, protect them from various stressors, and eventually remove aberrant or senescent proteins from the cell. The folding and stability of proteins are mainly supervised by so called chaperone proteins, while the efficient removal of unnecessary, damaged, or senescent proteins is handled by two machineries: the ubiquitin-proteasome system (UPS) and the autophagy-lysosome pathway.

Chaperones and Protein Quality Control

Chaperone proteins play an important role in the post-translational maturation of nascent proteins by facilitating their folding. They also function as protectors of mature proteins under various stressful conditions, by helping to maintain their natural conformation and by preventing aggregation. Actually, the first identified chaperones were named heat shock proteins (Hsp), because their expression was induced by elevated temperatures. Importantly, many of these stress responsive chaperones were reported to show reduced expression with aging (Calderwood et al., 2009), and genetic manipulations that affected the expression of certain heat shock proteins resulted in altered aging phenotypes in model organisms. Overexpression or upregulation of Hsp-s was shown to extend lifespan, together with providing increased stress resistance, in both worms and flies (Walker and Lithgow, 2003; Morrow et al., 2004; Chiang et al., 2012), while reduced chaperone function caused accelerated aging in mice (Min et al., 2008).

In humans, chaperones, together with other proteostasis maintenance mechanisms, were suggested to play important roles in neurodegenerative diseases (Morimoto, 2008). This role, however, may not be entirely protective, as some Hsp-s were actually indicated to augment propagation of malformed proteins in proteinopathies (Dickey et al., 2007; Luo et al., 2007).

In dogs, the few studies that investigated chaperone proteins in relation to aging reported similar age-related changes as in humans. For example, blood levels of the Hsp70 chaperone were shown to decrease with age in dogs (Alexander et al., 2018), similarly to what had been previously reported in humans (Deguchi et al., 1988). Interestingly, a research group that investigated the hippocampi of donated pet dogs from various breeds (Ghi et al., 2009) reported an age-related increase in Hsp90 levels. This finding could indicate both a compensatory response to the accumulation of damaged proteins and a more direct link between Hsp90 and age-related neural decline in dogs, similarly as it was suggested in humans, where Hsp90 was implicated as a factor that may actually drive spreading of taupathy (Dickey et al., 2007; Luo et al., 2007). Based on these possible similarities between canine and human chaperone functions in the brain, dogs can be suitable to test various pharmacological interventions and small molecular chaperones (Calamini et al., 2012), which modify or complement chaperone activity to support proteostasis and reduce neurodegenerative pathologies. Such interventions have already been successfully tested in rodents (Gehrig et al., 2012).

The Ubiquitin-Proteasome System

The UPS is responsible for the selective removal of misfolded and senescent proteins in cells. Mutations in genes that encode subunits of the proteasome and proteins responsible for proteasomal targeting can lead to accumulation of aberrant proteins, and have been actually linked to several types of neurodegenerative diseases, including Alzheimer's disease and Parkinson's disease (Zheng et al., 2016). Especially in the case of AD, causative links were described between disturbances in the UPS and progression of the disease (de Vrij et al., 2004; Liu et al., 2014).

Importantly, the UPS was also linked to longevity in model organisms. In flies, loss-of-function mutations in the ubiquitin activating enzyme E1 were shown to reduce lifespan and cause disturbances in motor function (Liu and Pfleger, 2013); meanwhile, extended lifespan in worms was associated with increased expression of a proteasome subunit (Vilchez et al., 2012).

In dogs, an increased density of ubiquitinated bodies was reported to be present in the brains of aged individuals (Ferrer et al., 1993; Borràs et al., 1999), and further signs of impaired proteostasis were also indicated (reviewed by Romanucci and Della Salda, 2015). The same group that reported age-related increase in the Hsp90 chaperone in dog brains also found incongruent changes in the abundance of various proteasomal proteins, suggesting complex impairments and compensatory mechanisms in the regulation of the UPS in aged dogs (Ghi et al., 2009).

Interestingly, a homozygous lethal mutation in the proteasome β2 subunit was reported as the possible causative variant behind the unique harlequin coat color of Great Dane dogs (Clark et al., 2011). Further studies may shed light on the possible health or longevity effects of this mutation.

Importantly, as proteasome activation by pharmacological agents has been proposed as a promising approach to delay aging and the development of age-related diseases (Chondrogianni et al., 2015), dogs may provide an appropriate large animal model for pre-clinical testing of these interventions, especially in the case of brain pathologies.

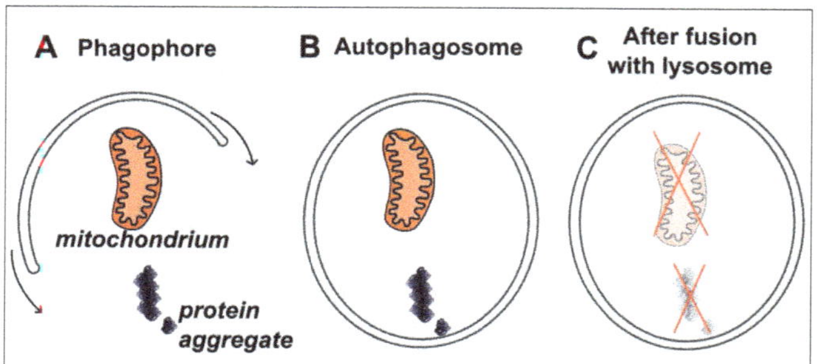

FIGURE 5 | Macroautophagy. This figure depicts macroautophagy, which is the only mechanism in cells able to remove aberrant mitochondria and large protein aggregates. **(A)** First, formation of a double membrane structure, the phagophore, is initiated around the target. **(B)** The expansion of the double membrane structure around the target will eventually form a vesicle, called autophagosome. **(C)** When the autophagosome fuses with a lysosome, degradation of the autophagosome's content can take place and resulting molecular compounds can be recycled thereafter.

Autophagy

While the UPS eliminates individual proteins or small aggregates tagged by ubiquitin, the autophagic machinery is capable of targeting greater amounts of cellular content for lysosomal degradation, including mitochondria and large protein aggregates. In fact, autophagy is a fundamental mechanism in eukaryotic cells and was often found indispensable for the ontogenesis of multicellular organisms, including the embryonic development of mice (Cecconi and Levine, 2008) and the metamorphosis of flies (Juhász et al., 2003). Three main types of autophagy have been described in the literature. In the case of macroautophagy, targeted cytoplasmic constituents get isolated by double membrane vesicles, called autophagosomes. These then fuse with lysosomes, leading to the degradation of their content into small molecular components (**Figure 5**), which can be recycled thereafter (Klionsky, 2005). The other two types, microautophagy and chaperone-mediated autophagy, utilize different targeting mechanisms and may be less capable for bulk degradation of intracellular content. Therefore, the name autophagy usually refers to macroautophagy in the literature. In general, all types of autophagy play a crucial role in cellular metabolism (Rabinowitz and White, 2010); pathogen resistance (Levine, 2005; Deretic, 2006); inflammation (Levine et al., 2011); and cleansing of macromolecular debris, like protein aggregates seen in Alzheimer's disease (Rubinsztein, 2006; Mizushima et al., 2008; Nixon and Yang, 2011) and in programmed cell death (Tsujimoto and Shimizu, 2005; Ouyang et al., 2012). Impairments in autophagy were linked to several disease phenotypes in model organisms, as well as in dogs (listed below) and humans (Levine and Kroemer, 2008). Importantly, reduced autophagic activity in the adult brain was shown to promote neurodegeneration in mice (Hara et al., 2006; Komatsu et al., 2006).

Based on these findings, it is not surprising that autophagy has been proposed as a major factor in aging regulation. In *C. elegans*, loss-of-function mutations in autophagy genes shortened lifespan, while disruption of signaling pathways that downregulate autophagy led to a significant increase in expected lifespan (Hars et al., 2007; Tóth et al., 2008). Similar findings were reported from yeast, flies, and mice (Juhász et al., 2007; Simonsen et al., 2008; Eisenberg et al., 2009; Pyo et al., 2013), although with a less pronounced lifespan extension in the latter. Importantly, the longevity effect of caloric restriction (CR)—which is discussed in the **Supplementary Section** "Beyond Genetics"—was shown to be dependent on the proper functioning of autophagy (Jia and Levine, 2007). Chaperon-mediated autophagy was also reported to directly affect cellular senescence through the selective elimination of soluble proteins (Cuervo and Dice, 2000; Massey et al., 2006;

Zhang and Cuervo, 2008). In the livers of aged mice, but not of young animals, impaired function of chaperone-mediated autophagy resulted in increased loss of proteostasis (Schneider et al., 2015).

Surprisingly, cohort studies have reported little or no association between autophagy linked genes and longevity in humans, implicating that the effects of mutations, which alter autophagic activity, are less pronounced, or that such mutations are not common in people. Nevertheless, the role autophagy has in neurodegenerative processes is indisputable in humans (Jiang and Mizushima, 2014). For example, mutations in the *WD repeat domain 45* (*WDR45*) gene, which functions in formation of the double membrane structures ("phagophores"), were shown to cause static encephalopathy of childhood with neurodegeneration in adulthood (SENDA). Also, both Alzheimer's and Parkinson's diseases were characterized by accumulation of autophagic vacuoles, indicating a disruption in their turnover (Nixon et al., 2005; Nixon and Yang, 2011). Consonantly, loss-of-function mutations in the *Parkinson's disease associated protein DJ-1* gene were linked to reduced basal levels of autophagy (Krebiehl et al., 2010). On the other hand, enhanced levels of autophagy have been linked to neuron loss in ALS (Sasaki, 2011; Chen et al., 2012), marking it as a possible driver of neurodegeneration in this case. Such controversial findings may result from the complex roles autophagy plays in cellular homeostasis, stress resistance, and also in programmed cell death (White and DiPaola, 2009; Tung et al., 2012), calling for further research to clarify its contribution to different types of neurodegeneration. In this regard, the dog could serve as a model more closely related to human physiology than rodents. Some canine hereditary diseases have already been linked to mutations in autophagy genes and many of these diseases have human homologs. For example, a polymorphism in the *Ras-Related Protein Rab-24* (*RAB24*) gene, a member of the RAS oncogene family, which encodes a protein necessary for autophagosome trafficking, was found responsible for juvenile onset ataxia in some breeds (Agler et al., 2014). A missense mutation in the *autophagy related 4D cysteine peptidase* (*ATG4D*) gene was linked to vacuolar storage deficiency and neurodegeneration in Lagotto Romagnolo dogs (Kyöstilä et al., 2015). A study investigating juvenile onset neuroaxonal dystrophy in Spanish Water Dogs identified a non-synonymous mutation in the *tectonin beta-propeller repeat containing 2* (*TECPR2*) gene, which had been linked to autophagosome formation (Hahn et al., 2015). A very similar type of neuroaxonal dystrophy exists in humans; hence, this finding could have actually suggested a possible genetic background to look for in affected people.

DM is another example of a naturally occurring neurodegenerative disease in dogs and shows a high degree of similarity to human ALS. Both DM and ALS have been linked to mutations in the ROS neutralizing *SOD1* gene, suggesting a shared genetic and metabolic background. Importantly, the possible contribution of autophagy to motor neuron loss was reported to be controversial both in DM (Ogawa et al., 2015) and in ALS (Chen et al., 2012). Autophagy also has a similarly controversial role in muscular atrophy in humans and dogs (Sandri, 2010; Pagano et al., 2015). Altogether, these findings indicate many homologies between dogs and humans regarding the regulation of autophagy in aging and disease.

Deregulation of Nutrient Sensing

Cellular metabolism, protein synthesis, and autophagy are strictly regulated by various signaling pathways (**Figure 6**) (Martindale and Holbrook, 2002; He and Klionsky, 2009). Most of these have evolved to synchronize cell growth and metabolism with nutrient availability; hence, they are often referred to as nutrient sensing pathways. Many of them converge on the target of rapamycin (TOR) kinase (**Figure 6A**), a main factor in determining rates of protein turnover and metabolism (Wullschleger et al., 2006). In mammals, the TOR kinase may function in different complexes, named mTORC1 or mTORC2, depending on its protein partners. The mTORC1 complex, which includes the regulatory associated protein of MTOR (RPTOR) protein, corresponds to the invertebrate TOR complex in its regulatory interactions, while mTORC2 controls other intracellular processes. Knock-down of TOR expression by RNA interference was shown to increase lifespan of *C. elegans* by threefold (Vellai et al., 2003). Later, similar effects of inhibiting TOR or its homologs were reported in *S. cerevisiae* (Kaeberlein et al., 2005), *D. melanogaster* (Kapahi et al., 2004), and laboratory mice (Wu et al., 2013), emphasizing its conserved role in the aging process (Kapahi et al., 2010).

Importantly, the function of mTOR can be efficiently inhibited by rapamycin, which is an already approved immunosuppressant in human medicine, and therefore has been proposed as a promising anti-aging compound to be used in humans. However, it was reported to cause severe side effects in medical dosages (Hartford and Ratain, 2007). Therefore, optimal dosages, which do not cause undesirable syndromes, yet still exert longevity promoting effects should be carefully determined in preclinical studies. Actually, pharmaceutical studies have already been initiated to investigate the effects of rapamycin on the lifespan of dogs (Kaeberlein et al., 2016; Urfer et al., 2017).

One of the main signaling pathways that regulate TOR activity is the insulin and IGF1 signaling (IIS) pathway (**Figure 6B**). It was first linked to aging when strains of *C. elegans* with doubled lifespan revealed a mutation in *daf-2*, the worm homologue of the *IGF1 receptor (IGF1R)* gene (Kenyon et al., 1993). Later, a threefold elongation in the non-replicative lifespan of *S. cerevisiae* was also linked to two genes that functioned in the glucose sensing pathway (Thevelein and de Winde, 1999). In flies and mice with hypomorphic alleles of *IGF1R* homologs, a significant increase in lifespan was observed together with characteristic pleiotropic effects (Tatar et al., 2001; Holzenberger et al., 2003). However, the longevity effect was less pronounced in mice, pointing at the possibility that the relative contribution of IIS to aging regulation may differ in various taxa.

Importantly, comparisons between centenarian and younger human cohorts also showed associations between expected lifespan and serum IGF1 levels or genetic polymorphisms in

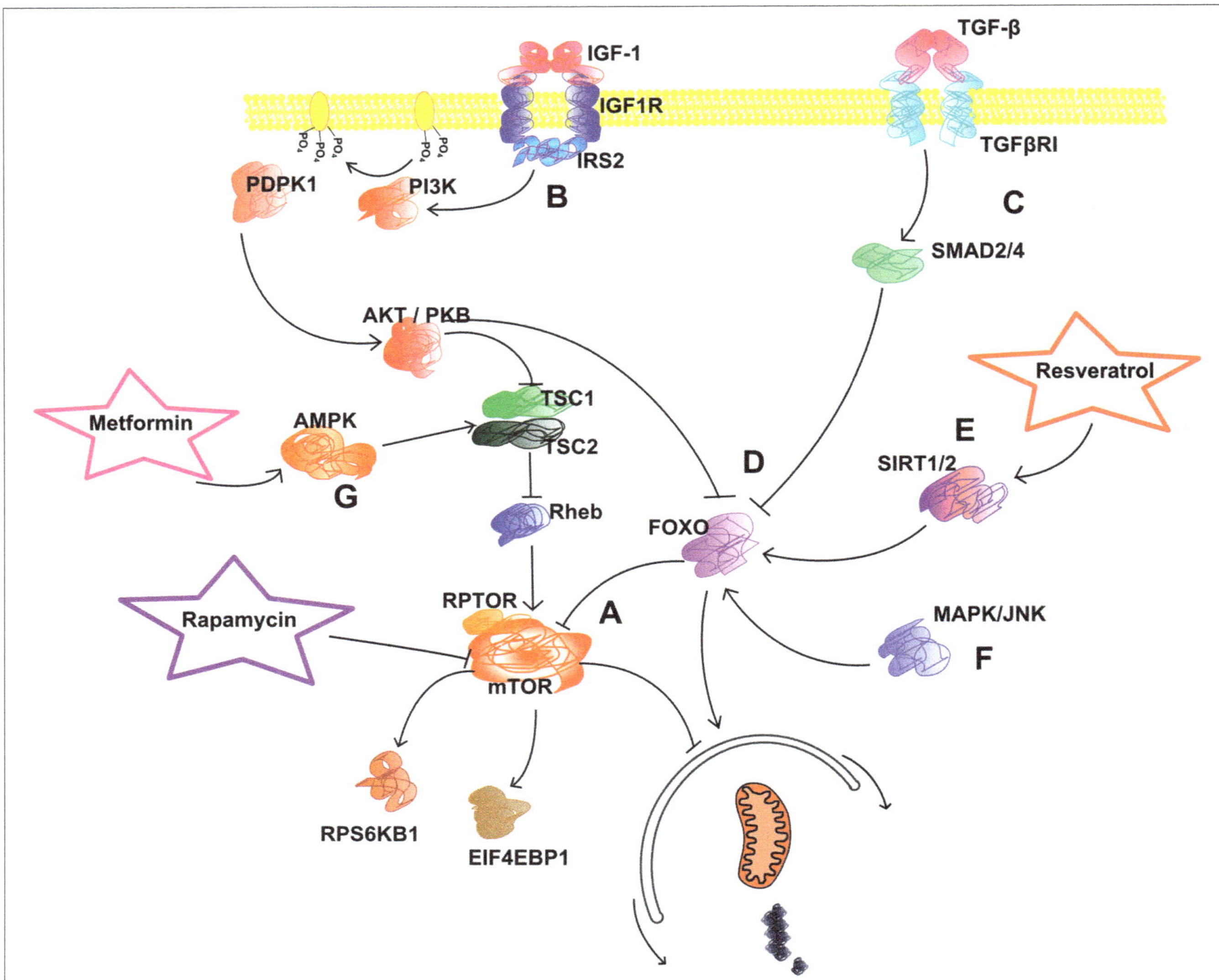

FIGURE 6 | Signaling pathways. This figure illustrates some of the many signaling pathways that have been connected to aging. Activating interactions are shown with arrows, while inhibiting interactions are represented by bar headed lines. **(A)** Almost all of the age-related signaling pathways converge on the metabolic signal integrator mTORC1 complex, which includes the mTOR kinase together with RPTOR and other proteins. mTORC1 integrates stimuli to fine-tune metabolic processes, protein synthesis, cell growth, and autophagy. Downstream targets of mTORC1 include ribosomal proteins and translation initiation factors, like RPS6KB1 and EIF4EBP1, as well as ULK1, which is an activator of autophagy. As its name indicates, mTOR is the main target of rapamycin, which inhibits its function. **(B)** The IGF1 signaling is considered to be the main modulator that links autophagy to aging. Upregulation of this pathway leads to repression of autophagy and activation of protein synthesis by mTOR. This pathway includes many proteins, most of which have kinase activity. The PI3K enzymes transmit the signal from the IGF1 receptor by phosphorylating phosphatidylinositol molecules in the membrane, which then activate PDPK1. From here, the signal is forwarded to AKT (also known as PKB) by phosphorylation. AKT then inhibits the function of the TSC1 and TSC2 proteins, and consequently releases RHEB from inhibition. RHEB directly binds and activates the mTORC1 complex. **(C)** Another signaling pathway, which acts parallel to IGF1, is the TGF-β signalization. It is implicated in cellular growth control and also in tumorigenesis and inhibits autophagy. SMAD proteins transduce the TGF-β signal to downstream targets. An important target of SMAD2/4 is the FOXO gene family. **(D)** FOXO transcription factors have an evolutionary conserved function in aging regulation and integrate several pathways to upregulate autophagy and inhibit mTORC1. **(E)** Sirtuins (SIRT1/2) act contrary to the TGF-β pathway as they upregulate FOXO and thus autophagy. Resveratrol and caloric restriction exert their anti-aging effect through the activation of sirtuins. **(F)** The MAPK proteins were also shown to play a role in aging by regulating FOXO. They serve as important early responsive elements of different cellular stimuli and also play a role in apoptotic cell death induction in the case of UV-light damage. **(G)** AMPK integrates metabolite sensing information and acts contrary to the IGF1 pathway: activation of AMPK leads to down-regulation of mTOR and activation of autophagy. AMPK is the main target of metformin. mTOR, mechanistic target of rapamycin; RPTOR, regulatory associated protein of MTOR; RPS6KB1, ribosomal protein S6 kinase, 70kD, polypeptide 1; EIF4EBP1, eukaryotic translation initiation factor 4E binding protein 1; ULK1, unc-51 like autophagy activating kinase 1; IGF1, insulin-like growth factor 1; PIK3, phosphatidylinositol-4,5-bisphosphate 3-kinase; PDPK1, 3-phosphoinositide dependent protein kinase 1; AKT, AKT serine/threonine kinase 1; TSC1, tuberous sclerosis 1; TSC2, tuberous sclerosis 2; RHEB, Ras homolog, mTORC1 binding protein b; complex 1; TGF-β, transforming growth factor β; SMAD, MAD, mothers against decapentaplegic; FOXO, forkhead box O; SIRT, sirtuin; MAPK, mitogen-activated protein kinase; AMPK, adenosine monophosphate kinase.

related genes (Barbieri et al., 2003; Van Heemst et al., 2005). Furthermore, functional variants in *IGF1R* were shown to be enriched in centenarians (Suh et al., 2008). Polymorphisms in other genes of the IIS pathway were also linked to longevity in GWAS, although not without contradictions (Soerensen et al., 2012a). In fact, some studies reported a decrease in GH and IGF1 plasma levels during normal aging (Breese et al., 1991; Sonntag et al., 1997). In this regard, it was hypothesized that the reduction in IGF1 levels may actually serve as a first line compensatory mechanism when age-related damage starts to accumulate in cells (Schumacher et al., 2008; López-Otín et al., 2013). Although low basic IIS signaling may delay aging, the overcompensation resulting from continuously accumulating damage in aged individuals may lead to insufficiencies in IGF1 signaling, and this can cause further decline. This effect may be particularly relevant in the case of neural aging, because the brain has special metabolic properties and a high need for optimal glucose levels. In support of this hypothesis, some age-related neurodegenerative states were linked to low IGF1 levels (Sonntag et al., 2000; Sonntag et al., 2005; Moloney et al., 2010). In addition, lower plasma IGF1 levels were shown to impair vascular maintenance in the brain (Sonntag et al., 1997). In this regard, dogs, which are more similar to humans in brain physiology and function than rodents, also seem promising to further unfold the relationship between IGF1 signaling and healthy aging.

Importantly, functional mutations in the *IGF1* and *IGF1R* genes have already been linked to body size variability in dogs (Sutter et al., 2007; Hoopes et al., 2012; Rimbault et al., 2013), similarly to humans and laboratory animals (Liu et al., 1993; Ishida et al., 1998; Perry and Dominy, 2009). The notion that small dog breeds usually live longer than large breeds (Galis et al., 2007; Greer et al., 2007; Kraus et al., 2013) also hints at the potential role of the IIS pathway in canine lifespan determination. In fact, the genomic region harboring the *IGF1* locus was linked to size and lifespan across different breeds (Jones et al., 2008) and serum IGF1 levels were shown to correlate with age and obesity (Greer et al., 2011) in individual dogs.

Some other pathways linked to body size in dogs (Rimbault et al., 2013; Schoenebeck and Ostrander, 2014) are also known to regulate TOR and autophagy. The *SMAD family member 2* (*SMAD2*) gene, which functions in the transforming growth factor beta (TGF-β) pathway (**Figure 6C**) (Vellai, 2009), was associated with body size (Rimbault et al., 2013) and was previously found to be in linkage with mortality of dog breeds (Jones et al., 2008). The *growth hormone receptor* (*GHR*) and *growth* hormone (*GH*) genes, which also modulate dogs' body size, were shown to affect longevity in humans (Soerensen et al., 2012a; van der Spoel et al., 2016), and in mice (Bartke et al., 2001; Flurkey et al., 2001; Kinney et al., 2001; Amador-Noguez et al., 2004).

Both IIS and TGF-β signaling have several targets beyond TOR, and many of them were implicated in aging. For example, the forkhead box O (FOXO) transcription factors are targeted by both IGF1 and TGF-β signaling (**Figure 6D**) and were shown to have an important role in tumor suppression (Greer and Brunet, 2005) and age-related diseases (Hesp et al., 2015). The worm homologue of the mammalian *FOXO* genes, *daf-16*, was one of the first genes linked to extreme longevity in *C. elegans*, as it was found necessary for the longevity effect observed in *daf-2* deficient worms (Kenyon et al., 1993; Larsen et al., 1995; Lin et al., 1997; Ruvkun et al., 1997). Out of the four mammalian orthologues, *FOXO3a* has been associated with aging in human cohort studies (Willcox et al., 2008; Anselmi et al., 2009; Soerensen et al., 2010). *FOXO1a* SNPs were also reported to affect longevity, however, in a gender-specific manner (Li et al., 2009). In addition, FOXO3 was shown to regulate autophagy in skeletal muscle and plays a role in muscular atrophy (Mammucari et al., 2007). Despite the emphasized role of *FOXOs* in disease and aging, the canine homologues have not yet been studied in detail.

Sirtuins (**Figure 6E**) and the 5' AMP-activated protein kinase (AMPK) also play an important role in nutrient sensing. Sirtuins function as nicotinamide adenine dinucleotide (NAD) dependent protein deacetylases, sensing the levels of NAD in cells. Decreased NAD levels were shown to reduce their activity, and thus NAD replacement therapies have been suggested as possible anti-aging interventions (Chini et al., 2017). AMPK detects the levels of adenosine monophosphate (AMP) in cells, and it is able to counteract IGF1 signaling by inhibiting TOR (Inoki et al., 2003; Gwinn et al., 2008) and activating FOXO3a (Sanchez et al., 2012). It was also suggested to play a major neuroprotective role by activating the UNC-51 Like 1 (ULK1) kinase (Kim et al., 2011), a key autophagy inducing protein (Wong et al., 2013).

Both sirtuins and AMPK are targets of several proposed anti-aging drugs. For example, the anti-diabetic drugs, metformin and acarbose, were both shown to exert an anti-aging effect in model animals (Anisimov et al., 2011; Cabreiro et al., 2013; Martin-Montalvo et al., 2013; Harrison et al., 2014) and to modulate various aging-related intracellular processes, including the activation of AMPK (Cho et al., 2015; Lu et al., 2015; Chan et al., 2016). Importantly, metformin was actually reported to decrease mortality of diabetic people in comparison to patients treated with other drugs in a retrospective large-scale study (Bannister et al., 2014). Consequently, metformin has been suggested as a promising candidate for anti-aging interventions (Barzilai et al., 2016). It may also be easily applied in family dogs to test its longevity enhancing potential, because it was already shown to have relatively mild side effects in dogs (Heller, 2007).

However, it is important to note that all of these drugs, including rapamycin, may exert pleiotropic effects in organisms through various cellular signaling and regulatory mechanisms. For example, metformin was implicated to modify the composition of the gut microbiome in diabetic patients (Forslund et al., 2015), which in turn can indirectly affect aging and neural function (see below in the section *Microbiome*). Such pleiotropic effects should be thoroughly considered in humans and family dogs, as both are exposed to variable environmental stimuli, have diverse genetic background, and may use other medications, which can alter the mechanisms of actions of anti-aging compounds through complex interactions.

A fairly recently emerged possible regulator of aging that interacts with IGF1 signaling and FOXO activity is the klotho hormone, which was first identified in mice as a longevity factor (Kuro-o et al., 1997; Kurosu et al., 2005). The *klotho* (*KL*)

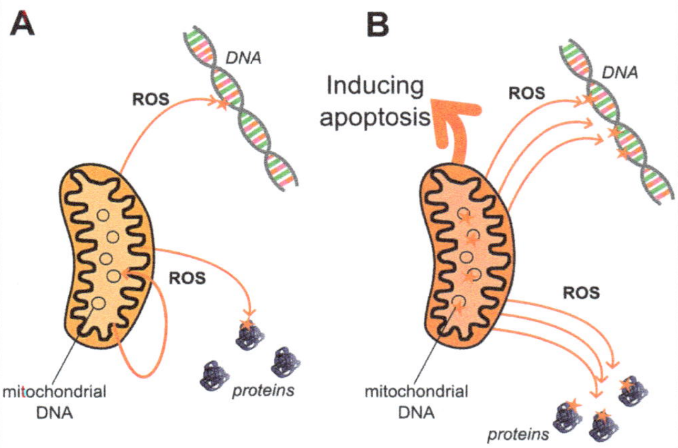

FIGURE 7 | Mitochondria and oxidative stress. **(A)** Mitochondria represent the main source for reactive oxygen species (ROS) within eukaryotic cells as the oxidative respiration processes take place in the inner membrane of mitochondria, utilizing a special electron transport chain. Increased respiration rate due to metabolic changes and reduced antioxidant accessibility may also increase generation of ROS, which can damage the mitochondrial genome as well (indicated by thick arrow). **(B)** Accumulation of mutations in the mitochondrial genome may lead to malfunction in the electron transport chain in aberrant mitochondria that consequently produce an elevated rate of ROS. Removal of aberrant mitochondria is a key process for maintaining oxidative balance in cells.

gene represents an example of longevity genes that are missing from invertebrate models, but show functional polymorphisms associated with human longevity (Arking et al., 2002).

Mitochondrial Dysfunction

Nutrient sensing pathways converge on the regulation of mitochondrial activity, as these organelles are the main sources of energy (in the form of adenosine triphosphate, ATP) in eukaryotic cells under normal circumstances, when enough oxygen is present. The availability of nutrients determines the rate of mitochondrial respiration, which, however, generates not only ATP but also chemical by-products, including ROS (**Figure 7A**). The oxidative burden created by mitochondria may be especially high in neurons, which solely depend on aerobic mitochondrial respiration as energy source. In accordance with this, associations between chronological age and a higher ROS production rate of mitochondria in brain cells were demonstrated in rodents (Navarro and Boveris, 2004; Petrosillo et al., 2008), humans (Mecocci et al., 1993), and also in dogs (Head et al., 2009). Oxidative DNA lesions could also occur in the mitochondrial genome and consequently modify gene expression and optimal function of mitochondria, possibly leading to a positive feedback mechanism in the generation of extensive levels of ROS. In fact, age-related changes in mitochondrial gene expression profiles were reported in mice (Manczak et al., 2005) and the accumulation of mitochondrial DNA mutations, mainly deletions, in certain brain regions was linked to impaired mitochondrial respiration in humans (Corral-Debrinski et al., 1992; Kraytsberg et al., 2006). Importantly, mitochondrial dysfunction is considered to be a main driver of the pathophysiology of neurodegenerative diseases, including Alzheimer's disease, Parkinson's disease, and ALS (Lin and Beal, 2006). For example, gain-of-function mutations in the *Leucine-rich repeat kinase 2 (LRRK2)* gene causing autosomal dominant form of PD (Di Fonzo et al., 2005) were shown to result in hampered mitochondrial function (Mortiboys et al., 2010). Although the generation of malfunctioning mitochondria may be counterbalanced by elevated levels of mitophagy, a form of macroautophagy that is able to degrade mitochondria, it is not yet clear in the literature how mitophagic activity is generally changed in affected cells of PD patients (Chu, 2019).

The role of mitochondrial dysfunction and increased oxidative burden in neural aging was also investigated in dogs. In general, dog brains were shown to accumulate oxidative damage with age (for more details, see the section *Genomic Instability*). In a study published by Head et al., 2009, mitochondrial ROS production and complex I driven respiration rate showed significant alterations between old and young laboratory Beagle dogs from the same colony, with aged dogs having higher ROS production and lower respiration rate. The same study reported that a diet enriched with antioxidants and mitochondrial cofactors improved mitochondrial respiration rate and reduced ROS production in aged dogs, and also had a positive effect on their cognitive performance. In another study, a ketosis-inducing diet was shown to modify mitochondrial function and, to some extent, reduce amyloid-β deposition in dog brains (Studzinski et al., 2008). Interestingly, Christie et al. reported in 2009 that short-term supplementation with lipoic acid (LA), which is both an important mitochondrial cofactor and a powerful antioxidant, did not improve cognitive function of aged Beagle dogs, contrary to their previous findings where LA had been used together with other antioxidants (Cotman et al., 2002; Milgram et al., 2002a; Milgram et al., 2002b). Furthermore, another mitochondrial cofactor, acetyl-L-carnitine (ALCAR), when supplemented in itself, was shown to decrease cognitive performance (Christie et al., 2009). In a paper, Snigdha et al., 2016 who also failed to replicate findings about the beneficial effects of antioxidant enriched diet on the cognition of aged Beagle dogs, suggested that these controversies could have resulted from differences in the baseline nutrition of dogs.

Nevertheless, such findings could also result from a more complicated interaction between ROS and aging, as it was suggested by several authors, who re-evaluated the classical theories about the connection between mitochondria, ROS, and general longevity, based on the increasing body of experimental evidences (Hekimi et al., 2011; López-Otín et al., 2013). Accordingly, the ambiguous results listed above could result from altered mitochondrial homeostasis (mithormesis) in cells and not solely from impaired mitochondrial respiration and ROS overproduction. The concept of mithormesis suggests that mild mitochondrial stressors may actually benefit cellular health and longevity (López-Otín et al., 2013). Such minor stress, which, for example, can be induced by pharmaceutical agents, can boost mitochondrial turnover and activate defensive mechanisms (Haigis and Yankner, 2010). As it was shown that malfunctioning mitochondria can also directly affect aging by other mechanisms than increased oxidative stress (Trifunovic et al., 2004; Vermulst et al., 2008; Edgar et al., 2009; Hiona et al., 2010), for example by inducing apoptosis (Kroemer et al., 2007) (**Figure 7B**), elevated mitochondrial turnover can actually protect cells from these deleterious effects. Since both resveratrol and metformin have been hypothesized to be mild mitochondrial toxins, they may also exert their anti-aging effect at least partly by inducing mithormesis (López-Otín et al., 2013).

Altogether, mitochondria-targeting interventions may require mindful considerations, especially in populations with high genetic variability. Genetic variants in mitochondrial genomes are known to cause disorders in humans (Koopman et al., 2012), and they may also substantially alter the capability of cells to cope with mitochondrial poisons (Finsterer and Frank, 2016). This means that interactions between mitochondrial genotypes and specific chemical compounds should also be considered in anti-aging intervention studies. In this regard, dogs can again become ideal models with good translatability. Several mitochondrial diseases are known in dogs, which have human homologs, such as the sensory ataxic neuropathy found in Golden Retriever dogs (Baranowska et al., 2009) or the familial dilated cardiomyopathy in Doberman Pinschers (Meurs et al., 2012). As several promising anti-aging drugs are likely to be tested in dogs in preclinical studies, looking into their effects on mitochondrial function and testing their possible interactions with mitochondrial genotypes can be highly relevant for humans.

Cellular Senescence

All the mechanisms discussed so far act congruently to modulate cellular metabolism, growth, proliferation, and, eventually, senescence, which is characterized by a permanent cell cycle arrest and stereotyped phenotypic changes (Campisi and d'Adda di Fagagna, 2007; Collado et al., 2007). Specific mechanisms serve as effectors of senescence in response to unrepaired DNA damage, mitochondrial malfunction, and other forms of excessive stress. Most famously, telomere attrition represents a somewhat genetically programmed route to cellular senescence as it was implied from experiments with human fibroblasts (Harley et al., 1990; Allsopp et al., 1992). However, the fact that cultured murine cells also reached senescence despite their telomerase positivity suggested that other mechanisms, like increased oxidative damage in cultured conditions, should have contributed to their limited proliferative potential (Sherr and DePinho, 2000).

Among other examples, the activation of the p16^{INK4a}/Rb and the p14^{ARF}/p53 signaling pathways is able to induce cellular senescence in response to time-dependent changes, including the accumulation of DNA damage (d'Adda di Fagagna, 2008). The expression of the *INK4/ARF* locus, which encodes the p16^{INK4}, p15^{INK4}, and p14^{ARF} proteins in humans, was reported to correlate with chronological age in various tissues of rodents and humans (Krishnamurthy et al., 2004; Krishnamurthy et al., 2006; Ressler et al., 2006; Liu et al., 2009b), nominating it as an ideal biomarker of aging. Importantly, the *INK4/ARF* locus can directly affect healthspan and longevity, as it was shown experimentally in mice (Matheu et al., 2009). Furthermore, simultaneous overexpression of *INK4/ARF* and *p53* caused extended lifespan in mice, accompanied by cancer resistance and reduced neural decline (Matheu et al., 2007; Carrasco-Garcia et al., 2015). The human *INK4/ARF* locus was also found to be the most strongly associated locus with several age-related pathologies in a meta-analysis of GWAS (Jeck et al., 2012), and it was associated with longevity in a smaller cohort study (Emanuele et al., 2010). Interestingly, the elevated expression and activity of p53 in itself did not increase longevity in experimental studies (García-Cao et al., 2002; Mendrysa et al., 2006). Actually, certain hyperactive variants of p53 were shown to reduce lifespan in mice, although with simultaneously prompting increased cancer resistance (Tyner et al., 2002; Dumble et al., 2007).

In this regard, it is important to note that the p14/p53 pathway, together with p16/pRb, are fundamental tumor suppressor mechanisms; therefore, they unquestionably contribute to healthy aging by forcing potentially malignant cells into a senescent state or into programmed cell death (Hickman et al., 2002).

This anti-tumor effect of induced cellular senescence can explain the contradictory findings regarding the role of p53 and other tumor suppressor mechanisms in aging (Rodier and Campisi, 2011), as a possible trade-off exists between longevity and cancer occurrence (Matheu et al., 2008).

So far, no studies have investigated the canine homologs of the *INK4/ARF* locus and *p53* in relation to aging. However, and not surprisingly, their role and regulation in tumorigenesis showed high similarities between dogs and humans (Rowell et al., 2011; Lutful Kabir et al., 2013), suggesting that their roles in aging, especially in healthy aging, are also conserved in dogs.

Accumulation of Senescent Cells in Tissues

The time-dependent upregulation of senescence inducing mechanisms means that the ratio of aged cells may gradually increase in the tissues of older individuals. Indeed, a marked elevation of senescent cell numbers was reported in old mice (Wang et al., 2009), although not in all tissues. Importantly, this accumulation process can result from both the increased generation of senescent cells and a decreased activity of macrophages that are able to eliminate aged or apoptotic cells from tissues. As the activity of the innate immune system was shown to decrease with age (Plowden et al., 2004; Mahbub et al., 2011), it is likely that reduced phagocytic capacity also contributes to organismal aging through the disrupted elimination of senescent cells (López-Otín et al., 2013). Furthermore, senescent cells were shown to produce inflammatory signals and create a special inflammatory microenvironment around themselves (Kuilman et al., 2010; Rodier and Campisi, 2011), which may directly contribute to tissue aging by creating a positive feedback loop and inducing cellular senescence in neighboring cells (Nelson et al., 2012). This so-called "bystander" effect was actually shown to modulate the number of senescent cells *in vivo* in mice (da Silva et al., 2019).

Little is known about the accumulation of senescent cells in canine tissues, although this phenomenon is also likely to show fundamental similarities with other mammalian species. As there is a growing interest toward pharmacological approaches to deplete senescent cells in tissues by specific apoptosis inducing agents (senolytic drugs) (Kirkland et al., 2017), dogs may eventually be involved in testing these types of anti-aging interventions.

Stem Cell Exhaustion

Tissue renewal depends on the abundance and replicative capacity of tissue-specific stem cells, which can replace cells lost by terminal senescence or apoptosis. Thus, the age-related increase in cellular senescence may also result in elevated stem cell activation and differentiation, eventually causing the depletion of stem cell pools. In fact, early exhaustion of stem cells in certain tissues was shown to accelerate aging in flies and mice (Cheng et al., 2000; Kippin et al., 2005; Rera et al., 2011). Furthermore, it was shown that increased basic fibroblast growth factor (FGF2) signaling in muscle tissues of aged mice accelerated depletion of stem cells by forcing them to leave quiescent state (Chakkalakal et al., 2012).

Importantly, senescence may also directly affect stem cells, depriving them from the ability to replicate and differentiate even if they are still present in tissues. For example, hematopoietic stem cells (HSCs) were reported to have reduced replicative capacity in both aged mice and humans, mainly because of accumulating DNA damage (de Haan and Lazare, 2018). This reduction can explain the old age anemia of elderly people (Patel, 2008). Importantly, similar forms of age-associated changes in blood parameters, including anemia, were reported in dogs (Strasser et al., 1993; Radakovich et al., 2017).

Stem cell quiescence and activation is regulated by many of the already discussed aging pathways, including p53 and IIS (Liu et al., 2009a; Xian et al., 2012). Thus, pharmacological interventions that act on these could also affect stem cell dynamics. In this regard, the inhibition of mTOR was shown to have beneficial effects on aging by promoting cellular rejuvenation (Castilho et al., 2009; Chen et al., 2009; Yilmaz et al., 2012). Furthermore, pharmacological inhibitors of the Cell Division Cycle 42 (CDC42) protein, which is an inducer of HSC senescence, were shown to promote rejuvenation of HSC pools in mice (Florian et al., 2012).

Besides pharmacological interventions, stem cell therapy has also been suggested as a possible anti-aging intervention, with highlighted promises to treat certain forms of neurodegeneration (Lindvall et al., 2004; Trounson and DeWitt, 2016). In this regard, stem cell therapy trials conducted on dogs affected with CCD or other forms of neurodegeneration could represent a crucial step before progressing to human trials. In the case of the Golden Retriever model for Duchenne muscular dystrophy, successful stem cell-based interventions had actually preceded human clinical trials (Pelatti et al., 2016). Other instances of dog stem cell therapy trials were discussed by Hoffman and Dow (2016).

Altered Intercellular Communication

In the course of evolution, several mechanisms have evolved to establish efficient communication between cells in multicellular organisms. Intercellular communication types include paracrine, endocrine, and neurocrine signaling, and all of these can be involved in the aging process. Especially hormones and other endocrine signal transducers can have a main role in systemic aging regulation. Actually, GH and the insulin/IGF1 signaling pathway belong to these main systemic regulators, most of which are supervised by the hypothalamic–pituitary–adrenal (HPA) and –thyroid axes. Endocrine signaling also involves hormones synthetized by the digestive system and reproductive glands. Furthermore, small molecules produced by gut bacteria can also have systemic effects on the host organism (Donia and Fischbach, 2015).

Neuroendocrine Signaling

The CNS mainly functions as conductor, coordinating various processes of the organism according to intrinsic and extrinsic stimuli. Signals provided by the CNS—together with the digestive system—can affect every part of the body. In this regard, "neural aging" has recently gained more focus as a central mechanism, which could impact the systemic aging of the whole organism (Weir and Mair, 2016). In support of this theory, both neuronal and intestinal genetic manipulations, which reduced mitochondrial electron transport chain function, were shown to extend lifespan in *C. elegans*, while similar manipulations in other tissues had no longevity effect (Durieux et al., 2011).

Importantly, several signaling pathways have been hypothesized to play fundamental roles in both neural senescence and systemic aging. For example, IGF1, together with the brain-derived neurotrophic factor (BDNF) and serotonin, were shown to affect brain aging and modulate metabolic changes linked to caloric restriction across the body (Mattson et al., 2004). The hypothalamus also has major implications in aging. For example, reproductive aging was shown to be controlled by the gonadotropin releasing hormone (GnRH), which is produced by special cells in the hypothalamus (Yin and Gore, 2006). Age-related reduction in GnRH levels, in response to activation of inflammatory pathways, was suggested to aggravate frailty and neurodegeneration in the elderly (Zhang et al., 2013). Altogether, age-related changes in the hypothalamus and, consequently, in HPA regulation seem to play a central role in the systemic regulation of aging (Deuschle et al., 1997; Kim and Choe, 2019). The activity of the hypothalamus and the HPA axis was reported to show similar general attributes in dogs as in humans and age-related changes in the HPA axis were already assessed in dogs (Reul et al., 1991; Rothuizen et al., 1991). However, further studies will be needed to investigate the function of GnRH and other hormones in canine aging.

Parabiosis Experiments and Systemic Factors of Aging

Most molecular effectors of systemic aging are excreted into the blood, by which they can reach every part of the body. This mediatory function of the blood was proven by parabiosis experiments in rodents, when the artificial connection of the circulatory systems of old and young animals resulted in beneficial effects on the cognitive performance of aged individuals (Katsimpardi et al., 2014; Villeda et al., 2014). Several of the possible effector molecules behind this phenomenon have been revealed since (Loffredo et al., 2013; Demontis et al., 2014; Elabd et al., 2014). Interestingly, some of the systemic factors present in human umbilical cord plasma were shown to beneficially influence brain aging when applied experimentally in mice (Castellano et al., 2017), indicating conserved functions for these molecules. It is important to note, however, that other blood-borne factors were shown to actually promote aging. For example, the β2 microglobulin was reported to negatively affect cognitive performance and regenerative potentials in aged mice (Smith et al., 2015). Although parabiosis is not really applicable in humans and in family dogs, the identified systemic factors seem promising as effectors or targets for anti-aging interventions in both species and may be introduced to preclinical studies conducted on dogs.

Extracellular Vesicles

In addition to hormones and metabolites, extracellular vesicles released by cells into the blood, called exosomes and ectosomes, have emerged as important transducers of various cellular signals (Meldolesi, 2018) and their content, including miRNAs, may provide diagnostic and prognostic measures for many diseases, including AD (Cheng et al., 2014; Cheng et al., 2015; Thind and Wilson, 2016; Van Giau and An, 2016). Consequently, exosomes may also modulate aging and neurodegeneration (Cheng et al., 2015). In support of this, it was recently demonstrated by Zhang et al. (2017) that the stem cells of the hypothalamus could affect the speed of aging by exosomal miRNAs secreted into the cerebrospinal fluid in mice.

Exosome research in dogs have been limited until recently. However, blood miRNA levels—which were hypothesized to be mainly found in exosomes—were reported to correlate with disease phenotypes in canine Duchenne muscular dystrophy (Mizuno et al., 2011). Similarly, miRNA content in circulating exosomes was shown to correlate with progression of secondary heart failure in cases of myxomatous mitral valve disease in dogs (Yang et al., 2017). Direct links were suggested between alterations in urinary exosome formation, miRNA content, and occurrence of kidney disease in dogs by Ichii et al., 2017. Furthermore, a recent study reported exosome derived miRNAs as biomarkers for canine mammary tumors (Fish et al., 2018). Altogether, investigations about the connections between exosome content and aging or age-related pathologies in dogs may lead to the identification of diagnostic markers with potential translational prospects into human studies.

Immunaging and Inflamm-Aging

Together with the CNS, the immune system has a main systemic regulatory function in the organism. Most immune cells synthesize various signaling molecules that act either in a paracrine or endocrine manner and can also provide defense against various pathogens. Macrophages, which are part of the innate immune system, can wander throughout the body and have important roles in tissue homeostasis by cleaning cellular debris and pathogens.

The human immune system is known to experience a general age-related decline in its function and in the abundance of some cell types, although the exact details of reported changes may vary between studies (Pawelec, 2018). In general, reduced numbers of naïve CD8+ T cells and moderately elevated numbers of memory T cells were found to be linked to aging. Importantly, bone marrow derived macrophages were also shown to lose phagocytic capacity with aging (Kim et al., 2017; Li et al., 2017), which can contribute to the accumulation of senescent cells in tissues.

In addition, it has long been hypothesized that systemic age-related changes in certain immune components linked to inflammation will lead to a so-called inflamm-aging phenomenon. Importantly, the exact interactions between immunosenescence and inflamm-aging have not yet been clarified (Fulop et al., 2018); hence, further studies using systems biology approaches may shed light on the detailed mechanisms that underlie them (Ostan et al., 2017).

Both immunosenescence and inflamm-aging were proposed as contributors to aging and age-related pathologies in dogs (Day, 2010). Large-scale hematologic and serum phenotyping studies done in various breeds (Faldyna et al., 2001; Lawrence et al., 2013; Chang et al., 2016) showed that several of the assessed blood parameters correlated with chronological age. Regarding the immune system, T and B lymphocytes were mainly affected in most cases; however, the directions of these changes were contradictory (Faldyna et al., 2001; Massimino et al., 2003; HogenEsch et al., 2004; Reis et al., 2005; Greeley et al., 2006). However, a recent study reported that changes in naïve and memory T cell numbers in old dogs were similar to those previously described in most human studies (Withers et al., 2018). Importantly, it was shown that lifelong calorie restriction positively affected lymphocyte numbers in aged dogs (Greeley et al., 2006). Taken together, the dog may become one of the most applicable model animals to study immunosenescence and inflamm-aging, and to test interventions that could attenuate the deterioration of the immune system.

Microbiome

Recent findings suggest that both systemic metabolism and immune function can be modulated by bacteria inhabiting the gut, termed gut microbiome (Tremaroli and Bäckhed, 2012). The microbiome can interact with the host organism through various chemical signals, and some of these may directly affect the function of distant organs, like the brain (Sharon et al., 2016). Therefore, the microbiome may fundamentally affect health and disease, and possibly aging (Zapata and Quagliarello, 2015). This was supported by findings that reported consistent changes in the composition of the microbiome in elderly people and centenarians (Biagi et al., 2010; Biagi et al., 2017). Although these correlations do not necessarily indicate causative links (Saraswati and Sitaraman, 2015), the theory of microbial modulation of aging has been gaining more and more scientific interest. Importantly, experimental evidences from rodents have already shown that the microbiome can affect the progression of neurodegeneration (Sampson et al., 2016). Furthermore, probiotics and prebiotics, which can beneficially alter the composition of the microbiome, were reported to positively influence the aging of the gut and systemic inflammation in people (Patel et al., 2014; Vaiserman et al., 2017).

Currently, not much is known about age-related changes in the canine gut microbiome; however, there is growing research interest in this field. Future findings may have direct implications to humans as well, because the composition of the canine microbiome was shown to be more similar to humans than that of mice and pigs (Coelho et al., 2018) and actual correlations between the

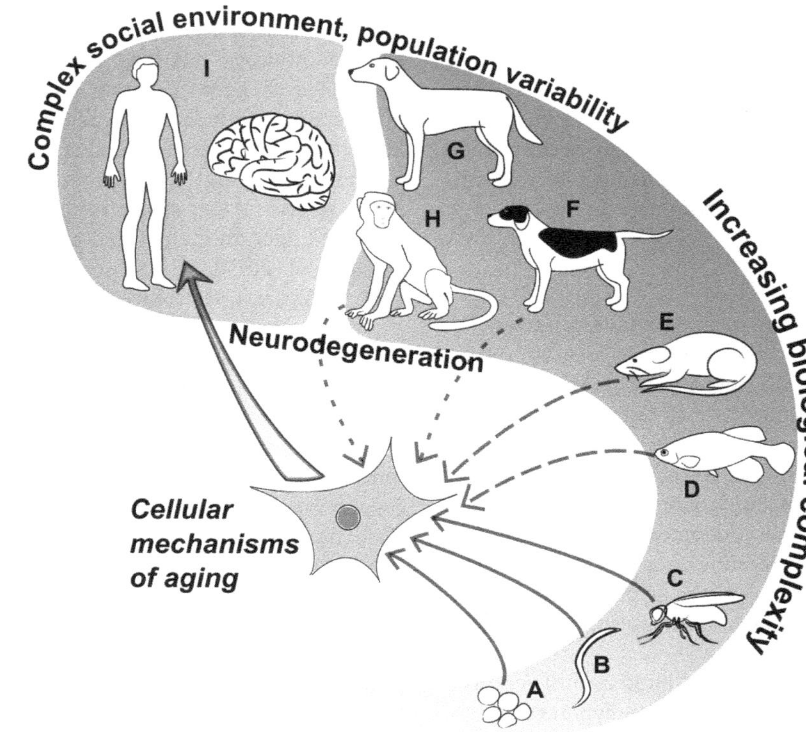

FIGURE 8 | Model organisms of aging. The figure illustrates common aging model organisms, including small animal models and large aninmal models used to study various aspetcs of aging. **(A–C)** Yeast (*Saccharomyces cerevisiae*) and the invertebrates *Caenorhabditis elegans* and *Drosophila melanogaster* are ideal to experimentally study the basic, conserved mechanisms of cellular – and organismal – aging. On the other hand, they show less biological complexity than vertebrates in many aspects, and they do not naturally develop neurodegeneration. **(D–E)** Vertebrate small animal models, like the turqoise killifish (*Nothobranchius furzeri*) and rodents (*Mus musculus* and *Rattus norvegicus*) are ideal to study the biological mechanisms that may be absent in invertebrates, and they can still be rather easily used in experimental studies, including genetic manipulations. However, they typically do not develop age-related neurodegeneration, and may lack many aspects of the complex social and environmental influencers of human aging. **(F–G)** Dogs show similarities to humans in their physiology and they tend to naturally develop age-related cognitive decline. Laboratory dogs **(F)** are traditional large animal models in pharmacology reserach. However, the same way as other laboratory models, they do not represent the natural genetic and environmental variability typical for human populations. Family dogs, **(G)** on the other hand, live in the same environment as humans do, and show a special population genetic stratification, with the presence of genetically isolated, diverse populations (breeds). **(H)** Primates are the closest related to humans, thus they may seem to be the most appropriate animals to study human aging. However, primates are not suited for large-scale sudies for many reasons, including ethical and financial ones. Although they tend to develop human-like age-related neurodegeneration, they still lack the genetic and environmental complexity (both in the laboratory and in their natural habitats), which may influence human aging phenotypes in human populations. **(I)** Human aging shows many unique attributes, including a high prevalence of neurodegeneration. Age-related neurodegeneration is hard to study in most animals, and translational experiments have had many limitations so far. Brain aging may be fundamentally affected by non-genetic factors, including diet, exercise and social environment, which seem challenging to be modelled under laboratory conditions to reflect the natural circumstances of human populations.

microbiomes of dogs and people living in the same household were also reported (Misic et al., 2015). Because dogs age faster than humans, they can be ideal models to test the potential aging effects of prebiotics and probiotics in longitudinal follow-up studies. Importantly, some probiotics used in humans were already suggested to promote health in dogs (Grześkowiak et al., 2015), and this can facilitate their adaptation for systemic anti-aging intervention trials.

It is important to note that other microbial niches on the human body may also affect aging and disease, as it was implicated when oral microbiota and inflammation were linked to the progression of Alzheimer's disease (Pritchard et al., 2017). As periodontitis is also a serious health issue in aged dogs (Albuquerque et al., 2012), this link between oral microbiome and neurodegeneration undoubtedly requires further focus in canine aging research and veterinary medicine and may also benefit humans by translational studies (An et al., 2018).

CONCLUSIONS AND PERSPECTIVES

Considering the remarkably complex nature of biological processes that underlie aging, it is not surprising that finding a biological model for aging that would unify all relevant aspects is challenging. Family dogs have been proposed as ideal models to complement findings from other model organisms (**Figure 8**); however, the still limited knowledge about the exact genetic and regulatory mechanisms that underlie their aging may restrict their applicability in translational studies. Although searching for links between genetic variants and aging phenotypes would be more challenging than in the case of other phenotypic parameters, which are easier to measure, such approaches seem indispensable to gain insight into the main genetic mechanisms that modulate aging variability in dogs. Actually, there have been some efforts along these lines (Jones et al., 2008); however, interbreed comparisons have a limited potential to reveal the exact variants responsible for longevity differences between individuals. Future studies should aim at intrabreed approaches, for which both genetic and aging related data should be available from the same animals. Furthermore, gene expression mapping could be a novel approach to pinpoint at pathways that show changes between young and old dogs or between dogs with short and long lifespan. Although it could be challenging to obtain good quality tissues from a large number of family dogs with known lifespan and other parameters, biobanks created following human examples may help to overcome this limitation in the long term.

As recent findings have increased the palette of possible anti-aging interventions, making almost all of the nine hallmarks of aging (López-Otín et al., 2013) targetable by drugs, a growing interest for preclinical testing of these compounds is expected. Consequently, the dog may gain more and more attention as a preclinical model species. Because family dogs are exposed to almost the same background effects, which can modify the outcome of interventions, as are people, they might even become inevitable to provide a suitable model to assess the effects of anti-aging interventions on natural populations.

It is important to emphasize that characterizing the aging process of dogs and establishing effective interventions within the species may benefit humans not only by clarifying scientific questions but also by making it possible to increase the healthy lifespan of companion and service animals. Owning a guide dog or service dog can lead to great improvements in the quality of life of disabled people. Also, service dogs may facilitate human–human interactions and contribute to the socio-emotional well-being of their owners. Caron-Lormier et al. (2016) reported that most guide dogs were retired due to age-related diseases or simply old age, after an average of 8.5 years of service. Increasing the lifespan and healthspan of working dogs could be emotionally beneficial for their owners, and also could be financially advantageous for societies, as the training of these animals is time consuming and expensive. Furthermore, providing average family dogs an elongated healthspan may also benefit their owners. Several studies have reported a positive correlation between dog walking, physical activity, and health variables in owners, although results were often controversial, suggesting the need for further research on this topic (Brown and Rhodes, 2006; Lentino et al., 2012; Christian et al., 2018). In some cases, improvements were most pronounced in older cohorts (Thorpe et al., 2006; Toohey et al., 2013; Garcia et al., 2015; Curl et al., 2016). Experiences from animal-assisted therapy also suggested that animal–human interactions may help the elderly to experience a successful aging course (Baun and Johnson, 2010). Therefore, providing a long and healthy life for companion animals may benefit the health and welfare of their owners as well.

Taken together, strong scientific evidence suggests that utilizing dogs as models of human aging and anti-aging interventions may hold prospects unattainable by other model organisms, if the complex interactions between genetics and environmental factors are taken into consideration. Thus, canine studies on aging may bring forward results that can eventually benefit the elderly as well as their pets.

AUTHOR CONTRIBUTIONS

SS collected literature and wrote manuscript parts regarding genetic pathways in aging and in dogs. EK collected literature and wrote manuscript parts regarding dogs as models in general, environmental, and cognitive factors. Both authors worked on reviewing the final text. EK provided funding.

FUNDING

This project has received funding from the European Research Council (ERC) under the European Unions Horizon 2020 research and innovation program (Grant Agreement No. 680040), the János Bolyai Research Scholarship of the Hungarian Academy of Sciences, the Bolyai+ ÚNKP-18-4 New National Excellence Program of the Ministry of Human Capacities, and the Hungarian Brain Research Program 2017-1.2.1-NKP-2017-00002.

REFERENCES

Agler, C., Nielsen, D. M., Urkasemsin, G., Singleton, A., Tonomura, N., Sigurdsson, S., et al. (2014). Canine hereditary ataxia in old English sheepdogs and Gordon Setters is associated with a defect in the autophagy gene encoding RAB24. *PLoS Genet.* 10, e1003991. doi: 10.1371/journal.pgen.1003991

Albani, D., Ateri, E., Mazzuco, S., Ghilardi, A., Rodilossi, S., Biella, G., et al. (2014). Modulation of human longevity by SIRT3 single nucleotide polymorphisms in the prospective study "Treviso Longeva (TRELONG)". *Age (Omaha)* 36, 469–478. doi: 10.1007/s11357-013-9559-2

Albuquerque, C., Morinha, F., Requicha, J., Martins, T., Dias, I., Guedes-Pinto, H., et al. (2012). Canine periodontitis: the dog as an important model for periodontal studies. *Vet. J.* 191, 299–305. doi: 10.1016/j.tvjl.2011.08.017

Alderete, K. S., Carlson, A., Grant, M., Sharkey, L., and Zordoky, B. (2017). The anti-cancer effects of resveratrol on canine hemangiosarcoma cells. *FASEB J.* 31, 996.15–996.15. doi: 10.1096/fasebj.31.1_supplement.996.15

Alexander, J. E., Colyer, A., Haydock, R. M., Hayek, M. G., and Park, J. (2018). Understanding how dogs age: longitudinal analysis of markers of inflammation, immune function, and oxidative stress. *J. Gerontol. Ser. A* 73, 720–728. doi: 10.1093/gerona/glx182

Allen, R., and Tresini, M. (2000). Oxidative stress and gene regulation. *Free Radic. Biol. Med.* 28, 463–499. doi: 10.1016/S0891-5849(99)00242-7

Allsopp, R. C., Vaziri, H., Patterson, C., Goldstein, S., Younglai, E. V., Futcher, A. B., et al. (1992). Telomere length predicts replicative capacity of human fibroblasts. *Proc. Natl. Acad. Sci.* 89, 10114–10118. doi: 10.1073/pnas.89.21.10114

Amador-Noguez, D., Yagi, K., Venable, S., and Darlington, G. (2004). Gene expression profile of long-lived Ames dwarf mice and little mice. *Aging Cell* 3, 423–441. doi: 10.1111/j.1474-9728.2004.00125.x

Amoasii, L., Hildyard, J. C. W., Li, H., Sanchez-Ortiz, E., Mireault, A., Caballero, D., et al. (2018). Gene editing restores dystrophin expression in a canine model of Duchenne muscular dystrophy. *Science* 362, 86–91. doi: 10.1126/science.aau1549

An, J. Y., Darveau, R., and Kaeberlein, M. (2018). Oral health in geroscience: animal models and the aging oral cavity. *GeroScience* 40, 1–10. doi: 10.1007/s11357-017-0004-9

Anisimov, V. N., Berstein, L. M., Popovich, I. G., Zabezhinski, M. A., Egormin, P. A., Piskunova, T. S., et al. (2011). If started early in life, metformin treatment increases life span and postpones tumors in female SHR mice. *Aging (Albany NY)* 3, 148–157. doi: 10.18632/aging.100273

Anon (2019). [ebook] Available at: (http://www.un.org/en/development/desa/population/publications/pdf/ageing/WPA2017_Highlights.pdf) (Accessed 19 Mar. 2019).

Anselmi, C. V., Malovini, A., Roncarati, R., Novelli, V., Villa, F., Condorelli, G., et al. (2009). Association of the *FOXO3A* locus with extreme longevity in a southern Italian centenarian study. *Rejuvenation Res.* 12, 95–104. doi: 10.1089/rej.2008.0827

Arking, D. E., Krebsova, A., Macek, M., Macek, M., Arking, A., Mian, I. S., et al. (2002). Association of human aging with a functional variant of klotho. *Proc. Natl. Acad. Sci. U. S. A.* 99, 856–861. doi: 10.1073/pnas.022484299

Arora, H., Chacon, A. H., Choudhary, S., McLeod, M. P., Meshkov, L., Nouri, K., et al. (2014). Bloom syndrome. *Int. J. Dermatol.* 53, 798–802. doi: 10.1111/ijd.12408

Atzmon, G., Cho, M., Cawthon, R. M., Budagov, T., Katz, M., Yang, X., et al. (2010). Genetic variation in human telomerase is associated with telomere length in Ashkenazi centenarians. *Proc. Natl. Acad. Sci.* 107, 1710 LP–1717. doi: 10.1073/pnas.0906191106

Awano, T., Johnson, G. S., Wade, C. M., Katz, M. L., Johnson, G. C., Taylor, J. F., et al. (2009). Genome-wide association analysis reveals a SOD1 mutation in canine degenerative myelopathy that resembles amyotrophic lateral sclerosis. *Proc. Natl. Acad. Sci. U. S. A.* 106, 2794–2799. doi: 10.1073/pnas.0812297106

Axelsson, E., Ratnakumar, A., Arendt, M.-L., Maqbool, K., Webster, M. T., Perloski, M., et al. (2013). The genomic signature of dog domestication reveals adaptation to a starch-rich diet. *Nature* 495, 360–364. doi: 10.1038/nature11837

Babior, B. M. (2004). NADPH oxidase. *Curr. Opin. Immunol.* 16, 42–47. doi: 10.1016/j.coi.2003.12.001

Banlaki, Z., Cimarelli, G., Viranyi, Z., Kubinyi, E., Sasvari-Szekely, M., and Ronai, Z. (2017). DNA methylation patterns of behavior-related gene promoter regions dissect the gray wolf from domestic dog breeds. *Mol. Genet. Genomics* 292, 685–697. doi: 10.1007/s00438-017-1305-5

Bannister, C. A., Holden, S. E., Jenkins-Jones, S., Morgan, C. L., Halcox, J. P., Schernthaner, G., et al. (2014). Can people with type 2 diabetes live longer than those without? A comparison of mortality in people initiated with metformin or sulphonylurea monotherapy and matched, non-diabetic controls. *Diabetes Obes. Metab.* 16, 1165–1173. doi: 10.1111/dom.12354

Baranowska, I., Jäderlund, K. H., Nennesmo, I., Holmqvist, E., Heidrich, N., Larsson, N.-G., et al. (2009). Sensory ataxic neuropathy in golden retriever dogs is caused by a deletion in the mitochondrial tRNATyr gene. *PLoS Genet.* 5, e1000499. doi: 10.1371/journal.pgen.1000499

Barbieri, M., Bonafè, M., Franceschi, C., and Paolisso, G. (2003). Insulin/IGF-I-signaling pathway: an evolutionarily conserved mechanism of longevity from yeast to humans. *Am. J. Physiol. - Endocrinol. Metab.* 285. doi: 10.1152/ajpendo.00296.2003

Bartke, A., Brown-Borg, H., Mattison, J., Kinney, B., Hauck, S., and Wright, C. (2001). Prolonged longevity of hypopituitary dwarf mice. *Exp. Gerontol.* 36, 21–28. doi: 10.1016/S0531-5565(00)00205-9

Barzilai, N., Crandall, J. P., Kritchevsky, S. B., and Espeland, M. A. (2016). Metformin as a tool to target aging. *Cell Metab.* 23, 1060–1065. doi: 10.1016/j.cmet.2016.05.011

Baun, M., and Johnson, R. (2010). Human/animal interaction and successful aging. *Handb. Anim. Ther.* 283–299. doi: 10.1016/B978-0-12-381453-1.10015-7

Baur, J. A., Pearson, K. J., Price, N. L., Jamieson, H. A., Lerin, C., Kalra, A., et al. (2006). Resveratrol improves health and survival of mice on a high-calorie diet. *Nature* 444, 337–342. doi: 10.1038/nature05354

Beekman, M., Blanché, H., Perola, M., Hervonen, A., Bezrukov, V., Sikora, E., et al. (2013). Genome-wide linkage analysis for human longevity: genetics of healthy aging study. *Aging Cell* 12, 184–193. doi: 10.1111/acel.12039

Ben-Zvi, A., Miller, E. A., and Morimoto, R. I. (2009). Collapse of proteostasis represents an early molecular event in *Caenorhabditis elegans* aging. *Proc. Natl. Acad. Sci.* 106, 14914–14919. doi: 10.1073/pnas.0902882106

Bensky, M. K., Gosling, S. D., and Sinn, D. L. (2013). The world from a dog's point of view: a review and synthesis of dog cognition research. *Adv. Study Behav.* 45, 209–406. doi: 10.1016/B978-0-12-407186-5.00005-7

Biagi, E., Nylund, L., Candela, M., Ostan, R., Bucci, L., Pini, E., et al. (2010). S AND CENTENARIANS. *PLoS One* 5, e10667. doi: 10.1371/journal.pone.0010667

Biagi, E., Rampelli, S., Turroni, S., Quercia, S., Candela, M., and Brigidi, P. (2017). The gut microbiota of centenarians: signatures of longevity in the gut microbiota profile. *Mech. Ageing Dev.* 165, 180–184. doi: 10.1016/j.mad.2016.12.013

Bird, A. (2002). DNA methylation patterns and epigenetic memory. *Genes Dev.* 16, 6–21. doi: 10.1101/gad.947102

Bitar, M. A., and Barry, G. (2017). Multiple innovations in genetic and epigenetic mechanisms cooperate to underpin human brain evolution. *Mol. Biol. Evol.* 35, 263–268. doi: 10.1093/molbev/msx303

Blasco, M. A. (2007). The epigenetic regulation of mammalian telomeres. *Nat. Rev. Genet.* 8, 299–309. doi: 10.1038/nrg2047

Borràs, D., Ferrer, I., and Pumarola, M. (1999). Age-related changes in the brain of the dog. *Vet. Pathol.* 36, 202–211. doi: 10.1354/vp.36-3-202

Botigué, L. R., Song, S., Scheu, A., Gopalan, S., Pendleton, A. L., Oetjens, M., and Bobo, D. (2017). Ancient European dog genomes reveal continuity since the early Neolithic. *Nat. Commun.* 8, 16082.

Boyko, A. R. (2011). The domestic dog: man's best friend in the genomic era. *Genome Biol.* 12, 216. doi: 10.1186/gb-2011-12-2-216

Breese, C. R., Ingram, R. L., and Sonntag, W. E. (1991). Influence of age and long-term dietary restriction on plasma insulin-like growth factor-1 (IGF-1), IGF-1 gene expression, and IGF-1 binding proteins. *J. Gerontol.* 46, B180–B187. doi: 10.1093/geronj/46.5.B180

Broer, L., Buchman, A. S., Deelen, J., Evans, D. S., Faul, J. D., Lunetta, K. L., et al. (2015). GWAS of longevity in CHARGE consortium confirms APOE and FOXO3 candidacy. *J. Gerontol. Ser. A Biol. Sci. Med. Sci.* 70, 110–118. doi: 10.1093/gerona/glu166

Brooks, C. L., and Gu, W. (2009). How does SIRT1 affect metabolism, senescence and cancer? *Nat. Rev. Cancer* 9, 123–128. doi: 10.1038/nrc2562

Brooks, M. B., Gu, W., Barnas, J. L., Ray, J., and Ray, K. (2003). A line 1 insertion in the factor IX gene segregates with mild hemophilia B in dogs. *Mamm. Genome* 14, 788–795. doi: 10.1007/s00335-003-2290-z

Brown, S. G., and Rhodes, R. E. (2006). Relationships among dog ownership and leisure-time walking in western Canadian adults. *Am. J. Prev. Med.* 30, 131–136. doi: 10.1016/j.amepre.2005.10.007

Cabanillas, R., Cadiñanos, J., Villameytide, J. A. F., Pérez, M., Longo, J., Richard, J. M., et al. (2011). Néstor-Guillermo progeria syndrome: a novel premature aging condition with early onset and chronic development caused by BANF1 mutations. *Am. J. Med. Genet. Part A* 155, 2617–2625. doi: 10.1002/ajmg.a.34249

Cabreiro, F., Au, C., Leung, K.-Y., Vergara-Irigaray, N., Cochemé, H. M., Noori, T., et al. (2013). Metformin retards aging in *C. elegans* by altering microbial folate and methionine metabolism. *Cell* 153, 228–239. doi: 10.1016/j.cell.2013.02.035

Calamini, B., Silva, M. C., Madoux, F., Hutt, D. M., Khanna, S., Chalfant, M. A., et al. (2012). Small-molecule proteostasis regulators for protein conformational diseases. *Nat. Chem. Biol.* 8, 185–196. doi: 10.1038/nchembio.763

Calderwood, S. K., Murshid, A., and Prince, T. (2009). The shock of aging: molecular chaperones and the heat shock response in longevity and aging–a mini-review. *Gerontology* 55, 550–558. doi: 10.1159/000225957

Calvanese, V., Lara, E., Kahn, A., and Fraga, M. F. (2009). The role of epigenetics in aging and age-related diseases. *Ageing Res. Rev.* 8, 268–276. doi: 10.1016/j.arr.2009.03.004

Campisi, J., and d'Adda di Fagagna, F. (2007). Cellular senescence: when bad things happen to good cells. *Nat. Rev. Mol. Cell Biol.* 8, 729–740. doi: 10.1038/nrm2233

Capy, P., Gasperi, G., Biémont, C., and Bazin, C. (2000). Stress and transposable elements: co-evolution or useful parasites? *Heredity (Edinb.)* 85, 101–106. doi: 10.1046/j.1365-2540.2000.00751.x

Caron-Lormier, G., England, G. C. W., Green, M. J., and Asher, L. (2016). Using the incidence and impact of health conditions in guide dogs to investigate healthy ageing in working dogs. *Vet. J.* 207, 124–130. doi: 10.1016/j.tvjl.2015.10.046

Carrasco-Garcia, E., Arrizabalaga, O., Serrano, M., Lovell-Badge, R., and Matheu, A. (2015). Increased gene dosage of *Ink4/Arf* and *p53* delays age-associated central nervous system functional decline. *Aging Cell* 14, 710–714. doi: 10.1111/acel.12343

Castellano, J. M., Mosher, K. I., Abbey, R. J., McBride, A. A., James, M. L., Berdnik, D., et al. (2017). Human umbilical cord plasma proteins revitalize hippocampal function in aged mice. *Nature* 544, 488–492. doi: 10.1038/nature22067

Castilho, R. M., Squarize, C. H., Chodosh, L. A., Williams, B. O., and Gutkind, J. S. (2009). mTOR mediates Wnt-induced epidermal stem cell exhaustion and aging. *Cell Stem Cell* 5, 279–289. doi: 10.1016/j.stem.2009.06.017

Cecconi, F., and Levine, B. (2008). The role of autophagy in mammalian development: cell makeover rather than cell death. *Dev. Cell* 15, 344–357. doi: 10.1016/j.devcel.2008.08.012

Chakkalakal, J. V., Jones, K. M., Basson, M. A., and Brack, A. S. (2012). The aged niche disrupts muscle stem cell quiescence. *Nature* 490, 355–360. doi: 10.1038/nature11438

Chan, K.-C., Yu, M.-H., Lin, M.-C., Huang, C.-N., Chung, D.-J., Lee, Y.-J., et al. (2016). Pleiotropic effects of acarbose on atherosclerosis development in rabbits are mediated *via* upregulating AMPK signals. *Sci. Rep.* 6, 38642. doi: 10.1038/srep38642

Chang, Y.-M., Hadox, E., Szladovits, B., and Garden, O. A. (2016). Serum biochemical phenotypes in the domestic dog. *PLoS One* 11, e0149650. doi: 10.1371/journal.pone.0149650

Chapagain, D., Range, F., Huber, L., and Virányi, Z. (2018). Cognitive aging in dogs. *Gerontology* 64, 165–171. doi: 10.1159/000481621

Chen, C., Liu, Y., Liu, Y., and Zheng, P. (2009). mTOR regulation and therapeutic rejuvenation of aging hematopoietic stem cells. *Sci. Signal.* 2, ra75. doi: 10.1126/scisignal.2000559

Chen, S., Zhang, X., Song, L., and Le, W. (2012). Autophagy dysregulation in amyotrophic lateral sclerosis. *Brain Pathol.* 22, 110–116. doi: 10.1111/j.1750-3639.2011.00546.x

Chénais, B., Caruso, A., Hiard, S., and Casse, N. (2012). The impact of transposable elements on eukaryotic genomes: from genome size increase to genetic adaptation to stressful environments. *Gene* 509, 7–15. doi: 10.1016/j.gene.2012.07.042

Cheng, L., Doecke, J. D., Sharples, R. A., Villemagne, V. L., Fowler, C. J., Rembach, A., et al. (2015). Prognostic serum miRNA biomarkers associated with Alzheimer's disease shows concordance with neuropsychological and neuroimaging assessment. *Mol. Psychiatry* 20, 1188–1196. doi: 10.1038/mp.2014.127

Cheng, L., Sharples, R. A., Scicluna, B. J., and Hill, A. F. (2014). Exosomes provide a protective and enriched source of miRNA for biomarker profiling compared to intracellular and cell-free blood. *J. Extracell. Vesicles* 3, 23743. doi: 10.3402/jev.v3.23743

Cheng, T., Rodrigues, N., Shen, H., Yang, Y., Dombkowski, D., Sykes, M., et al. (2000). Hematopoietic stem cell quiescence maintained by p21cip1/waf1. *Science* 287, 1804–1808. doi: 10.1126/science.287.5459.1804

Chiang, W.-C., Ching, T.-T., Lee, H. C., Mousigian, C., and Hsu, A.-L. (2012). HSF-1 regulators DDL-1/2 link insulin-like signaling to heat-shock responses and modulation of longevity. *Cell* 148, 322–334. doi: 10.1016/j.cell.2011.12.019

Chini, C. C. S., Tarragó, M. G., and Chini, E. N. (2017). NAD and the aging process: role in life, death and everything in between. *Mol. Cell. Endocrinol.* 455, 62–74. doi: 10.1016/j.mce.2016.11.003

Cho, K., Chung, J. Y., Cho, S. K., Shin, H.-W., Jang, I.-J., Park, J.-W., et al. (2015). Antihyperglycemic mechanism of metformin occurs *via* the AMPK/LXRα/POMC pathway. *Sci. Rep.* 5, 8145. doi: 10.1038/srep08145

Cho, M., and Suh, Y. (2014). Genome maintenance and human longevity. *Curr. Opin. Genet. Dev.* 26, 105–115. doi: 10.1016/j.gde.2014.07.002

Chondrogianni, N., Voutetakis, K., Kapetanou, M., Delitsikou, V., Papaevgeniou, N., Sakellari, M., et al. (2015). Proteasome activation: an innovative promising approach for delaying aging and retarding age-related diseases. *Ageing Res. Rev.* 23, 37–55. doi: 10.1016/j.arr.2014.12.003

Christian, H., Bauman, A., Epping, J. N., Levine, G. N., McCormack, G., Rhodes, R. E., et al. (2018). Encouraging dog walking for health promotion and disease prevention. *Am. J. Lifestyle Med* 12, 233–243. doi: 10.1177/1559827616643686

Christie, L.-A., Opii, W. O., Head, E., Araujo, J. A., de Rivera, C., Milgram, N. W., et al. (2009). Short-term supplementation with acetyl-l-carnitine and lipoic acid alters plasma protein carbonyl levels but does not improve cognition in aged beagles. *Exp. Gerontol.* 44, 752–759. doi: 10.1016/j.exger.2009.08.012

Chu, C. T. (2019). Multiple pathways for mitophagy: a neurodegenerative conundrum for Parkinson's disease. *Neurosci. Lett.* 697, 66–71. doi: 10.1016/j.neulet.2018.04.004

Cimarelli, G., Virányi, Z., Turcsán, B., Rónai, Z., Sasvári-Székely, M., and Bánlaki, Z. (2017). Social behavior of pet dogs is associated with peripheral OXTR methylation. *Front. Psychol.* 8, 549. doi: 10.3389/fpsyg.2017.00549

Clark, L. A., Tsai, K. L., Starr, A. N., Nowend, K. L., and Murphy, K. E. (2011). A missense mutation in the 20S proteasome β2 subunit of Great Danes having harlequin coat patterning. *Genomics* 97, 244–248. doi: 10.1016/j.ygeno.2011.01.003

Clark, L. A., Wahl, J. M., Rees, C. A., and Murphy, K. E. (2006). Retrotransposon insertion in SILV is responsible for merle patterning of the domestic dog. *Proc. Natl. Acad. Sci. U. S. A.* 103, 1376–1381. doi: 10.1073/pnas.0506940103

Codd, V., Nelson, C. P., Albrecht, E., Mangino, M., Deelen, J., Buxton, J. L., et al. (2013). Identification of seven loci affecting mean telomere length and their association with disease. *Nat. Genet.* 45, 422–427. doi: 10.1038/ng.2528

Coelho, L. P., Kultima, J. R., Costea, P. I., Fournier, C., Pan, Y., Czarnecki-Maulden, G., et al. (2018). Similarity of the dog and human gut microbiomes in gene content and response to diet. *Microbiome* 6, 72. doi: 10.1186/s40168-018-0450-3

Collado, M., Blasco, M. A., and Serrano, M. (2007). Cellular senescence in cancer and aging. *Cell* 130, 223–233. doi: 10.1016/j.cell.2007.07.003

Collier, L. S., and Largaespada, D. A. (2007). Transposable elements and the dynamic somatic genome. *Genome Biol.* 8, S5. doi: 10.1186/gb-2007-8-s1-s5

Corral-Debrinski, M., Horton, T., Lott, M. T., Shoffner, J. M., Flint Beal, M., and Wallace, D. C. (1992). Mitochondrial DNA deletions in human brain: regional variability and increase with advanced age. *Nat. Genet.* 2, 324–329. doi: 10.1038/ng1292-324

Cotman, C. W., and Head, E. (2008). The canine (dog) model of human aging and disease: dietary, environmental and immunotherapy approaches. *J. Alzheimer's Dis.* 15, 685–707. doi: 10.3233/JAD-2008-15413

Cotman, C. W., Head, E., Muggenburg, B. A., Zicker, S., and Milgram, N. W. (2002). Brain aging in the canine: a diet enriched in antioxidants reduces cognitive dysfunction. *Neurobiol. Aging* 23, 809–818. doi: 10.1016/S0197-4580(02)00073-8

Creevy, K. E., Austad, S. N., Hoffman, J. M., O'Neill, D. G., and Promislow, D. E. L. (2016). The companion dog as a model for the longevity dividend. *Cold Spring Harb. Perspect. Med.* 6, a026633. doi: 10.1101/cshperspect.a026633

Cuervo, A. M., and Dice, J. F. (2000). Age-related decline in chaperone-mediated autophagy. *J. Biol. Chem.* 275, 31505–31513. doi: 10.1074/jbc.M002102200

Cummings, B. J., Head, E., Ruehl, W., Milgram, N. W., and Cotman, C. W. (1996). The canine as an animal model of human aging and dementia. *Neurobiol. Aging* 17, 259–268. doi: 10.1016/0197-4580(95)02060-8

Curl, A. L., Bibbo, J., and Johnson, R. A (2016). Dog walking, the human–animal bond and older adults' physical health. *Gerontologist* 35, gnw051. doi: 10.1093/geront/gnw051

d'Adda di Fagagna, F. (2008). Living on a break: cellular senescence as a DNA-damage response. *Nat. Rev. Cancer* 8, 512–522. doi: 10.1038/nrc2440

da Silva, P. F. L., Ogrodnik, M., Kucheryavenko, O., Glibert, J., Miwa, S., Cameron, K., et al. (2019). The bystander effect contributes to the accumulation of senescent cells *in vivo*. *Aging Cell* 18, e12848. doi: 10.1111/acel.12848

Dai, H., Sinclair, D. A., Ellis, J. L., and Steegborn, C. (2018). Sirtuin activators and inhibitors: promises, achievements, and challenges. *Pharmacol. Ther.* 188, 140–154. doi: 10.1016/j.pharmthera.2018.03.004

Daniel, M., and Tollefsbol, T. O. (2015). Epigenetic linkage of aging, cancer and nutrition. *J. Exp. Biol.* 218, 59–70. doi: 10.1242/jeb.107110

Day, M. J. (2010). Ageing, immunosenescence and inflammageing in the dog and cat. *J. Comp. Pathol.* 142, S60–S69. doi: 10.1016/j.jcpa.2009.10.011

De Cecco, M., Criscione, S. W., Peterson, A. L., Neretti, N., Sedivy, J. M., and Kreiling, J. A. (2013). Transposable elements become active and mobile in the genomes of aging mammalian somatic tissues. *Aging (Albany NY)* 5, 867–883. doi: 10.18632/aging.100621

De Felice, F. G., and Munoz, D. P. (2016). Opportunities and challenges in developing relevant animal models for Alzheimer's disease. *Ageing Res. Rev.* 26, 112–114. doi: 10.1016/j.arr.2016.01.006

de Haan, G., and Lazare, S. S. (2018). Aging of hematopoietic stem cells. *Blood* 131, 479–487. doi: 10.1182/blood-2017-06-746412 de Jesus, B. B., Vera, E., Schneeberger, K., Tejera, A. M., Ayuso, E., Bosch, F., et al. (2012). Telomerase gene therapy in adult and old mice delays aging and increases longevity without increasing cancer. *EMBO Mol. Med.* 4, 691–704. doi: 10.1002/emmm.201200245

de Magalhães, J. P., Curado, J., and Church, G. M. (2009). Meta-analysis of age-related gene expression profiles identifies common signatures of aging. *Bioinformatics* 25, 875–881. doi: 10.1093/bioinformatics/btp073

De Sandre-Giovannoli, A., Bernard, R., Cau, P., Navarro, C., Amiel, J., Boccaccio, I., et al. (2003). Lamin a truncation in Hutchinson-Gilford progeria. *Science* 300, 2055. doi: 10.1126/science.1084125

de Vrij, F. M. S., Fischer, D. F., van Leeuwen, F. W., and Hol, E. M. (2004). Protein quality control in Alzheimer's disease by the ubiquitin proteasome system. *Prog. Neurobiol.* 74, 249–270. doi: 10.1016/j.pneurobio.2004.10.001

Deelen, J., Beekman, M., Uh, H.-W., Helmer, Q., Kuningas, M., Christiansen, L., et al. (2011). Genome-wide association study identifies a single major locus contributing to survival into old age; the APOE locus revisited. *Aging Cell* 10, 686–698. doi: 10.1111/j.1474-9726.2011.00705.x

Deguchi, Y., Negoro, S., and Kishimoto, S. (1988). Age-related changes of heat shock protein gene transcription in human peripheral blood mononuclear cells. *Biochem. Biophys. Res. Commun.* 157, 580–584. doi: 10.1016/S0006-291X(88)80289-4

Demontis, F., Patel, V. K., Swindell, W. R., and Perrimon, N. (2014). Intertissue control of the nucleolus *via a* myokine-dependent longevity pathway. *Cell Rep.* 7, 1481–1494. doi: 10.1016/j.celrep.2014.05.001

Deretic, V. (2006). Autophagy as an immune defense mechanism. *Curr. Opin. Immunol.* 18, 375–382. doi: 10.1016/j.coi.2006.05.019

Deuschle, M., Gotthardt, U., Schweiger, U., Weber, B., Körner, A., Schmider, J., et al. (1997). With aging in humans the activity of the hypothalamus–pituitary–adrenal system increases and its diurnal amplitude flattens. *Life Sci.* 61, 2239–2246. doi: 10.1016/S0024-3205(97)00926-0

Di Fonzo, A., Rohé, C. F., Ferreira, J., Chien, H. F., Vacca, L., Stocchi, F., et al. (2005). A frequent LRRK2 gene mutation associated with autosomal dominant Parkinson's disease. *Lancet* 365, 412–415. doi: 10.1016/S0140-6736(05)17829-5

Dias, J. N. R., Aguiar, S. I., Pereira, D. M., André, A. S., Gano, L., Correia, J. D. G., et al. (2018). The histone deacetylase inhibitor panobinostat is a potent antitumor agent in canine diffuse large B-cell lymphoma. *Oncotarget* 9, 28586–28598. doi: 10.18632/oncotarget.25580

Dickey, C. A., Kamal, A., Lundgren, K., Klosak, N., Bailey, R. M., Dunmore, J., et al. (2007). The high-affinity HSP90-CHIP complex recognizes and selectively degrades phosphorylated tau client proteins. *J. Clin. Invest.* 117, 648–658. doi: 10.1172/JCI29715

Donia, M. S., and Fischbach, M. A. (2015). Small molecules from the human microbiota. *Science (80-.).* 349, 1254766–1254766. doi: 10.1126/science.1254766

Doonan, R., McElwee, J. J., Matthijssens, F., Walker, G. A., Houthoofd, K., Back, P., et al. (2008). Against the oxidative damage theory of aging: superoxide dismutases protect against oxidative stress but have little or no effect on life span in *Caenorhabditis elegans*. *Genes Dev.* 22, 3236–3241. doi: 10.1101/gad.504808

Downs, L. M., Mellersh, C. S., Staden, R., Sivachenko, A., and Cibulskis, K. (2014). An intronic SINE insertion in FAM161A that causes exon-skipping is associated with progressive retinal atrophy in Tibetan spaniels and Tibetan terriers. *PLoS One* 9, e93990. doi: 10.1371/journal.pone.0093990

Dreger, D. L., Davis, B. W., Cocco, R., Sechi, S., Di Cerbo, A., Parker, H. G., et al. (2016a). Commonalities in development of pure breeds and population isolates revealed in the genome of the Sardinian Fonni's dog. *Genetics* 204, 737–755. doi: 10.1534/genetics.116.192427

Dreger, D. L., Rimbault, M., Davis, B. W., Bhatnagar, A., Parker, H. G., and Ostrander, E. A. (2016b). Whole-genome sequence, SNP chips and pedigree structure: building demographic profiles in domestic dog breeds to optimize genetic-trait mapping. *Dis. Model. Mech.* 9, 1445–1460. doi: 10.1242/dmm.027037

Dreger, D. L., and Schmutz, S. M. (2011). A SINE insertion causes the black-and-tan and saddle tan phenotypes in domestic dogs. *J. Hered.* 102, S11–S18. doi: 10.1093/jhered/esr042

Drummond, M. J., McCarthy, J. J., Sinha, M., Spratt, H. M., Volpi, E., Esser, K. A., et al. (2011). Aging and microRNA expression in human skeletal muscle: a microarray and bioinformatics analysis. *Physiol. Genomics* 43, 595–603. doi: 10.1152/physiolgenomics.00148.2010

Dumble, M., Moore, L., Chambers, S. M., Geiger, H., Van Zant, G., Goodell, M. A., et al. (2007). The impact of altered p53 dosage on hematopoietic stem cell dynamics during aging. *Blood* 109, 1736–1742. doi: 10.1182/blood-2006-03-010413

Durieux, J., Wolff, S., and Dillin, A. (2011). The cell-non-autonomous nature of electron transport chain-mediated longevity. *Cell* 144, 79–91. doi: 10.1016/j.cell.2010.12.016

Edens, W. A., Sharling, L., Cheng, G., Shapira, R., Kinkade, J. M., Lee, T., et al. (2001). Tyrosine cross-linking of extracellular matrix is catalyzed by Duox, a multidomain oxidase/peroxidase with homology to the phagocyte oxidase subunit gp91phox. *J. Cell Biol.* 154, 879–91. doi: 10.1083/jcb.200103132

Edgar, D., Shabalina, I., Camara, Y., Wredenberg, A., Calvaruso, M. A., Nijtmans, L., et al. (2009). Random point mutations with major effects on protein-coding genes are the driving force behind premature aging in mtDNA mutator mice. *Cell Metab.* 10, 131–138. doi: 10.1016/j.cmet.2009.06.010

Eisenberg, T., Knauer, H., Schauer, A., Büttner, S., Ruckenstuhl, C., Carmona-Gutierrez, D., et al. (2009). Induction of autophagy by spermidine promotes longevity. *Nat. Cell Biol.* 11, 1305–1314. doi: 10.1038/ncb1975

Elabd, C., Cousin, W., Upadhyayula, P., Chen, R. Y., Chooljian, M. S., Li, J., et al. (2014). Oxytocin is an age-specific circulating hormone that is necessary for muscle maintenance and regeneration. *Nat. Commun.* 5, 4082. doi: 10.1038/ncomms5082

Ellis, N. A., Groden, J., Ye, T.-Z., Straughen, J., Lennon, D. J., Ciocci, S., et al. (1995). The Bloom's syndrome gene product is homologous to RecQ helicases. *Cell* 83, 655–666. doi: 10.1016/0092-8674(95)90105-1

Elshafae, S. M., Kohart, N. A., Altstadt, L. A., Dirksen, W. P., and Rosol, T. J. (2017). The effect of a histone deacetylase inhibitor (AR-42) on canine prostate cancer growth and metastasis. *Prostate* 77, 776–793. doi: 10.1002/pros.23318

Emanuele, E., Fontana, J. M., Minoretti, P., and Geroldi, D. (2010). Preliminary evidence of a genetic association between chromosome 9p21.3 and human longevity. *Rejuvenation Res.* 13, 23–26. doi: 10.1089/rej.2009.0970

Eriksson, M., Brown, W. T., Gordon, L. B., Glynn, M. W., Singer, J., Scott, L., et al. (2003). Recurrent *de novo* point mutations in lamin A cause Hutchinson–Gilford progeria syndrome. *Nature* 423, 293–298. doi: 10.1038/nature01629

Faggioli, F., Wang, T., Vijg, J., and Montagna, C. (2012). Chromosome-specific accumulation of aneuploidy in the aging mouse brain. *Hum. Mol. Genet.* 21, 5246–5253. doi: 10.1093/hmg/dds375

Faldyna, M., Levá, L., Knötigová, P., and Toman, M. (2001). Lymphocyte subsets in peripheral blood of dogs—a flow cytometric study. *Vet. Immunol. Immunopathol.* 82, 23–37. doi: 10.1016/S0165-2427(01)00337-3

Ferrer, I., Pumarola, M., Rivera, R., Zújar, M. J., Cruz-Sánchez, F., and Vidal, A. (1993). Primary central white matter degeneration in old dogs. *Acta Neuropathol.* 86, 172–175. doi: 10.1007/BF00334884

Feuerbacher, E. N., and Wynne, C. D. L. (2011). A history of dogs as subjects in North American experimental psychological research. *Comp. Cogn. Behav. Rev.* 6, 46–71. doi: 10.3819/ccbr.2011.60001

Fick, L. J., Fick, G. H., Li, Z., Cao, E., Bao, B., Heffelfinger, D., et al. (2012). Telomere length correlates with life span of dog breeds. *Cell Rep.* 2, 1530–1536. doi: 10.1016/j.celrep.2012.11.021

Finsterer, J., and Frank, M. (2016). Propofol is mitochondrion-toxic and may unmask a mitochondrial disorder. *J. Child Neurol.* 31, 1489–1494. doi: 10.1177/0883073816661458

Fish, E. J., Irizarry, K. J., DeInnocentes, P., Ellis, C. J., Prasad, N., Moss, A. G., et al. (2018). Malignant canine mammary epithelial cells shed exosomes containing differentially expressed microRNA that regulate oncogenic networks. *BMC Cancer* 18, 832. doi: 10.1186/s12885-018-4750-6

Florian, M. C., Dörr, K., Niebel, A., Daria, D., Schrezenmeier, H., Rojewski, M., et al. (2012). Cdc42 activity regulates hematopoietic stem cell aging and rejuvenation. *Cell Stem Cell* 10, 520–530. doi: 10.1016/j.stem.2012.04.007

Flurkey, K., Papaconstantinou, J., Miller, R. A., and Harrison, D. E. (2001). Lifespan extension and delayed immune and collagen aging in mutant mice with defects in growth hormone production. *Proc. Natl. Acad. Sci.* 98, 6736–6741. doi: 10.1073/pnas.111158898

Forero, D. A., González-Giraldo, Y., López-Quintero, C., Castro-Vega, L. J., Barreto, G. E., and Perry, G. (2016). Meta-analysis of telomere length in

Alzheimer's disease. *J. Gerontol. Ser. A Biol. Sci. Med. Sci.* 71, 1069–1073. doi: 10.1093/gerona/glw053

Forsberg, L. A., Rasi, C., Razzaghian, H. R., Pakalapati, G., Waite, L., Thilbeault, K. S., et al. (2012). Age-related somatic structural changes in the nuclear genome of human blood cells. *Am. J. Hum. Genet.* 90, 217–228. doi: 10.1016/j.ajhg.2011.12.009

Forslund, K., Hildebrand, F., Nielsen, T., Falony, G., Le Chatelier, E., Sunagawa, S., et al. (2015). Disentangling type 2 diabetes and metformin treatment signatures in the human gut microbiota. *Nature* 528, 262–266. doi: 10.1038/nature15766

Fraga, C. G., Shigenaga, M. K., Park, J. W., Degan, P., and Ames, B. N. (1990). Oxidative damage to DNA during aging: 8-hydroxy-2'-deoxyguanosine in rat organ DNA and urine. *Proc. Natl. Acad. Sci. U. S. A.* 87, 4533–4537. doi: 10.1073/pnas.87.12.4533

Fraga, M. F., and Esteller, M. (2007). Epigenetics and aging: the targets and the marks. *Trends Genet.* 23, 413–418. doi: 10.1016/j.tig.2007.05.008

Frantz, L. A. F., Mullin, V. E., Pionnier-Capitan, M., Lebrasseur, O., Ollivier, M., Perri, A., et al. (2016). Genomic and archaeological evidence suggest a dual origin of domestic dogs. *Science (80-.).* 352, 1228–1231. doi: 10.1126/science.aaf3161

Freedman, A. H., Lohmueller, K. E., and Wayne, R. K. (2016). Evolutionary history, selective sweeps, and deleterious variation in the dog. *Annu. Rev. Ecol. Evol. Syst.* 47, 73–96. doi: 10.1146/annurev-ecolsys-121415-032155

Freund, A., Laberge, R.-M., Demaria, M., and Campisi, J. (2012). Lamin B1 loss is a senescence-associated biomarker. *Mol. Biol. Cell* 23, 2066–2075. doi: 10.1091/mbc.e11-10-0884

Fulop, T., Larbi, A., Dupuis, G., Le Page, A., Frost, E. H., Cohen, A. A., et al. (2018). Immunosenescence and inflamm-aging as two sides of the same coin: friends or foes? *Front. Immunol.* 8, 1960. doi: 10.3389/fimmu.2017.01960

Galis, F., Van Der Sluijs, I., Van Dooren, T. J. M., Metz, J. A. J., and Nussbaumer, M. (2007). Do large dogs die young? *J. Exp. Zool. Part B Mol. Dev. Evol.* 308B, 119–126. doi: 10.1002/jez.b.21116

García-Cao, I., García-Cao, M., Martín-Caballero, J., Criado, L. M., Klatt, P., Flores, J. M., et al. (2002). Super p53mice exhibit enhanced DNA damage response, are tumor resistant and age normallyc. *EMBO J.* 21, 6225–6235. doi: 10.1093/emboj/cdf595

Garcia, D. O., Wertheim, B. C., Manson, J. E., Chlebowski, R. T., Volpe, S. L., Howard, B. V., et al. (2015). Relationships between dog ownership and physical activity in postmenopausal women. *Prev. Med. (Baltim)* 70, 33–38. doi: 10.1016/j.ypmed.2014.10.030

Gaur, U., Tu, J., Li, D., Gao, Y., Lian, T., Sun, B., et al. (2017). Molecular evolutionary patterns of NAD+/Sirtuin aging signaling pathway across taxa. *PLoS One* 12, e0182306. doi: 10.1371/journal.pone.0182306

Gehrig, S. M., van der Poel, C., Sayer, T. A., Schertzer, J. D., Henstridge, D. C., Church, J. E., et al. (2012). Hsp72 preserves muscle function and slows progression of severe muscular dystrophy. *Nature* 484, 394–398. doi: 10.1038/nature10980

Geiman, T. M., and Muegge, K. (2009). DNA methylation in early development. *Mol. Reprod. Dev.* 77, n/a–n/a. doi: 10.1002/mrd.21118

Gelaleti, G. B., Granzotto, A., Leonel, C., Jardim, B. V., Moschetta, M. G., Carareto, C. M. A., et al. (2014). Short interspersed CAN SINE elements as prognostic markers in canine mammary neoplasia. *Oncol. Rep.* 31, 435–441. doi: 10.3892/or.2013.2827

Gentilini, D., Mari, D., Castaldi, D., Remondini, D., Ogliari, G., Ostan, R., et al. (2013). Role of epigenetics in human aging and longevity: genome-wide DNA methylation profile in centenarians and centenarians? Offspring. *Age (Omaha)* 35, 1961–1973. doi: 10.1007/s11357-012-9463-1

Gertz, M., Nguyen, G. T. T., Fischer, F., Suenkel, B., Schlicker, C., Fränzel, B., et al. (2012). A molecular mechanism for direct sirtuin activation by resveratrol. *PLoS One* 7, e49761. doi: 10.1371/journal.pone.0049761

Ghi, P., Di Brisco, F., Dallorto, D., Osella, M. C., and Orsetti, M. (2009). Age-related modifications of egr1 expression and ubiquitin-proteasome components in pet dog hippocampus. *Mech. Ageing Dev.* 130, 320–327. doi: 10.1016/j.mad.2009.01.007

Gilmore, K. M., and Greer, K. A. (2015). Why is the dog an ideal model for aging research? *Exp. Gerontol.* 71, 14–20. doi: 10.1016/j.exger.2015.08.008

Gocmez, S. S., Gacar, N., Utkan, T., Gacar, G., Scarpace, P. J., and Tumer, N. (2016). Protective effects of resveratrol on aging-induced cognitive impairment in rats. *Neurobiol. Learn. Mem.* 131, 131–136. doi: 10.1016/j.nlm.2016.03.022

Goldstein, O., Kukekova, A. V., Aguirre, G. D., and Acland, G. M. (2010). Exonic SINE insertion in STK38L causes canine early retinal degeneration (erd). *Genomics* 96, 362–368. doi: 10.1016/j.ygeno.2010.09.003

Golubtsova, N. N., Filippov, F. N., and Gunin, A. G. (2016). Lamin B1 and lamin B2 in human skin in the process of aging. *Adv. Gerontol.* 6, 275–281. doi: 10.1134/S2079057016040068

Gonskikh, Y., and Polacek, N. (2017). Alterations of the translation apparatus during aging and stress response. *Mech. Ageing Dev.* 168, 30–36. doi: 10.1016/j.mad.2017.04.003

Gonzalez-Suarez, I., Redwood, A. B., and Gonzalo, S. (2009). Loss of A-type lamins and genomic instability. *Cell Cycle* 8, 3860–3865. doi: 10.4161/cc.8.23.10092

Gorbunova, V., Boeke, J. D., Helfand, S. L., and Sedivy, J. M. (2014). Sleeping dogs of the genome. *Science* 346, 1187–1188. doi: 10.1126/science.aaa3177

Greeley, E. H., Spitznagel, E., Lawler, D. F., Kealy, R. D., and Segre, M. (2006). Modulation of canine immunosenescence by life-long caloric restriction. *Vet. Immunol. Immunopathol.* 111, 287–299. doi: 10.1016/j.vetimm.2006.02.002

Greenberg, R. A., Allsopp, R. C., Chin, L., Morin, G. B., and DePinho, R. A. (1998). Expression of mouse telomerase reverse transcriptase during development, differentiation and proliferation. *Oncogene* 16, 1723–1730. doi: 10.1038/sj.onc.1201933

Greer, E. L., and Brunet, A. (2005). FOXO transcription factors at the interface between longevity and tumor suppression. *Oncogene* 24, 7410–7425. doi: 10.1038/sj.onc.1209086

Greer, K. A., Canterberry, S. C., and Murphy, K. E. (2007). Statistical analysis regarding the effects of height and weight on life span of the domestic dog. *Res. Vet. Sci.* 82, 208–214. doi: 10.1016/j.rvsc.2006.06.005

Greer, K. A., Hughes, L. M., and Masternak, M. M. (2011). Connecting serum IGF-1, body size, and age in the domestic dog. *Age (Omaha)* 33, 475–483. doi: 10.1007/s11357-010-9182-4

Greiss, S., and Gartner, A. (2009). Sirtuin/Sir2 phylogeny, evolutionary considerations and structural conservation. *Mol. Cells* 28, 407–415. doi: 10.1007/s10059-009-0169-x

Grosse, N., Van Loon, B., and Bley, C. R. (2014). DNA damage response and DNA repair—dog as a model? *BMC Cancer* 14, 1–8. doi: 10.1186/1471-2407-14-203

Grześkowiak, Ł., Endo, A., Beasley, S., and Salminen, S. (2015). Microbiota and probiotics in canine and feline welfare. *Anaerobe* 34, 14–23. doi: 10.1016/j.anaerobe.2015.04.002

Guarente, L. (2011). Sirtuins, aging, and metabolism. *Cold Spring Harb. Symp. Quant. Biol.* 76, 81–90. doi: 10.1101/sqb.2011.76.010629

Gwinn, D. M., Shackelford, D. B., Egan, D. F., Mihaylova, M. M., Mery, A., Vasquez, D. S., et al. (2008). AMPK phosphorylation of raptor mediates a metabolic checkpoint. *Mol. Cell* 30, 214–226. doi: 10.1016/j.molcel.2008.03.003

Hahn, K., Rohdin, C., Jagannathan, V., Wohlsein, P., Baumgärtner, W., Seehusen, F., et al. (2015). TECPR2 associated neuroaxonal dystrophy in Spanish water dogs. *PLoS One* 10, 1–18. doi: 10.1371/journal.pone.0141824

Haigis, M. C., and Yankner, B. A. (2010). The aging stress response. *Mol. Cell* 40, 333–344. doi: 10.1016/j.molcel.2010.10.002

Halley-Stott, R. P., and Gurdon, J. B. (2013). Epigenetic memory in the context of nuclear reprogramming and cancer. *Brief. Funct. Genomics* 12, 164–173. doi: 10.1093/bfgp/elt011

Han, S., and Brunet, A. (2012). Histone methylation makes its mark on longevity. *Trends Cell Biol.* 22, 42–49. doi: 10.1016/j.tcb.2011.11.001

Hancks, D. C., and Kazazian, H. H. (2016). Roles for retrotransposon insertions in human disease. *Mob. DNA* 7, 9. doi: 10.1186/s13100-016-0065-9

Hannon, E., Spiers, H., Viana, J., Pidsley, R., Burrage, J., Murphy, T. M., et al. (2015). Methylation QTLs in the developing brain and their enrichment in schizophrenia risk loci. *Nat. Neurosci.* 19, 48–54. doi: 10.1038/nn.4182

Hara, T., Nakamura, K., Matsui, M., Yamamoto, A., Nakahara, Y., Suzuki-Migishima, R., et al. (2006). Suppression of basal autophagy in neural cells causes neurodegenerative disease in mice. *Nature* 441, 885–889. doi: 10.1038/nature04724

Harley, C. B., Futcher, B. A., and Greider, C. W. (1990). Telomeres shorten during ageing of human fibroblasts. *Nature* 345, 458–460. doi: 10.1038/345458a0

Harrison, D. E., Strong, R., Allison, D. B., Ames, B. N., Astle, C. M., Atamna, H., et al. (2014). Acarbose, 17-α-estradiol, and nordihydroguaiaretic acid extend mouse lifespan preferentially in males. *Aging Cell* 13, 273–282. doi: 10.1111/acel.12170

Hars, E. S., Qi, H., Jin, S. V., Cai, L., Hu, C., and Liu, L. F. (2007). Autophagy regulates ageing in *C. elegans*. *Autophagy* 3, 93–95. doi: 10.4161/auto.3636

Hartford, C. M., and Ratain, M. J. (2007). Rapamycin: something old, something new, sometimes borrowed and now renewed. *Clin. Pharmacol. Ther.* 82, 381–388. doi: 10.1038/sj.clpt.6100317

Hastie, N. D., Dempster, M., Dunlop, M. G., Thompson, A. M., Green, D. K., and Allshire, R. C. (1990). Telomere reduction in human colorectal carcinoma and with ageing. *Nature* 346, 866–868. doi: 10.1038/346866a0

Hayflick, L. (1976). The cell biology of Human aging. *N. Engl. J. Med.* 295, 1302–1308. doi: 10.1056/NEJM197612022952308

Hayward, J. J., Castelhano, M. G., Oliveira, K. C., Corey, E., Balkman, C., Baxter, T. L., et al. (2016). Complex disease and phenotype mapping in the domestic dog. *Nat. Commun.* 7, 10460. doi: 10.1038/ncomms10460

He, C., and Klionsky, D. J. (2009). Regulation mechanisms and signaling pathways of autophagy. *Annu. Rev. Genet.* 43, 67–93. doi: 10.1146/annurev-genet-102808-114910

Head, E., Liu, J., Hagen, T. M., Muggenburg, B. A., Milgram, N. W., Ames, B. N., et al. (2002). Oxidative damage increases with age in a canine model of human brain aging. *J. Neurochem.* 82, 375–381. doi: 10.1046/j.1471-4159.2002.00969.x

Head, E., Nukala, V. N., Fenoglio, K. A., Muggenburg, B. A., Cotman, C. W., and Sullivan, P. G. (2009). Effects of age, dietary, and behavioral enrichment on brain mitochondria in a canine model of human aging. *Exp. Neurol.* 220, 171–176. doi: 10.1016/j.expneurol.2009.08.014

Hecht, J., and Rice, E. S. (2015). Citizen science: a new direction in canine behavior research. *Behav. Processes* 110, 125–132. doi: 10.1016/j.beproc.2014.10.014

Hekimi, S., Lapointe, J., and Wen, Y. (2011). Taking a "good" look at free radicals in the aging process. *Trends Cell Biol.* 21, 569–576. doi: 10.1016/j.tcb.2011.06.008

Heller, J. B. (2007). Metformin overdose in dogs and cats. *Vet. Med.* 231–234.

Hesp, K., Smant, G., and Kammenga, J. E. (2015). Caenorhabditis elegans DAF-16/FOXO transcription factor and its mammalian homologs associate with age-related disease. *Exp. Gerontol.* 72, 1–7. doi: 10.1016/J.EXGER.2015.09.006

Hickman, E. S., Moroni, M. C., and Helin, K. (2002). The role of p53 and pRB in apoptosis and cancer. *Curr. Opin. Genet. Dev.* 12, 60–66. doi: 10.1016/S0959-437X(01)00265-9

Hilton, B. A., Liu, J., Cartwright, B. M., Liu, Y., Breitman, M., Wang, Y., et al. (2017). Progerin sequestration of PCNA promotes replication fork collapse and mislocalization of XPA in laminopathy-related progeroid syndromes. *FASEB J.* 31, 3882–3893. doi: 10.1096/fj.201700014R

Hiona, A., Sanz, A., Kujoth, G. C., Pamplona, R., Seo, A. Y., Hofer, T., et al. (2010). Mitochondrial DNA mutations induce mitochondrial dysfunction, apoptosis and sarcopenia in skeletal muscle of mitochondrial DNA mutator mice. *PLoS One* 5, e11468. doi: 10.1371/journal.pone.0011468

Hoffman, A. M., and Dow, S. W. (2016). Concise review: stem cell trials using companion animal disease models. *Stem Cells* 34, 1709–1729. doi: 10.1002/stem.2377

Hoffman, J. M., Creevy, K. E., Franks, A., O'Neill, D. G., and Promislow, D. E. L. (2018). The companion dog as a model for human aging and mortality. *Aging Cell* 17, e12737. doi: 10.1111/acel.12737

HogenEsch, H., Thompson, S., Dunham, A., Ceddia, M., and Hayek, M. (2004). Effect of age on immune parameters and the immune response of dogs to vaccines: a cross-sectional study. *Vet. Immunol. Immunopathol.* 97, 77–85. doi: 10.1016/j.vetimm.2003.08.010

Holzenberger, M., Dupont, J., Ducos, B., Leneuve, P., Géloën, A., Even, P. C., et al. (2003). IGF-1 receptor regulates lifespan and resistance to oxidative stress in mice. *Nature* 421, 182–187. doi: 10.1038/nature01298

Hoopes, B. C., Rimbault, M., Liebers, D., Ostrander, E. A., and Sutter, N. B. (2012). The insulin-like growth factor 1 receptor (IGF1R) contributes to reduced size in dogs. *Mamm. Genome* 23, 780–790. doi: 10.1007/s00335-012-9417-z

Hu, C.-K., and Brunet, A. (2018). The African turquoise killifish: a research organism to study vertebrate aging and diapause. *Aging Cell* 17, e12757. doi: 10.1111/acel.12757

Hua, J., Hoummady, S., Muller, C., Pouchelon, J.-L., Blondot, M., Gilbert, C., et al. (2016). Assessment of frailty in aged dogs. *Am. J. Vet. Res.* 77, 1357–1365. doi: 10.2460/ajvr.77.12.1357

Hunter, R. G., Gagnidze, K., McEwen, B. S., and Pfaff, D. W. (2015). Stress and the dynamic genome: steroids, epigenetics, and the transposome. *Proc. Natl. Acad. Sci. U. S. A.* 112, 6828–6833. doi: 10.1073/pnas.1411260111

Hwang, I. K., Yoon, Y. S., Yoo, K.-Y., Li, H., Choi, J. H., KIM, D. W., et al. (2008). Differences in lipid peroxidation and Cu,Zn-superoxide dismutase in the hippocampal CA1 region between adult and aged dogs. *J. Vet. Med. Sci.* 70, 273–277. doi: 10.1292/jvms.70.273

Ichii, O., Ohta, H., Horino, T., Nakamura, T., Hosotani, M., Mizoguchi, T., et al. (2017). Urinary exosome-derived microRNAs reflecting the changes of renal function and histopathology in dogs. *Sci. Rep.* 7, 40340. doi: 10.1038/srep40340

Ilska, J., Haskell, M. J., Blott, S. C., Sánchez-Molano, E., Polgar, Z., Lofgren, S. E., et al. (2017). Genetic characterization of dog personality traits. *Genetics* 206, 1101–1111. doi: 10.1534/genetics.116.192674

Inoki, K., Zhu, T., and Guan, K.-L. (2003). TSC2 mediates cellular energy response to control cell growth and survival. *Cell* 115, 577–590. doi: 10.1016/S0092-8674(03)00929-2

Inoue, M., Kwan, N. C. L., and Sugiura, K. (2018). Estimating the life expectancy of companion dogs in Japan using pet cemetery data. *J. Vet. Med. Sci.* 80, 1153–1158. doi: 10.1292/jvms.17-0384

Insua, D., Suárez, M.-L., Santamarina, G., Sarasa, M., and Pesini, P. (2010). Dogs with canine counterpart of Alzheimer's disease lose noradrenergic neurons. *Neurobiol. Aging* 31, 625–635. doi: 10.1016/j.neurobiolaging.2008.05.014

Inukai, S., de Lencastre, A., Turner, M., and Slack, F. (2012). Novel MicroRNAs differentially expressed during aging in the mouse brain. *PLoS One* 7, e40028. doi: 10.1371/journal.pone.0040028

Ishida, T., Suzuki, J., Duangchan, P., and Settheetham-Ishida, W. (1998). Preliminary report on the short stature of Southeast Asian forest dwellers, the Manni, in southern Thailand: lack of an adolescent spurt in plasma IGF-I concentration. *Southeast Asian J. Trop. Med. Public Heal.* 29, 62–65.

Jeck, W. R., Siebold, A. P., and Sharpless, N. E. (2012). Review: a meta-analysis of GWAS and age-associated diseases. *Aging Cell* 11, 727–731. doi: 10.1111/j.1474-9726.2012.00871.x

Jeggo, P. A., Pearl, L. H., and Carr, A. M. (2016). DNA repair, genome stability and cancer: a historical perspective. *Nat. Rev. Cancer* 16, 35–42. doi: 10.1038/nrc.2015.4

Jia, G., Su, L., Singhal, S., and Liu, X. (2012). Emerging roles of SIRT6 on telomere maintenance, DNA repair, metabolism and mammalian aging. *Mol. Cell. Biochem.* 364, 345–350. doi: 10.1007/s11010-012-1236-8

Jia, K., and Levine, B. (2007). Autophagy is required for dietary restriction-mediated life span extension in *C. elegans*. *Autophagy* 3, 597–599. doi: 10.4161/auto.4989

Jiang, P., and Mizushima, N. (2014). Autophagy and human diseases. *Cell Res.* 24, 69–79. doi: 10.1038/cr.2013.161

Jimenez, A. G. (2016). Physiological underpinnings in life-history trade-offs in man's most popular selection experiment: the dog. *J. Comp. Physiol. B* 186, 813–827. doi: 10.1007/s00360-016-1002-4

Jin, C., Li, J., Green, C. D., Yu, X., Tang, X., Han, D., et al. (2011). Histone demethylase UTX-1 regulates *C. elegans* life span by targeting the insulin/IGF-1 signaling pathway. *Cell Metab.* 14, 161–172. doi: 10.1016/j.cmet.2011.07.001

Jones, P., Chase, K., Martin, A., Davern, P., Ostrander, E. A., and Lark, K. G. (2008). Single-nucleotide-polymorphism-based association mapping of dog stereotypes. *Genetics* 179, 1033–1044. doi: 10.1534/genetics.108.087866

Jucker, M. (2010). The benefits and limitations of animal models for translational research in neurodegenerative diseases. *Nat. Med.* 16, 1210–1214. doi: 10.1038/nm.2224

Juhász, G., Csikós, G., Sinka, R., Erdélyi, M., and Sass, M. (2003). The Drosophila homolog of Aut1 is essential for autophagy and development. *FEBS Lett.* 543, 154–158. doi: 10.1016/S0014-5793(03)00431-9

Juhász, G., Erdi, B., Sass, M., and Neufeld, T. P. (2007). Atg7-dependent autophagy promotes neuronal health, stress tolerance, and longevity but is dispensable for metamorphosis in Drosophila. *Genes Dev.* 21, 3061–3066. doi: 10.1101/gad.1600707

Kaeberlein, M. (2016). The biology of aging: citizen scientists and their pets as a bridge between research on model organisms and human subjects. *Vet. Pathol.* 53, 291–298. doi: 10.1177/0300985815591082

Kaeberlein, M., Creevy, K. E., and Promislow, D. E. L. (2016). The dog aging project: translational geroscience in companion animals. *Mamm. Genome* 27, 279–288. doi: 10.1007/s00335-016-9638-7

Kaeberlein, M., McVey, M., and Guarente, L. (1999). The SIR2/3/4 complex and SIR2 alone promote longevity in *Saccharomyces cerevisiae* by two different mechanisms. *Genes Dev.* 13, 2570–2580. doi: 10.1101/gad.13.19.2570

Kaeberlein, M., Powers, R. W., Steffen, K. K., Westman, E. A., Hu, D., Dang, N., et al. (2005). Regulation of yeast replicative life span by TOR and Sch9 in response to nutrients. *Science* 310, 1193–6. doi: 10.1126/science.1115535

Kapahi, P., Chen, D., Rogers, A. N., Katewa, S. D., Li, P. W.-L., Thomas, E. L., et al. (2010). With TOR, less is more: a key role for the conserved nutrient-sensing TOR pathway in aging. *Cell Metab.* 11, 453–465. doi: 10.1016/j.cmet.2010.05.001

Kapahi, P., Zid, B. M., Harper, T., Koslover, D., Sapin, V., and Benzer, S. (2004). Regulation of lifespan in drosophila by modulation of genes in the TOR signaling pathway. *Curr. Biol.* 14, 885–890. doi: 10.1016/J.CUB.2004.03.059

Katsimpardi, L., Litterman, N. K., Schein, P. A., Miller, C. M., Loffredo, F. S., Wojtkiewicz, G. R., et al. (2014). Vascular and neurogenic rejuvenation of the aging mouse brain by young systemic factors. *Science (80-.).* 344, 630–634. doi: 10.1126/science.1251141

Kazazian, H. H. (2004). Mobile elements: drivers of genome evolution. *Science* 303 (5664), 1626–1632. doi: 10.1126/science.1089670

Kenyon, C., Chang, J., Gensch, E., Rudner, A., and Tabtiang, R. (1993). A *C. elegans* mutant that lives twice as long as wild type. *Nature* 366, 461–464. doi: 10.1038/366461a0

Kiatipattanasakul, W., Nakamura, S., Hossain, M. M., Nakayama, H., Uchino, T., Shumiya, S., et al. (1996). Apoptosis in the aged dog brain. *Acta Neuropathol.* 92, 242–248. doi: 10.1007/s004010050514

Kim, J., Kundu, M., Viollet, B., and Guan, K.-L. (2011). AMPK and mTOR regulate autophagy through direct phosphorylation of Ulk1. *Nat. Cell Biol.* 13, 132–141. doi: 10.1038/ncb2152

Kim, J., Williams, F. J., Dreger, D. L., Plassais, J., Davis, B. W., Parker, H. G., et al. (2018). Genetic selection of athletic success in sport-hunting dogs. *Proc. Natl. Acad. Sci. U. S. A.* 115, E7212–E7221. doi: 10.1073/pnas.1800455115

Kim, K., and Choe, H. K. (2019). Role of hypothalamus in aging and its underlying cellular mechanisms. *Mech. Ageing Dev.* 177, 74–79. doi: 10.1016/j.mad.2018.04.008

Kim, O.-H., Kim, H., Kang, J., Yang, D., Kang, Y.-H., Lee, D. H., et al. (2017). Impaired phagocytosis of apoptotic cells causes accumulation of bone marrow-derived macrophages in aged mice. *BMB Rep.* 50, 43–48. doi: 10.5483/BMBRep.2017.50.1.167

Kim, S., Bi, X., Czarny-Ratajczak, M., Dai, J., Welsh, D. A., Myers, L., et al. (2012). Telomere maintenance genes SIRT1 and XRCC6 impact age-related decline in telomere length but only SIRT1 is associated with human longevity. *Biogerontology* 13, 119–131. doi: 10.1007/s10522-011-9360-5

Kinney, B. A., Meliska, C. J., Steger, R. W., and Bartke, A. (2001). Evidence that Ames dwarf mice age differently from their normal siblings in behavioral and learning and memory parameters. *Horm. Behav.* 39, 277–284. doi: 10.1006/hbeh.2001.1654

Kipling, D., and Cooke, H. J. (1990). Hypervariable ultra-long telomeres in mice. *Nature* 347, 400–402. doi: 10.1038/347400a0

Kippin, T. E., Martens, D. J., and van der Kooy, D. (2005). p21 loss compromises the relative quiescence of forebrain stem cell proliferation leading to exhaustion of their proliferation capacity. *Genes Dev.* 19, 756–767. doi: 10.1101/gad.1272305

Kirkland, J. L., Tchkonia, T., Zhu, Y., Niedernhofer, L. J., and Robbins, P. D. (2017). The clinical potential of senolytic drugs. *J. Am. Geriatr. Soc.* 65, 2297–2301. doi: 10.1111/jgs.14969

Kirpensteijn, J., Kik, M., Teske, E., and Rutteman, G. R. (2008). TP53 gene mutations in canine osteosarcoma. *Vet. Surg.* 37, 454–460. doi: 10.1111/j.1532-950X.2008.00407.x

Klionsky, D. J. (2005). Autophagy. *Curr. Biol.* 15, R282–R283. doi: 10.1016/j.cub.2005.04.013

Koch, I. J., Clark, M. M., Thompson, M. J., Deere-Machemer, K. A., Wang, J., Duarte, L., et al. (2016). The concerted impact of domestication and transposon insertions on methylation patterns between dogs and grey wolves. *Mol. Ecol.* 25, 1838–1855. doi: 10.1111/mec.13480

Koenig, E. M., Fisher, C., Bernard, H., Wolenski, F. S., Gerrein, J., Carsillo, M., et al. (2016). The beagle dog MicroRNA tissue atlas: identifying translatable biomarkers of organ toxicity. *BMC Genomics* 17, 649. doi: 10.1186/s12864-016-2958-x

Koga, H., Kaushik, S., and Cuervo, A. M. (2011). Protein homeostasis and aging: the importance of exquisite quality control. *Ageing Res. Rev.* 10, 205–215. doi: 10.1016/j.arr.2010.02.001

Komatsu, M., Waguri, S., Chiba, T., Murata, S., Iwata, J., Tanida, I., et al. (2006). Loss of autophagy in the central nervous system causes neurodegeneration in mice. *Nature* 441, 880–884. doi: 10.1038/nature04723

Koopman, W. J. H., Willems, P. H. G. M., and Smeitink, J. A. M. (2012). Monogenic mitochondrial disorders. *N. Engl. J. Med.* 366, 1132–1141. doi: 10.1056/NEJMra1012478

Kraus, C., Pavard, S., and Promislow, D. E. L. (2013). The size–life span trade-off decomposed: why large dogs die young. *Am. Nat.* 181, 492–505. doi: 10.1086/669665

Kraytsberg, Y., Kudryavtseva, E., McKee, A. C., Geula, C., Kowall, N. W., and Khrapko, K. (2006). Mitochondrial DNA deletions are abundant and cause functional impairment in aged human substantia nigra neurons. *Nat. Genet.* 38, 518–520. doi: 10.1038/ng1778

Krebiehl, G., Ruckerbauer, S., Burbulla, L. F., Kieper, N., Maurer, B., Waak, J., et al. (2010). Reduced basal autophagy and impaired mitochondrial dynamics due to loss of Parkinson's disease-associated protein DJ-1. *PLoS One* 5, e9367. doi: 10.1371/journal.pone.0009367

Krishnamurthy, J., Ramsey, M. R., Ligon, K. L., Torrice, C., Koh, A., Bonner Weir, S., et al. (2006). p16INK4a induces an age-dependent decline in islet regenerative potential. *Nature* 443, 453–457. doi: 10.1038/nature05092

Krishnamurthy, J., Torrice, C., Ramsey, M. R., Kovalev, G. I., Al-Regaiey, K., Su, L., et al. (2004). Ink4a/Arf expression is a biomarker of aging. *J. Clin. Invest.* 114, 1299–1307. doi: 10.1172/JCI22475

Kroemer, G., Galluzzi, L., and Brenner, C. (2007). Mitochondrial membrane permeabilization in cell death. *Physiol. Rev.* 87, 99–163. doi: 10.1152/physrev.00013.2006

Kuilman, T., Michaloglou, C., Mooi, W. J., and Peeper, D. S. (2010). The essence of senescence. *Genes Dev.* 24, 2463–2479. doi: 10.1101/gad.1971610

Kuro-o, M., Nabeshima, Y., Matsumura, Y., Aizawa, H., Kawaguchi, H., Suga, T., et al. (1997). Mutation of the mouse klotho gene leads to a syndrome resembling ageing. *Nature* 390, 45–51. doi: 10.1038/36285

Kurosu, H., Yamamoto, M., Clark, J. D., Pastor, J. V., Nandi, A., Gurnani, P., et al. (2005). Suppression of aging in mice by the hormone Klotho. *Science (80-.).* 309, 1829–1833. doi: 10.1126/science.1112766

Kyöstilä, K., Syrjä, P., Jagannathan, V., Chandrasekar, G., Jokinen, T. S., Seppälä, E. H., et al. (2015). A missense change in the ATG4D gene links aberrant autophagy to a neurodegenerative vacuolar storage disease. *PLoS Genet.* 11, 1–22. doi: 10.1371/journal.pgen.1005169

Lagouge, M., Argmann, C., Gerhart-Hines, Z., Meziane, H., Lerin, C., Daussin, F., et al. (2006). Resveratrol improves mitochondrial function and protects against metabolic disease by activating SIRT1 and PGC-1α. *Cell* 127, 1109–1122. doi: 10.1016/j.cell.2006.11.013

Lamb, R., Ozsvari, B., Bonuccelli, G., Smith, D. L., Pestell, R. G., Martinez-Outschoorn, U. E., et al. (2015). Dissecting tumor metabolic heterogeneity: telomerase and large cell size metabolically define a sub-population of stem-like, mitochondrial-rich, cancer cells. *Oncotarget* 6, 21892–21905. doi: 10.18632/oncotarget.5260

Landsberg, G. M., Nichol, J., and Araujo, J. A. (2012). Cognitive dysfunction syndrome. a disease of canine and feline brain aging. *Vet. Clin. North Am. - Small Anim. Pract.* 42, 749–768. doi: 10.1016/j.cvsm.2012.04.003

Larsen, P. L., Albert, P. S., and Riddle D. L. (1995). Genes that regulate both development and longevity in *Caenorhabditis elegans. Genetics* 139, 1567–1583.

Larson, G., Karlsson, E. K., Perri, A., Webster, M. T., Ho, S. Y. W., Peters, J., et al. (2012). Rethinking dog domestication by integrating genetics, archeology, and biogeography. *Proc. Natl. Acad. Sci.* 109, 8878–8883. doi: 10.1073/pnas.1203005109

Lawrence, J., Chang, Y.-M. R., Szladovits, B., Davison, L. J., and Garden, O. A. (2013). Breed-specific hematological phenotypes in the dog: a natural resource for the genetic dissection of hematological parameters in a mammalian species. *PLoS One* 8, e81288. doi: 10.1371/journal.pone.0081288

Lee, C.-K., Klopp, R. G., Weindruch, R., and Prolla, T. A. (1999). Gene expression profile of aging and its retardation by caloric restriction. *Science (80-.).* 285, 1390–1393. doi: 10.1126/science.285.5432.1390

Lee, C.-K., Weindruch, R., and Prolla, T. A. (2000). Gene-expression profile of the ageing brain in mice. *Nat. Genet.* 25, 294–297. doi: 10.1038/77046

Lentino, C., Visek, A. J., McDonnell, K., and DiPietro, L. (2012). Dog walking is associated with a favorable risk profile independent of a moderate to high volume of physical activity. *J. Phys. Act. Heal.* 9, 414–420. doi: 10.1123/jpah.9.3.414

Levin, H. L., and Moran, J. V. (2011). Dynamic interactions between transposable elements and their hosts. *Nat. Rev. Genet.* 12, 615–627. doi: 10.1038/nrg3030

Levine, B. (2005). Eating oneself and uninvited guests: autophagy-related pathways in cellular defense. *Cell* 120, 159–162. doi: 10.1016/j.cell.2005.01.005

Levine, B., and Kroemer, G. (2008). Autophagy in the pathogenesis of disease. *Cell* 132, 27–42. doi: 10.1016/j.cell.2007.12.018

Levine, B., Mizushima, N., and Virgin, H. W. (2011). Autophagy in immunity and inflammation. *Nature* 469, 323–335. doi: 10.1038/nature09782

Levis, R. W., Ganesan, R., Houtchens, K., Tolar, L. A., and Sheen, F. (1993). Transposons in place of telomeric repeats at a Drosophila telomere. *Cell* 75, 1083–1093. doi: 10.1016/0092-8674(93)90318-K

Li, Y., Wang, W.-J., Cao, H., Lu, J., Wu, C., Hu, F.-Y., et al. (2009). Genetic association of FOXO1A and FOXO3A with longevity trait in Han Chinese populations. *Hum. Mol. Genet.* 18, 4897–4904. doi: 10.1093/hmg/ddp459

Li, Z., Jiao, Y., Fan, E. K., Scott, M. J., Li, Y., Li, S., et al. (2017). Aging-impaired filamentous actin polymerization signaling reduces alveolar macrophage phagocytosis of bacteria. *J. Immunol.* 199, 3176–3186. doi: 10.4049/jimmunol.1700140

Lin, K., Dorman, J. B., Rodan, A., and Kenyon, C. (1997). daf-16: An HNF-3/forkhead family member that can function to double the life-span of *Caenorhabditis elegans*. *Science* 278 (5341), 1319–1322. doi: 10.1126/science.278.5341.1319

Lin, L., Faraco, J., Li, R., Kadotani, H., Rogers, W., Lin, X., et al. (1999). The sleep disorder canine narcolepsy is caused by a mutation in the hypocretin (orexin) receptor 2 gene. *Cell* 98, 365–376. doi: 10.1016/S0092-8674(00)81965-0

Lin, M. T., and Beal, M. F. (2006). Mitochondrial dysfunction and oxidative stress in neurodegenerative diseases. *Nature* 443, 787–795. doi: 10.1038/nature05292

Lindblad-Toh, K., Wade, C. M., Mikkelsen, T. S., Karlsson, E. K., Jaffe, D. B., Kamal, M., et al. (2005). Genome sequence, comparative analysis and haplotype structure of the domestic dog. *Nature* 438, 803–819. doi: 10.1038/nature04338

Lindsey, J., McGill, N. I., Lindsey, L. A., Green, D. K., and Cooke, H. J. (1991). In vivo loss of telomeric repeats with age in humans. *Mutat. Res.* 256, 45–48. doi: 10.1016/0921-8734(91)90032-7

Lindvall, O., Kokaia, Z., and Martinez-Serrano, A. (2004). Stem cell therapy for human neurodegenerative disorders–how to make it work. *Nat. Med.* 10, S42–S50. doi: 10.1038/nm1064

Liu, H.-Y., and Pfleger, C. M. (2013). Mutation in E1, the ubiquitin activating enzyme, reduces Drosophila lifespan and results in motor impairment. *PLoS One* 8, e32835. doi: 10.1371/journal.pone.0032835

Liu, J.-P., Baker, J., Perkins, A. S., Robertson, E. J., and Efstratiadis, A. (1993). Mice carrying null mutations of the genes encoding insulin-like growth factor I (Igf-1) and type 1 IGF receptor (Igf1r). *Cell* 75, 59–72. doi: 10.1016/S0092-8674(05)80084-4

Liu, Y., Elf, S. E., Miyata, Y., Sashida, G., Liu, Y., Huang, G., et al. (2009a). p53 regulates hematopoietic stem cell quiescence. *Cell Stem Cell* 4, 37–48. doi: 10.1016/j.stem.2008.11.006

Liu, Y., Fiskum, G., and Schubert, D. (2002). Generation of reactive oxygen species by the mitochondrial electron transport chain. *J. Neurochem.* 80, 780–787. doi: 10.1046/j.0022-3042.2002.00744.x

Liu, Y., Hettinger, C. L., Zhang, D., Rezvani, K., Wang, X., and Wang, H. (2014). The proteasome function reporter GFPu accumulates in young brains of the APPswe/PS1dE9 Alzheimer's disease mouse model. *Cell. Mol. Neurobiol.* 34, 315–322. doi: 10.1007/s10571-013-0022-9

Liu, Y., Sanoff, H. K., Cho, H., Burd, C. E., Torrice, C., Ibrahim, J. G., et al. (2009b). Expression of *p16* INK4a in peripheral blood T-cells is a biomarker of human aging. *Aging Cell* 8, 439–448. doi: 10.1111/j.1474-9726.2009.00489.x

Loffredo, F. S., Steinhauser, M. L., Jay, S. M., Gannon, J., Pancoast, J. R., Yalamanchi, P., et al. (2013). Growth differentiation factor 11 is a circulating factor that reverses age-related cardiac hypertrophy. *Cell* 153, 828–839. doi: 10.1016/j.cell.2013.04.015

Lombard, D. B., Chua, K. F., Mostoslavsky, R., Franco, S., Gostissa, M., and Alt, F. W. (2005). DNA repair, genome stability, and aging. *Cell* 120, 497–512. doi: 10.1016/j.cell.2005.01.028

Longo, V. D., and Kennedy, B. K. (2006). Sirtuins in aging and age-related disease. *Cell* 126, 257–268. doi: 10.1016/j.cell.2006.07.002

López-Otín, C., Blasco, M. A., Partridge, L., Serrano, M., and Kroemer, G. (2013). The hallmarks of aging. *Cell* 153, 1194–1217. doi: 10.1016/j.cell.2013.05.039

Lu, J., Shi, J., Li, M., Gui, B., Fu, R., Yao, G., et al. (2015). Activation of AMPK by metformin inhibits TGF-β-induced collagen production in mouse renal fibroblasts. *Life Sci.* 127, 59–65. doi: 10.1016/j.lfs.2015.01.042

Lu, T., Pan, Y., Kao, S.-Y., Li, C., Kohane, I., Chan, J., et al. (2004). Gene regulation and DNA damage in the ageing human brain. *Nature* 429, 883–891. doi: 10.1038/nature02661

Lundberg, J. O., Weitzberg, E., and Gladwin, M. T. (2008). The nitrate–nitrite–nitric oxide pathway in physiology and therapeutics. *Nat. Rev. Drug Discov.* 7, 156–167. doi: 10.1038/nrd2466

Luo, W., Dou, F., Rodina, A., Chip, S., Kim, J., Zhao, Q., et al. (2007). Roles of heat-shock protein 90 in maintaining and facilitating the neurodegenerative phenotype in tauopathies. *Proc. Natl. Acad. Sci.* 104, 9511–9516. doi: 10.1073/pnas.0701055104

Luo, Y., Lu, X., and Xie, H. (2014). Dynamic Alu methylation during normal development, aging, and tumorigenesis. *Biomed Res. Int.* 2014, 784706. doi: 10.1155/2014/784706

Lutful Kabir, F. M., Agarwal, P., DeInnocentes, P., Zaman, J., Bird, A. C., and Bird, R. C. (2013). Novel frameshift mutation in the p16/INK4A tumor suppressor gene in canine breast cancer alters expression from the p16/INK4A/p14ARF locus. *J. Cell. Biochem.* 114, 56–66. doi: 10.1002/jcb.24300

Maegawa, S., Hinkal, G., Kim, H. S., Shen, L., Zhang, L., Zhang, J., et al. (2010). Widespread and tissue specific age-related DNA methylation changes in mice. *Genome Res.* 20, 332–340. doi: 10.1101/gr.096826.109

Mahbub, S., Brubaker, A. L., and Kovacs, J. (2011). Aging of the innate immune system: an update. *Curr. Immunol. Rev.* 7, 104–115, E. doi: 10.2174/157339511794474181

Mammucari, C., Milan, G., Romanello, V., Masiero, E., Rudolf, R., Del Piccolo, P., et al. (2007). FoxO3 controls autophagy in skeletal muscle *in vivo*. *Cell Metab.* 6, 458–471. doi: 10.1016/j.cmet.2007.11.001

Manczak, M., Jung, Y., Park, B. S., Partovi, D., and Reddy, P. H. (2005). Time-course of mitochondrial gene expressions in mice brains: implications for mitochondrial dysfunction, oxidative damage, and cytochrome c in aging. *J. Neurochem.* 92, 494–504. doi: 10.1111/j.1471-4159.2004.02884.x

Mandal, P. K., and Kazazian, H. H. (2008). SnapShot: vertebrate transposons. *Cell* 135, 192–192.e1. doi: 10.1016/j.cell.2008.09.028

Marchant, T. W., Johnson, E. J., McTeir, L., Johnson, C. I., Gow, A., Liuti, T., et al. (2017). Canine brachycephaly is associated with a retrotransposon-mediated missplicing of SMOC2. *Curr. Biol.* 27, 1573–1584.e6. doi: 10.1016/j.cub.2017.04.057

Marfe, G., De Martino, L., Tafani, M., Irno-Consalvo, M., Pasolini, M. P., Navas, L., et al. (2012). A multicancer-like syndrome in a dog characterized by p53 and cell cycle-checkpoint kinase 2 (CHK2) mutations and Sirtuin gene (SIRT1) down-regulation. *Res. Vet. Sci.* 93, 240–245. doi: 10.1016/j.rvsc.2011.07.030

Martin-Montalvo, A., Mercken, E. M., Mitchell, S. J., Palacios, H. H., Mote, P. L., Scheibye-Knudsen, M., et al. (2013). Metformin improves healthspan and lifespan in mice. *Nat. Commun.* 4, 2192. doi: 10.1038/ncomms3192

Martín-Rivera, L., Herrera, E., Albar, J. P., and Blasco, M. A. (1998). Expression of mouse telomerase catalytic subunit in embryos and adult tissues. *Proc. Natl. Acad. Sci.* 95 (18), 10471–10476. doi: 10.1073/pnas.95.18.10471

Martin, G. M. (2005). Genetic modulation of senescent phenotypes in *Homo sapiens*. *Cell* 120, 523–532. doi: 10.1016/j.cell.2005.01.031

Martindale, J. L., and Holbrook, N. J. (2002). Cellular response to oxidative stress: signaling for suicide and survival. *J. Cell. Physiol.* 192, 1–15. doi: 10.1002/jcp.10119

Massey, A. C., Zhang, C., and Cuervo, A. M. (2006). Chaperone-mediated autophagy in aging and disease. *Curr. Top. Dev. Biol.* 73, 205–235. doi: 10.1016/S0070-2153(05)73007-6

Massimino, S., Kearns, R. J., Loos, K. M., Burr, J., Park, J. S., Chew, B., et al. (2003). Effects of age and dietary β-carotene on immunological variables in dogs. *J. Vet. Intern. Med.* 17, 835–842. doi: 10.1111/j.1939-1676.2003.tb02523.x

Masutomi, K., Possemato, R., Wong, J. M. Y., Currier, J. L., Tothova, Z., Manola, J. B., et al. (2005). The telomerase reverse transcriptase regulates chromatin state and DNA damage responses. *Proc. Natl. Acad. Sci. U. S. A.* 102, 8222–8227. doi: 10.1073/pnas.0503095102

Matheu, A., Maraver, A., Collado, M., Garcia-Cao, I., Cañamero, M., Borras, C., et al. (2009). Anti-aging activity of the *Ink4/Arf* locus. *Aging Cell* 8, 152–161. doi: 10.1111/j.1474-9726.2009.00458.x

Matheu, A., Maraver, A., Klatt, P., Flores, I., Garcia-Cao, I., Borras, C., et al. (2007). Delayed ageing through damage protection by the Arf/p53 pathway. *Nature* 448, 375–379. doi: 10.1038/nature05949

Matheu, A., Maraver, A., and Serrano, M. (2008). The Arf/p53 pathway in cancer and aging. *Cancer Res.* 68, 6031–6034. doi: 10.1158/0008-5472.CAN-07-6851

Mathew, L. M., Woode, R. A., Axiak-Bechtel, S. M., Amorim, J. R., and DeClue, A. E. (2018). Resveratrol administration increases phagocytosis, decreases oxidative burst, and promotes pro-inflammatory cytokine production in healthy dogs. *Vet. Immunol. Immunopathol.* 203, 21–29. doi: 10.1016/j.vetimm.2018.07.013

Mattson, M. P., Maudsley, S., and Martin, B. (2004). A neural signaling triumvirate that influences ageing and age-related disease: insulin/IGF-1, BDNF and serotonin. *Ageing Res. Rev.* 3, 445–464. doi: 10.1016/j.arr.2004.08.001

Maxwell, P. H., Burhans, W. C., and Curcio, M. J. (2011). Retrotransposition is associated with genome instability during chronological aging. *Proc. Natl. Acad. Sci. U. S. A.* 108 (51), 20376–20381. doi: 10.1073/pnas.1100271108

Mazzatenta, A., Carluccio, A., Robbe, D., and Giulio, C. Di (2017). The companion dog as a unique translational model for aging. *Semin. Cell Dev. Biol.* 70, 141–153. doi: 10.1016/J.SEMCDB.2017.08.024

Mech, L. D. (2006). Estimated age structure of wolves in Northeastern Minnesota. *J. Wildl. Manage.* 70, 1481–1483. doi: 10.2193/0022-541X(2006)70[1481:EASOWI]2.0.CO;2

Mecocci, P., MacGarvey, U., Kaufman, A. E., Koontz, D., Shoffner, J. M., Wallace, D. C., et al. (1993). Oxidative damage to mitochondrial DNA shows marked age-dependent increases in human brain. *Ann. Neurol.* 34, 609–616. doi: 10.1002/ana.410340416

Meldolesi, J. (2018). Exosomes and ectosomes in intercellular communication. *Curr. Biol.* 28, R435–R444. doi: 10.1016/j.cub.2018.01.059

Mendrysa, S. M., O'Leary, K. A., McElwee, M. K., Michalowski, J., Eisenman, R. N., Powell, D. A., et al. (2006). Tumor suppression and normal aging in mice with constitutively high p53 activity. *Genes Dev.* 20, 16–21. doi: 10.1101/gad.1378506

Merry, T. L., and Ristow, M. (2016). Do antioxidant supplements interfere with skeletal muscle adaptation to exercise training? *J. Physiol.* 594, 5135–5147. doi: 10.1113/JP270654

Mesquita, A., Weinberger, M., Silva, A., Sampaio-Marques, B., Almeida, B., Leão, C., et al. (2010). Caloric restriction or catalase inactivation extends yeast chronological lifespan by inducing H2O2 and superoxide dismutase activity. *Proc. Natl. Acad. Sci.* 107, 15123–15128. doi: 10.1073/pnas.1004432107

Meurs, K. M., Hendrix, K. P., and Norgard, M. M. (2008). Molecular evaluation of five cardiac genes in Doberman Pinschers with dilated cardiomyopathy. *Am. J. Vet. Res.* 69, 1050–1053. doi: 10.2460/ajvr.69.8.1050

Meurs, K. M., Lahmers, S., Keene, B. W., White, S. N., Oyama, M. A., Mauceli, E., et al. (2012). A splice site mutation in a gene encoding for PDK4, a mitochondrial protein, is associated with the development of dilated cardiomyopathy in the Doberman pinscher. *Hum. Genet.* 131, 1319–1325. doi: 10.1007/s00439-012-1158-2

Michell, A. R. (1999). Longevity of British breeds of dog and its relationships with sex, size, cardiovascular variables and disease. *Vet. Rec.* 145, 625–629. doi: 10.1136/vr.145.22.625

Miklósi, Á. (2014). *Dog behaviour, evolution, and cognition.* (Oxford: Oxford University Press). doi: 10.1093/acprof:oso/9780199646661.001.0001

Miklósi, Á., and Kubinyi, E. (2016). Current trends in canine problem-solving and cognition. *Curr. Dir. Psychol. Sci.* 25, 300–306. doi: 10.1177/0963721416666061

Milgram, N. W., Head, E., Muggenburg, B., Holowachuk, D., Murphey, H., Estrada, J., et al. (2002a). Landmark discrimination learning in the dog: effects of age, an antioxidant fortified food, and cognitive strategy. *Neurosci. Biobehav. Rev.* 26, 679–695. doi: 10.1016/S0149-7634(02)00039-8

Milgram, N. W., Zicker, S. C., Head, E., Muggenburg, B. A., Murphey, H., Ikeda-Douglas, C. J., et al. (2002b). Dietary enrichment counteracts age-associated cognitive dysfunction in canines. *Neurobiol. Aging* 23, 737–745. doi: 10.1016/S0197-4580(02)00020-9

Min, J.-N., Whaley, R. A., Sharpless, N. E., Lockyer, P., Portbury, A. L., and Patterson, C. (2008). CHIP deficiency decreases longevity, with accelerated aging phenotypes accompanied by altered protein quality control. *Mol. Cell. Biol.* 28, 4018–4025. doi: 10.1128/MCB.00296-08

Misic, A. M., Davis, M. F., Tyldsley, A. S., Hodkinson, B. P., Tolomeo, P., Hu, B., et al. (2015). The shared microbiota of humans and companion animals as evaluated from Staphylococcus carriage sites. *Microbiome* 3, 2. doi: 10.1186/s40168-014-0052-7

Mizuno, H., Nakamura, A., Aoki, Y., Ito, N., Kishi, S., Yamamoto, K., et al. (2011). Identification of muscle-specific MicroRNAs in serum of muscular dystrophy animal models: promising novel blood-based markers for muscular dystrophy. *PLoS One* 6, e18388. doi: 10.1371/journal.pone.0018388

Mizushima, N., Levine, B., Cuervo, A. M., and Klionsky, D. J. (2008). Autophagy fights disease through cellular self-digestion. *Nature* 451, 1069–1075. doi: 10.1038/nature06639

Moloney, A. M., Griffin, R. J., Timmons, S , O'Connor, R., Ravid, R., and O'Neill, C. (2010). Defects in IGF-1 receptor, insulin receptor and IRS-1/2 in Alzheimer's disease indicate possible resistance to IGF-1 and insulin signalling. *Neurobiol. Aging* 31, 224–243. doi: 10.1016/j.neurobiolaging.2008.04.002

Morales, M. E., Servant, G., Ade, C., and Roy-Engel, A. M. (2015). Altering genomic integrity: heavy metal exposure promotes transposable element-mediated damage. *Biol. Trace Elem. Res.* 166, 24–33. doi: 10.1007/s12011-015-0298-3

Morimoto, R. I. (2008). Proteotoxic stress and inducible chaperone networks in neurodegenerative disease and aging. *Genes Dev.* 22, 1427–1438. doi: 10.1101/gad.1657108

Morrow, G., Samson, M., Michaud, S., and Tanguay, R. M. (2004). Overexpression of the small mitochondrial Hsp22 extends Drosophila life span and increases resistance to oxidative stress. *FASEB J.* 18, 598–599. doi: 10.1096/fj.03-0860fje

Mortiboys, H., Johansen, K. K., Aasly, J. O., and Bandmann, O. (2010). Mitochondrial impairment in patients with Parkinson disease with the G2019S mutation in LRRK2. *Neurology* 75, 2017–2020. doi: 10.1212/WNL.0b013e3181ff9685

Moskalev, A. A., Shaposhnikov, M. V., Plyusnina, E. N., Zhavoronkov, A., Budovsky, A., Yanai, H., et al. (2013). The role of DNA damage and repair in aging through the prism of Koch-like criteria. *Ageing Res. Rev.* 12, 661–684. doi: 10.1016/j.arr.2012.02.001

Murphy, M. P. (2009). How mitochondria produce reactive oxygen species. *Biochem. J.* 417, 1–13. doi: 10.1042/BJ20081386

Murray, V. (1990). Are transposons a cause of ageing? *Mutat. Res.* 237, 59–63. doi: 10.1016/0921-8734(90)90011-F

Nasir, L., Devlin, P., Mckevitt, T., Rutteman, G., and Argyle, D. J. (2001). Telomere lengths and telomerase activity in dog tissues: a potential model system to study human telomere and telomerase biology. *Neoplasia* 3, 351–359. doi: 10.1038/sj.neo.7900173

Navarro, A., and Boveris, A. (2004). Rat brain and liver mitochondria develop oxidative stress and lose enzymatic activities on aging. *Am. J. Physiol. Integr. Comp. Physiol.* 287, R1244–R1249. doi: 10.1152/ajpregu.00226.2004

Nebel, A., Kleindorp, R., Caliebe, A., Nothnagel, M., Blanché, H., Junge, O., et al. (2011). A genome-wide association study confirms APOE as the major gene influencing survival in long-lived individuals. *Mech. Ageing Dev.* 132, 324–330. doi: 10.1016/j.mad.2011.06.008

Neilson, J. C., Hart, B. L., Cliff, K. D., and Ruehl, W. W. (2001). Prevalence of behavioral changes associated with age-related cognitive impairment in dogs. *J. Am. Vet. Med. Assoc.* 218, 1787–1791. doi: 10.2460/javma.2001.218.1787

Nelson, G., Wordsworth, J., Wang, C., Jurk, D., Lawless, C., Martin-Ruiz, C., et al. (2012). A senescent cell bystander effect: senescence-induced senescence. *Aging Cell* 11, 345–349. doi: 10.1111/j.1474-9726.2012.00795.x

Nixon, R. A., Wegiel, J., Kumar, A., Yu, W. H., Peterhoff, C., Cataldo, A., et al. (2005). Extensive involvement of autophagy in Alzheimer disease: an immuno-electron microscopy study. *J. Neuropathol. Exp. Neurol.* 64, 113–122. doi: 10.1093/jnen/64.2.113

Nixon, R. A., and Yang, D.-S. (2011). Autophagy failure in Alzheimer's disease—locating the primary defect. *Neurobiol. Dis.* 43, 38–45. doi: 10.1016/j.nbd.2011.01.021

O'Neill, D. G., Church, D. B., Mcgreevy, P D., Thomson, P. C., and Brodbelt, D. C. (2013). Longevity and mortality of owned dogs in England. *Vet. J.* 198, 638–643. doi: 10.1016/j.tvjl.2013.09.020

Ogawa, M., Uchida, K., Yamato, O., Mizukami, K., Chambers, J. K., and Nakayama, H. (2015). Expression of autophagy-related proteins in the spinal cord of Pembroke Welsh Corgi dogs with canine degenerative myelopathy. *Vet. Pathol.* 52, 1099–1107. doi: 10.1177/0300985815570070

Orrell, R. W. (2000). Amyotrophic lateral sclerosis: copper/zinc superoxide dismutase (SOD1) gene mutations. *Neuromuscul. Disord.* 10, 63–68. doi: 10.1016/S0960-8966(99)00071-1

Ostan, R., Borelli, V., and Castellani, G. (2017). Inflammaging and human longevity in the omics era. *Mech. Ageing Dev.* 165, 129–138. doi: 10.1016/j.mad.2016.12.008

Ouyang, L., Shi, Z., Zhao, S., Wang, F.-T., Zhou, T.-T., Liu, B., et al. (2012). Programmed cell death pathways in cancer: a review of apoptosis, autophagy and programmed necrosis. *Cell Prolif.* 45, 487–498. doi: 10.1111/j.1365-2184.2012.00845.x

Pace, J. K., and Feschotte, C. (2007). The evolutionary history of human DNA transposons: evidence for intense activity in the primate lineage. *Genome Res.* 17, 422–432. doi: 10.1101/gr.5826307

Pagano, T. B., Wojcik, S., Costagliola, A., De Biase, D., Iovino, S., Iovane, V., et al. (2015). Age related skeletal muscle atrophy and upregulation of autophagy in dogs. *Vet. J.* 206, 54–60. doi: 10.1016/j.tvjl.2015.07.005

Pal, S., and Tyler, J. K. (2016). Epigenetics and aging. *Sci. Adv.* 2, 1–20. doi: 10.1126/sciadv.1600584

Papaioannou, N., Tooten, P. C. J., van Ederen, A. M., Bohl, J. R. E., Rofina, J., Tsangaris, T., et al. (2001). Immunohistochemical investigation of the brain of aged dogs. I. Detection of neurofibrillary tangles and of 4-hydroxynonenal protein, an oxidative damage product, in senile plaques. *Amyloid* 8, 11–21. doi: 10.3109/13506120108993810

Parker, H. G., VonHoldt, B. M., Quignon, P., Margulies, E. H., Shao, S., Mosher, D. S., et al. (2009). An expressed fgf4 retrogene is associated with breed-defining Chondrodysplasia in domestic dogs. *Science* (80-). 325, 995–998. doi: 10.1126/SCIENCE.1173275

Parker, H. G., Dreger, D. L., Rimbault, M., Davis, B. W., Mullen, A. B., Carpintero-Ramirez, G., and Ostrander, E. A. (2017). Genomic analyses reveal the influence of geographic origin, migration, and hybridization on modern dog breed development. *Cell Reports* 19 (4), 697–708. doi: 10.1016/j.celrep.2017.03.079

Patel, P. J., Singh, S. K., Panaich, S., and Cardozo, L. (2014). The aging gut and the role of prebiotics, probiotics, and synbiotics: A review. *J. Clin. Gerontol. Geriatr.* 5, 3–6. doi: 10.1016/j.jcgg.2013.08.003

Patel, K. V. (2008). Epidemiology of anemia in older adults. *Semin. Hematol.* 45, 210–217. doi: 10.1053/j.seminhematol.2008.06.006

Pawelec, G. (2018). Age and immunity: what is "immunosenescence"? *Exp. Gerontol.* 105, 4–9. doi: 10.1016/j.exger.2017.10.024

Pelatti, M. V., Gomes, J. P. A., Vieira, N. M. S., Cangussu, E., Landini, V., Andrade, T., et al. (2016). Transplantation of human adipose mesenchymal stem cells in non-immunosuppressed GRMD dogs is a safe procedure. *Stem Cell Rev. Reports* 12, 448–453. doi: 10.1007/s12015-016-9659-3

Penso-Dolfin, L., Swofford, R., Johnson, J., Alföldi, J., Lindblad-Toh, K., Swarbreck, D., et al. (2016). An improved microRNA annotation of the canine genome. *PLoS One* 11, e0153453. doi: 10.1371/journal.pone.0153453

Perry, G. H., and Dominy, N. J. (2009). Evolution of the human pygmy phenotype. *Trends Ecol. Evol.* 24, 218–225. doi: 10.1016/j.tree.2008.11.008

Petrosillo, G., Matera, M., Casanova, G., Ruggiero, F., and Paradies, G. (2008). Mitochondrial dysfunction in rat brain with aging. Involvement of complex I, reactive oxygen species and cardiolipin. *Neurochem. Int.* 53, 126–131. doi: 10.1016/j.neuint.2008.07.001

Pfahler, S., and Distl, O. (2012). Identification of quantitative trait loci (QTL) for canine hip dysplasia and canine elbow dysplasia in Bernese Mountain dogs. *PLoS One* 7, e49782. doi: 10.1371/journal.pone.0049782

Pievani, M., Filippini, N., van den Heuvel, M. P., Cappa, S. F., and Frisoni, G. B. (2014). Brain connectivity in neurodegenerative diseases—from phenotype to proteinopathy. *Nat. Rev. Neurol.* 10, 620–633. doi: 10.1038/nrneurol.2014.178

Pizarro, J. G., and Cristofari, G. (2016). Post-transcriptional control of LINE-1 retrotransposition by cellular host factors in somatic cells. *Front. Cell Dev. Biol.* 4, 14. doi: 10.3389/fcell.2016.00014

Plassais, J., Rimbault, M., Williams, F. J., Davis, B. W., Schoenebeck, J. J., and Ostrander, E. A. (2017). Analysis of large versus small dogs reveals three genes on the canine X chromosome associated with body weight, muscling and back fat thickness. *PLOS Genet.* 13, e1006661. doi: 10.1371/journal.pgen.1006661

Plowden, J., Renshaw-Hoelscher, M., Engleman, C., Katz, J., and Sambhara, S. (2004). Innate immunity in aging: impact on macrophage function. *Aging Cell* 3, 161–167. doi: 10.1111/j.1474-9728.2004.00102.x

Pritchard, A. B., Crean, S., Olsen, I., and Singhrao, S. K. (2017). Periodontitis, microbiomes and their role in Alzheimer's disease. *Front. Aging Neurosci.* 9, 336. doi: 10.3389/fnagi.2017.00336

Proschowsky, H. F., Rugbjerg, H., and Ersbøll, A. K. (2003). Mortality of purebred and mixed-breed dogs in Denmark. *Prev. Vet. Med.* 58, 63–74. doi: 10.1016/S0167-5877(03)00010-2

Prowse, K. R., and Greidert, C. W. (1995). Developmental and tissue-specific regulation of mouse telomerase and telomere length. *Cell Biol.* 92, 4818–4822. doi: 10.1073/pnas.92.11.4818

Puzzo, D., Gulisano, W., Palmeri, A., and Arancio, O. (2015). Rodent models for Alzheimer's disease drug discovery. *Expert Opin. Drug Discov.* 10, 703–711. doi: 10.1517/17460441.2015.1041913

Pyo, J.-O., Yoo, S.-M., Ahn, H.-H., Nah, J., Hong, S.-H., Kam, T.-I., et al. (2013). Overexpression of Atg5 in mice activates autophagy and extends lifespan. *Nat. Commun.* 4, 2300. doi: 10.1038/ncomms3300

Rabinowitz, J. D., and White, E. (2010). Autophagy and metabolism. *Science* 330, 1344–1348. doi: 10.1126/science.1193497

Radakovich, L. B., Pannone, S. C., Truelove, M. P., Olver, C. S., and Santangelo, K. S. (2017). Hematology and biochemistry of aging-evidence of "anemia of the elderly" in old dogs. *Vet. Clin. Pathol.* 46, 34–45. doi: 10.1111/vcp.12459

Raposo-Ferreira, T. M. M., Bueno, R. C., Terra, E. M., Avante, M. L., Tinucci-Costa, M., Carvalho, M., et al. (2016). Downregulation of *ATM* gene and protein expression in canine mammary tumors. *Vet. Pathol.* 53, 1154–1159. doi: 10.1177/0300985816643367

Reis, A. B., Carneiro, C. M., Carvalho, M., das, G., Teixeira-Carvalho, A., Giunchetti, R. C., et al., et al. (2005). Establishment of a microplate assay for flow cytometric assessment and it is use for the evaluation of age-related phenotypic changes in canine whole blood leukocytes. *Vet. Immunol. Immunopathol.* 103, 173–185. doi: 10.1016/j.vetimm.2004.08.014

Rera, M., Bahadorani, S., Cho, J., Koehler, C. L., Ulgherait, M., Hur, J. H., et al. (2011). Modulation of longevity and tissue homeostasis by the Drosophila PGC-1 homolog. *Cell Metab.* 14, 623–634. doi: 10.1016/j.cmet.2011.09.013

Ressler, S., Bartkova, J., Niederegger, H., Bartek, J., Scharffetter-Kochanek, K., Jansen-Durr, P., et al. (2006). p16 INK4A is a robust *in vivo* biomarker of cellular aging in human skin. *Aging Cell* 5, 379–389. doi: 10.1111/j.1474-9726.2006.00231.x

Reul, J. M. H. M., Rothuizen, J., and de Kloet, E. R. (1991). Age-related changes in the dog hypothalamic–pituitary–adrenocortical system: neuroendocrine activity and corticosteroid receptors. *J. Steroid Biochem. Mol. Biol.* 40, 63–69. doi: 10.1016/0960-0760(91)90168-5

Riley, P. A. (1994). Free radicals in biology: oxidative stress and the effects of ionizing radiation. *Int. J. Radiat. Biol.* 65, 27–33. doi: 10.1080/09553009414550041

Rimbault, M., Beale, H. C., Schoenebeck, J. J., Hoopes, B. C., Allen, J. J., Kilroy-Glynn, P., et al. (2013). Derived variants at six genes explain nearly half of size reduction in dog breeds. *Genome Res.* 23, 1985–1995. doi: 10.1101/GR.157339.113

Ristow, M., Zarse, K., Oberbach, A., Klöting, N., Birringer, M., Kiehntopf, M., et al. (2009). Antioxidants prevent health-promoting effects of physical exercise in humans. *Proc. Natl. Acad. Sci. U. S. A.* 106, 8665–8670. doi: 10.1073/pnas.0903485106

Rivera, P., Melin, M., Biagi, T., Fall, T., Häggström, J., Lindblad-Toh, K., et al. (2009). Mammary tumor development in dogs is associated with BRCA1 and BRCA2. *Cancer Res.* 69, 8770–8774. doi: 10.1158/0008-5472.CAN-09-1725

Rodier, F., and Campisi, J. (2011). Four faces of cellular senescence. *J. Cell Biol.* 192, 547–556. doi: 10.1083/jcb.201009094

Rofina, J. E., Singh, K., Skoumalova-Vesela, A., van Ederen, A. M., van Asten, A. J., Wilhelm, J., et al. (2004). Histochemical accumulation of oxidative damage products is associated with Alzheimer-like pathology in the canine. *Amyloid* 11, 90–100. doi: 10.1080/13506120412331285779

Rogina, B., and Helfand, S. L. (2004). Sir2 mediates longevity in the fly through a pathway related to calorie restriction. *PNAS* 101, 15998–16003. doi: 10.1073/pnas.0404184101

Romanucci, M., and Della Salda, L. (2015). Oxidative stress and protein quality control systems in the aged canine brain as a model for human neurodegenerative disorders. *Oxid. Med. Cell. Longev.* 2015, 1–8. doi: 10.1155/2015/940131

Rothuizen, J., Reul, J. M., Rijnberk, A., Mol, J. A., and de Kloet, E. R. (1991). Aging and the hypothalamus–pituitary–adrenocortical axis, with special reference to the dog. *Acta Endocrinol. (Copenh)* 125 Suppl 1, 73–76.

Roudebush, P., Zicker, S. C., Cotman, C. W., Milgram, N. W., Muggenburg, B. A., and Head, E. (2005). Nutritional management of brain aging in dogs. *J. Am. Vet. Med. Assoc.* 227, 722–728. doi: 10.2460/javma.2005.227.722

Rowe, J., and Kahn, R. (1987). Human aging: usual and successful. *Science (80-.).* 237, 143–149. doi: 10.1126/science.3299702

Rowe, J. W., and Kahn, R. L. (2015). Successful aging 2.0: conceptual expansions for the 21st century. *Journals Gerontol. Ser. B Psychol. Sci. Soc. Sci.* 70, 593–596. doi: 10.1093/geronb/gbv025

Rowell, J. L., McCarthy, D. O., and Alvarez, C. E. (2011). Dog models of naturally occurring cancer. *Trends Mol. Med.* 17, 380–388. doi: 10.1016/j.molmed.2011.02.004

Rubbo, H., Radi, R., Trujillo, M., Telleri, R., Kalyanaraman, B., Barnes, S., et al. (1994). Nitric oxide regulation of superoxide and peroxynitrite-dependent lipid peroxidation. Formation of novel nitrogen-containing oxidized lipid derivatives*. *J. Biol. Chem.* 269, 26066–26075.

Rubinsztein, D. C. (2006). The roles of intracellular protein-degradation pathways in neurodegeneration. *Nature* 443, 780–786. doi: 10.1038/nature05291

Ruvkun, G., Ogg, S., Paradis, S., Gottlieb, S., Patterson, G. I., Lee, L., et al. (1997). The Fork head transcription factor DAF-16 transduces insulin-like metabolic and longevity signals in C. elegans. *Nature* 389, 994–999. doi: 10.1038/40194

Salt, C., Morris, P. J., Wilson, D., Lund, E. M., and German, A. J. (2018). Association between life span and body condition in neutered client-owned dogs. *J. Vet. Intern. Med.* 33, jvim.15367. doi: 10.1111/jvim.15367

Sampson, T. R., Debelius, J. W., Thron, T., Janssen, S., Shastri, G. G., Ilhan, Z. E., et al. (2016). Gut microbiota regulate motor deficits and neuroinflammation in a model of Parkinson's disease. *Cell* 167, 1469–1480.e12. doi: 10.1016/j.cell.2016.11.018

Sanchez, A. M., Csibi, A., Raibon, A., Cornille, K., Gay, S., Bernardi, H., et al. (2012). AMPK promotes skeletal muscle autophagy through activation of forkhead FoxO3a and interaction with Ulk1. *J. Cell Biochem.* 113, 695–710. doi: 10.1002/jcb.23399

Sandri, M. (2010). Autophagy in skeletal muscle. *FEBS Lett.* 584, 1411–1416. doi: 10.1016/j.febslet.2010.01.056

Sarasa, L., Gallego, C., Monleón, I., Olvera, A., Canudas, J., Montañés, M., et al. (2010). Cloning, sequencing and expression in the dog of the main amyloid precursor protein isoforms and some of the enzymes related with their processing. *Neuroscience* 171, 1091–1101. doi: 10.1016/j.neuroscience.2010.09.042

Saraswati, S., and Sitaraman, R. (2015). Aging and the human gut microbiota—from correlation to causality. *Front. Microbiol.* 5, 764. doi: 10.3389/fmicb.2014.00764

Sasaki, S. (2011). Autophagy in spinal cord motor neurons in sporadic amyotrophic lateral sclerosis. *J. Neuropathol. Exp. Neurol.* 70, 349–359. doi: 10.1097/NEN.0b013e3182160690

Schieber, M., and Chandel, N. S. (2014). ROS function in redox signaling and oxidative stress. *Curr. Biol.* 24, R453–R462. doi: 10.1016/j.cub.2014.03.034

Schmidt, F., Boltze, J., Jäger, C., Hofmann, S., Willems, N., Seeger, J., et al. (2015). Detection and quantification of β-amyloid, pyroglutamyl Aβ, and tau in aged canines. *J. Neuropathol. Exp. Neurol.* 74, 912–923. doi: 10.1097/NEN.0000000000000230

Schneider, J. L., Villarroya, J., Diaz-Carretero, A., Patel, B., Urbanska, A. M., Thi, M. M., et al. (2015). Loss of hepatic chaperone-mediated autophagy accelerates proteostasis failure in aging. *Aging Cell* 14, 249–264. doi: 10.1111/acel.12310

Schoenebeck, J. J., and Ostrander, E. A. (2014). Insights into morphology and disease from the dog genome project. *Annu. Rev. Cell Dev. Biol.* 30, 535–560. doi: 10.1146/annurev-cellbio-100913-012927

Schulz, T. J., Zarse, K., Voigt, A., Urban, N., Birringer, M., and Ristow, M. (2007). Glucose restriction extends *Caenorhabditis elegans* life span by inducing mitochondrial respiration and increasing oxidative stress. *Cell Metab.* 6, 280–293. doi: 10.1016/j.cmet.2007.08.011

Schumacher, B., van der Pluijm, I., Moorhouse, M. J., Kosteas, T., Robinson, A. R., Suh, Y., et al. (2008). Delayed and accelerated aging share common longevity assurance mechanisms. *PLoS Genet.* 4, e1000161. doi: 10.1371/journal.pgen.1000161

Sebastiani, P., and Perls, T. T. (2012). The genetics of extreme longevity : lessons from the New England Centenarian study. *Front. Genet.* 3, 1–7. doi: 10.3389/fgene.2012.00277

Sebastiani, P., Solovieff, N., DeWan, A. T., Walsh, K. M., Puca, A., Hartley, S. W., et al. (2012). Genetic signatures of exceptional longevity in humans. *PLoS One* 7, e29848. doi: 10.1371/journal.pone.0029848

Seisenberger, S., Andrews, S., Krueger, F., Arand, J., Walter, J., Santos, F., et al. (2012). The Dynamics of genome-wide DNA methylation reprogramming in mouse primordial germ cells. *Mol. Cell* 48, 849–862. doi: 10.1016/j.molcel.2012.11.001

Shadel, G. S., and Horvath, T. L. (2015). Mitochondrial ROS signaling in organismal homeostasis. *Cell* 163, 560–569. doi: 10.1016/j.cell.2015.10.001

Shampay, J., and Blackburn, E. H. (1988). Generation of telomere-length heterogeneity in *Saccharomyces cerevisiae. Genetics* 85, 534–538. doi: 10.1073/pnas.85.2.534

Sharon, G., Sampson, T. R., Geschwind, D. H., and Mazmanian, S. K. (2016). The central nervous system and the gut microbiome. *Cell* 167, 915–932. doi: 10.1016/j.cell.2016.10.027

Shearin, A. L., Hedan, B., Cadieu, E., Erich, S. A., Schmidt, E. V., Faden, D. L., et al. (2012). The MTAP-CDKN2A locus confers susceptibility to a naturally occurring canine cancer. *Cancer Epidemiol. Biomarkers Prev.* 21, 1019–1027. doi: 10.1158/1055-9965.EPI-12-0190-T

Sherr, C. J., and DePinho, R. A. (2000). Cellular senescence: mitotic clock or culture shock? *Cell* 102, 407–410. doi: 10.1016/S0092-8674(00)00046-5

Simonsen, A., Cumming, R. C., Brech, A., Isakson, P., Schubert, D. R., and Finley, K. D. (2008). Promoting basal levels of autophagy in the nervous system enhances longevity and oxidant resistance in adult Drosophila. *Autophagy* 4, 176–184. doi: 10.4161/auto.5269

Singhal, R. P., Mays-Hoopes, L. L., and Eichhorn, G. L. (1987). DNA methylation in aging of mice. *Mech. Ageing Dev.* 41, 199–210. doi: 10.1016/0047-6374(87)90040-6

Skoglund, P., Ersmark, E., Palkopoulou, E. and Dalén, L. (2015). Ancient wolf genome reveals an early divergence of domestic dog ancestors and admixture into high-latitude breeds. *Curr. Biol.* 25 (11), 1515–1519. doi: 10.1016/j.cub.2015.04.019

Skoumalova, A., Rofina, J., Schwippelova, Z., Gruys, E., and Wilhelm, J. (2003). The role of free radicals in canine counterpart of senile dementia of the Alzheimer type. *Exp. Gerontol.* 38, 711–719. doi: 10.1016/S0531-5565(03)00071-8

Smith, B. F., Yue, Y., Woods, P. R., Kornegay, J. N., Shin, J.-H., Williams, R. R., et al. (2011). An intronic LINE-1 element insertion in the dystrophin gene aborts dystrophin expression and results in Duchenne-like muscular dystrophy in the corgi breed. *Lab. Investig.* 91, 216–231. doi: 10.1038/labinvest.2010.146

Smith, L. K., He, Y., Park, J.-S., Bieri, G , Snethlage, C. E., Lin, K., et al. (2015). β2-microglobulin is a systemic pro-aging factor that impairs cognitive function and neurogenesis. *Nat. Med.* 21, 932–937. doi: 10.1038/nm.3898

Smith, Z. D., Chan, M. M., Mikkelsen, T. S., Gu, H., Gnirke, A., Regev, A., et al. (2012). A unique regulatory phase of DNA methylation in the early mammalian embryo. *Nature* 484, 339–344. doi: 10 1038/nature10960

Smogorzewska, A., and De Lange, T. (2002). Different telomere damage signaling pathways in human and mouse cells *EMBO J.* 21, 4338–4348. doi: 10.1093/emboj/cdf433

Smolek, T., Madari, A., Farbakova, J., Kandrac, O., Jadhav, S., Cente, M., et al. (2016). Tau hyperphosphorylation in synaptosomes and neuroinflammation are associated with canine cognitive impairment. *J. Comp. Neurol.* 524, 874–895. doi: 10.1002/cne.23877

Snigdha, S., de Rivera, C., Milgram, N. W., and Cotman, C. W. (2016). Effect of mitochondrial cofactors and antioxidants supplementation on cognition in the aged canine. *Neurobiol. Aging* 37, 171–178. doi: 10.1016/j.neurobiolaging.2015.09.015

Soerensen, M., Dato, S., Christensen, K., McGue, M., Stevnsner, T., Bohr, V. A., et al. (2010). Replication of an association of variation in the FOXO3A gene with human longevity using both case-control and longitudinal data. *Aging Cell* 9, 1010–1017. doi: 10.1111/j.1474-9726.2010.00627.x

Soerensen, M., Dato, S., Tan, Q., Thinggaard, M., Kleindorp, R., Beekman, M., et al. (2012a). Human longevity and variation in GH/IGF-1/insulin signaling, DNA damage signaling and repair and pro/antioxidant pathway genes: Cross sectional and longitudinal studies. *Exp. Gerontol.* 47, 379–387. doi: 10.1016/j.exger.2012.02.010

Soerensen, M., Thinggaard, M., Nygaard, M., Dato, S., Tan, Q., Hjelmborg, J., et al. (2012b). Genetic variation in TERT and TERC and human leukocyte telomere length and longevity: a cross-sectional and longitudinal analysis. *Aging Cell* 11, 223–227. doi: 10.1111/j.1474-9726.2011.00775.x

Somel, M., Guo, S., Fu, N., Yan, Z., Hu, H. Y., Xu, Y., et al. (2010). MicroRNA, mRNA, and protein expression link development and aging in human and macaque brain. *Genome Res.* 20, 1207–1218. doi: 10.1101/gr.106849.110

Sonntag, W. E., Lynch, C. D., Cooney, P. T., and Hutchins, P. M. (1997). Decreases in cerebral microvasculature with age are associated with the decline in growth hormone and insulin-like growth factor 1*. *Endocrinology* 138, 3515–3520. doi: 10.1210/endo.138.8.5330

Sonntag, W. E., Lynch, C., Thornton, P., Khan, A., Bennet, S., and Ingram, R. (2000). The effects of growth hormone and IGF-1 deficiency on cerebrovascular and brain ageing. *J. Anat.* 197, 575–585. doi: 10.1017/S002187829900713X

Sonntag, W. E., Ramsey, M., and Carter, C. S. (2005). Growth hormone and insulin-like growth factor-1 (IGF-1) and their influence on cognitive aging. *Ageing Res. Rev.* 4, 195–212. doi: 10.1016/j.arr.2005.02.001

Stadtman, E. R., and Levine, R. L. (2006). Protein Oxidation. *Ann. N. Y. Acad. Sci.* 899, 191–208. doi: 10.1111/j.1749-6632.2000.tb06187.x

Stewart, L., MacLean, E. L., Ivy, D., Woods, V., Cohen, E., Rodriguez, K., et al. (2015). Citizen science as a new tool in dog cognition research. *PLoS One* 10, e0135176. doi: 10.1371/journal.pone.0135176

Stone, R. C., Horvath, K., Kark, J. D., Susser, E., Tishkoff, S. A., and Aviv, A. (2016). Telomere length and the cancer–atherosclerosis trade-off. *PLOS Genet.* 12, e1006144. doi: 10.1371/journal.pgen.1006144

Strasser, A., Niedermüller, H., Hofecker, G., and Laber, G. (1993). The effect of aging on laboratory values in dogs. *J. Vet. Med. Ser. A* 40, 720–730. doi: 10.1111/j.1439-0442.1993.tb00689.x

Stribinskis, V., and Ramos, K. S. (2006). Activation of human long interspersed nuclear element 1 retrotransposition by benzo(*a*)pyrene, an ubiquitous environmental carcinogen. *Cancer Res.* 66, 2616–2620. doi: 10.1158/0008-5472.CAN-05-3478

Studzinski, C. M., MacKay, W. A., Beckett, T. L., Henderson, S. T., Murphy, M. P., Sullivan, P. G., et al. (2008). Induction of ketosis may improve mitochondrial function and decrease steady-state amyloid-β precursor protein (APP) levels in the aged dog. *Brain Res.* 1226, 209–217. doi: 10.1016/j.brainres.2008.06.005

Sturm, Á., Ivics, Z., and Vellai, T. (2015). The mechanism of ageing: primary role of transposable elements in genome disintegration. *Cell. Mol. Life Sci.* 72, 1839–1847. doi: 10.1007/s00018-015-1896-0

Su, M.-Y., Tapp, P. D., Vu, L., Chen, Y.-F., Chu, Y., Muggenburg, B., et al. (2005). A longitudinal study of brain morphometrics using serial magnetic resonance imaging analysis in a canine model of aging. *Prog. Neuropsychopharmacol. Biol. Psychiatry* 29, 389–397. doi: 10.1016/j.pnpbp.2004.12.005

Suh, Y., Atzmon, G., Cho, M.-O., Hwang, D., Liu, B., Leahy, D. J., et al. (2008). Functionally significant insulin-like growth factor I receptor mutations in centenarians. *Proc. Natl. Acad. Sci. U. S. A.* 105, 3438–3442. doi: 10.1073/pnas.0705467105

Sundaram, V., Cheng, Y., Ma, Z., Li, D., Xing, X., Edge, P., et al. (2014). Widespread contribution of transposable elements to the innovation of gene regulatory networks. *Genome Res.* 24, 1963–1976. doi: 10.1101/gr.168872.113

Sutter, N. B., Bustamante, C. D., Chase, K., Gray, M. M., Zhao, K., Zhu, L., et al. (2007). A single IGF1 allele is a major determinant of small size in dogs. *Science* 316, 112–115. doi: 10.1126/science.1137045

Swanson, K. S., Vester, B. M., Apanavicius, C. J., Kirby, N. A., and Schook, L. B. (2009). Implications of age and diet on canine cerebral cortex transcription. *Neurobiol. Aging* 30, 1314–1326. doi: 10.1016/j.neurobiolaging.2007.10.017

Swindell, W. R., Masternak, M. M., Kopchick, J. J., Conover, C. A., Bartke, A., and Miller, R. A. (2009). Endocrine regulation of heat shock protein mRNA levels in long-lived dwarf mice. *Mech. Ageing Dev.* 130, 393–400. doi: 10.1016/j.mad.2009.03.004

Szabó, D., Gee, N. R., and Miklósi, Á. (2016). Natural or pathologic? Discrepancies in the study of behavioral and cognitive signs in aging family dogs. *J. Vet. Behav.* 11, 86–98. doi: 10.1016/j.jveb.2015.08.003

Tatar, M., Kopelman, A., Epstein, D., Tu, M.-P., Yin, C.-M., and Garofalo, R. S. (2001). A mutant Drosophila insulin receptor homolog that extends life-span and impairs neuroendocrine function. *Science* 292, 107–110. doi: 10.1126/science.1057987

Thalmann, O., Shapiro, B., Cui, P., Schuenemann, V. J., Sawyer, S. K., Greenfield, D. L., et al. (2013). Complete mitochondrial genomes of ancient canids suggest a European origin of domestic dogs. *Science (80-.).* 342, 871–874. doi: 10.1126/science.1243650

Thamm, D. H., Grunerud, K. K., Rose, B. J., Vail, D. M., and Bailey, S. M. (2013). DNA repair deficiency as a susceptibility marker for spontaneous lymphoma in Golden Retriever dogs: a case-control study. *PLoS One* 8, 1–8. doi: 10.1371/journal.pone.0069192

Thevelein, J. M., and de Winde, J. H. (1999). Novel sensing mechanisms and targets for the cAMP-protein kinase A pathway in the yeast *Saccharomyces cerevisiae. Mol. Microbiol.* 33, 904–918. doi: 10.1046/j.1365-2958.1999.01538.x

Thind, A., and Wilson, C. (2016). Exosomal miRNAs as cancer biomarkers and therapeutic targets. *J. Extracell. Vesicles* 5, 31292. doi: 10.3402/jev.v5.31292

Thompson, M. J., vonHoldt, B., Horvath, S., and Pellegrini, M. (2017). An epigenetic aging clock for dogs and wolves. *Aging (Albany NY)* 9, 1055–1068. doi: 10.18632/aging.101211

Thorpe, R. J., Simonsick, E. M., Brach, J. S., Ayonayon, H., Satterfield, S., Harris, T. B., et al. (2006). Dog ownership, walking behavior, and maintained mobility in late life. *J. Am. Geriatr. Soc.* 54, 1419–1424. doi: 10.1111/j.1532-5415.2006.00856.x

Tiret, L., Kessler, J., Pele, M., Tiret, L., Kessler, J., Blot, S., et al. (2005). SINE exonic insertion in the PTPLA gene leads to multiple splicing defects and segregates with the autosomal recessive centronuclear myopathy in dogs. *Hum. Mol. Genet.* 14, 1417–1427. doi: 10.1093/hmg/ddi151

Tissenbaum, H. A., and Guarente, L. (2001). Increased dosage of a sir-2 gene extends lifespan in *Caenorhabditis elegans*. *Nature* 410, 227–230. doi: 10.1038/35065638

Tokudome, S., Hashimoto, S., and Igata, A. (2016). Life expectancy and healthy life expectancy of Japan: the fastest graying society in the world. *BMC Res. Notes* 9, 482. doi: 10.1186/s13104-016-2281-2

Toohey, A. M., McCormack, G. R., Doyle-Baker, P. K., Adams, C. L., and Rock, M. J. (2013). Dog-walking and sense of community in neighborhoods: implications for promoting regular physical activity in adults 50 years and older. *Health Place* 22, 75–81. doi: 10.1016/j.healthplace.2013.03.007

Topál, J., Miklósi, Á., Gácsi, M., Dóka, A., Pongrácz, P., Kubinyi, E., et al. (2009). Chapter 3: The dog as a model for understanding human social behavior. *Adv. Study Behav.* 39, 71–116. doi: 10.1016/S0065-3454(09)39003-8

Tóth, M. L., Sigmond, T., Borsos, É., Barna, J., Erdélyi, P., Takács-Vellai, K., et al. (2008). Longevity pathways converge on autophagy genes to regulate life span in *Caenorhabditis elegans. Autophagy* 4, 330–338. doi: 10.4161/auto.5618

Tremaroli, V., and Bäckhed, F. (2012). Functional interactions between the gut microbiota and host metabolism. *Nature* 489, 242–249. doi: 10.1038/nature11552

Trifunovic, A., Wredenberg, A., Falkenberg, M., Spelbrink, J. N., Rovio, A. T., Bruder, C. E., et al. (2004). Premature ageing in mice expressing defective mitochondrial DNA polymerase. *Nature* 429, 417–423. doi: 10.1038/nature02517

Trounson, A., and DeWitt, N. D. (2016). Pluripotent stem cells progressing to the clinic. *Nat. Rev. Mol. Cell Biol.* 17, 194–200. doi: 10.1038/nrm.2016.10

Tsujimoto, Y., and Shimizu, S. (2005). Another way to die: autophagic programmed cell death. *Cell Death Differ.* 12, 1528–1534. doi: 10.1038/sj.cdd.4401777

Tung, Y.-T., Wang, B.-J., Hu, M.-K., Hsu, W.-M., Lee, H., Huang, W.-P., et al. (2012). Autophagy: A double-edged sword in Alzheimer's disease. *J. Biosci.* 37, 157–165. doi: 10.1007/s12038-011-9176-0

Tyner, S. D., Venkatachalam, S., Choi, J., Jones, S., Ghebranious, N., Igelmann, H., et al. (2002). p53 mutant mice that display early ageing-associated phenotypes. *Nature* 415, 45–53. doi: 10.1038/415045a

Ukraintseva, S., Yashin, A., Arbeev, K., Kulminski, A., Akushevich, I., Wu, D., et al. (2016). Puzzling role of genetic risk factors in human longevity: "risk alleles" as pro-longevity variants. *Biogerontology* 17, 109–127. doi: 10.1007/s10522-015-9600-1

Urfer, S. R., Kaeberlein, T. L., Mailheau, S., Bergman, P. J., Creevy, K. E., Promislow, D. E. L., et al. (2017). A randomized controlled trial to establish effects of short-term rapamycin treatment in 24 middle-aged companion dogs. *GeroScience* 39, 117–127. doi: 10.1007/s11357-017-9972-z

Vaiserman, A. M., Koliada, A. K., and Marotta, F. (2017). Gut microbiota: a player in aging and a target for anti-aging intervention. *Ageing Res. Rev.* 35, 36–45. doi: 10.1016/j.arr.2017.01.001

van der Spoel, E., Jansen, S. W., Akintola, A. A., Ballieux, B. E., Cobbaert, C. M., Slagboom, P. E., et al. (2016). Growth hormone secretion is diminished and tightly controlled in humans enriched for familial longevity. *Aging Cell* 15, 1126–1131. doi: 10.1111/acel.12519

Van Giau, V., and An, S. S. A. (2016). Emergence of exosomal miRNAs as a diagnostic biomarker for Alzheimer's disease. *J. Neurol. Sci.* 360, 141–152. doi: 10.1016/j.jns.2015.12.005

Van Heemst, D., Beekman, M., Mooijaart, S. P., Heijmans, B. T., Brandt, B. W., Zwaan, B. J., et al. (2005). Reduced insulin/IGF-1 signalling and human longevity. *Aging Cell* 4, 79–85. doi: 10.1111/j.1474-9728.2005.00148.x

Van Raamsdonk, J. M., and Hekimi, S. (2009). Deletion of the mitochondrial superoxide dismutase sod-2 extends lifespan in *Caenorhabditis elegans*. *PLoS Genet.* 5, e1000361. doi: 10.1371/journal.pgen.1000361

Van Remmen, H., Ikeno, Y., Hamilton, M., Pahlavani, M., Wolf, N., Thorpe, S. R., et al. (2003). Life-long reduction in MnSOD activity results in increased DNA damage and higher incidence of cancer but does not accelerate aging. *Physiol. Genomics* 16, 29–37. doi: 10.1152/physiolgenomics.00122.2003

Vaysse, A., Ratnakumar, A., Derrien, T., Axelsson, E., Rosengren Pielberg, G., Sigurdsson, S., et al. (2011). Identification of genomic regions associated with phenotypic variation between dog breeds using selection mapping. *PLoS Genet.* 7, e1002316. doi: 10.1371/journal.pgen.1002316

Vellai, T. (2009). Autophagy genes and ageing. *Cell Death Differ.* 16, 94–102. doi: 10.1038/cdd.2008.126

Vellai, T., Takacs-Vellai, K., Zhang, Y., Kovacs, A. L., Orosz, L., and Müller, F. (2003). Influence of TOR kinase on lifespan in *C. elegans. Nature* 426, 620–620. doi: 10.1038/426620a

Vermulst, M., Wanagat, J., Kujoth, G. C., Bielas, J. H., Rabinovitch, P. S., Prolla, T. A., et al. (2008). DNA deletions and clonal mutations drive premature aging in mitochondrial mutator mice. *Nat. Genet.* 40, 392–394. doi: 10.1038/ng.95

Vila, C. (1997). Multiple and ancient origins of the domestic dog. *Science* 276, 1687–1689. doi: 10.1126/science.276.5319.1687

Vilchez, D., Morantte, I., Liu, Z., Douglas, P. M., Merkwirth, C., Rodrigues, A. P. C., et al. (2012). RPN-6 determines *C. elegans* longevity under proteotoxic stress conditions. *Nature* 489, 263–268. doi: 10.1038/nature11315

Villeda, S. A., Plambeck, K. E., Middeldorp, J., Castellano, J. M., Mosher, K. I., Luo, J., et al. (2014). Young blood reverses age-related impairments in cognitive function and synaptic plasticity in mice. *Nat. Med.* 20, 659–663. doi: 10.1038/nm.3569

Vonderheide, R. H., Hahn, W. C., Schultze, J. L., and Nadler, L. M. (1999). The telomerase catalytic subunit is a widely expressed tumor-associated antigen recognized by cytotoxic T lymphocytes. *Immunity* 10, 673–679. doi: 10.1016/S1074-7613(00)80066-7

vonHoldt, B. M., Pollinger, J. P., Lohmueller, K. E., Han, E., Parker, H. G., Quignon, P., et al. (2010). Genome-wide SNP and haplotype analyses reveal a rich history underlying dog domestication. *Nature* 464, 898–902. doi: 10.1038/nature08837

Walker, G. A., and Lithgow, G. J. (2003). Lifespan extension in *C. elegans* by a molecular chaperone dependent upon insulin-like signals. *Aging Cell* 2, 131–139. doi: 10.1046/j.1474-9728.2003.00045.x

Wang, C., Jurk, D., Maddick, M., Nelson, G., Martin-Ruiz, C., and Von Zglinicki, T. (2009). DNA damage response and cellular senescence in tissues of aging mice. *Aging Cell* 8, 311–323. doi: 10.1111/j.1474-9726.2009.00481.x

Wang, G.-D., Zhai, W., Yang, H.-C., Wang, L., Zhong, L., Liu, Y.-H., et al. (2016). Out of southern East Asia: the natural history of domestic dogs across the world. *Cell Res.* 26, 21–33. doi: 10.1038/cr.2015.147

Wang, W., and Kirkness, E. F. (2005). Short interspersed elements (SINEs) are a major source of canine genomic diversity. *Genome Res.* 15, 1798–1808. doi: 10.1101/gr.3765505

Waterland, R. A., and Jirtle, R. L. (2003). Transposable elements: targets for early nutritional effects on epigenetic gene regulation. *Mol. Cell. Biol.* 23, 5293–5300. doi: 10.1128/MCB.23.15.5293-5300.2003

Waters, D. J. (2011). Aging research 2011: exploring the pet dog paradigm. *ILAR J.* 52, 97–105. doi: 10.1093/ilar.52.1.97

Weir, H. J., and Mair, W. B. (2016). SnapShot: neuronal regulation of aging. *Cell* 166, 784–784.e1. doi: 10.1016/j.cell.2016.07.022

White, E., and DiPaola, R. S. (2009). The double-edged sword of autophagy modulation in cancer. *Clin. Cancer Res.* 15, 5308–5316. doi: 10.1158/1078-0432.CCR-07-5023

Whittemore, K., Vera, E., Martínez-Nevado, E., Sanpera, C., and Blasco, M. A. (2019). Telomere shortening rate predicts species life span. *Proc. Natl. Acad. Sci.* 116, 15122–15127. doi: 10.1073/pnas.1902452116

Wicker, T., Sabot, F., Hua-Van, A., Bennetzen, J. L., Capy, P., Chalhoub, B., et al. (2007). A unified classification system for eukaryotic transposable elements. *Nat. Rev. Genet.* 8, 973–982. doi: 10.1038/nrg2165

Wiersma, A. C., Stabej, P., Leegwater, P. A. J., Van Oost, B. A., Ollier, W. E., and Dukes-McEwan, J. (2007). Evaluation of 15 candidate genes for dilated cardiomyopathy in the Newfoundland dog. *J. Hered.* 99, 73–80. doi: 10.1093/jhered/esm090

Willcox, B. J., Donlon, T. A., He, Q., Chen, R., Grove, J. S., Yano, K., et al. (2008). FOXO3A genotype is strongly associated with human longevity. *Proc. Natl. Acad. Sci. U. S. A.* 105, 13987–13992. doi: 10.1073/pnas.0801030105

Wilson, C. H., Shalini, S., Filipovska, A., Richman, T. R., Davies, S., Martin, S. D., et al. (2015). Age-related proteostasis and metabolic alterations in Caspase-2-deficient mice. *Cell Death Dis.* 6, e1615–e1615. doi: 10.1038/cddis.2014.567

Wilson, V. L., and Jones, P. A. (1983). DNA methylation decreases in aging but not in immortal cells. *Science* 220, 1055–1057. doi: 10.1126/science.6844925

Withers, S. S., Moore, P. F., Chang, H., Choi, J. W., McSorley, S. J., Kent, M. S., et al. (2018). Multi-color flow cytometry for evaluating age-related changes in memory lymphocyte subsets in dogs. *Dev. Comp. Immunol.* 87, 64–74. doi: 10.1016/j.dci.2018.05.022

Wockner, L. F., Morris, C. P., Noble, E. P., Lawford, B. R., Whitehall, V. L. J., Young, R. M., et al. (2015). Brain-specific epigenetic markers of schizophrenia. *Transl. Psychiatry* 5, e680. doi: 10.1038/tp.2015.177

Wong, P.-M., Puente, C., Ganley, I. G., and Jiang, X. (2013). The ULK1 complex. *Autophagy* 9, 124–137. doi: 10.4161/auto.23323

Wood, Z. A., Poole, L. B., and Karplus, P. A. (2003). Peroxiredoxin evolution and the regulation of hydrogen peroxide signaling. *Science (80-.)* 300, 650 LP–65 653. doi: 10.1126/science.1080405

Wright, W. E., and Shay, J. W. (2000). Telomere dynamics in cancer progression and prevention: fundamental differences in human and mouse telomere biology. *Nat. Med.* 6, 849–851. doi: 10.1038/78592

Wu, J. J., Liu, J., Chen, E. B., Wang, J. J., Cao, L., Narayan, N., et al. (2013). Increased mammalian lifespan and a segmental and tissue-specific slowing of aging after genetic reduction of mTOR expression. *Cell Rep.* 4, 913–920. doi: 10.1016/J.CELREP.2013.07.030

Wullschleger, S., Loewith, R., and Hall, M. N. (2006). TOR signaling in growth and metabolism. *Cell* 124, 471–484. doi: 10.1016/j.cell.2006.01.016

Xian, L., Wu, X., Pang, L., Lou, M., Rosen, C. J., Qiu, T., et al. (2012). Matrix IGF-1 maintains bone mass by activation of mTOR in mesenchymal stem cells. *Nat. Med.* 18, 1095–1101. doi: 10.1038/nm 2793

Yang, V. K., Loughran, K. A., Meola, D. M., Juhr, C. M., Thane, K. E., Davis, A. M., et al. (2017). Circulating exosome microRNA associated with heart failure secondary to myxomatous mitral valve disease in a naturally occurring canine model. *J. Extracell. Vesicles* 6, 1350088. doi: 10.1080/20013078.2017.1350088

Yazawa, M., Okuda, M., Setoguchi, A., Iwabuchi, S., Nishimura, R., Sasaki, N., et al. (2001). Telomere length and telomerase activity in canine mammary gland tumors. *Am. J. Vet. Res.* 62, 1539–1543. doi: 10.2460/ajvr.2001.62.1539

Yazawa, M., Okuda, M., Setoguchi, A., Nishimura, R., Sasaki, N., Hasegawa, A., et al. (1999). Measurement of telomerase activity in dog tumors. *J. Vet. Med. Sci.* 61, 1125–1129. doi: 10.1292/jvms 61.1125

Yilmaz, Ö. H., Katajisto, P., Lamming, D. W., Gültekin, Y., Bauer-Rowe, K. E., Sengupta, S., et al. (2012). mTORC1 in the Paneth cell niche couples intestinal stem-cell function to calorie intake. *Nature* 486, 490–495. doi: 10.1038/nature11163

Yin, W., and Gore, A. C. (2006). Neuroendocrine control of reproductive aging: roles of GnRH neurons. *Reproduction* 131, 403–414. doi: 10.1530/rep.1.00617

Yu, C. E., Oshima, J., Fu, Y. H., Wijsman, E. M., Hisama, F., Alisch, R., et al. (1996). Positional cloning of the Werner's syndrome gene. *Science* 272, 258–62. doi: 10.1126/science.272.5259.258

Zahn, J. M., Poosala, S., Owen, A. B., Ingram, D. K., Lustig, A., Carter, A., et al. (2007). AGEMAP: a gene expression database for aging in mice. *PLoS Genet.* 3, e201. doi: 10.1371/journal.pgen.0030201

Zapata, H. J., and Quagliarello, V. J. (2015). The microbiota and microbiome in aging: potential implications in health and age-related diseases. *J. Am. Geriatr. Soc.* 63, 776–781. doi: 10.1111/jgs.13310

Zeng, R., Farias, F. H. G., Johnson, G. S., McKay, S. D., Schnabel, R. D., Decker, J. E., et al. (2011). A truncated retrotransposon disrupts the GRM1 coding sequence in Coton de Tulear dogs with Bandera's neonatal ataxia. *J. Vet. Intern. Med.* 25, 267–272. doi: 10.1111/j.1939-1676.2010.0666.x

Zhang, C., and Cuervo, A. M. (2008). Restoration of chaperone-mediated autophagy in aging liver improves cellular maintenance and hepatic function. *Nat. Med.* 14, 959–965. doi: 10.1038/nm.1851

Zhang, C., Doherty, J. A., Burgess, S., Hung, R. J., Lindström, S., Kraft, P., et al. (2015). Genetic determinants of telomere length and risk of common cancers: a Mendelian randomization study. *Hum. Mol. Genet.* 24, 5356–5366. doi: 10.1093/hmg/ddv252

Zhang, G., Li, J., Purkayastha, S., Tang, Y., Zhang, H., Yin, Y., et al. (2013). Hypothalamic programming of systemic ageing involving IKK-β, NF-κB and GnRH. *Nature* 497, 211–216. doi: 10.1038/nature12143

Zhang, X., Azhar, G., and Wei, J. Y. (2012). The expression of microRNA and microRNA clusters in the aging heart. *PLoS One* 7, e34688. doi: 10.1371/journal.pone.0034688

Zhang, Y., Ikeno, Y., Qi, W., Chaudhuri, A., Li, Y., Bokov, A., et al. (2009). Mice deficient in both Mn superoxide dismutase and glutathione peroxidase-1 have increased oxidative damage and a greater incidence of pathology but no reduction in longevity. *Journals Gerontol. Ser. A Biol. Sci. Med. Sci.* 64A, 1212–1220. doi: 10.1093/gerona/glp132

Zhang, Y., Kim, M. S., Jia, B., Yan, J., Zuniga-Hertz, J. P., Han, C., et al. (2017). Hypothalamic stem cells control ageing speed partly through exosomal miRNAs. *Nature* 548, 52–57. doi: 10.1038/nature23282

Zheng, Q., Huang, T., Zhang, L., Zhou, Y., Luo, H., Xu, H., et al. (2016). Dysregulation of ubiquitin-proteasome system in neurodegenerative diseases. *Front. Aging Neurosci.* 8, 303. doi: 10.3389/fnagi.2016.00303

Zhu, Z.-Z., Sparrow, D., Hou, L., Tarantini, L., Bollati, V., Litonjua, A. A., et al. (2011). Repetitive element hypomethylation in blood leukocyte DNA and cancer incidence, prevalence, and mortality in elderly individuals: the Normative Aging Study. *Cancer Causes Control* 22, 437–447. doi: 10.1007/s10552-010-9715-2

Zimmermann, F. K. (1971). Genetic aspects of carcinogenesis. *Biochem. Pharmacol.* 20, 985–995. doi: 10.1016/0006-2952(71)90322-4

Zou, Q., Wang, X., Liu, Y., Ouyang, Z., Long, H., Wei, S., et al. (2015). Generation of gene-target dogs using CRISPR/Cas9 system. *J. Mol. Cell Biol.* 7, 580–583. doi: 10.1093/jmcb/mjv061

10

Can the Geriatric Day Hospital Act as a Hub for Services for Older People across the Spectrum of Ageing from Active Ageing to Advanced Frailty?

Rónán O'Caoimh[1,2], Siobhán Kennelly[2,3] and Diamuid O'Shea[2,4]*

[1] Clinical Sciences Institute, National University of Ireland, Galway, Galway, Ireland, [2] National Clinical Programme for Older People, Royal College of Physicians of Ireland, Dublin, Ireland, [3] Department of Medicine for the Elderly, Connolly Hospital, Blanchardstown, Dublin, Ireland, [4] Department of Geriatric Medicine, St Vincent's University Hospital, Dublin, Ireland

Edited by:
Helena Canhao,
Unidade EpiDoC, Epidemiologia de doenças crônicas, Portugal

Reviewed by:
Antony Bayer,
Cardiff University, United Kingdom
Lisa Robinson,
Newcastle upon Tyne Hospitals NHS Foundation Trust, United Kingdom

****Correspondence:***
Rónán O'Caoimh
rocaoimh@hotmail.com

Keywords: Day Hospital, frailty, pre-frailty, Comprehensive Geriatric Assessment, geriatrics, ageing

This article examines the potential of the Geriatric Day Hospital to address the challenge of an aging society, which has begun to place an emphasis on the promotion of active and healthy aging, yet faces rising numbers of pre-frail and frail older adults with complex care needs. Can the Day Hospital model become a hub for the care of older adults across the spectrum of aging? This article explores its origins and traditional role in delivering Comprehensive Geriatric Assessment (CGA), assesses how it is currently being used to identify, triage and manage frailty, providing reablement, chronic disease management and anticipatory care planning, and discusses future models focused on the prevention, surveillance, and monitoring of frailty. It will examine how such approaches could increasingly deploy information communication technologies (ICT) using the Geriatric Day Hospital as a hub to maintain older adults in their home environment, to promote active aging, while both preventing and managing frailty.

A consequence of population aging worldwide, but particularly in the European Union (1), is high rates of frailty (2) and multi-morbidity (3) among older people. This has directed health polices toward prevention and the pursuit of active and healthy aging (4, 5) but has nevertheless resulted in increasing numbers of older patients who could benefit from specialist geriatric services, meaning that limited resources must be stretched further. A fundamental challenge now faced in the management of older adults with multiple interacting medical and social problems is how to move from a single system, unidimensional construct to a more holistic and multidimensional model of care (6) that promotes preventative approaches and reablement as well as providing long-term management and rehabilitation. In this evolving environment, established ambulatory models of care for older people with complex needs that traditionally focused on the latter such as the Geriatric Day Hospital could be leveraged to find an additional purpose, to promote active and healthy aging and manage pre-frailty, while continuing to support the care of frail older adults.

The Geriatric Day Hospital, which originated in the United Kingdom in the 1950s, is a dedicated outpatient service providing specialized, interdisciplinary, ambulatory, and usually rapid access geriatric medical, nursing, and rehabilitation care to community-dwelling older patients, whose primary strength is arguably the flexibility it offers (7). Day Hospitals represented an evolution in primary and secondary level ambulatory care models for older people with complex needs. Those attending Day Hospitals receive and benefit from CGA, individualized multi-domain assessment by a multidisciplinary team using validated scales and interventions that reduce adverse outcomes, hospital admission, and length of hospitalization (8). CGA is, however, labor intensive and economically costly; the Day Hospital rationalizes and targets this limited resource "under one roof" (9) in an effective (10) and cost-effective manner (11). A recent systematic review summarizing evidence from 16 studies comparing Geriatric Day Hospitals to non-integrated, non-comprehensive services suggests that it is superior, reducing the risk of functional impairment, institutionalization and death, albeit the evidence remains limited, and no cost benefit has been established (9). Further, there is much heterogeneity in terms of what is offered and to whom with studies varying in their sampling strategies; the strongest evidence being for models focusing on geriatric rehabilitation and subspecialty diseases such as stroke, dementia, and heart failure (12). There is limited evidence for its use in prevention and health promotion.

The most recent change in Day Hospitals is a shift toward specialty services, clinics, and ambulatory investigations. Paralleling this change, the relatively new construct of frailty has begun to replace historical models of geriatric care and is increasingly being used in Day Hospitals to select and risk-stratify attendees. Frailty is a multi-factorial state correlating with vulnerability, disability, comorbidity, and self-reported health status with a recognized prodrome, pre-frailty (13). This construct recognizes that the stereotypical characteristics of community-dwelling older patients such as age are insufficient to identify older adults deemed most at risk of adverse healthcare outcomes and hence most in need of CGA (14). Given the current ageing demographic (1), the construct of frailty can help to identify those most likely to benefit from the Day Hospital (15). However, few studies have been conducted to examine the role of the Day Hospital in identifying frail older adults. A study using the SHARE Frailty Index to examine the prevalence of frailty among community-dwelling attendees at a University Hospital affiliated Day Hospital in Ireland found that the prevalence of frailty in this transitional care sample was high at 32% (16). In France, another observational cross sectional study applying consecutive sampling using Fried's criteria, to a similar sample referred to a single geriatric unit, found a higher prevalence of 51% (17). Levels of pre-frailty were also high in both samples at 26 and 41%, respectively. These data represent values between those in community and inpatient settings (2, 18, 19), suggesting that most attendees at Day Hospitals have high-care requirements, but also represent an ideal population to target for measures designed to tackle, prevent, and reverse frailty, including those that promote active and health aging at population-level.

The Geriatric Day Hospital is also increasingly being used as a coordination center to deliver integrated care (20) between acute services (emergency departments, acute medicine assessment units, and inpatient wards) (21), rehabilitation services (formal inpatient and early supported discharge teams), community services (primary care teams and general practitioners), and public health services designed to promote active and healthy aging in place, the person's own community (implementation of local, national, and transnational population-level preventative healthcare strategies). A consistent approach to identify frailty across primary, secondary, and social care, e.g., coordinated by case managers, community public health nurses, or primary care physicians can promote equity of access to CGA services (22). Identifying pre-frailty and frailty in people attending for Day Hospital assessment services may be looked on as a form of case finding and an opportunity for health promotion (23). This, in turn, allows for comprehensive proactive management of conditions that result in high levels of acute care episodes. Models that reflect mutual goal setting in determining outcomes (e.g., Goal Attainment Scores) will be increasingly used and will provide a key element of person-centered support in the Day Hospital (20). Screening for complexity and pre-frailty also may have the additional benefit of taking on a much more proactive approach to the planning of care needs and potentially impact on transitions of care given that most of the CGA has taken place beforehand (24). In essence, the Day Hospital is a "hub" or "command center" to integrate the delivery of CGA services, subspecialty clinics, and preventative healthcare to those most in need.

The Day Hospital may be the ideal location to encourage anticipatory care planning including end-of-life care and cancer survivorship care planning, which help people think about their future health and social care needs. When aligned with CGA, the development of a person-centered care plan to promote this way of thinking about the future in a non-acute care setting enables the older person, their family members, and the multidisciplinary team to address changing needs, complexity, and requirement for support, surveillance, and monitoring from health and social care systems (24). Advanced and personalized care planning is most sustainable when incorporated into routine care in a specialized, dedicated environment where patient trajectories can be predicted and followed (25, 26). Similarly, cancer survivorship care is poorly coordinated in general practice, with little evidence for its integration into routine care (27). Older patients with chronic conditions such as dementia (20) and older cancer survivors (28), whose care needs are markedly different from younger patients could benefit from the CGA, monitoring and advanced care planning delivered in a Day Hospital setting offered in an arguably more appropriate, unhurried and timely manner than in primary or secondary care.

Interventions to target frailty transitions and potentially reverse or prevent onset of frailty may also be best delivered in a Geriatric Day Hospital. A randomized controlled trial that assessed the effectiveness of CGA and subsequent intervention in pre-frail and frail community-dwelling older adults based on the Fried's criteria found that CGA and subsequent intervention showed a favorable outcome based on frailty status and the Barthel Index of activities of daily living (29). More recently, randomized trial data have shown that targeting pre-frailty using two-staged frailty screening followed by more detailed assessment with tailored multi-factorial interventions may slow progression to frailty (30) and is acceptable to community-dwelling older adults (31). Similarly, programs that promote active and healthy aging that improve outcomes in randomized trials such as the "I am active program" (32) could be coordinated or delivered in Day Hospitals.

The use of innovative ICT solutions to improve care for older adults attending the Day Hospital may represent the next step in re-purposing the construct. There is a growing consensus that these new approaches can drive active and healthy aging (33), and it is argued that the use of ICT in ambulatory care settings (including Geriatric Day Hospitals) could be used to promote this through improved diagnostics, individualized telemedicine, and by enhancing connectivity, social engagement, and continued learning (eHealth literacy) among older adults (34). This use of "silver innovations" to support active aging and healthcare strategies has already proven useful in community-based samples in countries ranging from the Netherlands (35) and Italy (36) to the United States (37) and Japan (38), though these innovations require educational, financial, and policy supports to succeed (38). Although the extent to which ICT can be promoted and implemented in a Day Hospital setting is unknown, its success is likely to be similar to its use in a home care setting (39). The expected shift to greater use of remote monitoring using mobile ICT health technologies is predicted to require more infrastructure (40), particularly for older adults who will require greater support to utilize these services. Traditional services like the Geriatric Day Hospital could be leveraged to this new purpose by providing a "hub" to assist and supervise this for appropriate patients rather than require the building of new and likely commercial infrastructure, which may not have the means or interest to serve this distinct and specialized group. Given that older adults attending a Geriatric Day Hospital in Ireland rated their experience with ICT as limited (41), eHealth literacy would also need to be fostered in this setting. This is echoed by evidence that a supportive environment attuned to the needs of older adults is required for them to effectively use ICT (42).

In a time of limited resources, the Geriatric Day Hospital is as important as ever. Current healthcare systems, under pressure from aging demographics, should re-examine its role and the evidence base for the care it provides, which has arguably not received the attention and recognition that it deserves. Day Hospitals have the potential to evolve and manage the care of older adults with complex care needs across the spectrum from active aging to pre-frailty and from established frailty to end-of-life care. While they should continue to focus on providing CGA, capitalizing on the growing evidence for a frailty syndrome has helped rationalize this limited resource more appropriately (43), Day Hospitals should focus increasingly on providing innovative and proactive, preventative approaches including those that use new mobile ICT technologies to promote healthy aging, address pre-frailty and prevent or reverse frailty at an early stage, before the onset of functional decline (33). Day Hospitals can also be used to promote a system's wide integrated program of care and education for older adults and healthcare professionals. Thus, although in the future the Day Hospital is likely to remain clinically focused, given its flexibility, it should be able take on new role as a connector "hub" to link primary, secondary, social, and public healthcare; to promote the use of new ICT developments to screen, monitor, and manage the care of community-dwelling older adults; and to advance educational initiatives and eHealth literacy to encourage active and healthy aging well into the twenty-first century.

AUTHOR CONTRIBUTIONS

All the authors (ROC, SK, DOS) contributed equally to the planning and writing of the manuscript.

REFERENCES

1. Rechel B, Grundy E, Robine JM, Cylus J, Mackenbach JP, Knai C, et al. Ageing in the European Union. *Lancet* (2013) 381(9874):1312–22. doi:10.1016/S0140-6736(12)62087-X
2. Collard RM, Boter H, Schoevers RA, Oude Voshaar RC. Prevalence of frailty in community-dwelling older persons: a systematic review. *J Am Geriatr Soc* (2012) 60(8):1487–92. doi:10.1111/j.1532-5415.2012.04054.x
3. Prince MJ, Wu F, Guo Y, Gutierrez Robledo LM, O'Donnell M, Sullivan R, et al. The burden of disease in older people and implications for health policy and practice. *Lancet* (2015) 385:549–62. doi:10.1016/S0140-6736(14)61347-7
4. O'Caoimh R, Sweeney C, Hynes H, McGlade C, Cornally N, Daly E, et al. COLLaboration on AGEing-COLLAGE: Ireland's three star reference site for the European Innovation Partnership on Active and Healthy Ageing (EIP on AHA). *Eur Geriatr Med* (2015) 6(5):505–11. doi:10.1016/j.eurger.2015.04.009
5. Michel JP, Dreux C, Vacheron A. Healthy ageing: evidence that improvement is possible at every age. *Eur Geriatr Med* (2016) 7(4):298–305.
6. Lacas A, Rockwood K. Frailty in primary care: a review of its conceptualisation and implications for practice. *BMC Med* (2012) 10:4. doi:10.1186/1741-7015-10-4
7. Black DA. The Geriatric Day Hospital. *Age Ageing* (2005) 34:427–9. doi:10.1093/ageing/afi149
8. Ellis G, Whitehead MA, O'Neill D, Langhorne P, Robinson D. Comprehensive geriatric assessment for older adults admitted to hospital. *Cochrane Database Syst Rev* (2011) 7:CD006211. doi:10.1002/14651858.CD006211.pub2
9. Brown L, Forster A, Young J, Crocker T, Benham A, Langhorne P, et al. Medical day hospital care for older people versus alternative forms of care. *Cochrane Database Syst Rev* (2015) (6):CD001730. doi:10.1002/14651858.CD001730.pub3
10. Forster A, Young J, Langhorne P. Systematic review of day hospital care for elderly people. *BMJ* (1999) 318:837–40. doi:10.1136/bmj.318.7187.837
11. Tousignant M, Hebert R, Desrosiers J, Hollander MJ. Economic evaluation of a Geriatric Day Hospital: cost-benefit analysis based on functional autonomy changes. *Age Ageing* (2003) 32:53–9. doi:10.1093/ageing/32.1.53
12. Petermans J, Velghe A, Gillain D, Boman X, Van den Noortgate N. Geriatric Day Hospital: what evidence? A systematic review. *Geriatr Psychol Neuropsychiatr Vieil* (2011) 9(3):295–303.
13. Rodríguez-Mañas L, Féart C, Mann G, Viña J, Chatterji S, Chodzko-Zajko W, et al. Searching for an operational definition of frailty: a Delphi method based consensus statement. The frailty operative definition-consensus conference project. *J Gerontol A Biol Sci Med Sci* (2013) 68(1):62–7. doi:10.1093/gerona/gls119
14. O'Caoimh R, Gao Y, Svendrovski A, Healy E, O'Connell E, O'Keeffe G, et al. The risk instrument for screening in the community (RISC): a new instrument for predicting risk of adverse outcomes in community dwelling older adults. *BMC Geriatr* (2015) 15:92. doi:10.1186/s12877-015-0095-z
15. Pereira SR, Chiu W, Turner A, Chevalier S, Joseph L, Huang AR, et al. How can we improve targeting of frail elderly patients to a Geriatric Day-Hospital rehabilitation program? *BMC Geriatr* (2010) 10(1):82. doi:10.1186/1471-2318-10-82
16. Ntlholang O, Kelly RE, Romero-Ortuno R, Cosgrave S, Kelly D, Crowe M, et al. The role the frailty syndrome can play in advocacy and resource allocation for our ageing population – findings in a Dublin Day Hospital. *J Frailty Aging* (2013) 3(1):21–4. doi:10.14283/jfa.2014.5
17. Soler V, Sourdet S, Balardy L, Abellan van Kan G, Brechemier D, Rouge-Bugat ME, et al. Visual impairment screening at the geriatric frailty clinic for assessment of frailty and prevention of disability at the gerontopole. *J Nutr Health Aging* (2016) 20(8):870–7. doi:10.1007/s12603-015-0648-z
18. Andela RM, Dijkstra A, Slaets JP, Sanderman R. Prevalence of frailty on clinical wards: description and implications. *Int J Nurs Pract* (2010) 16(1):14–9. doi:10.1111/j.1440-172X.2009.01807.x
19. Clegg A, Young J, Iliffe S, Rikkert MO, Rockwood K. Frailty in elderly people. *Lancet* (2013) 381(9868):752–62. doi:10.1016/S0140-6736(12)62167-9
20. Moorhouse P, Theou O, Fay S, McMillan M, Moffatt H, Rockwood K. Treatment in a Geriatric Day Hospital improve individualized outcome

measures using Goal Attainment Scaling. *BMC Geriatr* (2017) 17(1):9. doi:10.1186/s12877-016-0397-9

21. Jones S, Maxwell M. Ambulatory care for older people living with frailty: an innovative use of the medical day hospital. *Future Hosp J* (2016) 3(2):106–8. doi:10.7861/futurehosp.3-2-106
22. Liotta G, O'Caoimh R, Gilardi F, Proietti MG, Rocco G, Alvaro R, et al. Assessment of frailty in community-dwelling older adults residents in the Lazio region (Italy): a model to plan regional community-based services. *Arch Gerontol Geriatr* (2017) 68:1–7. doi:10.1016/j.archger.2016.08.004
23. Roberts J, Browne GB, Streiner D, Gafni A, Pallister R, Hoxby H, et al. The effectiveness and efficiency of health promotion in specialty clinic care. *Med Care* (1995) 33(9):892–905. doi:10.1097/00005650-199509000-00002
24. Baker A, Leak P, Ritchie LD, Lee A, Fielding S. Anticipatory care planning and integration: a primary care pilot study aimed at reducing unplanned hospitalisation. *Br J Gen Pract* (2012) 62(595):e113–20. doi:10.3399/bjgp12X625175
25. Coulter A, Entwistle VA, Eccles A, Ryan S, Shepperd S, Perera R. Personalised care planning for adults with chronic or long-term health conditions. *Cochrane Database Syst Rev* (2015) (3):CD010523. doi:10.1002/14651858.CD010523
26. Lund S, Richardson A, May C. Barriers to advance care planning at the end of life: an explanatory systematic review of implementation studies. *PLoS One* (2015) 10(2):e0116629. doi:10.1371/journal.pone.0116629
27. Rubinstein EB, Miller WL, Hudson SV, Howard J, O'Malley D, Tsui J, et al. Cancer survivorship care in advanced primary care practices: a qualitative study of challenges and opportunities. *JAMA Intern Med* (2017) 177(12):1726–32. doi:10.1001/jamainternmed.2017.4747
28. O'Caoimh R, Cornally N, O'Sullivan R, Hally R, Weathers E, Lavan AH, et al. Advance care planning within survivorship care plans for older cancer survivors: a systematic review. *Maturitas* (2017) 105:52–7. doi:10.1016/j.maturitas.2017.06.027
29. Li CM, Chen CY, Li CY, Wang WD, Wu SC. The effectiveness of a comprehensive geriatric assessment intervention program for frailty in community-dwelling older people: a randomized, controlled trial. *Arch Gerontol Geriatr* (2010) 50(1):S39–42. doi:10.1016/S0167-4943(10)70011-X
30. Serra-Prat M, Sist X, Domenich R, Jurado L, Saiz A, Roces A, et al. Effectiveness of an intervention to prevent frailty in pre-frail community-dwelling older people consulting in primary care: a randomised controlled trial. *Age Ageing* (2017) 46(3):401–7. doi:10.1093/ageing/afw242
31. Van Velsen L, Illario M, Jansen-Kosterink S, Crola C, Di Somma C, Colao A, et al. A community-based, technology-supported health service for detecting and preventing frailty among older adults: a participatory design development process. *J Aging Res* (2015) 2015:216084. doi:10.1155/2015/216084
32. Mendoza-Ruvalcaba NM, Arias-Merino ED. "I am active": effects of a program to promote active aging. *Clin Interv Aging* (2015) 10:829. doi:10.2147/CIA.S79511
33. Illario M, Vollenbroek-Hutten MM, Molloy DW, Menditto E, Iaccarino G, Eklund P. Active and healthy ageing and independent living 2016. *J Aging Res* (2016) 2016:8062079. doi:10.1155/2016/8062079
34. Beard HPJR, Bloom DE. Towards a comprehensive public health response to population ageing. *Lancet* (2015) 385(9968):658. doi:10.1016/S0140-6736(14)61461-6
35. O'Caoimh R, Molloy DW, Fitzgerald C, Van Velsen L, Cabrita M, Nassabi MH, et al. Healthcare recommendations from the personalised ICT supported service for independent living and active ageing (PERSSILAA) study. *ICT4Ageing Well 2017*; 2017 Apr 28–29. Porto, Portugal (2017).
36. Lattanzio F, Abbatecola AM, Bevilacqua R, Chiatti C, Corsonello A, Rossi L, et al. Advanced technology care innovation for older people in Italy: necessity and opportunity to promote health and wellbeing. *J Am Med Dir Assoc* (2014) 15(7):457–66. doi:10.1016/j.jamda.2014.04.003
37. Gardner PJ, Kamber T, Netherland J. "Getting turned on": using ICT training to promote active ageing in New York city. *J Commun Inf* (2012) 8(1):1–16.
38. Obi T, Ishmatova D, Iwasaki N. Promoting ICT innovations for the ageing population in Japan. *Int J Med Inform* (2013) 82(4):47–62. doi:10.1016/j.ijmedinf.2012.05.004
39. Lindberg B, Nilsson C, Zotterman D, Söderberg S, Skär L. Using information and communication technology in home care for communication between patients, family members, and healthcare professionals: a systematic review. *Int J Telemed Appl* (2013) 2013:461829. doi:10.1155/2013/461829
40. Helbostad JL, Vereijken B, Becker C, Todd C, Taraldsen K, Pijnappels M, et al. Mobile health applications to promote active and healthy ageing. *Sensors* (2017) 17(3):622. doi:10.3390/s17030622
41. Scanlon L, O'Shea E, O'Caoimh R, Timmons S. Technology use and frequency and self-rated skills: a survey of community-dwelling older adults. *J Am Geriatr Soc* (2015) 63(7):1483–4. doi:10.1111/jgs.13507
42. Hickman JM, Rogers WA, Fisk AD. Training older adults to use new technology. *J Gerontol B Psychol Sci Soc Sci* (2007) 62(Special_Issue_1):77–84. doi:10.1093/geronb/62.special_issue_1.77
43. Romero-Ortuno R, O'Shea D. Fitness and frailty; opposite ends of a challenging continuum? Will the end of age discrimination make frailty assessments an imperative? *Age Ageing* (2013) 42(3):279–80. doi:10.1093/ageing/afs189

11

Neuropsychological Correlates of Pre-Frailty in Neurocognitive Disorders: A Possible Role for Metacognitive Dysfunction and Mood Changes

Martina Amanzio[1,2]*, Sara Palermo*[1]**, Milena Zucca*[3]*, Rosalba Rosato*[1,4]*, Elisa Rubino*[3]*, Daniela Leotta*[5]*, Massimo Bartoli*[1] *and Innocenzo Rainero*[3]

[1] *Department of Psychology, University of Turin, Turin, Italy,* [2]*European Innovation Partnership on Active and Healthy Ageing, Brussels, Belgium,* [3] *Department of Neuroscience "Rita Levi Montalcini", University of Turin, Turin, Italy,* [4] *Unit of Cancer Epidemiology, "Città della Salute e della Scienza" Hospital and CPO Piemonte, Turin, Italy,* [5] *Neurology Division, Martini Hospital, Turin, Italy*

Edited by:
Giuseppe Liotta,
Università degli Studi di Roma Tor Vergata, Italy

Reviewed by:
Marco Canevelli,
Sapienza Università di Roma, Italy
Giuseppe Bellelli,
Università degli studi di Milano Bicocca, Italy

****Correspondence:***
Sara Palermo
sara.palermo@unito.it

Background: Recent studies have suggested that cognitive functions in patients with neurocognitive disorders have a significant role in the pathogenic mechanisms of frailty. Although pre-frailty is considered an intermediate, preclinical state, epidemiological research has begun to dislodge cognition and frailty into their specific subcomponents to understand the relationship among them. We aim to analyse the possible association between pre-frailty and neuropsychological variables to outline which factors can contribute to minor and major neurocognitive disorders.

Methods: 60 subjects complaining of different cognitive deficits underwent a deep-in-wide frailty and neuropsychological assessment. We conducted three multiple linear regression analyses adjusted for a combination of demographic measures and involving several neuropsychological–behavioural parameters selected by the literature on physical frailty.

Results: We found a significant association between frailty—as measured by the multi-dimensional prognostic index (MPI)—and action monitoring and monetary gain (cognitive domain), depression and disinhibition (behavioural domain). Moreover, an association between MPI and impaired awareness for instrumental activities disabilities exists.

Conclusion: We propose a novel framework for understanding frailty associated with metacognitive–executive dysfunction.

Keywords: pre-frailty, mild cognitive impairment, comprehensive geriatric assessment, Alzheimer's disease, executive dysfunction

INTRODUCTION

Frailty is a complex and heterogeneous clinical syndrome. It is described by augmented vulnerability resulting from age-related decline across several body organs and physiological systems (1, 2). Frailty leads to a decrease in the ability to remain independent and to maintain a good quality of life (3). Moreover, it increases the risk of disability and mortality (3). The frailty syndrome has principally been explored by focussing on the physical domain, mostly relying on signs and symptoms such as muscle weakness, sedentary behaviour, slow gait speed, and weight loss (1). Frailty has also been involved in general cognitive decline and impaired global cognition (4).

Canevelli and colleagues (5) have recently emphasised some criticalities of these studies: (a) the overwhelming majority of them have assessed frailty using the criteria proposed by Fried and colleagues (1), primarily aimed at describing the physical dimension of frailty; (b) most of these researches adopted only a measure of global cognitive functioning, mostly assessed by the Mini Mental State Examination [MMSE; (6)] to assess cognition, in absence of a comprehensive neuropsychological evaluation; (c) finally, the sample populations were mainly composed of community-dwelling older adults, preventing the applicability of results to other types of patients. The limitations of those studies have also been previously reported (7).

The overall concept of examining the specific cognitive correlates of frailty is interesting and may indeed shed light on a more comprehensive model of frailty that details a specific neuropsychological profile. Interestingly, the most novel evidence comes from a small number of studies aimed at examining the association between specific cognitive functions and physical frailty (5). In particular, Canevelli and colleagues (5) pointed out a significant impairment of attention and executive functions. Importantly, literature has shown that the executive function and attention domains are related to frailty, while gait speed or grip strength are the components of frailty most strongly associated with cognition (8–20). O'Halloran and colleagues (8) recently stated that pre-frail and frail individuals seem less able than robust subjects in the "Sustained Attention to Response Task" (SART). Even if these studies represent a first important attempt to describe the association between cognitive functions and physical frailty, there is still the need to assess frailty with a multidimensional approach (21–23).

Although executive function and attention domains may be related to physical frailty, no previous studies have investigated the role of different neuropsychological domains by carrying out a multidimensional assessment of frailty. In line with this, the multidimensional prognostic index (MPI) currently represents one of the suggested methods for a comprehensive assessment of frailty (24–26).

The aim of this study is to investigate whether pre-frailty, measured through the MPI, might be influenced by cognitive–behavioural measures in individuals with minor and major neurocognitive disorders [DSM-5; (27)], from mild cognitive impairment (MCI) likely due to Alzheimer's disease (AD), to mild AD patients (28). For this reason, we conducted three multiple linear regression analyses to study: (1) the role of global cognitive functioning and specific cognitive variables (selective attention, episodic memory, language comprehension, and reasoning in the visual modality); (2) the role of metacognitive executive functions, such as response monitoring; and (3) the relationship with mood changes, quality of life, and awareness of independence for daily living instrumental activities.

MATERIALS AND METHODS

Participants

All the outpatients were enrolled at the Neurology Division of the "Città della Scienza e della Salute" Hospital and the Martini Hospital, both in Turin (Italy).

Participants were included in the study if they had: (a) minor or major neurocognitive disorders (27), such as MCI-likely due to AD and mild AD. On the other hand, participants were excluded from the study if they had: (a) dysthymia or major depressive disorder, based on DSM-5 criteria (27); (b) A MMSE score <20, given that the neuropsychological measurement is not as reliable when problems of language comprehension occur; (c) were taking medications that could substantially impact cognitive functioning. CSF diagnosis that did not provide *in vivo* evidence of Alzheimer's pathology was considered exclusion criterion.

The patients underwent a complete neurological examination and neuroradiological investigations (MRI and FDG-PET). All the patients underwent lumbar puncture with cerebrospinal fluid measurement of 1-42 beta-amyloid, phospho-Tau, and total-Tau (Innogenetics kits, Ghent, Belgium).

Assessment of Frailty

Several operational definitions have been proposed to assess frailty in the elderly (29). Although this variability might be acceptable from a public health perspective, the identification of a gold standard measure might still be important to obtain. To date, frailty is still detected using different instruments and none of them has been able to prevail as superior to the others (29).

An index originally conceived and designed in the Italian general practice setting for the evaluation of chronic multipathological conditions was initially used to screen the participants' levels of frailty (30). The scale for the Evaluation of the frailty elderly (Scheda di Valutazione dell'Anziano Fragile,[1] SVAFRA) is a "multiaxial" score, interpreted according to the principles of the complexity theory in medicine and healthcare (30). This scale is a useful tool in case of multiaxial assessment in the setting of primary care (31), especially for its ability to combine technical skills, synthesis of information, and care-management suggestions (30, 31). SVAFRA was used for the first "Cognitive survey on the frailty of elderly people in Italy," which was attended by 34 Primary Care Physicians and 521 elderly recruited in Veneto, Lazio, and Sicily (32).

According to the authors, frailty is determined by issues pertaining at least one of the following evaluative dimensions (30): physical and mental health; physical and cognitive–behavioural disabilities; patient management considering the care burden; family and socio-environmental background. For each axis, determinants can assume a value between 0 (no deficiencies) and 3 (very serious problems). The level of frailty is then classified based on a combination of these four dimensions. A synthetic value—regardless of the value previously assigned to the four determinants—can also be assigned: F0 (absence of frailty, typical

[1] Frailty in the elderly evaluation sheet.

of healthy patients); F1 (pre-frailty); F2 (medium frailty); F3 (severe frailty, typical of severely ill patients); T (extreme frailty, typical of *terminally ill* patients).

Since clinicians needed an outcome instrument with sound clinimetric properties (33), frailty was assessed using a comprehensive geriatric assessment (CGA), which was considered the first-choice tool for evaluating biological, functional, cognitive, social, and clinical aspects of elderly subjects, as expressed by the Italian Society of Gerontology and Geriatrics (34, 35). The MPI was developed from a standardised CGA (26, 35, 36). It was originally conceived as a prognostic index of mortality in the short- and long-term period based on information obtained through the CGA in hospitalised (37) and outpatient settings (38). With this index, the prognostic value of negative outcomes and related severity are even higher than with the indices calculated in the single domains of the rating. The MPI is also considered suitable for assessing frailty in the elderly (34–36). Moreover, as a cumulative multidimensional index, the MPI allows professionals to develop a treatment plan (22). In 2013, the European Innovation Partnership on Active and Healthy Ageing identified 98 "good practices" involved in research to reverse or prevent frailty (24). As demonstrated by the Marco Polo Initiative, the MPI is helpful in identifying frailty elders, providing personalised interventions, avoiding drug prescriptions and adverse hospital admissions (24, 39).

The MPI includes information on clinical, functional, nutritional, and neuropsychological aspects, as well as polypathology, pharmacological treatment, and the social support network (22, 25, 26, 35–40). Specifically, the MPI is calculated using a mathematical algorithm that includes scores of individual profiles obtained from the eight evaluation tools that make up the CGA: 1. *activity of daily living scale* (ADL); 2. *instrumental activity of daily living* scale (iADL); 3. *short portable mental status questionnaire* (to assess cognitive status); 4. *cumulative illness rating scale—comorbidity index* (CIRS-CI, to explore comorbidity); 5. *Mini Nutritional Assessment* scale (MNA, to assess nutritional status); 6. *Exton Smith Scale* (to evaluate the risk of developing pressure sores); 7. polypharmacy; 8. social condition (22, 25, 26, 35–40).

The numerical index obtained has a value between 0.0 (lowest risk) and 1.0 (highest risk of mortality) and reports three grades of risk of severe prognosis: low risk (MPI value $\leq$ 0.33), moderate risk (MPI value between 0.34 and 0.66), and severe risk (MPI $\geq$ 0.67) (22, 26, 36, 37, 40). Importantly, the effectiveness of the MPI has recently been verified in population-based cohorts. Higher MPI risk scores were associated with more days in hospital and with fewer years of survival, across a broad and stratified age range (25, 40).

Neuropsychological Assessment

The neuropsychological evaluation involved a wide assessment of global cognitive deterioration using: the CDR (41), the Addenbrooke's Cognitive Examination-Revised version [ACE-R; (42)] and, finally, the MMSE (6). Other cognitive domains were also assessed with the use of different scales: selective attention with Attentional Matrices [AM; (43)], divided attention and cognitive shifting with the Trial Making Test [TMT; (43, 44)], episodic memory with the Recall of a Short Story test [Babcock; (37)], reasoning in the visual modality with Coloured Progressive Matrices [CPM-36; (43)], comprehension of spoken language with the Token Test [TT; (43, 45)].

Executive functions were analysed with the metacognitive version of the Wisconsin Card Sorting Test [m-WCST; (46, 47)]. This test is aimed to assess "on-line" metacognitive monitoring and control during the execution of the test (46, 47). For each card of the test, two questions evaluated "on-line" metacognitive monitoring ("What is your degree of confidence in this answer?") and control ("Do you want to take this response into account in your total score?") (46–48). In the original version of Koren's protocol, the participants were assigned a dollar value for each correct response (46–48). In this study, the patients received a monetary gain of 10 cents for each correct answer and they were deprived of 10 cents for every wrong answer (49). As described in our previous work that used the same procedure (49), a set of metacognitive indices were evaluated: "(1) accuracy score (AS), the number of correct voluntary answers/ number of voluntary responses; (2) free choice improvement (FCI) (accuracy—number of correct responses from forced responses)/number of cards presented; (3) global monitoring (GM), the number of correct responses—the total number of sorts required in the final score; (4) monitoring resolution (MR), the gamma correlation calculated between the confidence and correctness of the sorts in the entire test; (5) control sensitivity (CS), to what extent the control process depended on the monitoring process, indexed by the gamma correlation calculated across all sorts between the level of confidence and the decision to gamble; (6) monetary gains (MG), given by the number of correct voluntary responses—incorrect number of voluntary responses" [(49), p. 138].

We verified the subjects' level of autonomy in basic and instrumental activities of daily living (50, 51) and accordingly, their quality of life with the Quality of life scale in Alzheimer's disease (QoL-AD)—patient's subscale (52). Patients were also assessed using specific neuropsychiatric rating scales of mood changes: apathy and depression with Hamilton Depression Rating Scale [HDR-S; (53)], disinhibition and hypomania with the Disinhibition Scale and the Mania Scale [DIS-S (54); MAS (55)].

Finally, in accordance with what we did in our previous work (56), "we followed the classification of Starkstein and colleagues (57) who used principal component analysis to subdivide the Awareness of Deficit Questionnaire—Dementia scale [AQD (58)] into four domains taking into consideration the factors loading on each item. One of these factors, identified in terms of impaired awareness in instrumental activities of daily living (AQD_iADL), was designated as factor 1 by the authors. Factor 1 embraces 12 items: 'recalling the date, orienting to new places, recalling telephone calls, remembering the location of objects at home, understanding conversation and the plot of a movie, keeping belongings in order, handling money, doing mental calculations, remembering shopping lists and appointments, performing clerical work.' Thus it accounted for most of the variance and also rated as the earliest functional deficit in patients with cognitive impairment" [(56), p. 65]. Since disabilities in instrumental activities of daily living were one of the descriptors of frailty used in the Canadian Study on Health and Ageing (59), we decided to take it into consideration in our analyses.

Procedures

We implemented a cross-sectional study to explore data collected from our clinical population. Patients were evaluated by performing a neuropsychological assessment during a week in hospital. The participants were assessed in three experimental sessions held 1 day apart and each lasting 1 h, with a view to preventing fatigue and lack of adherence to the tasks.

Statistical Analysis

We performed statistical analyses using SAS/STAT® 9.3 (60, 61). The *post hoc* power was determined using the formula for sample size with continuous measures through G*Power 3, which is a stand-alone power analysis tool for statistical tests commonly used in social and behavioural research (62). The achieved power with a sample size of 60 was estimated to provide a minimum of 70% power at a 5% level of significance (two-sided) to detect a medium effect ($r^2 = 0.2$).

To study whether the level of the MPI index could be associated with cognitive and behavioural measurements, we conducted three multiple linear regression analyses adjusted for age, gender, and schooling. Normality assumption distribution of linear regression model residuals was evaluated by means of the Kolmogorov–Smirnov test.

Importantly, the selection of the three models was performed in line with the results obtained in the literature on physical frailty. In particular, frailty has been previously associated with general cognitive decline, impaired global cognition, and memory (5, 8, 18). Moreover, executive function and attention domains have been consistently related to frailty (8–10, 12–20). Finally, the association between physical frailty and the performance at the SART test (8) seems to suggest that pre-frail and frail people might be impaired in response monitoring.

The final selected models considered the MPI as the dependent variable and the following as independent variables:

- Model (1) to address the role of global cognitive functioning and specific cognitive variables (selective attention, episodic memory, language comprehension, and reasoning in the visual modality): ACE-R, MA, BABCOCK, TT and CPM-36;
- Model (2) to study the role of metacognitive executive functions with m-WCST: FCI, GM, MR, and MG;
- Model (3) to investigate the relationship with mood changes, quality of life and awareness of autonomy in instrumental activities of daily living: HDR-S, MAS, DIS-S, QOL-AD, and AQD_iADL.

RESULTS

Over a 24-month period, 72 patients—complaining of different cognitive deficits and presenting for the first time at the out-dep of our clinics—were evaluated with the overall neuropsychological assessment. After a month, based on CSF analysis results, only subjects with an AD-compatible liquor were included in the experimental sample. As a result, 12 patients were excluded, while 60 subjects were enrolled. Based on the exclusion criterion, 12 patients were excluded, while 60 subjects (M/F = 22/38; mean age ± SD = 69.6 ± 6.8 years) were enrolled (see **Table 1** for demographic and clinical data). In particular, 24 MCI due to AD patients according to the CSF analysis, were included in the study. For those patients with major neurocognitive disorders, the CSF diagnosis provided *in vivo* evidence of Alzheimer's pathology for 36 patients. The neuropsychological assessment reflected the diagnoses made by the CSF (see **Table 2** and Table S1 in Supplementary Material), biomarkers and neurological exams. Fifty-six of the 60 patients obtained a CDR score of between 0 and 1 attesting a low level of cognitive impairment.

Prevalence of Frailty Status

As regard the CGA evaluation, the patients fell within the lowest MPI range, attesting a low risk of severe prognosis. Considering the SVAFRA index, 97% of all patients were classified as pre-frail, and 3% with medium frailty.

Association between Frailty and Neuropsychological Variables

After adjusting the analysis for age, gender, and schooling, the MPI index scores were influenced by MR and MONEY in model 2, and by HDR-S, DIS-S, and AQD_iADL in model 3. On the contrary, the level of pre-frailty measured through the MPI index was not influenced by global cognition, memory,

TABLE 1 | Demographic characteristics and frailty evaluation by a comprehensive geriatric assessment.

	Maximum scores	Mean ± SD	Cutoff
Demographic characteristics			
Gender (male/female)		22/38	
Age (years)		66.62 ± 6.80	
Schooling (years)		9.28 ± 3.86	
Early cognitive symptoms complaints (months)		31.15 ± 27.82	
Clinical dementia rating scale		0.78 ± 0.44	
Multidimentional prognostic index			
Activity of daily living scale	8	5.70 ± 0.53	≥4
Instrumental activity of daily living scale	6	6.63 ± 1.55	≥6
Short portable mental state questionnaire	10	2.46 ± 1.63	≤2
Cumulative illness rating scale—comorbidity index	13	1.43 ± 1.42	
Mini nutritional assessment	30	21.32 ± 3.62	≥24
Exton Smith Scale	20	18.80 ± 1.47	≥15
Polypharmacy		4.12 ± 2.46	
Social condition		Household	
Multidimensional prognostic index	1	0.19 ± 0.12	
SVAFRA[a]			
F1		% = 97	
F2		% = 3	

Wherever there is a normative value, the cutoff scores are given in the statistical normal direction. Cells in grey indicate the absence of a normative cutoff.
[a]Scheda di Valutazione dell'Anziano Fragile.

TABLE 2 | Neuropsychological and neuropsychiatric assessment synopsis.

	Maximum scores	Mean ± SD	Cutoff
Neuropsychological assessment			
Mini-mental state examination	30	25.02 ± 2.85	≥24
Addenbrooke's cognitive examination—revised version	100	69.57 ± 12.60	≥82
Attentional matrices	60	30.52 ± 9.91	≥31
Trial making test A	500	110.73 ± 82.92	≤94
Trial making test B	500	297.18 ± 158.12	≤283
Trial making test B-A		194.92 ± 127.11	≤187
Babcock	16	6.22 ± 3.72	≥4.75
Coloured progressive matrices-36	36	22.17 ± 7.26	≥18.96
Token test	36	30.21 ± 3.61	≥32.69
Wisconsin card sorting test % correct answers		52.59 ± 15.44	≥37.1
Wisconsin card sorting test % perseverative errors		34.34 ± 14.95	≤42.7
Wisconsin card sorting test—metacognitive version			
Accuracy score		0.03 ± 0.11	
Free choice improvement		−1.17 ± 4.98	
Global monitoring		−20.13 ± 14.29	
Monitoring resolution		0.19 ± 0.24	
Control sensitivity		−0.04 ± 0.58	
Monetary gains		2.37 ± 1.93	
Neuropsychiatric assessment			
Quality of life scale in Alzheimer's disease—patient module	39	17.90 ± 8.01	
Hamilton depression rating scale	67	10.95 ± 7.47	≤7
Disinhibition scale	96	9.40 ± 6.95	≤16.9
Mania scale	44	2.62 ± 3.57	≤15
Awareness of deficit questionnaire—dementia scale for instrumental activity domain	16	3.20 ± 8.22	≤4

Wherever there is a normative value, the cutoff scores are given in the statistical normal direction. Cells in grey indicate the absence of a normative cutoff.

language comprehension, non-verbal reasoning (in model 1), or by QOL-AD (in model 3, see **Table 3**).

The normality distribution assumption of residuals in each model is fulfilled (Kolmogorov–Smirnov test > 0.05).

DISCUSSION

The aim of this study was to analyse the association among a multidimensional assessment of frailty, executive dysfunction and specific cognitive and behavioural variables using an overall neuropsychological battery. Our findings suggested that pre-frailty was associated with metacognitive executive dysfunction, in terms of action monitoring in MCI-likely due to AD and AD patients. Specifically, we observed a significant association between the MPI index and MR underlying the role of MR, where patients fail to distinguish between correct and incorrect sorts. The results obtained were specific and not influenced by other cognitive functions such as global cognition, memory, language comprehension, and non-verbal reasoning, with the exception of the selective attention task that reached a near significance level. Moreover, taking the MPI scores into account, we observed an involvement of mood changes in terms of depression, apathy, and disinhibition and a reduced awareness of iADL, while the relationship with hypomania was near to the significance value.

Although we considered patients with different degrees of cognitive impairment, our sample was homogeneous in terms of the etiopathogenesis, MPI level of risk, comorbidity with physical illness, somatic complaints, laboratory tests, and the level of mood changes. Moreover, we excluded all patients with neurological diseases other than AD. Most importantly, our attempt to consider these kinds of patients in the same sample was justified by the regression analysis approach we used and by

TABLE 3 | Effect of the independent variables on the multidimensional prognostic index estimated by the univariate and multiple linear regression analyses.

		Crude estimates			Adjusted estimates		
Model	**Independent variables**	**β**	***p***	**SE**	**β**	***p***	**SE**
1	Addenbrooke's cognitive examination—revised version	−0.20	0.18	0.001	−0.03	0.87	0.001
	Attentional matrices	−0.36	0.02	0.002	−0.29	0.11	0.002
	Babcock	−0.05	0.75	0.005	0.09	0.60	0.006
	Token test	−0.12	0.43	0.005	−0.01	0.95	0.005
	Coloured progressive matrices-36	−0.27	0.06	0.002	−0.14	0.44	0.003
	Model significance	$R^2 = 0.2056$, $F = 1.42$ $p = 0.2137$					
2	Free choice improvement	0.07	0.60	0.003	0.03	0.84	0.003
	Global monitoring	−0.07	0.60	0.001	0.11	0.42	0.001
	Monitoring resolution	0.33	0.02	0.075	***0.37***	***0.01***	0.073
	Monetary gains	−0.21	0.14	0.009	***−0.30***	***0.04***	0.009
	Model significance	$R^2 = 0.2863$, $F = 2.46$ $p = 0.0322$					
3	Hamilton depression rating scale	0.49	<0.00	0.002	***0.41***	***<0.00***	0.002
	Mania scale	0.09	0.52	0.005	−0.25	0.07	0.005
	Disinhibition scale	0.50	<0.00	0.002	***0.52***	***<0.00***	0.003
	Quality of life scale in Alzheimer's disease	−0.21	0.17	0.002	−0.01	0.91	0.002
	AQ-D scale for instrumental activity domain	−0.14	0.35	0.002	***−0.30***	***0.02***	0.002
	Model significance	$R^2 = 0.4980$, $F = 5.46$ $p < 0.0001$					

In multivariable analyses standardised coefficients are adjusted for age, gender, and schooling. Values in bold italics showed a statistically significant association (p < 0.05).
AQ-D, Awareness Questionnaire in Dementia.

the international guidelines on ageing that consider patients with cognitive impairment to lie on a continuum between MCI and mild AD (28, 63, 64).

Based on the results we obtained, there appear to be no straightforward associations between pre-frailty and specific aspects of neuropsychological functioning such as global cognition, long-term verbal memory, language comprehension, and non-verbal reasoning. As underlined by a review on cognitive impairment and frailty, not all cognitive domains may become impaired simultaneously (7). Although Canevelli et al. (5) have described a possible association between memory and physical frailty, other studies have found that memory does not seem to be clearly associated with frailty [i.e., Ref. (17, 65)]. As far as we are aware, no previous studies have addressed the association between frailty and language comprehension on the one hand, and frailty and non-verbal reasoning on the other (18). Moreover, we found no generalised cognitive impairment as a prerequisite of pre-frailty in our patients. Nevertheless, previously researches have reported a substantial association between frailty and cognitive deterioration (5, 7, 18, 66), although the phenotype model often used in these does not include cognitive function in its definition (1). Despite these evidences—as previously suggested by Robertson and colleagues (7)—statistical analyses of the proposed components of frailty suggest that, while energy, mobility, mood, physical activity, and strength aggregate as one concept, cognitive function does not clearly correlate with this and therefore may not be part of the frailty syndrome (67, 68). Furthermore, a study of AD patients found that 22% had no indications of frailty (69, 70). Indeed, Fougère and colleagues in their review concluded that "it seems most useful, therefore, to treat frailty and cognitive impairment as related but distinct concepts that frequently co-occur" [(71), p. 3].

Notably, the assessment of executive dysfunction should be seen as an important early predictor of cognitive frailty (9), since these problems may appear as the first cognitive changes in MCI patients (72), with concomitant iADL difficulties (73). Indeed, the early identification of executive impairments may be helpful for predicting the long-term functional outcome (74). Interestingly, O'Halloran and colleagues (8) recently stated that pre-frail and frail individuals seem to make more commission errors and omissions than robust subjects on the SART that evaluates the ability to sustain attention for a long time with a response-suppression element (75, 76). This fact suggests that they may be impaired in response monitoring, as we have demonstrated through the association between pre-frailty and action monitoring using the m-WCST. Indeed, the main predictor at this level has been MR, expressed by Koren and colleagues as the correlation between the level of confidence expected from the response and correctness of the sorts in the entire WCST (46–48). In particular, our patients have shown failure to monitor their own performance considering the errors made during task execution, in terms of low metacognitive self-awareness. Moreover, we have found an association between the MPI and monetary gain, which can be interpreted as subjects' ability to benefit from environmental feedback, anticipate the consequences of their future actions and make decisions accordingly. In addition, we have also found pre-frailty to be associated with an inability to report unsuccessful experiences in iADL through the Awareness Questionnaire in Dementia (AQ-D) (56). In our previous article concerning impaired awareness of deficits in AD and the role of everyday executive dysfunction (56), mood orientation changes, inhibition, self-monitoring, and set shifting appeared to be important skills for awareness of iADL (AQD_iADL) (56). According to this and considering the neural substrate, AD patients with impaired awareness showed reduced activation in the Mid Cingulate Cortex during an event-related fMRI response-inhibition paradigm, compared to subjects aware of their deficits (77).

Through our current results we hypothesise that pre-frailty may arise by a disruption of the comparator mechanisms responsible for monitoring behavioural mood changes and cognitive disturbances (56). If the executive system does not function properly, as frequently described in MCI-likely due to AD and AD patients (78), the comparator mechanism does not detect incongruities between the previous and the actual state of behaviour/performance. This phenomenon has been observed as an inability: (1) to monitor one's own performance with reference to the impact of errors made during task execution, in terms of a reduction in metacognitive self-awareness; and (2) to relate fruitless experiences in one's everyday living through the AQ-D.

The few studies investigating the neuropsychiatric factors (79–81) have suggested that "one mechanism underlying the link between frailty and cognition may be due to psychological factors such as mood. Indeed, mood disorders such as depression have been found to be both a risk factor for and a consequence of frailty" [(7), p. 847]. In line with this, we observed a role of HDR-S scores in pre-frailty condition. The HDR-S actually measures mood changes, in terms of apathetic behaviour and depressive mood possibly related to prefrontal dysfunctions (82). This evidence also suggests a possible role of apathy in pre-frailty conditions (83). Interestingly, apathy, disinhibition, and metacognitive executive dysfunction appear to be neurally inscribed in the same network (84–87). The results we obtained proposed the suggestive hypothesis that pre-frailty may be due to a possible dysfunction of the medial prefrontal–ventral striatal network observed throughout action-monitoring disability, mood changes, and reduced awareness of iADL. These findings ask for new neuroimaging investigations and replication in a larger group of patients.

Limitations Section

The study here presented has been carefully designed and reached its aims; however, some critical aspects have to be outlined. The first aspect regards the tools used to assess frailty, which could represent a possible confounding factor. In particular, pre-frailty is defined by adopting the SVAFRA that may not be considered appropriate for stratifying the frailty status of the older person and it has been rarely adopted for these purposes. Moreover, the MPI was originally conceived as a prognostic index of mortality in the short- and long-term period (37) and a recent international survey among clinical practitioners on the methods to assess frailty in their daily practice (29) did not include MPI as a tool to assess frailty. However, as previously expressed by Bruyére and colleagues (29), frailty is still detected using different instruments and none of them has been able to prevail as superior to the others (29). Second, the results we obtained are not generalisable for patients with different etiopathogenesis other than AD. However, our study is a first attempt to investigate possible association between pre-frailty and neuropsychological variables in a selected patient population, on the basis of liquor examination and may be limited to identify pathogenetic mechanisms of frailty. This is a cross-sectional study aimed to evaluate a possible association between frailty and neuropsychological variables in MCI-likely due to AD and AD patients. A longitudinal study may be the most correct approach to assess for the presence of cognitive disorders many years before the development of frailty itself. Further studies will be important to better characterised this association over time and replicate these findings in a larger group of patients.

CONCLUSION

This study represents a first important attempt to extend the frailty issue to neuropsychological correlates taking in consideration a multidimensional approach These findings suggest that the assessment of pre-frailty conditions must be achieved quantitatively by means of a multidimensional approach to clarify the nature and correlates of this multifaceted phenomenon. In particular, the impact of everyday executive dysfunction, early changes in mood and the awareness of iADL disabilities must be considered. Our results benefit from the homogeneity of the experimental sample in terms of etiopathogenetic mechanisms, disease severity (CDR) and functionality in daily life (ADL/iADL). The evaluation of pre-frailty conditions and their neuropsychological correlates is clinically relevant. Indeed, this multifaceted phenomenon has diagnostic, nosological, and prognostic implications that may affect patients' wellbeing in the continuum from MCI to AD.

AUTHOR CONTRIBUTIONS

The study is based on a concept developed by MA who wrote the paper and took part in the review and critique processes as PI. She also organised the study and participated in the statistical analyses (execution and organisation, review, and critique). SP performed the neuropsychological assessment (execution and organisation), participated in the statistical analyses, participated in writing the paper and created the infographics. RR conducted the statistical analyses (execution), participated in interpretation of results and in writing the paper. ER performed the neurological assessment (execution) and took part in the organisation of the study and in the diagnostic phase (organisation and diagnosis). MZ and MB performed the neuropsychological assessment (execution), participated in writing the paper and in drafting the work. DL and IR supervised the neurological assessment, took part in the organisation of the study and participated in writing the paper (organisation, review, and critique). All the contributors gave their approval of this version of the manuscript to be submitted.

ACKNOWLEDGMENTS

The study was approved by the Ethics Committee "*A.O.U. Città della Salute e della Scienza di Torino—A.O. Ordine Mauriziano—A.S.L. Città di Torino*" as part of the core research criteria followed by the Neurological Units. All the implemented procedures ensured the safety, integrity, and privacy of patients. All subjects gave their informed written consent to participate in the study. As far as data regarding human biological samples are concerned, the cerebrospinal fluid acquisition procedures used are safe and fall within the scope of ordinary clinical–diagnostic routine practice. Finally, any critical aspects, neither with regard to the functional–neurocognitive assessment phase nor to the neuropsychological assessment could be noticed. Importantly, the study has been conducted according to the principles set forth by the Declaration of Helsinki (59th WMA General Assembly, Seoul, October 2008) and in accordance with the Medical Research Involving Human Subjects Act (WMO).

REFERENCES

1. Fried LP, Tangen CM, Walston J, Newman AB, Hirsch C, Gottdiener J, et al. Frailty in older adults: evidence for a phenotype. *J Gerontol A Biol Sci Med Sci* (2001) 56:M146–56. doi:10.1093/gerona/56.3.M146
2. Rockwood K, Mitnitski A. Frailty in relation to the accumulation of deficits. *J Gerontol A Biol Sci Med Sci* (2007) 62:722–7. doi:10.1093/gerona/62.7.722
3. Heuberger RA. The frailty syndrome: a comprehensive review. *J Nutr Gerontol Geriatr* (2011) 30:315–68. doi:10.1080/21551197.2011.623931
4. Matusik P, Tomaszewski K, Chmielowska K, Nowak J, Nowak W, Parnicka A, et al. Severe frailty and cognitive impairment are related to higher mortality in 12-month follow-up of nursing home residents. *Arch Gerontol Geriatr* (2012) 55:22–4. doi:10.1016/j.archger.2011.06.034
5. Canevelli M, Cesari M, van Kan GA. Frailty and cognitive decline: how do they relate? *Curr Opin Clin Nutr Metab Care* (2015) 18:43–50. doi:10.1097/MCO.0000000000000133
6. Folstein MF, Folstein SE, McHugh PR. "Mini-mental state". A practical method for grading the cognitive state of patients for the clinician. *J Psychiatr Res* (1975) 12:189–98. doi:10.1016/0022-3956(75)90026-6
7. Robertson DA, Savva GM, Kenny RA. Frailty and cognitive impairment. A review of the evidence and causal mechanisms. *Ageing Res Rev* (2013) 12:840–51. doi:10.1016/j.arr.2013.06.004
8. O'Halloran AM, Finucane C, Savva GM, Robertson IH, Kenny RA. Sustained attention and frailty in the older adult population. *J Gerontol B Psychol Sci Soc Sci* (2014) 69:147–56. doi:10.1093/geronb/gbt009
9. Delrieu J, Andrieu S, Pahor M, Cantet C, Cesari M, Ousset PJ, et al. Neuropsychological profile of "cognitive frailty" subjects in MAPT study. *J Prev Alzheimers Dis* (2016) 3:151. doi:10.14283/jpad.2016.94
10. Harley C, Wilkie RM, Wann JP. Stepping over obstacles: attention demands and aging. *Gait Posture* (2009) 29:428–32. doi:10.1016/j.gaitpost.2008.10.063
11. Hooghiemstra AM, Ramakers IHGB, Sistermans N, Pijnenburg YAL, Aalten P, Hamel REG, et al. Gait speed and grip strength reflect cognitive impairment and are modestly related to incident cognitive decline in memory clinic

patients with subjective cognitive decline and mild cognitive impairment: findings from the 4C study. *J Gerontol A Biol Sci Med Sci* (2017) 72:846–54. doi:10.1093/gerona/glx003
12. Kang HG, Costa MD, Priplata AA, Starobinets OV, Goldberger AL, Peng CK, et al. Frailty and the degradation of complex balance dynamics during a dual-task protocol. *J Gerontol A Biol Sci Med Sci* (2009) 64:1304–11. doi:10.1093/gerona/glp113
13. Langlois F, Vu TT, Kergoat MJ, Chassé K, Dupuis G, Bherer L. The multiple dimensions of frailty: physical capacity, cognition, and quality of life. *Int Psychogeriatr* (2012) 24:1429–36. doi:10.1017/S1041610212000634
14. Lundin-Olsson L, Nyberg L, Gustafson Y. Attention, frailty, and falls: the effect of a manual task on basic mobility. *J Am Geriatr Soc* (1998) 46:758–61. doi:10.1111/j.1532-5415.1998.tb03813.x
15. McGough EL, Cochrane BB, Pike KC, Logsdon RG, McCurry SM, Teri L. Dimensions of physical frailty and cognitive function in older adults with amnestic mild cognitive impairment. *Ann Phys Rehabil Med* (2013) 56:329–41. doi:10.1016/j.rehab.2013.02.005
16. O'Halloran AM, Fan CW, Kenny RA, Pénard N, Galli A, Robertson IH. Variability in sustained attention and risk of frailty. *J Am Geriatr Soc* (2011) 59:2390–2. doi:10.1111/j.1532-5415.2011.03706.x
17. Patrick L, Gaskovski P, Rexroth D. Cumulative illness and neuropsychological decline in hospitalized geriatric patients. *Clin Neuropsychol* (2002) 16:145–56. doi:10.1076/clin.16.2.145.13239
18. Sargent L, Brown R. Assessing the current state of cognitive frailty: measurement properties. *J Nutr Health Aging* (2017) 21:152–60. doi:10.1007/s12603-016-0735-9
19. Shimada H, Makizako H, Doi T, Yoshida D, Tsutsumimoto K, Anan Y, et al. Combined prevalence of frailty and mild cognitive impairment in a population of elderly Japanese people. *J Am Med Dir Assoc* (2013) 14:518–24. doi:10.1016/j.jamda.2013.03.010
20. Woollacott M, Shumway-Cook A. Attention and the control of posture and gait: a review of an emerging area of research. *Gait Posture* (2002) 16:1–14. doi:10.1016/S0966-6362(01)00156-4
21. Avelino-Silva TJ, Farfel JM, Curiati JA, Amaral JR, Campora F, Jacob-Filho W. Comprehensive geriatric assessment predicts mortality and adverse outcomes in hospitalized older adults. *BMC Geriatr* (2014) 14:129. doi:10.1186/1471-2318-14-129
22. Pilotto A, Ferrucci LA. A clinical definition of frailty: usefulness of the multidimensional assessment. *G Gerontol* (2011) 59:125–9. (Italian).
23. Sternberg SA, Bentur N. The contribution of comprehensive geriatric assessment to primary care physicians. *Isr J Health Policy Res* (2014) 3:44. doi:10.1186/2045-4015-3-44
24. European Innovation Partnership on Active and Healthy Ageing (EIP-AHA). *A Compilation of Good Practices – Prevention and Early Diagnosis of Frailty and Functional Decline, both Physical and Cognitive in Older People*. Action Group A3, European Commission (2013). Available from: https://ec.europa.eu/research/innovation-union/pdf/active-healthy-ageing/gp_a3.pdf
25. Angleman SB, Santoni G, Pilotto A, Fratiglioni L, Welmer AK; MPI_AGE Project Investigators. Multidimensional prognostic index in association with future mortality and number of hospital days in a population-based sample of older adults: results of the EU funded MPI_AGE project. *PLoS One* (2015) 10:e0133789. doi:10.1371/journal.pone.0133789
26. Pilotto A, Gallina P, Fontana A, Sancarlo D, Bazzano S, Copetti M, et al. Development and validation of a multidimensional prognostic index for mortality based on a standardized multidimensional assessment schedule (MPI-SVaMA) in community-dwelling older subjects. *J Am Med Dir Assoc* (2013) 14:287–92. doi:10.1016/j.jamda.2013.01.005
27. American Psychiatric Association (APA). *Diagnostic and Statistical Manual of Mental Disorders*. 5th ed. Washington, DC: American Psychiatric Association Publishing (2013).
28. Albert MS, DeKosky ST, Dickson D, Dobois B, Feldman HH, Fox NC, et al. The diagnosis of mild cognitive impairment due to Alzheimer's disease: recommendations from the National Institute on Aging-Alzheimer's Association workgroups on diagnostic guidelines for Alzheimer's disease. *Alzheimers Dement* (2011) 7:270–9. doi:10.1016/j.jalz.2011.03.008
29. Bruyère O, Buckinx F, Beaudart C, Reginster JY, Bauer J, Cederholm T, et al. How clinical practitioners assess frailty in their daily practice: an international survey. *Aging Clin Exp Res* (2017) 29:905–12. doi:10.1007/s40520-017-0806-8
30. De Toni AF, Giacomelli F, Ivis S. *Il mondo invisibile dei pazienti anziani. La fragilità interpretata dalla medicina di famiglia mediante la teoria della complessità*. Torino, Italy: UTET Università (2010). 480 p. (Italian).
31. De Gobbi R, Fassina R, Tonon R, Benetti G. Il paziente anziano fragile: strumenti di valutazione cognitivo-funzionale in Medicina Generale. *Rivista SIMG* (2012) 5:14–9. (Italian).
32. Forum Ania Consumatori, CENSIS. Indagine conoscitiva sullo stato di fragilità della popolazione anziana in Italia. In: Gli scenari del welfare. editor. *Verso uno stato sociale sostenibile*. Milano, Italy: Franco Angeli (2015). 288. p. (Italian).
33. De Vries NM, Staal JB, Van Ravensberg CD, Hobbelen JSM, Rikkert MO, Nijhuis-Van der Sanden MWG. Outcome instruments to measure frailty: a systematic review. *Ageing Res Rev* (2011) 10:104–14. doi:10.1016/j.arr.2010.09.001
34. Giordano A, Rozzini M, Trabucchi M. Frailty in elderly: a clinical view. *G Gerontol* (2007) 55:2–6. (Italian).
35. Pilotto A, Franceschi M, Ferrucci L. A multidimensional prognostic index (MPI) for the evaluation of the hospitalized frail older patient. *G Gerontol* (2007) 55:7–10. (Italian).
36. Pilotto A, Ferrucci L, Franceschi M, D'Ambrosio LP, Scarcelli C, Cascavilla L, et al. Development and validation of a multidimensional prognostic index for one-year mortality from comprehensive geriatric assessment in hospitalized older patients. *Rejuvenation Res* (2008) 11:151–61. doi:10.1089/rej.2007.0569
37. Pilotto A, Sancarlo D, Panza F, Paris F, D'Onofrio G, Cascavilla L, et al. The multidimensional prognostic index (MPI), based on a comprehensive geriatric assessment predicts short- and long-term mortality in hospitalized older patients with dementia. *J Alzheimers Dis* (2009) 18:191–9. doi:10.3233/JAD-2009-1139
38. Gallucci M, Battistella G, Bergamelli C, Spagnolo P, Mazzuco S, Carlini A, et al. Multidimensional prognostic index in a cognitive impairment outpatient setting: mortality and hospitalizations. The Treviso Dementia (TREDEM) study. *J Alzheimers Dis* (2014) 42:1461–8. doi:10.3233/JAD-140516
39. Maggi S, Pilotto A. The challenge of the clinical decisions in frail multimorbid older subjects: results and recommendations from the European MPI_AGE PROJECT. *International Congress of the European Union Geriatric Medicine Society*; Sep 20–22; Nice, France (2017).
40. Volpato S, Bazzano S, Fontana A, Ferrucci L, Pilotto A; MPI-TriVeneto Study Group. Multidimensional prognostic index predicts mortality and length of stay during hospitalization in the older patients: a multicenter prospective study. *J Gerontol A Biol Sci Med Sci* (2015) 70:325–31. doi:10.1093/gerona/glu167
41. Hughes CP, Berg L, Danziger WL, Coben LA, Martin RL. A new clinical scale for the staging of dementia. *Br J Psychiatry* (1982) 140:566–72. doi:10.1192/bjp.140.6.566
42. Mioshi E, Dawson K, Mitchell J, Arnold R, Hodges JR. The Addenbrooke's cognitive examination revised (ACE-R): a brief cognitive test battery for dementia screening. *Int J Geriatr Psychiatry* (2006) 21:1078–85. doi:10.1002/gps.1610
43. Spinnler H, Tognoni G. *Standardizzazione italiana e taratura di test neuropsicologici. Italian Journal of Neurological Sciences*. (Vol. 6). Milano, Italy: Masson Italiana Periodici (1987). 120 p. (Italian).
44. Reitan RM, Wolfson D. A selective and critical review of neuropsychological deficits and the frontal lobes. *Neuropsychol Rev* (1994) 4:161–98. doi:10.1007/BF01874891
45. De Renzi E, Vignolo LA. The token test: a sensitive test to detect receptive disturbances in aphasics. *Brain* (1962) 85:665–78. doi:10.1093/brain/85.4.665
46. Koren D, Seidman LJ, Poyurovsky M, Goldsmith M, Viksman P, Zichel S, et al. The neuropsychological basis of insight in first-episode schizophrenia: a pilot metacognitive study. *Schizophr Res* (2004) 70:195–202. doi:10.1016/j.schres.2004.02.004
47. Koren D, Seidman LJ, Goldsmith M, Harvey PD. Real-world cognitive- and metacognitive-dysfunction in schizophrenia: a new approach for measuring (and remediating) more "right stuff". *Schizophr Bull* (2006) 32:310–26. doi:10.1093/schbul/sbj035
48. Quiles C, Verdoux H, Prouteau A. Assessing metacognition during a cognitive task: impact of "on-line" metacognitive questions on neuropsychological performances in a non-clinical sample. *J Int Neuropsychol Soc* (2014) 20:547–54. doi:10.1017/S1355617714000290

49. Amanzio M, Palermo S, Zibetti M, Leotta D, Rosato R, Geminiani G, et al. Self-unawareness of levodopa induced dyskinesias in patients with Parkinson's disease. *Brain Cogn* (2014) 90:135–41. doi:10.1016/j.bandc.2014.06.014
50. Katz S, Ford AB, Moskowitz RW, Jackson BA, Jaffe MW. Studies of illness in the aged. The index of Adl: a standardized measure of biological and psychosocial function. *JAMA* (1963) 185:914–9. doi:10.1001/jama.1963.03060120024016
51. Lawton MP, Brody EM. Assessment of older people: self-maintaining and instrumental activities of daily living. *Gerontologist* (1969) 9:179–86. doi:10.1093/geront/9.3_Part_1.179
52. Logsdon RG, Gibbons LE, McCurry SM, Teri L. Assessing quality of life in older adults with cognitive impairment. *Psychosom Med* (2002) 64:510–9. doi:10.1097/00006842-200205000-00016
53. Hamilton M. A rating scale for depression. *J Neurol Neurosurg Psychiatry* (1960) 23:56–62. doi:10.1136/jnnp.23.1.56
54. Starkstein SE, Garau ML, Cao A. Prevalence and clinical correlates of disinhibition in dementia. *Cogn Behav Neurol* (2004) 17:139–47. doi:10.1097/01.wnn.0000119241.65522.90
55. Bech P, Rafaelsen OJ, Kramp P, Bolwig TG. The mania rating scale: scale construction and inter-observer agreement. *Neuropharmacology* (1978) 17:430–1. doi:10.1016/0028-3908(78)90022-9
56. Amanzio M, Vase L, Leotta D, Miceli R, Palermo S, Geminiani G. Impaired awareness of deficits in Alzheimer's disease: the role of everyday executive dysfunction. *J Int Neuropsychol Soc* (2013) 19:63–72. doi:10.1017/S1355617712000896
57. Starkstein SE, Jorge R, Mizrahi R, Robinson RG. A diagnostic formulation for anosognosia in Alzheimer's disease. *J Neurol Neurosurg Psychiatry* (2006) 77:719–25. doi:10.1136/jnnp.2005.085373
58. Migliorelli R, Tesón A, Sabe L, Petracca G, Petracchi M, Leiguarda R, et al. Anosognosia in Alzheimer's disease: a study of associated factors. *J Neuropsychiatry Clin Neurosci* (1995) 7:338–44. doi:10.1176/jnp.7.3.338
59. Rockwood K, Song X, MacKnight C, Bergman H, Hogan DB, Mitnitski A, et al. A global clinical measure of fitness and frailty in elderly people. *CMAJ* (2005) 173:489–95. doi:10.1503/cmaj.050051
60. Freund RJ, Littell RC, Spector PC. *SAS System for Linear Models*. 3rd ed. Cary, NC: SAS Institute Inc. (1991). 352 p.
61. Schlotzhauer SD, Littell RC. *SAS System for Elementary Statistical Analysis*. Cary, NC: SAS Institute Inc. (1987). 416 p.
62. Faul F, Erdfelder E, Lang AG, Buchner A. G*Power 3: a flexible statistical power analysis program for the social, behavioral, and biomedical sciences. *Behav Res Methods* (2007) 39:175–91. doi:10.3758/BF03193146
63. Dubois B, Feldman HH, Jacova C, Hampel H, Molinuevo JL, Blennow K, et al. Advancing research diagnostic criteria for Alzheimer's disease: the IWG-2 criteria. *Lancet Neurol* (2014) 13:614–29. doi:10.1016/S1474-4422(14)70090-0
64. Petersen RC, Negash S. Mild cognitive impairment: an overview. *CNS Spectr* (2008) 13:45–53. doi:10.1017/S1092852900016151
65. Yassuda MS, Lopes A, Cachioni M, Falcao DV, Batistoni SS, Guimaraes VV, et al. Frailty criteria and cognitive performance are related: data from the FIBRA study in Ermelino Matarazzo, São Paulo, Brazil. *J Nutr Health Aging* (2012) 16:55–61. doi:10.1007/s12603-012-0003-6
66. Samper-Ternent R, Al Snih S, Raji MA, Markides KS, Ottenbacher KJ. Relationship between frailty and cognitive decline in older Mexican Americans. *J Am Geriatr Soc* (2008) 56:1845–52. doi:10.1111/j.1532-5415.2008.01947.x
67. Sourial N, Bergman H, Karunananthan S, Wolfson C, Guralnik J, Payette H, et al. Contribution of frailty markers in explaining differences among individuals in five samples of older persons. *J Gerontol A Biol Sci Med Sci* (2012) 67:1197–204. doi:10.1093/gerona/gls084
68. Sourial N, Wolfson C, Bergman H, Zhu B, Karunananthan S, Quail J, et al. A correspondence analysis revealed frailty deficits aggregate and are multidimensional. *J Clin Epidemiol* (2010) 63:647–54. doi:10.1016/j.jclinepi.2009.08.007
69. Bilotta C, Bergamaschini L, Nicolini P, Casè A, Pina G, Rossi S, et al. Frailty syndrome diagnosed according to the study of osteoporotic fractures criteria and mortality in older outpatients suffering from Alzheimer's disease: a one-year prospective cohort study. *Aging Ment Health* (2012) 16:273–80. doi:10.1080/13607863.2011.609534
70. Bilotta C, Nicolini P, Casè A, Pina G, Rossi S, Vergani C. Frailty syndrome diagnosed according to the study of osteoporotic fractures (SOF) criteria and adverse health outcomes among community-dwelling older outpatients in Italy. A one-year prospective cohort study. *Arch Gerontol Geriatr* (2012) 54:e23–8. doi:10.1016/j.archger.2011.06.037
71. Fougère B, Delrieu J, Del Campo N, Soriano G, Sourdet S, Vellas B. Cognitive frailty: mechanisms, tools to measure, prevention and controversy. *Clin Geriatr Med* (2017) 33:339–55. doi:10.1016/j.cger.2017.03.001
72. Johns EK, Phillips NA, Belleville S, Goupil D, Babins L, Kelner N, et al. The profile of executive functioning in amnestic mild cognitive impairment: disproportionate deficits in inhibitory control. *J Int Neuropsychol Soc* (2012) 18:541–55. doi:10.1017/S1355617712000069
73. Jekel K, Damian M, Wattmo C, Hausner L, Bullock R, Connelly PJ, et al. Mild cognitive impairment and deficits in instrumental activities of daily living: a systematic review. *Alzheimers Res Ther* (2015) 7:17. doi:10.1186/s13195-015-0099-0
74. Gothe NP, Fanning J, Awick E, Chung D, Wójcicki TR, Olson EA, et al. Executive function processes predict mobility outcomes in older adults. *J Am Geriatr Soc* (2014) 62:285–90. doi:10.1111/jgs.12654
75. Robertson DA, Savva G, Coen RF, Kenny RA. Cognitive function in the pre-frailty and frailty syndrome. *J Am Geriatr Soc* (2014) 62:2118–24. doi:10.1111/jgs.13111
76. Langner R, Eickhoff SB. Sustaining attention to simple tasks: a meta-analytic review of the neural mechanisms of vigilant attention. *Psychol Bull* (2013) 139:870–900. doi:10.1037/a0030694
77. Amanzio M, Torta DM, Sacco K, Cauda F, D'Agata F, Duca F, et al. Unawareness of deficits in Alzheimer's disease: role of the cingulate cortex. *Brain* (2011) 134:1061–76. doi:10.1093/brain/awr020
78. Espinosa A, Alegret M, Boada M, Vinyes G, Valero S, Martínez-Lage P, et al. Ecological assessment of executive functions in mild cognitive impairment and mild Alzheimer's disease. *J Int Neuropsychol Soc* (2009) 15:751–7. doi:10.1017/S135561770999035X
79. Espinoza SE, Jung I, Hazuda H. The Hispanic paradox and predictors of mortality in an aging biethnic cohort of Mexican Americans and European Americans: the San Antonio longitudinal study of aging. *J Am Geriatr Soc* (2013) 61:1522–9. doi:10.1111/jgs.12421
80. Mezuk B, Edwards L, Lohman M, Choi M, Lapane K. Depression and frailty in later life: a synthetic review. *Int J Geriatr Psychiatry* (2012) 27:879–92. doi:10.1002/gps.2807
81. Paulson D, Lichtenberg PA. Vascular depression: an early warning sign of frailty. *Aging Ment Health* (2013) 17:85–93. doi:10.1080/13607863.2012.692767
82. Assal F, Cummings JL. Neuropsychiatric symptoms in the dementias. *Curr Opin Neurol* (2002) 15:445–50. doi:10.1097/00019052-200208000-00007
83. Semprini R, Lubrano A, Misaggi G, Martorana A. Apathy as marker of frail status. *J Aging Res* (2012) 2012:436251. doi:10.1155/2012/436251
84. Bonelli RM, Cummings JL. Frontal-subcortical circuitry and behavior. *Dialogues Clin Neurosci* (2007) 9:141–51.
85. Cummings JL. Anatomic and behavioral aspects of frontal-subcortical circuits. *Ann N Y Acad Sci* (1995) 769:1–13. doi:10.1111/j.1749-6632.1995.tb38127.x
86. Masterman DL, Cummings JL. Frontal-subcortical circuits: the anatomic basis of executive, social and motivated behaviors. *J Psychopharmacol* (1997) 11:107–14. doi:10.1177/026988119701100203
87. Tekin S, Cummings JL. Frontal-subcortical neuronal circuits and clinical neuropsychiatry: an update. *J Psychosom Res* (2002) 53:647–54. doi:10.1016/S0022-3999(02)00428-2

12

Is the Retina a Mirror of the Aging Brain? Aging of Neural Retina Layers and Primary Visual Cortex across the Lifespan

Lília Jorge[1,2], *Nádia Canário*[1,2], *Hugo Quental*[1,2], *Rui Bernardes*[1,2,3] *and Miguel Castelo-Branco*[1,2,3]*

[1]Coimbra Institute for Biomedical Imaging and Translational Research (CIBIT), University of Coimbra, Coimbra, Portugal, [2]Institute for Nuclear Sciences Applied to Health (ICNAS), University of Coimbra, Coimbra, Portugal, [3]Faculty of Medicine, University of Coimbra, Coimbra, Portugal

Edited by:
Ashok Kumar,
University of Florida, United States

Reviewed by:
Rongqiao He,
Institute of Biophysics (CAS), China
Eszter Farkas,
University of Szeged, Hungary

***Correspondence:**
Miguel Castelo-Branco
mcbranco@fmed.uc.pt

How aging concomitantly modulates the structural integrity of the brain and retina in healthy individuals remains an outstanding question. Given the strong bottom-up retinocortical connectivity, it is important to study how these structures co-evolve during healthy aging in order to unravel mechanisms that may affect the physiological integrity of both structures. For the 56 participants in the study, primary visual cortex (BA17), as well as frontal, parietal and temporal regions thicknesses were measured in T1-weighted magnetic resonance imaging (MRI), and retinal macular thickness (10 neuroretinal layers) was measured by optical coherence tomography (OCT) imaging. We investigated the statistical association of these measures and their age dependence. We found an age-related decay of primary visual cortical thickness that was significantly correlated with a decrease in global and multiple layer retinal thicknesses. The atrophy of both structures might jointly account for the decline of various visual capacities that accompany the aging process. Furthermore, associations with other cortical regions suggest that retinal status may index cortical integrity in general.

Keywords: healthy aging, optical coherence tomography (OCT), magnetic resonance imaging (MRI), primary visual cortex (BA17), retinal segmentation, ganglion cell layer (GCL), outer segment photoreceptor/RPE complex (OPR)

INTRODUCTION

The primary visual cortex, Broadman area 17 (BA17), receives direct sensory input through the lateral geniculate nucleus (LGN), conveyed from the retina and is the cortical area where retinotopic information processing begins. This region may undergo considerable neurodevelopmental reorganization in response to retinal input changes (d'Almeida et al., 2013; Ferreira et al., 2017).

Concerning retinocortical changes in response to disease-related degeneration, Barcella et al. (2010) resorting to voxel-based morphometry (VBM) demonstrated that patients with clinically installed Leber Hereditary Optic Neuropathy (LOHN)—marked by a predominant central macular ganglion cell degeneration and death—had reduced gray matter volume in the respective lesion projection zones of the primary visual cortex, compared to healthy controls.

In fact, alterations in the thickness of this region are already present in asymptomatic patients suffering from the same disease, although in early stages changes are still compensatory (increased thickness in extrastriate visual cortex; d'Almeida et al., 2013). Moreover, also age-related retinal diseases, such as late-stage macular degeneration have an impact on cortical morphology. For example, Burge et al. (2016) found that the regions of the striate cortex that usually sample the visual input from the injured area of the retina were thinner in participants with macular disease when compared to controls. On the contrary, regions corresponding to non-damaged areas demonstrated a significant increase in cortical thickness. Overall, these findings suggest a strong retinocortical coupling of structural and functional changes in retinal disorders.

Healthy aging is characterized by diverse structural changes in both brain and retina, which association remains to be studied. Concerning the former, there is substantial evidence suggesting that widespread cortical shrinkage takes place with increasing aging (Courchesne et al., 2000; Good et al., 2001; Lemaître et al., 2005). The nature of such effects in early visual areas remains controversial. Whereas some studies have shown volume loss or cortical thinning of visual cortices (Resnick et al., 2003; Salat et al., 2004; Fjell et al., 2009), others have reported a certain sparing of these areas during aging (Allen et al., 2005; Grieve et al., 2005; Raz et al., 2005). Specifically to the primary visual cortex, according to Griffis et al. (2016), such discrepancy in the literature could be explained by methodological issues, since they demonstrated that different sub-regions of primary visual cortex were unequally affected by aging, depending on their retinotopic eccentricity. Nonetheless, studies directly examining the structure and function of primary visual areas are scarce in healthy aging, in spite of the fact that the organization of early visual areas is well documented in young adults.

Moreover, some studies have suggested that cortical alterations might contribute to age-related visual deficits, but the lack of studies on the visual cortex in healthy old individuals makes it difficult to know what changes actually occur.

The retina also undergoes substantial modifications throughout the lifespan. Histological studies have reported a reduction in the density of photoreceptors, ganglion cells, and pigment epithelial cells with age (Dolman et al., 1980; Quigley et al., 1989). Overall, retinal thickness studies using optical coherence tomography (OCT) imaging have revealed regional age-dependent differences in global macular integrity (Alamouti and Funk, 2003; Eriksson and Alm, 2009; Neuville et al., 2009; Sung et al., 2009; Song et al., 2010). The improvement of OCT image processing techniques has now allowed for the automatic segmentation of retinal individual layers, which provides a more detailed and specific perspective on such alterations. For instance, Demirkaya et al. (2013) measured the mean thickness of seven macular layers across different regions in subjects with different ages, and they found that the thickness of the pericentral ganglion cell layer (GCL), peripheral inner plexiform layer (IPL) and foveal outer segment layer (OS) were negatively correlated with age. Conversely, foveal retinal pigment epithelium (RPE) thickness was positively correlated with age.

The study of Won et al. (2016) addressed nine retinal layers and also found evidence of age-related morphologic changes. They compared a younger (<30) vs. an older group (>60) and found that the thickness and volume of peripheral retinal nuclear fiber layer (RNFL), GCL, and pericentral and peripheral IPL were superior in the first group, whereas the thickness and volume of foveal inner nuclear layer (INL) and inner retina (IR) were higher in the older group.

Furthermore, retinal alterations have been reported in patients with neurological disorders such as Stroke, Multiple Sclerosis, Parkinson and Alzheimer diseases (Grzybowski and Barboni, 2016; Alves et al., 2018). On the other hand, Satue et al. (2016) demonstrated that Alzheimer's disease (AD) might share degenerative mechanisms that may be difficult to disentangle from ocular diseases, as for example glaucoma and age-related macular degeneration.

Given that the retina exhibits similarities to the brain in terms of functional, anatomic and immunological properties (London et al., 2013), it is not surprising that common degenerative mechanisms might affect both in health and disease. Consequently, there is a strong need to investigate the interdependence of both the brain and retina during healthy aging. This will also facilitate the identification of specific alterations resulting from age-dependent pathological mechanisms.

Thus, despite previous work on the impact of aging on the anatomic-physiology of each structure individually (retina and primary visual cortex), as far as we know, no efforts were made in order to investigate their integrity in the same study simultaneously. This is critical to directly investigate their concomitant aging. Therefore, we aimed to investigate the association of retinal layer and cortical integrity, in a healthy cohort aged between 20–80 years old. To that end, we performed MR structural data imaging measurements of cortical thickness in the primary visual cortex—BA17—the cortical area that receives direct retinal input—and OCT to measure the thickness of the macula and their individual layers, in the same set of participants. In parallel, we have also searched for correlations between the retina and other cortical regions—frontal, temporal and parietal lobes—in order to investigate whether associations between brain and retina go beyond the occipital lobe.

MATERIALS AND METHODS

Participants

MR structural data acquisitions were obtained from 56 normally sighted controls (28 females, 28 males; with age ranging from 23 to 79 years old) without cognitive impairment, as assessed by the Montreal Cognitive Assessment (MoCA; Freitas et al., 2011) and with no clinical history of psychiatric or neurological disorders.

After excluding the history of any ocular disease or ocular clinical intervention, all participants underwent a comprehensive ophthalmological examination to check the absence of any visual complication, which included: visual acuity assessment with Snellen chart, ocular tension (Goldmann applanation tonometer), slit-lamp biomicroscopy and OCT imaging. Only subjects with normal or corrected to normal vision (visual acuity $\geq$ 8/10) were included, with the refractive error between $\pm$ 5 diopters, and with intraocular pressure $\leq$21 mmHg.

Images of the retina were obtained from the same set of participants with spectral-domain OCT (Cirrus HD-OCT 5000, Carl Zeiss Meditec, Dublin, CA, USA) and only participants without any abnormalities of the optic disc or macula were included. Additionally, we used as exclusion criteria family history of glaucoma, or any other hereditary eye disease; diabetes, because conditions of the vascular system may concomitantly impact on cortical and retinal health (Patton et al., 2005) or other systemic disease that could affect the eye.

The study was approved by the Ethics Committee of the University of Coimbra, and all subjects participated voluntarily and gave their informed written consent for the study, according to the Declaration of Helsinki.

Retinal Imaging

For each participant, the retinal images from both eyes were acquired using OCT resorting to the HD-OCT Cirrus 5000 system with the macular cube 512 × 128 protocol. This protocol creates a cube of data through a 6 mm square grid around the fovea centralis by acquiring a series of 128 horizontal B-scans lines each composed of 512 A-scans, with an axial resolution of 5 μm. Two experienced technicians performed all the acquisitions.

MRI Imaging

Magnetic resonance imaging (MRI) data were acquired in a 3 Tesla Siemens Magnetom Trio Scanner, using a whole-brain approach, with a 12-channel head coil. Two 3D anatomical MPRAGE (rapid gradient-echo) T1-weighted sequence were acquired with the following acquisition parameters: 1.0 × 1.0 × 1.0 mm^3 voxel resolution, repetition time (TR) 2,530 ms, echo time (TE) 3.42 ms, and a field of view (FOV) of 256 × 256 mm. The anatomical sequence comprised 176 slices, a flip angle of 7° and an inversion time of 1,100 ms.

MRI Data Analysis

Brain image processing was conducted using BrainVoyager QX software (version 2.8.2), which allows largely automatically cortex segmentation through the application of a set of advanced tools, and reliable cortical thickness measurements resorting to the second-order partial differential Laplace's equation. To each anatomic data set, the following pre-processing steps were executed in all subjects: a bias-field mask (Dale et al., 1999) was applied in order to diminish the intensity variations caused by magnetic field and RF-field inhomogeneities, before the inhomogeneity correction a mask was applied to extract the skull and remove the extra-cerebral voxels (Goebel et al., 2006). The two structural data acquisitions of each subject were then averaged, to increase the signal-to-noise ratio, re-oriented into the AC-PC plane and then transformed into the Talairach reference system. Later on, the anatomical data were submitted through the advanced automatic segmentation routines for later cortical thickness measures. Simultaneously, the same anatomical volumes were segmented using automatic routines (Kriegeskorte and Goebel, 2001) to create surface representations (meshes) of each hemisphere for further measurements on surface space.

Cortical Thickness Assessment

Cortical thickness measurements were obtained using the BrainVoyager software pipeline, which starts with the automatic cortex segmentation in volume space of white matter-gray matter (WM-GM) and gray matter-cerebrospinal fluid (GM-CSF) boundaries. In a preliminary stage, the anatomical images were transformed to 0.5 × 0.5 × 0.5 mm iso-voxels using sync interpolation. Thereon, the ventricles and subcortical structures were masked and, as the final preparatory step, a sigma filter was used to enhance the contrast between the GM and WM tissue types.

Thereafter, an adaptive region growing step relying on locally computed intensity histograms and gradient information was used to split white from gray matter voxels. The resulting noisy WM-GM border was smoothed by computing a magnitude map build upon computed gradient maps of the binary segmentation outcomes. After that, a dilatation process starting at the WM-GM border enabled the CM-CSF border segmentation.

At the end of the automatic segmentation process, a dataset consisting of two intensity values was obtained, one representing the WM and the other the GM. This dataset was then used for the cortical thickness measurements. The software uses an automatic algorithm that applies the second-order partial differential Laplace's equation, as described in Jones et al. (2000). After the thickness calculation, a cortical thickness map was shown overlaying on the volumetric data set (VMR).

Since we aimed to compare the thickness values from a specific area, the primary visual area BA17, between all subjects and examine aging effects, it was necessary to guarantee an exact correspondence of this area among the different participants. Since the Talairach normalization produces only a rough alignment between subject's cortices, the subsequent analyses were conducted in the surface space (previously created cortical meshes) in order to benefit from the cortex-based alignment (CBA), as described in Geuze et al. (2008), of the different subject's brains.

Thus, after the cortical measurements in volume space, the volumetric maps were interpolated to the individual cortex meshes that resulted from a former CBA, creating the subsequent surface cortical maps (SMPs). After the SMPs were made to all subjects, they were provided to the software along with a Patch-Of-Interest (POI) file containing the BA17 surface patch (**Figure 1**), and the information describing the alignment of the individual cortex to the target cortex. Additionally, we have also measured the thickness values from frontal, temporal and parietal lobes following the same methodology. Thus, we provided to the software the POIs files containing the frontal, temporal and parietal anatomically delineated regions (BV mask) along with the information describing the alignment of the individual cortex to the target cortex, for thickness measurements inside these regions.

Afterward, the thickness values averaged over all POIs vertices for each subject were calculated for the right and left hemisphere

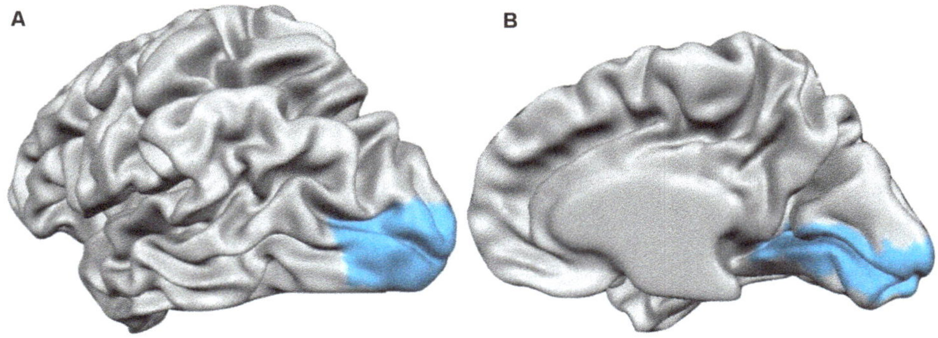

FIGURE 1 | Cortex surface view of the anatomically outlined BA17 used to measure the cortical thickness [**(A)** left hemisphere **(B)** right hemisphere].

individually, and exported for further statistical analyses on SPSS software.

Retinal Thickness Assessment

For each participant's eye, the OCT acquisition went through an automatic segmentation routine resorting to the *Iowa Reference Algorithms* (Retinal Image Analysis Lab, Iowa Institute for Biomedical Imaging, Iowa City, IA, USA; Li et al., 2006; Garvin et al., 2009; Abràmoff et al., 2010) that allows significantly accurate segmentation up to 10 retinal layers.

From each macular volume, 11 surfaces, outlining the 10 retinal layers, were automatically segmented by the algorithm mentioned above. Consequently, the layers investigated in this study were: RNFL; GCL; IPL; INL; outer plexiform layer (OPL); outer nuclear layer (ONL); inner segment/outer segment junction (IS/OS); outer segment (OS); outer segment photoreceptor/RPE complex (OPR), retinal pigment epithelium (RPE), see **Figure 2**. All B-scans and surface layers were visually assessed, and manual corrections on the segmentation were introduced wherever required. The thickness of each layer was computed as the distance (in voxels) between the two surfaces delimiting the layer, multiplied by the voxel size in that direction. This value was provided by the segmentation software based on the number of voxels and imaging depth.

The thickness of the all lamina (global retinal thickness), as well as of each macular layer, were calculated as the average from the complete macular area.

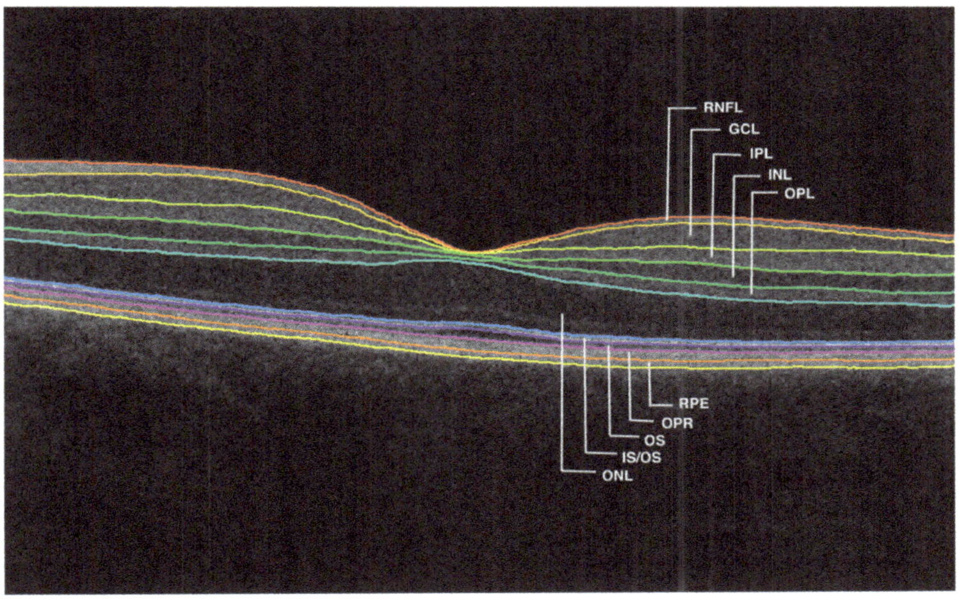

FIGURE 2 | Segmented retinal layers: retinal nerve fiber layer (RNFL); ganglion cell layer (GCL); inner plexiform layer (IPL); inner nuclear layer (INL); outer plexiform layer (OPL); outer nuclear layer (ONL); inner segment/outer segment junction (IS/OS); outer segment (OS); outer segment photoreceptor/RPE complex (OPR); retinal pigment epithelium (RPE).

Statistical Analyses

Overall, 56 subjects were considered for cortical thickness analysis and only 52 were considered for the retinal thickness analysis (four OCT acquisitions were excluded due to acquisition problems). Brain/retina correlation analyses were consequently limited to 52 cases.

The mean cortical thickness values of BA17, frontal, temporal and parietal regions were obtained for each participant calculated as the average of all vertices inside these regions, and a mean value from both hemispheres was calculated for each participant.

Concerning the retina, the mean thickness value was calculated for each retinal layer and all lamina (global retinal thickness), by averaging the values from both eyes to each individual.

Pearson correlation coefficients were computed between age and thickness measurements to investigate the relationship of both structures with age, as well as between BA17 and all lamina thicknesses to study the interplay between both. Additionally, a multivariate ANOVA (MANOVA) analysis including the 10 segmented layers followed by *post hoc* univariate analysis was performed to study the individual behavior of each layer with age.

Thereafter, a multiple regression analysis was run to inspect whether retina integrity indices and age can predict cortical integrity, to further assess the relationship between the retina and cortex integrity.

In a final analysis, we also searched for associations between other cerebral areas—frontal, temporal and parietal areas—and retina.

Data analysis was conducted in IBM SPSS Statistics (version 22.0), and for graphs, GraphPad Prism (version 6.0) was used. The tests were performed two-tailed and $p < 0.05$ was used as a threshold for statistical significance.

RESULTS

For the cortical measurements, 56 subjects were considered, gender-balanced, with age ranging from 23 and 79 years, and average ± standard deviation (SD) of 47.03 ± 16.89 years (see **Table 1**).

Regarding the macular measurements, 52 subjects were considered, also gender-balanced, with age ranging from 23 to 79 years, as above, and average ± SD of 46.77 ± 17.27 years.

The subject's average ± SD of BA17 cortical thickness was 2.337 ± 0.246 mm. The corresponding regression plot is depicted in **Figure 3**. Simultaneously the correlation test demonstrated a strong negative statistically significant correlation between age and BA17 average cortical thickness ($r = -0.724$, $p < 0.0001$), showing that the primary visual cortex becomes significantly thinner as people get older (about 106 μm per decade, based on the regression equation).

TABLE 1 | Age distribution of the participants included in the study and the number of smokers by group of ages.

Age range	Participants (n = 56)	Light Smokers
20–29	11	3
30–39	9	1
40–49	10	2
50–59	10	3
60–69	10	0
70–79	6	0

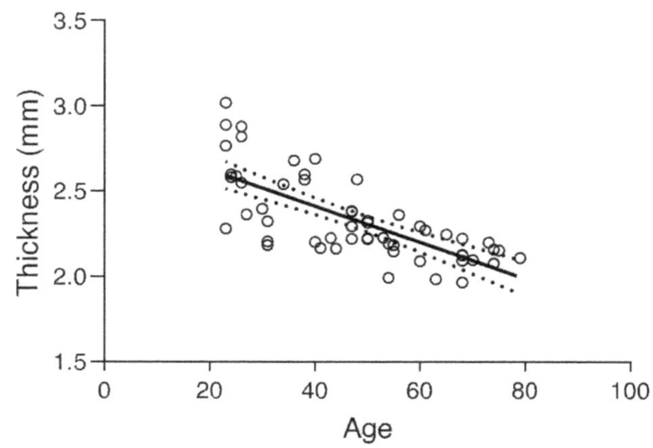

FIGURE 3 | Regression plot of the BA17 thickness vs. age and 95% confidence of the regression slope ($Y = -0.01062 \times X + 2.836$; $r = -0.724$; $p < 0.0001$).

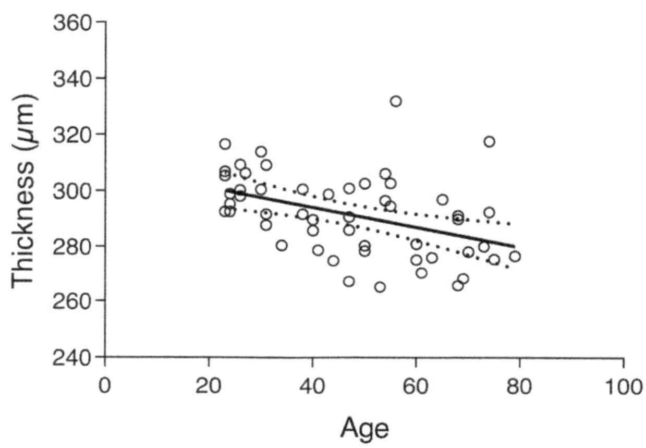

FIGURE 4 | Regression plot of the total retinal thickness vs. age and 95% confidence of the regression slop ($Y = -0.3566 \times X + 308.3$; $r = -0.4186$; $p < 0.0020$).

The subject's global thickness average was 291.6 ± 14.71 μm. A similar finding as above was found between the global thickness and age since the correlation test shows a statistically significant negative association between the two variables ($r = -0.4186, p < 0.0020$). The correspondent regression plot can be seen in **Figure 4**. The decrease of macular thickness with age is 3.6 μm per decade.

To investigate general and specific effects at the retinal level, we have computed a multivariate ANOVA (MANOVA), using age as a predictor and the individual layers as dependent variables. Overall we found that age significantly predicts the macular thickness, Pillai's Trace = 0.456, $F_{(10,41)} = 3.44, p = 0.002$. *Post hoc* analysis showed that GCL: $F_{(1)}$ = 9.483, p = 0.003;

IPL: $F_{(1)} = 8.453$, $p = 0.005$; INL: $F_{(1)} = 9.218$, $p = 0.004$; ONL: $F_{(1)} = 7.813$, $p = 0.007$; OS: $F_{(1)} = 8.970$, $p < 0.004$ and OPR: $F_{(1)} = 14.54$, $p < 0.001$ were significantly predicted by age.

Plots in **Figure 5**, along with results from the multivariate analysis, show that the thickness of the GCL, IPL, INL, ONL, and OPR layers decreased with age, whereas the thickness of OS layer increased. The RNFL, OPL, IS/OS, and RPE layers, on its turn, showed no significant alterations with age.

The results from the correlation tests performed to measure the association between cortical and retinal thickness showed a positive association between BA17 and the overall thickness of all lamina ($r = 0.277$, $p < 0.047$). The respective regression plot is presented in **Figure 6**, showing that the primary visual cortex is positively associated with macular thickness; a decrease of macular thickness is significantly associated with a decrease in BA17 thickness (about 0.0047 mm per unit of macular thickness change, according to the regression equation).

Considering the association between global macular thickness and BA17, we have posteriorly run a multiple linear regression analysis to verify whether age and all lamina thickness are potentially predictive of BA17's thickness. These variables statistically significantly predicted BA17, $F_{(2,49)} = 27.018$, $p < 0.0001$, $R^2 = 0.52$. Age was the only variable that contributed significantly to the prediction ($\beta = -0.737$, $p < 0.0001$) Thus, when adjusting for age we can see that the relation between cortex and retina is disrupted. Therefore, we can conclude that age is the main responsible for the association between the two structures.

Considering the emerging literature relating GC-IPL to putative cortical integrity we have also computed the correlation with GC-IPL and results show a significant positive correlation between both ($r = 0.300$, $p < 0.030$).

We have further computed a multiple linear regression, using all the individual layers and age as predictors for BA17 integrity.

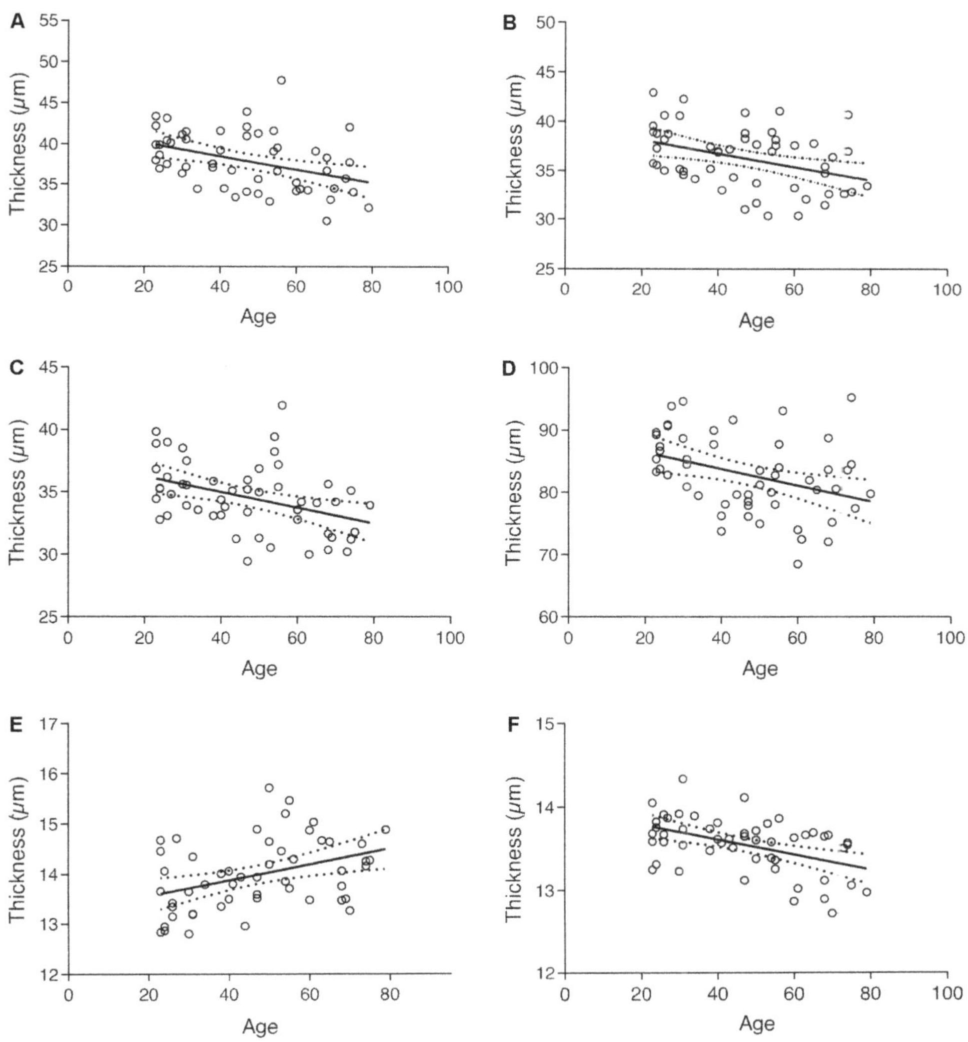

FIGURE 5 | Regression plot of **(A)** GCL; **(B)** IPL; **(C)** INL; **(D)** ONL; **(E)** OS and **(F)** OPR thickness vs. age and 95% confidence intervals for the regression line.

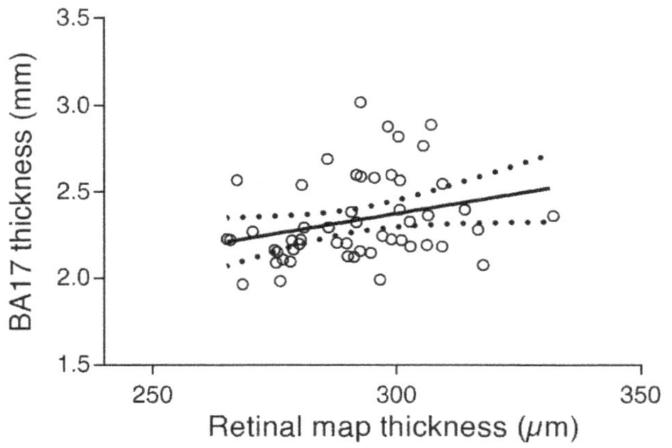

FIGURE 6 | Regression plot of the BA17 thickness vs. all lamina macular thickness and 95% confidence of the regression slope ($Y = 0.004687 \times X + 0.9676$; $r = 0.277$; $p < 0.047$).

The results have shown that these variables statistically significantly predicted the interaction between age and BA17 $F_{(11,40)} = 6.438$, $p < 0.0001$, $R^2 = 0.6391$. We found that OPR ($\beta = -0.272, p < 0.05$) and age ($\beta = -0.895, p < 0.0001$) were the only variables that significantly interact to explain the variance of BA17 thickness. Thus, we can conclude that age *per se* is the main responsible for the interplay between cortex and retina.

In addition, correlations between other cortical regions and retina showed a significant association between frontal ($r = 0.351$, $p = 0.011$), parietal ($r = 0.350, p = 0.011$) and temporal ($r = 0.335$, $p = 0.015$) lobes. Therefore, this link between brain and retina might not be limited to the occipital region, suggesting that retinal thickness may be indicative or an accessible read-out of cortical structure in general.

DISCUSSION

This study is, to the best of our knowledge, the first that attempted to evaluate, in the same sample of healthy individuals, structural changes in both cortex and retina as a function of age in anatomically defined primary visual cortex (BA17) and in 10 different macular layers, and its associations. Our results provide evidence of a positive relationship between the thicknesses of these structures and a concomitant negative correlation with age. While it is in general well accepted that a heterogeneous global age-related loss of cortical tissue occurs, results across studies regarding the primary visual cortex have been inconsistent. Nonetheless, several groups have indeed reported a decrease in gray matter thickness of this region, as we found in the present study. For instance Salat et al. (2004), Fjell et al. (2009), Ziegler et al. (2010) and McGinnis et al. (2011), who performed whole-brain approaches measures, that model the impact of aging at each surface vertex, found evidence of an age-related decline in primary visual cortex thickness. Brewer and Barton (2016) found that healthy aging subjects do have the reduced surface area and increased pRF sizes in the foveal representations (0° to 3° eccentricity) of V1 (primary visual cortex) as compared with healthy young control subjects. Moreover, Sowell et al. (2003) suggested that occipital cortex surrounding the calcarine sulcus exhibits a linear pattern of gray matter density loss with age.

It is worth to mention that our results are not consistent with some whole-brain studies suggesting a certain sparing of the occipital cortex during the aging process when compared to parietal-temporal regions (Thambisetty et al., 2010) since we found evident atrophy of BA17 across age. However, our results might be explained by the fact that we have conducted a region-based analysis in a relatively large sample.

On its turn, Lemaitre et al. (2012) in a whole-brain approach did not find significant age-related reduction in volume, thickness or surface area in the occipital cortex. They pointed out as a possible explanation for their results, the fact of their sample had only 17% of individuals with age above 60 years, and they hypothesized that it is above that age that this area possible suffers a more significant reduction. In fact, McGinnis et al. (2011) found that thinning in the primary visual cortex was highest in their older sample. Raz et al. (2004), who traced ROIs manually, did not find age-related differences in the volume of this region. Likewise, Crossland et al. (2008) found no changes in the overall size of V1.

Despite the incongruities in the existing literature, overall, our data corroborate the notion that this visual area does become thinner with advancing aging. Nevertheless, such discrepancies between studies could derive from differences in analytic techniques, where measures of cortical thickness and volume are detecting different degenerative processes with distinct sensitivity (Ziegler et al., 2010), differences in the population characteristics (Lemaitre et al., 2012), or in the way that this region is defined (Griffis et al., 2016). In the present study, and in addition to a well-distributed sample across ages, we resorted to surface-based thickness tools, known to be more sensitive for the detection of age-related morphological decline (Hutton et al., 2009).

Concerning the retina, during lifetime the macula undergoes significant degenerative changes, causing visual decline and often visual loss. In a healthy population, our data revealed a significant decrease in the total macular thickness with increasing age. Overall, there is a broad consensus about retinal loss with age (Alamouti and Funk, 2003; Eriksson and Alm, 2009; Sung et al., 2009; Casaletto et al., 2017), possibly resulting from the loss of retinal cells such as bipolar, ganglion cells, as well as photoreceptor cells (Gao and Hollyfield, 1992; Curcio et al., 1993; Harman et al., 2000; Aggarwal et al., 2007). Moreover, vascular compartments may also decrease over time (Klein, 2006; Sun et al., 2008).

Imaging studies with the segmentation of retinal layers are scarce. To the best of our knowledge, this is the first study to differentiate the retina in 10 distinct layers addressing the effect of aging on thickness. In the previous study of Won et al. (2016) (only addressing the retina and not the cortex), nine retinal layers were individualized using the same algorithm as ours.

Our measurement outcomes revealed that while some layers remained stable with age (RNFL, OPL, IS/OS, and RPE), others decreased (GCL, IPL, INL, ONL, and OPR), and only one of them appeared to be increased in terms of thickness (OS). In particular, our results demonstrated a GCL age-related thinning, similarly to other findings (Ooto et al., 2011; Demirkaya et al., 2013; Won et al., 2016). In fact, this layer seems to be one of the most prone to be affected by aging mechanisms, being in agreement a significant decline of the number of ganglion cells across age (Balazsi et al., 1984; Gao and Hollyfield, 1992; Harman et al., 2000; Kerrigan-Baumrind et al., 2000; Nag and Wadhwa, 2012).

We also found evidence of IPL and INL reduction being in accordance with previous studies (Ooto et al., 2011; Demirkaya et al., 2013; Won et al., 2016). Evidence about how INL cells change with age and respond to different pathological conditions is scarce (Nag and Wadhwa, 2012). This decrease could, however, result from the loss of some neurons or glial cells, as it is known to occur with bipolar cells (Aggarwal et al., 2007). Regarding IPL, since it comprises synapses between the amacrine and bipolar cells with ganglion cells dendrites, it seems feasible that the shrinkage of this layer could be attributed to a loss of both bipolar and ganglion synapses. The studies of Demirkaya et al. (2013) and Ooto et al. (2011) also found an age-related decrease of this layer across age.

Likewise, ONL and OPR showed to be affected negatively by aging. Gartner and Henkind (1981) were the first to report a thinning of the ONL with aging, as a result of photoreceptor loss. Subsequent studies have shown substantial loss of rods, but not cones, from the periphery (Gao and Hollyfield, 1992) and macula with aging (Curcio et al., 1993; Jackson et al., 2002). This age-related photoreceptor loss might also contribute to the OPR thinning, as found in the current study.

Conversely, RNFL, OPL, IS/OS, and RPE did not show differences with our morphologic metrics with increasing age. Despite the considerable evidence pointing out to a decrease in retinal neuron fibers, resulting from ganglion cell loss (Balazsi et al., 1984; Harman et al., 2000; Kerrigan-Baumrind et al., 2000; Nag and Wadhwa, 2012), the majority of the studies have focused on peripapillary measures, around the optic disk, rather than on macular RNFL (Alamouti and Funk, 2003; Eriksson and Alm, 2009; Sung et al., 2009). For instance, Demirkaya et al. (2013) indeed found a thinning in peripapillary RNFL, but their results did not reveal a significant decrease in the whole macular RNFL thickness. Instead, a slight increase was verified in the pericentral ring. Won et al. (2016), in turn, when comparing a young group with an older one, found a significantly lower thickness and volume in the RNFL peripheral region in the latter. Also, Neuville et al. (2009) have reported only an age-related decreasing of this layer thickness in the more peripheral nasal region. Thus, one might assume that an age-related decrease probably occurs, however just detectable in regions where the axons are denser, yet when the full thickness is analyzed this subtle effect might become undetected.

The fact that may explain the consistently reported decrease of axons in the region of the optic disc is that it corresponds to the region where axons of the GCL converge, including those from the extramacular area. As such, it is not surprising that this region presents a higher GCL decrease (Harman et al., 2000) compared with the macular area. Nonetheless, Ooto et al. (2011) found a significant decrease in the RNFL thickness in the macula.

Concerning the OPL, our results are in line with the works of Ooto et al. (2011), Demirkaya et al. (2013), and Won et al. (2016), who studied the same layer in their sample. With regard to the RPE, it undergoes considerable changes through age, including loss of melanin granules, accumulation of lipofuscin, basal deposits, and thickened Bruch's membrane (Bonilha, 2008). As a result, there are claims that the RPE thickens with age, at least in its central area (Staurenghi et al., 2014). However, and in accordance with Demirkaya et al.'s (2013) and Won et al.'s (2016) results, we did not find an increase in the total macular RPE thickness although we do find the change mentioned above in the OS, which is tightly related with age-related changes in RPE. Thus, it seems likely that the thickness of this layer might increase with age only in specific sub-regions, namely in the more central macula. For example, Demirkaya et al.'s (2013) results show that as a whole the RPE thickness did not change, but increased significantly in the foveal region. Besides, there are arguments about a reduction in the number of pigment epithelium cells (Gao and Hollyfield, 1992; Watzke et al., 1993; Panda-Jonas et al., 1996), which might balance the cell deposits, perhaps explaining the absence of structural changes in our results. Similarly, Won et al. (2016) did not find differences between groups (younger and adults) in the RPE in any of the regions analyzed.

Results pertaining to the only macular layer that revealed increased with age, that is, the OS, are in agreement with Ooto et al. (2011). One should note, however, that their OS definition also included the RPE, precluding direct comparisons. These structures show an intimate functional relationship. Moreover, segmentation beyond the ONL, in the outer macula, has been more uneven across studies. The OS is known to be the locus of high membrane turnover with the accumulation of its products as aging progress, which might explain its increases with age. Thus, we do believe that a higher OS thickness could derive from the excessive metabolic strain that accumulates with aging. In fact, the RPE is responsible for the OS phagocytosis (Hogan et al., 1974; Anderson et al., 1978; Bok, 1985; Holtkamp et al., 2001; Strauss, 2005), a process that is known to deteriorate with age (Dorey et al., 1989; Bonnel et al., 2003).

In convergence with the concept that the primary visual cortex goes through considerable modifications in response to retinal changes, in the current work, we were able to show that aging *per se* is associated with such effect. When a multivariate analysis was carried out, our results showed that apparently, OPR is the only layer that explains the variance of BA17 thickness through an interaction term, e.g., changes are not solely justified by age. The atrophy of both structures might account for the decline of various visual capacities that accompany the aging process. For instance,

Weale (1975, 1978, 1982) suggested that the decline in acuity results from a random loss of neurons in the retina or in central visual pathways. In turn, Brewer and Barton (2016) suggest that the functionally detected alterations in PRF's and visual field maps as well as surface reduction in foveal V1 might account for the age-related alterations in vision such as reduced visual acuity and decreased contrast sensitivity at medium and high spatial frequencies.

In fact, normal aging leads to a decline of several visual abilities that cannot be attributed only to optical changes, and also derive from neuronal changes in the retina and/or brain (Elliott, 1987; Whitaker and Elliott, 1992; Spear, 1993). Nevertheless, the relative roles of each one are still unclear. For example, while some researchers have suggested that the decline in spatial-frequency contrast sensitivity is due to retinal changes (Sloane et al., 1988), others have related it to cortical mechanisms (Crassini et al., 1988). Thus, our results shed some light on this issue, since they demonstrate that there are morphologic changes in both structures, which probably account for the loss of visual functions that have been repeatedly reported by psychophysical studies studying a broad range of visual channels (Mateus et al., 2013; Silva et al., 2014). Such age-related changes in healthy population are of critical importance to understand the ones emerging in pathological neurodegeneration (Silva et al., 2005; Castelo-Branco et al., 2009; Lemos et al., 2012, 2016; Graewe et al., 2013), including regions beyond visual areas, as demonstrated here.

Despite the focus of the present work on studying the impact of age in the visual system, by assessing the structural integrity of both retina and primary visual cortex (the cortical area that receives direct projections from the retina) and their relationship, other regions were also investigated. We have therefore additionally searched for associations between the retina and other cortical regions—frontal, parietal and temporal lobes.

In fact, recent reports have suggested that retina is an approachable window to neurodegenerative diseases (Yu et al., 2014; Thomson et al., 2015; den Haan et al., 2018) and in healthy brain aging (Liu et al., 2016; Casaletto et al., 2017). Accordingly, we identified that associations between retina and brain exist beyond the visual areas. This finding suggests that the retina indexes cerebral cortical changes irrespective of retinocortical connectivity. Brain and retina, since their similarities, might share the same neurodegenerative mechanisms that occur in parallel across the lifetime.

Other studies had also searched for associations between the retina and cortical integrity in healthy individuals. For instance, Casaletto et al. (2017) in neurologically normal older adults, have found evidence of an association between medial temporal lobe volume (encompassing bilateral entorhinal, parahippocampal, and hippocampal volumes) with peripapillary RNFL thickness, macular volume, and macular ganglion cell volumes, while associations between other regions such as parietal-temporal regions, precuneus or basal ganglia were not found.

Liu et al. (2016), in a whole-brain approach, searched for associations between GCL-IPL and whole cortex white matter (WM) integrity as well as gray matter volumes (GMV) in three distinct groups of participants, a group of healthy individuals, a group of mild cognitive impairment subjects and other of AD patients. For subjects with no cognitive impairment (healthy aging), they found that a GC-IPL loss of integrity was related to a lower WM microstructure integrity in several regions as for example in frontal, parietal, and cingulum regions, and was weakly associated with GMV reduction in occipital lobe and cerebellum. Interestingly, this association was lost in the other two groups.

In addition, in a recent study, an association between a decrease in GC-IPL thickness and a decrease in GMV of the occipital and temporal lobes was found in an elderly heterogeneous sample composed by three demented subjects, 36 with no cognitive impairment (healthy subjects) and 125 with cognitive impairment (Ong et al., 2015). On its turn, den Haan et al. (2018) found a significant correlation between retinal thickness and cortical parietal atrophy in healthy controls and a cohort of AD patients, suggesting an association between the two structures that is independent of amyloid.

CONCLUSION

The present study enables a better understanding of how the visual system ages, by providing concomitant measurements of neuroretinal layers and cortical thickness. We provide evidence suggesting that the primary visual cortex suffers an age-related loss that leads to its shrinkage, a finding that it is not consensual yet and is highly debated. Second, we demonstrate how 10 different individual layers anatomically change with increasing aging and identify novel and distinct patterns of change in different layers. Finally, associations between brain and retina were found beyond visual cortices (frontal, parietal and temporal regions), suggesting that retinal health may indeed be a potential read-out of cortical structure in general.

AUTHOR CONTRIBUTIONS

LJ designed the study, performed data acquisition and analysis and wrote the article. NC performed data acquisition and analysis and revised the article. HQ performed data acquisition and analysis. RB performed data acquisition and analysis. MC-B designed the study, performed data analysis and wrote the article.

REFERENCES

Abràmoff, M. D., Garvin, M. K., and Sonka, M. (2010). Retinal imaging and image analysis. *IEEE Rev. Biomed. Eng.* 3, 169–208. doi: 10.1109/RBME.2010.2084567

Aggarwal, P., Nag, T. C., and Wadhwa, S. (2007). Age-related decrease in rod bipolar cell density of the human retina: an immunohistochemical study. *J. Biosci.* 32, 293–298. doi: 10.1007/s12038-007-0029-9

Alamouti, B., and Funk, J. (2003). Retinal thickness decreases with age: an OCT study. *Br. J. Ophthalmol.* 87, 899–901. doi: 10.1136/bjo.87.7.899

Allen, J. S., Bruss, J., Brown, C. K., and Damasio, H. (2005). Normal neuroanatomical variation due to age: the major lobes and a parcellation of the temporal region. *Neurobiol. Aging* 26, 1245–1260. doi: 10.1016/j.neurobiolaging.2005.05.023

Alves, C., Batista, S., d'Almeida, O. C., Sousa, L., Cunha, L., Bernardes, R., et al. (2018). The retinal ganglion cell layer predicts normal-appearing white matter tract integrity in multiple sclerosis: a combined diffusion tensor imaging and optical coherence tomography approach. *Hum. Brain Mapp.* 39, 1712–1720. doi: 10.1002/hbm.23946

Anderson, D. H., Fisher, S. K., and Steinberg, R. H. (1978). Mammalian cones: disc shedding, phagocytosis, and renewal. *Invest. Ophthalmol. Vis. Sci.* 17, 117–133.

Balazsi, A. G., Rootman, J., Drance, S. M., Schulzer, M., and Douglas, G. R. (1984). The effect of age on the nerve fiber population of the human optic nerve. *Am. J. Ophthalmol.* 97, 760–766. doi: 10.1016/0002-9394(84)90509-9

Barcella, V., Rocca, M. A., Bianchi-Marzoli, S., Milesi, J., Melzi, L., Falini, A., et al. (2010). Evidence for retrochiasmatic tissue loss in Leber's hereditary optic neuropathy. *Hum. Brain Mapp.* 31, 1900–1906. doi: 10.1002/hbm.20985

Bok, D. (1985). Retinal photorecepfor-pigment epithelium interactions. *Invest. Ophthalmol. Vis. Sci.* 26, 1659–1694.

Bonilha, V. L. (2008). Age and disease-related structural changes in the retinal pigment epithelium. *Clin. Ophthalmol.* 2, 413–424. doi: 10.2147/opth.s2151

Bonnel, S., Mohand-Said, S., and Sahel, J. A. (2003). The aging of the retina. *Exp. Gerontol.* 38, 825–831. doi: 10.1016/s0531-5565(03)00093-7

Brewer, A. A., and Barton, B. (2016). Effects of healthy aging on human primary visual cortex. *Health* 4, 695–702. doi: 10.4236/health.2012.429109

Burge, W. K., Griffis, J. C., Nenert, R., Elkhetali, A., DeCarlo, D. K., ver Hoef, L. W., et al. (2016). Cortical thickness in human V1 associated with central vision loss. *Sci. Rep.* 6:23268. doi: 10.1038/srep23268

Casaletto, K. B., Ward, M. E., Baker, N. S., Bettcher, B. M., Gelfand, J. M., Li, Y., et al. (2017). Retinal thinning is uniquely associated with medial temporal lobe atrophy in neurologically normal older adults. *Neurobiol. Aging* 51, 141–147. doi: 10.1016/j.neurobiolaging.2016.12.011

Castelo-Branco, M., Mendes, M., Silva, F., Massano, J., Januário, G., Januário, C., et al. (2009). Motion integration deficits are independent of magnocellular impairment in Parkinson's disease. *Neuropsychologia* 47, 314–320. doi: 10.1016/j.neuropsychologia.2008.09.003

Courchesne, E., Chisum, H. J., Townsend, J., Cowles, A., Covington, J., Egaas, B., et al. (2000). Normal brain development and aging: quantitative analysis at *in vivo* MR imaging in healthy volunteers. *Radiology* 216, 672–682. doi: 10.1148/radiology.216.3.r00au37672

Crassini, B., Brown, B., and Bowman, K. (1988). Age-related changes in contrast sensitivity in central and peripheral retina. *Perception* 17, 315–332. doi: 10.1068/p170315

Crossland, M. D., Morland, A. B., Feely, M. P., von dem Hagen, E., and Rubin, G. S. (2008). The effect of age and fixation instability on retinotopic mapping of primary visual cortex. *Invest. Ophthalmol. Vis. Sci.* 49, 3734–3739. doi: 10.1167/iovs.07-1621

Curcio, C. A., Millican, C. L., Allen, K. A., and Kalina, R. E. (1993). Aging of the human photoreceptor mosaic: evidence for selective vulnerability of rods in central retina. *Invest. Ophthalmol. Vis. Sci.* 34, 3278–3296.

d'Almeida, O. C., Mateus, C., Reis, A., Grazina, M. M., and Castelo-Branco, M. (2013). Long term cortical plasticity in visual retinotopic areas in humans with silent retinal ganglion cell loss. *Neuroimage* 81, 222–230. doi: 10.1016/j.neuroimage.2013.05.032

Dale, A. M., Fischl, B., and Sereno, M. I. (1999). Cortical surface-based analysis I. Segmentation and surface reconstruction. *Neuroimage* 9, 179–194. doi: 10.1006/nimg.1998.0395

Demirkaya, N., van Dijk, H. W., van Schuppen, S. M., Abràmoff, M. D., Garvin, M. K., Sonka, M., et al. (2013) Effect of age on individual retinal layer thickness in normal eyes as measured with spectral-domain optical coherence tomography. *Invest. Ophthalmol. Vis. Sci.* 54, 4934–4940. doi: 10.1167/iovs.13-11913

den Haan, J., Janssen, S. F., van de Kreeke, J. A., Scheltens, P., Verbraak, F. D., and Bouwman, F. H. (2018). Retinal thickness correlates with parietal cortical atrophy in early-onset alzheimer's disease and controls. *Alzheimers Dement.* 10, 49–55. doi: 10.1016/j.dadm.2017.10.005

Dolman, C. L., McCormick, A. Q., and Drance, S. M. (1980). Aging of the optic nerve. *Arch. Ophthalmol.* 98, 2053–2058. doi: 10.1001/archopht.1980.01020040905024

Dorey, K., Wu, G., Ebensrein, D., Garsd, A., and Weiter, J. J. (1989). Cell loss in the aging retina. Relationship to lipofuscin accumulation and macular degeneration. *Invest. Ophthalmol. Vis. Sci.* 30, 1691–1699.

Elliott, D. B. (1987). Contrast sensitivity decline with ageing: a neural or optical phenomenon? *Ophthalmic Physiol. Opt.* 7, 415–419. doi: 10.1016/0275-5408(87)90065-2

Eriksson, U., and Alm, A. (2009). Macular thickness decreases with age in normal eyes: a study on the macular thickness map protocol in the Stratus OCT. *Br. J. Ophthalmol.* 93, 1448–1452. doi: 10.1136/bjo.2007.131094

Ferreira, S., Pereira, A. C., Quendera, B., Reis, A., Silva, E. D., and Castelo-Branco, M. (2017). Primary visual cortical remapping in patients with inherited peripheral retinal degeneration. *Neuroimage Clin.* 13, 428–438. doi: 10.1016/j.nicl.2016.12.013

Fjell, A. M., Westlye, L. T., Amlien, I., Espeseth, T., Reinvang, I., Raz, N., et al. (2009). High consistency of regional cortical thinning in aging across multiple samples. *Cereb. Cortex* 19, 2001–2012. doi: 10.1093/cercor/bhn232

Freitas, S., Simões, M. R., Alves, L., and Santana, I. (2011). Montreal cognitive assessment (MoCA): normative study for the Portuguese population. *J. Clin. Exp. Neuropsychol.* 33, 989–996. doi: 10.1080/13803395.2011.589374

Gao, H., and Hollyfield, J. G. (1992). Aging of the human retina. Differential loss of neurons and retinal pigment epithelial cells. *Invest. Ophthalmol. Vis. Sci.* 33, 1–17.

Gartner, S., and Henkind, P. (1981). Aging and degeneration of the human macula. 1. Outer nuclear layer and photoreceptors. *Br. J. Ophthalmol.* 65, 23–28. doi: 10.1136/bjo.65.1.23

Garvin, M. K., Abràmoff, M. D., Wu, X., Russell, S. R., Burns, T. L., and Sonka, M. (2009). Automated 3-D intraretinal layer segmentation of macular spectral-domain optical coherence tomography images. *IEEE Trans. Med. Imaging* 28, 1436–1447. doi: 10.1109/tmi.2009.2016958

Geuze, E., Westenberg, H. G. M., Heinecke, A., De Kloet, C. S., Goebel, R., and Vermetten, E. (2008). Thinner prefrontal cortex in veterans with posttraumatic stress disorder. *Neuroimage* 41, 675–681. doi: 10.1016/j.neuroimage.2008.03.007

Goebel, R., Esposito, F., and Formisano, E. (2006). Analysis of functional image analysis contest (FIAC) data with brainvoyager QX: from single-subject to cortically aligned group general linear model analysis and self-organizing group independent component analysis. *Hum. Brain Mapp.* 27, 392–401. doi: 10.1002/hbm.20249

Good, C. D., Johnsrude, I. S., Ashburner, J., Henson, R. N. A., Friston, K. J., and Frackowiak, R. S. J. (2001). A voxel-based morphometric study of ageing in 465 normal adult human brains. *Neuroimage* 14, 21–36. doi: 10.1006/nimg.2001.0786

Graewe, B., Lemos, R., Ferreira, C., Santana, I., Farivar, R., De Weerd, P., et al. (2013). Impaired processing of 3D motion-defined faces in mild cognitive impairment and healthy aging: an fMRI study. *Cereb. Cortex* 23, 2489–2499. doi: 10.1093/cercor/bhs246

Grieve, S. M., Clark, C. R., Williams, L. M., Peduto, A. J., and Gordon, E. (2005). Preservation of limbic and paralimbic structures in aging. *Hum. Brain Mapp.* 25, 391–401. doi: 10.1002/hbm.20115

Griffis, J. C., Burge, W. K., and Visscher, K. M. (2016). Age-dependent cortical thinning of peripheral visual field representations in primary visual cortex. *Front. Aging Neurosci.* 8:248. doi: 10.3389/fnagi.2016.00248

Grzybowski, A., and Barboni, P. (2016). "Introduction: retina imaging—past and present," in *OCT in Central Nervous System Diseases*, eds A. Grzybowski and P. Barboni (Cham: Springer), 1–7.

Harman, A., Abrahams, B., Moore, S., and Hoskins, R. (2000). Neuronal density in the human retinal ganglion cell layer from 16–77 years. *Anat. Rec.* 260, 124–131. doi: 10.1002/1097-0185(20001001)260:2<124::AID-AR20>3.0.CO;2-D

Hogan, M. J., Wood, I., and Steiberg, R. H. (1974). Phagocytosis by pigment epithelium of human retinal cones. *Nature* 252, 305–307. doi: 10.1038/252305a0

Holtkamp, G. M., Kijlstra, A., Peek, R., and de Vos, A. F. (2001). Retinal pigment epithelium-immune system interactions: cytokine production and cytokine-induced changes. *Prog. Retin. Eye Res.* 20, 29–48. doi: 10.1016/s1350-9462(00)00017-3

Hutton, C., Draganski, B., Ashburner, J., and Weiskopf, N. (2009). A comparison between voxel-based cortical thickness and voxel-based morphometry in normal aging. *Neuroimage* 48, 371–380. doi: 10.1016/j.neuroimage.2009.06.043

Jackson, G. R., Owsley, C., and Curcio, C. A. (2002). Photoreceptor degeneration and dysfunction in aging and age-related maculopathy. *Ageing Res. Rev.* 1, 381–396. doi: 10.1016/s1568-1637(02)00007-7

Jones, S. E., Buchbinder, B. R., and Aharon, I. (2000). Three-dimensional mapping of cortical thickness using Laplace's equation. *Hum. Brain Mapp.* 11, 12–32. doi: 10.1002/1097-0193(200009)11:1<12::aid-hbm20>3.0.co;2-k

Kerrigan-Baumrind, L. A., Quigley, H. A., Pease, M. E., Kerrigan, D. F., and Mitchell, R. S. (2000). Number of ganglion cells in glaucoma eyes compared with threshold visual field tests in the same persons. *Invest. Ophthalmol. Vis. Sci.* 41, 741–748.

Klein, R. (2006). Are inflammatory factors related to retinal vessel caliber? *Arch. Ophthalmol.* 124, 87–94. doi: 10.1001/archopht.124.1.87

Kriegeskorte, N., and Goebel, R. (2001). An efficient algorithm for topologically correct segmentation of the cortical sheet in anatomical MR volumes. *Neuroimage* 14, 329–346. doi: 10.1006/nimg.2001.0831

Lemaître, H., Crivello, F., Grassiot, B., Alpérovitch, A., Tzourio, C., and Mazoyer, B. (2005). Age-and sex-related effects on the neuroanatomy of healthy elderly. *Neuroimage* 26, 900–911. doi: 10.1016/j.neuroimage.2005.02.042

Lemaitre, H., Goldman, A. L., Sambataro, F., Verchinski, B. A., Meyer-Lindenberg, A., Weinberger, D. R., et al. (2012). Normal age-related brain morphometric changes: nonuniformity across cortical thickness, surface area and gray matter volume? *Neurobiol. Aging* 33, 617.e1–617.e9. doi: 10.1016/j.neurobiolaging.2010.07.013

Lemos, R., Figueiredo, P., Santana, I., Simões, M. R., and Castelo-Branco, M. (2012). Temporal integration of 3D coherent motion cues defining visual objects of unknown orientation is impaired in amnestic mild cognitive impairment and Alzheimer's disease. *J. Alzheimers Dis.* 28, 885–896. doi: 10.3233/jad-2011-110719

Lemos, R., Santana, I., Caetano, G., Bernardino, I., Morais, R., Farivar, R., et al. (2016). Three-dimensional face recognition in mild cognitive impairment: a psychophysical and structural MR study. *J. Int. Neuropsychol. Soc.* 22, 744–754. doi: 10.1017/s135561771600059x

Li, K., Wu, X., Chen, D. Z., and Sonka, M. (2006). Optimal surface segmentation in volumetric images—a graph-theoretic approach. *IEEE Trans. Pattern Anal. Mach. Intell.* 28, 119–134. doi: 10.1109/TPAMI.2006.19

Liu, S., Ong, Y. T., Hilal, S., Loke, Y. M., Wong, T. Y., Chen, C. L. H., et al. (2016). The association between retinal neuronal layer and brain structure is disrupted in patients with cognitive impairment and Alzheimer's disease. *J. Alzheimers Dis.* 54, 585–595. doi: 10.3233/jad-160067

London, A., Benhar, I., and Schwartz, M. (2013). The retina as a window to the brain-from eye research to CNS disorders. *Nat. Rev. Neurol.* 9, 44–53. doi: 10.1038/nrneurol.2012.227

Mateus, C., Lemos, R., Silva, M. F., Reis, A., Fonseca, P., Oliveiros, B., et al. (2013). Aging of low and high level vision: from chromatic and achromatic contrast sensitivity to local and 3D object motion perception. *PLoS One* 8:e55348. doi: 10.1371/journal.pone.0055348

McGinnis, S. M., Brickhouse, M., Pascual, B., and Dickerson, B. C. (2011). Age-Related changes in the thickness of cortical zones in humans. *Brain Topogr.* 24, 279–291. doi: 10.1007/s10548-011-0198-6

Nag, T. C., and Wadhwa, S. (2012). Ultrastructure of the human retina in aging and various pathological states. *Micron* 43, 759–781. doi: 10.1016/j.micron.2012.01.011

Neuville, J. M., Bronson-Castain, K., Bearse, M. A. Jr., Ng, J. S., Harrison, W. W., Schneck, M. E., et al. (2009). Optical coherence tomography reveals regional differences in macular thickness with age. *Optom. Vis. Sci.* 86, E810–E816. doi: 10.1097/OPX.0b013e3181adff59

Ong, Y.-T., Hilal, S., Cheung, C. Y., Venketasubramanian, N., Niessen, W. J., Vrooman, H., et al. (2015). Retinal neurodegeneration on optical coherence tomography and cerebral atrophy. *Neurosci. Lett.* 584, 12–16. doi: 10.1016/j.neulet.2014.10.010

Ooto, S., Hangai, M., Tomidokoro, A., Saito, H., Araie, M., Otani, T., et al. (2011). Effects of age, sex, and axial length on the three-dimensional profile of normal macular layer structures. *Invest. Ophthalmol. Vis. Sci.* 52, 8769–8779. doi: 10.1167/iovs.11-8388

Panda-Jonas, S., Jonas, J. B., and Jakobczyk-Zmija, M. (1996). Retinal pigment epithelial cell count, distribution and correlations in normal human eyes. *Am. J. Ophthalmol.* 121, 181–189. doi: 10.1016/s0002-9394(14)70583-5

Patton, N., Aslam, T., MacGillivray, T., Pattie, A., Deary, I. J., and Dhillon, B. (2005). Retinal vascular image analysis as a potential screening tool for cerebrovascular disease: a rationale based on homology between cerebral and retinal microvasculatures. *J. Anat.* 206, 319–348. doi: 10.1111/j.1469-7580.2005.00395.x

Quigley, H. A., Dunkelberger, G. R., and Green, W. R. (1989). Retinal ganglion cell atrophy correlated with automated perimetry in human eyes with glaucoma. *Am. J. Ophthalmol.* 107, 453–464. doi: 10.1016/0002-9394(89)90488-1

Raz, N., Gunning-Dixon, F., Head, D., Rodrigue, K. M., Williamson, A., and Acker, J. D. (2004). Aging, sexual dimorphism and hemispheric asymmetry of the cerebral cortex: replicability of regional differences in volume. *Neurobiol. Aging* 25, 377–396. doi: 10.1016/s0197-4580(03)00118-0

Raz, N., Lindenberger, U., Rodrigue, K. M., Kennedy, K. M., Head, D., Williamson, A., et al. (2005). Regional brain changes in aging healthy adults: general trends, individual differences and modifiers. *Cereb. Cortex* 15, 1676–1689. doi: 10.1093/cercor/bhi044

Resnick, S. M., Pham, D. L., Kraut, M. A., Zonderman, A. B., and Davatzikos, C. (2003). Longitudinal magnetic resonance imaging studies of older adults: a shrinking brain. *J. Neurosci.* 23, 3295–3301. doi: 10.1523/jneurosci.23-08-03295.2003

Salat, D. H., Buckner, R. L., Snyder, A. Z., Greve, D. N., Desikan, R. S. R., Busa, E., et al. (2004). Thinning of the cerebral cortex in aging. *Cereb. Cortex* 14, 721–730. doi: 10.1093/cercor/bhh032

Satue, M., Obis, J., Rodrigo, M. J., Otin, S., Fuertes, M. I., Vilades, E., et al. (2016). Optical coherence tomography as a biomarker for diagnosis, progression and prognosis of neurodegenerative diseases. *J. Ophthalmol.* 2016:8503859. doi: 10.1155/2016/8503859

Silva, M. F., d'Almeida, O. C., Oliveiros, B., Mateus, C., and Castelo-Branco, M. (2014). Development and aging of visual hemifield asymmetries in contrast sensitivity. *J. Vis.* 14:19. doi: 10.1167/14.12.19

Silva, M. F., Faria, P., Regateiro, F. S., Forjaz, V., Januário, C., Freire, A., et al. (2005). Independent patterns of damage within magno-, parvo- and koniocellular pathways in Parkinson's disease. *Brain* 128, 2260–2271. doi: 10.1093/brain/awh581

Sloane, M. E., Owsley, C., and Jackson, C. A. (1988). Aging and luminance-adaptation effects on spatial contrast sensitivity. *J. Opt. Soc. Am. A* 5, 2181–2190. doi: 10.1364/josaa.5.002181

Song, W. K., Lee, S. C., Lee, E. S., Kim, C. Y., and kim, S. S. (2010). Macular thickness variations with sex, age, and axial length in healthy subjects: a spectral domain-optical coherence tomography study. *Invest. Ophthalmol. Vis. Sci.* 51, 3913–3918. doi: 10.1167/iovs.09-4189

Sowell, E. R., Peterson, B. S., Thompson, P. M., Welcome, S. E., Henkenius, A. L., and Toga, A. W. (2003). Mapping cortical change across the human lifespan. *Nat. Neurosci.* 6, 309–315. doi: 10.1038/nn1008

Spear, P. D. (1993). Neural bases of visual deficits during aging. *Vision Res.* 33, 2589–2609. doi: 10.1016/0042-6989(93)90218-l

Staurenghi, G., Sadda, S., Chakravarthy, U., and Spaide, R. F. (2014). Proposed lexicon for anatomic landmarks in normal posterior segment spectral-domain optical coherence tomography. *Ophthalmology* 121, 1572–1578. doi: 10.1016/j.ophtha.2014.02.023

Strauss, O. (2005). The retinal pigment epithelium in visual function. *Physiol. Rev.* 85, 845–881. doi: 10.1152/physrev.00021.2004

Sun, C., Liew, G., Wang, J. J., Mitchell, P., Saw, S. M., Aung, T., et al. (2008). Retinal vascular caliber, blood pressure and cardiovascular risk factors in an asian population: the Singapore malay eye study. *Invest. Ophthalmol. Vis. Sci.* 49, 1784–1790. doi: 10.1167/iovs.07-1450

Sung, R. K., Wollstein, G., Bilonick, R. A., Townsend, K. A., Ishikawa, H., Kagemann, L., et al. (2009). Effects of age on optical coherence tomography measurements of healthy retinal nerve fiber layer, macula, and optic nerve head. *Ophthalmology* 116, 1119–1124. doi: 10.1016/j.ophtha.2009.01.004

Thambisetty, M., Wan, J., Carass, A., An, Y., Prince, J. L., and Resnick, S. M. (2010). Longitudinal changes in cortical thickness associated with normal aging. *Neuroimage* 52, 1215–1223. doi: 10.1016/j.neuroimage.2010.04.258

Thomson, K. L., Yeo, M., Waddell, B., Cameron, J. R., and Pal, S. (2015). A systematic review and meta-analysis of retinal nerve fiber layer change in dementia, using optical coherence tomography. *Alzheimers Dement.* 1, 136–143. doi: 10.1016/j.dadm.2015.03.001

Watzke, R. C., Soldevilla, J. D., and Trune, D. R. (1993). Morphometric analysis of human retinal pigment epithelium: correlation with age and location. *Curr. Eye Res.* 12, 133–142. doi: 10.3109/02713689308999481

Weale, R. A. (1975). Senile changes in visual acuity. *Trans. Ophthalmol. Soc. U K* 95, 36–38.

Weale, R. A. (1978). The eye and aging. *Interdiscip. Top. Gerontol.* 13, 1–13.

Weale, R. A. (1982). "Senile ocular changes, cell death and vision," in *Aging and Human Visual Function*, eds K. Sekuler, R. Kline and D. Dismukes (New York, NY: Liss), 161–171.

Whitaker, D., and Elliott, D. B. (1992). Simulating age-related optical changes in the human eye. *Doc. Ophthalmol.* 82, 307–316. doi: 10.1007/bf00161018

Won, J. Y., Kim, S. E., and Park, Y.-H. (2016). Effect of age and sex on retinal layer thickness and volume in normal eyes. *Medicine* 95:e5441. doi: 10.1097/md.0000000000005441

Yu, J., Feng, Y., Xiang, Y., Huang, J., Savini, G., Parisi, V., et al. (2014). Retinal nerve fiber layer thickness changes in parkinson disease: a meta-analysis. *PLoS One* 9:e85718. doi: 10.1371/journal.pone.0085718

Ziegler, D. A., Piguet, O., Salat, D. H., Prince, K., Connally, E., and Corkin, S. (2010). Cognition in healthy aging is related to regional white matter integrity, but not cortical thickness. *Neurobiol. Aging* 31, 1912–1926. doi: 10.1016/j.neurobiolaging.2008.10.015

13

Active Ageing in Europe: Adding Healthy Life to Years

Giuseppe Liotta[1], Helena Canhao[2], Fabian Cenko[3], Rita Cutini[4], Ercole Vellone[1], Maddalena Illario[5], Przemyslaw Kardas[6], Andrea Poscia[7], Rute Dinis Sousa[2], Leonardo Palombi[1] and Maria Cristina Marazzi[8]*

[1] Department of Biomedicine and Prevention, University of Rome "Tor Vergata", Rome, Italy, [2] CEDOC, EpiDoC Unit, NOVA Medical School, Nova University of Lisbon, Lisbon, Portugal, [3] Catholic University "Our Lady of Good Counsel", Tirana, Albania, [4] Sociology, University for Foreigners "Dante Alighieri", Reggio Calabria, Italy, [5] UOD Health Innovation, Campania Region, Naples, Italy, [6] Department of Family Medicine, Medical University of Lodz, Lodz, Poland, [7] Institute of Hygiene, University of Sacred Heart, Rome, Italy, [8] LUMSA University, Rome, Italy

Edited by:
Gary Sinoff,
University of Haifa, Israel

Reviewed by:
Anna Zisberg,
University of Haifa, Israel
Mario Ulises Pérez-Zepeda,
Instituto Nacional de Geriatría, Mexico

***Correspondence:**
Giuseppe Liotta
giuseppeliotta@hotmail.com

Keywords: active and healthy ageing, Europe, healthy life years, blue print initiative, frailty

BACKGROUND

The European Union (EU) is a conglomerate of more than 500 million people, 19.2% (approximately 100 million) of whom are older adults (1). The ageing population is triggering dramatic demographic, epidemiological, and anthropological changes, highlighting the importance of active and healthy ageing (AHA). In Europe, the most common household type is single occupancy (33.4% of the total number of households) (2). This household type also recorded the highest increase from 2005 to 2015 (3). These findings highlight several questions from both an individual and public perspective. Who will take care of the current generation as we become older? What types of health and social organisations should we develop to preserve the quality of life of an ageing population and sustain our health care systems over the medium and long term? Supporting AHA is one answer to these questions: an AHA population is a resource that benefits all of society. Maintaining a healthy ageing population may also lower demands for health care services. In addition, in many cases, older adults in good health are able to support their fellow generation and represent a strength dedicated to the common well-being.

ACTIVE AGEING AND HEALTHY LIFE YEARS

Active ageing is a multidimensional concept affected by several factors, including physical functionality, lifestyle, urban environment, and social inclusion (4, 5). In 2015, the World Health Organisation defined active ageing as "...the process of optimizing opportunities for health, participation and security in order to enhance quality of life as people age" and healthy ageing as "...the process of developing and maintaining the functional ability that enables well-being in older age" (6). The World Health Report on ageing underlined the role of public health strategies in building and maintaining health in older adults.

An operational definition of healthy ageing is still being debated, however, and consensus has not yet been achieved. McLaughlin and colleagues, who analysed the impact of different definitions of healthy ageing, concluded that a functional definition of health, i.e., free from symptomatic diseases and disabilities, may be acceptable (7). The valuable pragmatic approach supported by these researchers, however, does not account for the social dimension of "active" ageing. This social dimension is considered to be crucial because of its impact on developing and maintaining health at all ages. For example, the role played by social isolation as a risk factor for negative events in the older adult population, such as death, is well known (8–11). A more comprehensive approach to assess the process of AHA at the population level, therefore, should take into account several domains, including health status, income security, capability, and environment (12). This concept is consistent with the approach recently proposed by WHO, that describes healthy ageing as the result of the interaction between the physical and mental capacity of an individual (the intrinsic capacity), and the context of each individual's life (the environment) (13).

Several models have been proposed to measure AHA, however, consensus is needed to be able to implement specific actions (14, 15). The healthy life year (HLY) expectancy, which accounts for the interaction of psychophysical and socioeconomic factors during the individual's life course, could be considered a marker of AHA (16). In this view, HLY expectancy could be used as a measure to guide the development of the AHA process at the population level (17).

Although life expectancy at birth has increased by approximately 3 years over the past decade, disability-free life expectancy (i.e., the HLY expectancy) has not increased over this same time period (18). This phenomenon is not consistent across European countries, since in 12 countries out of 28 the HLY expectancy at 65 years is decreased from 2010 to 2014 (19). Moreover, the gap between life expectancy and healthy life expectancy is increasing. HLY expectancy is determined primarily by progressive impairment in performing activities of daily life (ADL), a measure of functional decline that is associated with frailty (20, 21). Frailty is associated with loss of autonomy in performing ADLs as well as health-related problems, institutionalisation, and/or hospitalisation, with negative influences on quality of life. From a public health perspective, frailty is a multidimensional issue resulting from changes in physical and mental health and functional status as well as lack of social and economic resources. There is evidence that functional decline is associated with lower psychosocial status, namely social isolation, malnutrition, and comorbidity (22–26), which are all determinants of frailty.

A number of initiatives are ongoing at the EU level to increase HLY expectancy at the population level *via* management of frailty at the community level. For example, the European Innovation Partnership on AHA gathers hundreds of public and private stakeholders from different backgrounds (e.g., academic and regulatory bodies, private entrepreneurs, non-government organisations, civil society) to brainstorm and execute innovative solutions for AHA to be exchanged and implemented across different settings within Europe (27). As another example, the Joint Action on Frailty witnesses the commitment of the European governments to set up common instruments and approaches to manage frailty in the community (28).

ACTIVE AGEING AND PREVENTION IN EUROPE

Prevention is the likely key to increasing HLY expectancy (29). For example, approximately 50% of the reduction in mortality due to cardiovascular disease is the result of prevention-based activities, such as a change in lifestyle or smoking cessation (30, 31). Unfortunately, prevention programmes that are targeted to older adults are limited and chaotic, and not implemented in the framework of programmes with measurable outcomes. The European project "Pro Health 65+," which seeks to determine effective methods for promoting a healthy lifestyle among older individuals, experienced some difficulties in collecting information on prevention programmes targeted to the older population. In many European countries, such as Italy, the public administration provides only a generic regulatory framework for promoting and facilitating such programmes (32). Even in countries with a national plan for the elderly, gathering data about either the implementation of different programmes or their impact is difficult (33), suggesting that more effort is needed to determine the impact of prevention programmes on the quality of life and demand of care among the older adult population in Europe.

Some communities within Europe have already developed successful programmes. In Barcelona, the Institut d'Investigació en Atenció Primària (IDIAP) Jordi Gol has developed a programme working with community nurses who provides elderly community members with advice on physical activities, diet, and medication schedule and also hold memory workshops: this programme reduced the use of health care services as well as the mortality rate of individuals over 65 years old in this community (34). The University Federico II in Naples has developed a programme that provides both information and communication technology (ICT) literacy and suggestions on diet and physical activities to the elderly community with positive outcomes among the over-65 population (35). In Rome, the Community of Sant'Egidio, a catholic NGO, has been running a programme called "Long Live the Elderly!" for the past 14 years. This programme, which applies social interventions to counteract social isolation in the over-75 population, was associated with a reduction in the use of health care services, health care costs, and mortality rate among this population (36). In addition, a study from the Campania Region of Italy has shown an improvement in bone health among older individuals who adhered to a Mediterranean diet (37). Thus, interventions aimed at lifestyle changes or counteracting social isolation are associated with reduced risk of death and reduced use of hospital services among older populations in Europe.

OCCUPATIONAL PERSPECTIVE ON ACTIVE AGEING

The European Commission is strongly committed to connecting digitalization to AHA. The "Blueprint" initiative, a framework for strategic cooperation between key stakeholders (e.g., business, trade unions, research, education and training institutions, public authorities), outlined how digital innovation enabled by a functioning Digital Single Market can transform demographic changes into opportunities for Europe's economy and society (38, 39) providing also the increase of job opportunities. The Digital Single Market is a strategy of the European Commission adopted in May 2015, to ensure access to online activities for individuals and businesses under conditions of fair competition and consumer and data protection. The grey digital gap (i.e., the lower proclivity of older adults to use personal computers or to communicate *via* the Internet), however, is deep; only approximately 45% of the over-65 population across Europe use the Internet at least once per week (40), and in 19 out of 28 countries in the EU, less than 50% of older adult citizens use the Internet at least once per week. Low Internet usage is due in part to lower education levels of older European citizens in these countries. In Portugal, for example, 77.3% of individuals over 65 years old have 4 or less years of education, and 84.5% have never used computers, videogames, or tablets (41). The "Blueprint" initiative, which aims to implement prevention programmes among European older adults, will, therefore, take significant time (e.g., 5–10 years) to implement among elderly EU citizens. It is likely that parallel efforts, aimed at health promotion and education and targeted at robust and pre-frail individuals, will be needed to maximise the impact of the "Blueprint" initiative over the next several years.

The health care market has not declined over the past 10 years despite the presence of a general economic crisis. The need for care has continued to increase as the population ages, and households are likely to invest more of their resources into this sector over the coming years. There is a window of opportunity, therefore, to implement programmes that proactively target the population at highest risk of frailty and functional decline, namely those over 75 years old. A large investment in health promotion and education that centres on strengthening health, ICT literacy, and social integration not only would serve as insurance for healthier old age and support for the sustainability of the European Health Systems, but also would offer significant occupational benefits to those who are interested in care services. Such programmes would require reorganisation of current models of care at the community level, and would also require individuals to change their view of AHA to that of a long-life approach based on health promotion and education.

CONCLUSION

This debate emphasizes the key role of the determinants of health in AHA. In nineteenth century Europe, an improvement in socioeconomic conditions was the starting point for the most revolutionary demographic and epidemiologic transition in the contemporary age. Environmental sanitation and improved nutrition were the most important factors leading to this revolution at the population level. During this time, life expectancy increased from an average of 45 years to an average of approximately 80 years in most European countries. Europe was the first geographical area in the world to experience this success in life expectancy. Today, Europe continues to experience more advantages and more challenges with its ageing population than any other region in the world. Strengthening the social dimension of prevention programmes and changing the life styles represent key elements in improving quality of life and reducing the risk of loss of physical autonomy, especially among the over-75 population. These programmes can also provide occupational advantages across many European countries.

A strong effort is needed to improve the integration of the growing number of older adults to avoid the negative consequences of social isolation, malnutrition, and reduced physical activity. In the era of technological development and personalised medicine, environmental and nutritional factors together with healthy lifestyles represent the most powerful factors that determine the health of a population, which is encouraging because these are factors that can be influenced by health promotion and educational intervention. The current weakness of the public health approach to the promotion of AHA which threatens the quality of life of European older adults as well as the medium- and long-term sustainability of the health systems. However, Europe is well-poised to play a leading role worldwide in facing the challenges of increasing HLY expectancy by taking advantage of its assets in knowledge and innovation.

AUTHOR CONTRIBUTIONS

GL wrote the text. HC, MI, AP, and PK revised the text. FC, RC, EV, LP, MM, and RS contributed to the text with suggestions, comments, and proposals.

REFERENCES

1. Eurostat. *Population Structure and Ageing*. Available from: https://ec.europa.eu/eurostat/statistics-explained/index.php/Population_structure_and_ageing (Accessed: July 20, 2017).
2. Eurostat. *Households Composition Statistics*. Available from: https://ec.europa.eu/eurostat/statistics-explained/index.php/Household_composition_statistics (Accessed: July 20, 2017).
3. Eurostat. *Population by Age Group*. Available from: https://ec.europa.eu/eurostat/tgm/refreshTableAction.do?tab=table&plugin=1&pcode=tps00010&language=en (Accessed: May 10, 2017).
4. Illario M, Vollenbroek-Hutten MMR, Molloy DW, Menditto E, Iaccarino G, Eklund P. Active and healthy ageing and independent living 2016. *J Aging Res* (2016) 2016:8062079. doi:10.1155/2016/8062079
5. World Health Organization. *Ageing and Life-Course*. Available from: https://www.who.int/ageing/active_ageing/en/ (Accessed: August 01, 2017).
6. World Health Organization. *World Report on Ageing and Health*. Luxembourg (2015).
7. McLaughlin SJ, Jette AM, Connell CM. An examination of healthy aging across a conceptual continuum: prevalence estimates, demographic patterns, and validity. *J Gerontol A Biol Sci Med Sci* (2012) 67(7):783–9. doi:10.1093/gerona/glr234
8. Stolz E, Mayerl H, Waxenegger A, Rásky É, Freidl W. Impact of socioeconomic position on frailty trajectories in 10 European countries: evidence from the survey of health, ageing and retirement in Europe (2004-2013). *J Epidemiol Community Health* (2017) 71(1):73–80. doi:10.1136/jech-2016-207712
9. Tabue Teguo M, Simo-Tabue N, Stoykova R, Meillon C, Cogne M, Amiéva H, et al. Feelings of loneliness and living alone as predictors of mortality in the elderly: the PAQUID study. *Psychosom Med* (2016) 78(8):904–9. doi:10.1097/PSY.0000000000000386
10. Shankar A, McMunn A, Demakakos P, Hamer M, Steptoe A. Social isolation and loneliness: prospective associations with functional status in older adults. *Health Psychol* (2017) 36(2):179–87. doi:10.1037/hea0000437
11. Steptoe A, Shankar A, Demakakos P, Wardle J. Social isolation, loneliness, and all-cause mortality in older men and women. *Proc Natl Acad Sci U S A* (2013) 110(15):5797–801. doi:10.1073/pnas.1219686110
12. HelpAge International. *The Global Watch Age index*. Available from: https://www.helpage.org/global-agewatch/about/about-global-agewatch/ (Accessed: October 31, 2017).
13. Cesari M, Araujo de Carvalho I, Amuthavalli Thiyagarajan J, Cooper C, Martin FC, Reginster JY, et al. Evidence for the domains supporting the construct of intrinsic capacity. *J Gerontol A Biol Sci Med Sci* (2018). doi:10.1093/gerona/gly011
14. Bousquet J, Kuh D, Bewick M, Standberg T, Farrell J, Pengelly R, et al. Operational definition of active and healthy ageing (AHA): a conceptual framework. *J Nutr Health Aging* (2015) 19(9):955–60. doi:10.1007/s12603-015-0589-6

15. Malva JO, Bousquet J. Operational definition of active and healthy ageing: roadmap from concept to change of management. *Maturitas* (2016) 84:3–4. doi:10.1016/j.maturitas.2015.11.004
16. European Commission – DG Health and Food Safety. *Health Indicators*. Available from: https://ec.europa.eu/health/indicators/healthy_life_years/hly_en (Accessed: August 01, 2017).
17. Lagiewka K. European innovation partnership on active and healthy ageing: triggers of setting the headline target of 2 additional healthy life years at birth at EU average by 2020. *Arch Public Health* (2012) 70(1):23. doi:10.1186/0778-7367-70-23
18. The MOPACT Coordination Team. *Declining Trends of Healthy Life Years Expectancy (HLYE) in EUROPE*. Available from: https://docplayer.net/5031483-Mobilising-the-potential-of-active-ageing-in-europe-trends-in-healthy-life-expectancy-and-health-indicators-among-older-people-in-27-eu-countries.html (Accessed: May 10, 2017).
19. Eurostat. *Healthy Life Years and Life Expectancy at Age 65 by Sex*. Available from: https://ec.europa.eu/eurostat/web/health/health-status-determinants/data/main-tables (Accessed: November 11, 2017).
20. Lawton MP. Instrumental activities of daily living. *Gerontologist* (1969) 9: 179. doi:10.1093/geront/9.3_Part_1.179
21. Katz TF. A.D.L. activities of daily living. *JAMA* (1963) 185:914. doi:10.1001/jama.1963.03060120024016
22. Mulasso A, Roppolo M, Giannotta F, Rabaglietti E. Associations of frailty and psychosocial factors with autonomy in daily activities: a cross-sectional study in Italian community-dwelling older adults. *Clin Interv Aging* (2016) 11:37–45. doi:10.2147/CIA.S95162
23. Dent E, Hoogendijk EO. Psychosocial factors modify the association of frailty with adverse outcomes: a prospective study of hospitalised older people. *BMC Geriatr* (2014) 14:108. doi:10.1186/1471-2318-14-108
24. Lorenzo-López L, Maseda A, de Labra C, Regueiro-Folgueira L, Rodríguez-Villamil JL, Millán-Calenti JC. Nutritional determinants of frailty in older adults: a systematic review. *BMC Geriatr* (2017) 17:108. doi:10.1186/s12877-017-0496-2
25. Kelaiditi E, Guyonnet S, Cesari M. Is nutrition important to postpone frailty? *Curr Opin Clin Nutr Metab Care* (2015) 18(1):37. doi:10.1097/MCO.0000000000000129
26. Le Cossec C, Perrine AL, Beltzer N, Fuhrman C, Carcaillon-Bentata L. Pre-frailty, frailty, and multimorbidity: prevalences and associated characteristics from two french national surveys. *J Nutr Health Aging* (2016) 20(8):860–9. doi:10.1007/s12603-016-0802-2
27. European Commission. *European Innovation Partnership on Active and Healthy Ageing Portal*. Available from: https://ec.europa.eu/eip/ageing/home_en (Accessed: August 01, 2017).
28. Advantage Joint Action on Prevention of Frailty. Available from: https://chrodis.eu/advantage-joint-action-prevention-frailty-kicks-off-madrid/ (Accessed: August 01, 2017).
29. Lopreite M, Mauro M. The effects of population ageing on health care expenditure: a Bayesian VAR analysis using data from Italy. *Health Policy* (2017) 121(6):663–74. doi:10.1016/j.healthpol.2017.03.015
30. World Health Organzation. *Cardiovascular Diseases: Fact Sheet*. Available from: https://www.who.int/mediacentre/factsheets/fs317/en/ (Accessed: November 29, 2017).
31. White MC, Holman DM, Boehm JE, Peipins LA, Grossman M, Henley SJ. Age and cancer risk: a potentially modifiable relationship. *Am J Prev Med* (2014) 46(3 Suppl 1):S7–15. doi:10.1016/j.amepre.2013.10.029
32. Poscia A, Falvo R, La Milia DI, Collamati A, Pelliccia F, Kowalska-Bobko I, et al. Healthy ageing–happy ageing: health promotion for older people in Italy. *Zdrowie Publiczne i Zarzadzanie* (2017) 1:34–48. doi:10.4467/2084262 7OZ.17.005.6231
33. Falvo R, Poscia A, Magnavita N, La Milia DI, Collamati A, Moscato U, et al. Health promotion for older people in Portugal. *Zdrowie Publiczne i Zarzadzanie* (2017) 1:49–61. doi:10.4467/20842627OZ.17.006.6232
34. Romera L, Orfila F, Segura JM, Ramirez A, Möller M, Fabra ML, et al. Effectiveness of a primary care based multifactorial intervention to improve frailty parameters in the elderly: a randomised clinical trial: rationale and study design. *BMC Geriatr* (2014) 14:125. doi:10.1186/1471-2318-14-125
35. Barrea L, Muscogiuri G, Di Somma C, Tramontano G, De Luca V, Illario M, et al. Association between Mediterranean diet and hand grip strength in older adult women. *Clin Nutr* (2018). doi:10.1016/j.clnu.2018.03.012
36. Marazzi MC, Inzerilli MC, Madaro O, Palombi L, Scarcella P, Orlando S, et al. Impact of the community-based active monitoring program on the long term care services use and in-patient admissions of the over-74 population. *Adv Aging Res* (2015) 4(06):187. doi:10.4236/aar.2015.46020
37. Vuolo L, Barrea L, Savanelli MC, Savastano S, Rubino M, Scarano E, et al. Nutrition and Osteoporosis: preliminary data of Campania region of European PERsonalised ICT supported service for independent living and active ageing. *Transl Med UniSa* (2016) 31(13):13–8.
38. Oettinger G. *Keynote Speech at the Official Opening of the 4th Conference of Partners*; 2015 December 9; Brussels: EIPonAHA. (2015). Available from: https://ec.europa.eu/research/innovation-union/pdf/active-healthy-ageing/oettinger_cop_2015.pdf (Accessed: January 25, 2018).
39. Kardas P. *Europe Opens a New Era in Digital Revolution: The Blueprint on Digital Transformation of Health and Care for Aging Society has Been Launched*. Available from: https://www.digitmedicine.com (Accessed: July 19, 2017).
40. Eurostat. *What is the Share of the Elderly Who Use Internet at Least Once a Week?* Available from: https://ec.europa.eu/eurostat/cache/infographs/elderly/index.html (Accessed: April 03, 2017).
41. Rodrigues AM, Gregório MJ, Sousa RD, Dias SS, Santos MJ, Mendes JM, et al. Challenges of ageing in Portugal: data from the EpiDoC cohort. *Acta Med Port* (2018) 31(2):80–93. doi:10.20344/amp.9817

14

Food Insecurity in Older Adults: Results From the Epidemiology of Chronic Diseases Cohort Study 3

*Simone G. Fernandes[1], Ana M. Rodrigues[2], Carla Nunes[1,3], Osvaldo Santos[4,5], Maria J. Gregório[2], Rute Dinis de Sousa[2], Sara Dias[2] and Helena Canhão[1,2]**

[1] Escola Nacional de Saúde Pública, Universidade Nova de Lisboa, Lisbon, Portugal, [2] CEDOC, EpiDoc Unit – Unidade de Epidemiologia em Doenças Crónicas, NOVA Medical School, Universidade Nova de Lisboa, Lisbon, Portugal, [3] Centro de Investigação em Saúde Pública, Escola Nacional de Saúde Pública, Universidade Nova de Lisboa, Lisbon, Portugal, [4] Instituto de Medicina Preventiva e Saúde Pública, Faculdade de Medicina, Universidade de Lisboa, Lisbon, Portugal, [5] Instituto de Saúde Ambiental, Faculdade de Medicina, Universidade de Lisboa, Lisbon, Portugal

Edited by:
Maw Pin Tan,
University of Malaya, Malaysia

Reviewed by:
Somnath Chatterji,
World Health Organization, Switzerland
Martin Caraher,
City University of London, United Kingdom

Correspondence:
Helena Canhão
helena.canhao@nms.unl.pt

Introduction: The public health problem of food insecurity also affects the elderly population. This study aimed to estimate the prevalence of household food insecurity and its associations with chronic disease and health-related quality of life characteristics in individuals ≥65 years of age living in the community in Portugal.

Methods: The data were collected from the Epidemiology of Chronic Diseases Cohort Study 3 (EpiDoC3)—Promoting Food Security Study (2015–2016), which was the third evaluation wave of the EpiDoC and represented the Portuguese adult population. Food insecurity was assessed using a psychometric scale adapted from the Brazilian Food Insecurity Scale. The data on sociodemographic variables, chronic disease, and management of chronic disease were self-reported. Health-related quality of life were assessed using the European Quality of Life Survey (version validated for the Portuguese population). Logistic regression models were used to determine crude and adjusted odds ratios (for age group, gender, region, and education). The dependent variable was the perceived level of food security.

Results: Among older adults, 23% were living in a food-insecure household. The odds of living in a food-insecure household were higher for individuals in the 70–74 years age group (odds ratio (OR) = 1.405, 95% confidence interval (CI) 1.392–1.417), females (OR = 1.545, 95% CI 1.534–1.556), those with less education (OR = 3.355, 95% CI 3.306–3.404), low income (OR = 4,150, 95% CI 4.091–4.210), and those reporting it was very difficult to live with the current income (OR = 16.665, 95% CI 16.482–16.851). The odds of having a chronic disease were also greater among individuals living in food-insecure households: diabetes mellitus (OR = 1.832, 95% CI 1.818–1.846), pulmonary diseases (OR = 1.628, 95% CI 1.606–1.651), cardiac disease (OR = 1.329, 95% CI 1.319–1.340), obesity (OR = 1.493, 95% CI 1.477–1.508), those who reduced their frequency of medical visits (OR = 4.381, 95% CI 4.334–4.428), and who stopped taking medication due to economic difficulties (OR = 5.477, 95% CI 5.422–5.532). Older adults in food-insecure households had lower health-related quality of life (OR = 0.212, 95% CI 0.210–0.214).

Conclusions: Our findings indicated that food insecurity was significantly associated with economic factors, higher values for prevalence of chronic diseases, poor management of chronic diseases, and decreased health-related quality of life in older adults living in the community.

Keywords: food insecurity, chronic diseases, quality of life, older adults, management of chronic diseases

INTRODUCTION

Populations worldwide are undergoing unprecedented changes in age demographics. In Portugal and other European countries, more than 19% of the individuals are ≥65 years of age (1, 2). Age is the most powerful predictor of morbidity and mortality. Multifaceted and numerous mechanisms link age to health status (1). To maximize health and well-being, healthcare systems should be responsive to the diversity and heterogeneity of the health status of older adults (1).

The increasing proportions of countries' oldest populations are associated with greater vulnerability and high-risk of development of chronic diseases and disabilities. These negative health outcomes have direct effects on access to adequate food and result in food insecurity (3). Food security is the condition where *"all people, at all times, have physical and economic access to sufficient, safe and nutritious food to meet their dietary needs and food preferences for an active and healthy life"* (4). This broad concept encompasses the availability of food and the accessibility and proper use of food. Food insecurity can affect the health and well-being of individuals (4–8). Nutrition is one of the main determinants of healthy and active aging. Consumption of nutritious food is crucial for physiological well-being and better health and quality of life (9).

The health characteristics of older adults differ from other age groups. The multidimensional phenomenon of food insecurity is also different in this population (10, 11). In older populations, food insecurity results from more than financial resource constraints. Functional impairment, not owning a home, isolation, gender, financial vulnerability, and poor health have statistically significant associations with food insecurity. These associations suggest that differences in food use between older and younger populations should be considered. These important risk factors for food insecurity tend to occur together, which results in a much higher risk for food insecurity in older populations (8, 10–13). As older populations increase in size, accurate assessments of the extension of food insecurity become more essential for public health (14). Previous studies of food insecurity have mostly examined populations of children and non-elderly adults. Little is known about the characteristics of food insecurity in older adults and associations with health outcomes (11, 15).

Approximately 23% of the global burden of disease is attributable to conditions that affect older people; the main conditions that contribute to this excessive burden are chronic diseases (16). Chronic disease can negatively affect the ability to shop for food, carry foodstuffs home, and prepare meals, which can affect older adults' food security as much as financial vulnerability (5). A poor diet also has severe effects on quality of life and health. Older adults who adopt poor dietary patterns have higher risks of malnutrition, frailty, deteriorating health conditions, and disability compared with those that consume a healthy diet (9, 12). Previous findings indicate that food insecurity is particularly prevalent among older adults (11, 12, 17) and is associated with poor health (5, 12), increased depression, disability (18), and poor quality of life (5, 19).

National and international initiatives promote active and healthy aging, but there are still opportunities for the results of this approach to be reflected in increased quality of life and health of older adults. Rethinking aging implies a true transverse commitment and reconsideration of the entire set of associated factors (20). One of the main objectives of the Healthy People 2020 Report is to *"improve the health, function, and quality of life"* (21), so understanding the associations between food insecurity, chronic diseases, and quality of life is fundamental for improvement of health policies and resulting successful promotion of active and healthy aging populations. The purpose of this study was to estimate the prevalence of household food insecurity and its associations with chronic diseases and health-related quality of life (HRQoL) factors in individuals ≥65 years of age living in the community.

MATERIALS AND METHODS

This observational study used a cross-sectional analysis of data from a national ongoing prospective cohort study, the Epidemiology of Chronic Diseases Cohort Study (EpiDoC). The data from this population-based study represent the Portuguese adult non-institutionalized (i.e., live in private homes) population in Portugal (Mainland, Madeira, and Azores Islands). The EpiDoC cohort began with the EpiDoC 1 study (EpiReumaPt); two subsequent evaluations have been performed using data from the same subjects [EpiDoC 2 (CoReumaPt) and EpiDoC 3 (Promoting Food Security)] studies. The sampling method used for the EpiDoc 1 study followed a cross-country random route procedure; sampling was stratified by region (North, Centre, Lisbon, Alentejo, Algarve, Madeira, and Azores) and size of locality. Data collection was performed using a computer-assisted telephone interview method. The number of interviews conducted for each stratum was proportional to

Abbreviations: EpiDoC3, Promoting Food Security Study; EpiDoC cohort, Epidemiology of Chronic Diseases Cohort Study; BMI, Body mass index; HRQoL, Health-related quality of life; EQ-5D-3L, European Quality of Life Survey with five dimensions and three levels; EQ VAS, thermometer scale from the EQ5D-3L questionnaire.

the actual distribution of the population. Census 2001 results indicated that the eligible Portuguese population ≥18 years old was $N = 7{,}719{,}986$. Therefore, a sample of 10,661 participants was randomly selected (random route method) (22). All 10,661 participants in the EpiDoC 1 study signed an informed consent form for follow-up, and those who provided their telephone number were included in the subsequent EpiDoC cohort follow-up evaluations (EpiDoC 2 and EpiDoC 3). In the EpiDoC 2 and EpiDoC 3 studies, all participants were contacted by telephone (23, 24). Of the 9,003 participants eligible for the EpiDoC 3 (Promoting Food Security) study, 2,366 were lost due to unsuccessful contact and 1,004 participants were lost to follow-up for other reasons; there were 5,653 participants in the third wave of the study. A total of 1,885 individuals in this Portuguese noninstitutionalised population were ≥65 years of age; the data from these participants were included in the analyses described in this article.

Instruments and Variables

Sociodemographic (age, gender, years of education, and health region) and socioeconomic (income and information on perception of family income) data were collected. Data on self-reported diseases (high cholesterol levels, hypertension, diabetes, gastrointestinal disease, mental disease, cardiac disease, pulmonary disease, cancer, neurological disease, hyperuricemia, and urinary disease) were also assessed. HRQoL was assessed using the European Quality of Life Survey (version validated for the Portuguese population) (25) with five dimensions and three levels (EQ-5D-3L). The EQ-5D descriptive system was converted into a single index using a formula that assigned values to each of the levels in each dimension. These value-sets were derived for use of the EQ-5D for the Portuguese population (25). A higher EQ-5D index score corresponded to a higher quality of life. Self-perception of general health status at the time of the survey was also assessed by adapting the original EQ5D-3L visual analog scale to the question *"Considering a scale on which the best state of health you can imagine is 100 and the worst state of health you can imagine is 0, we would like you to tell us how good or bad it is, in your opinion, your state of health today?"*.

Data on whether there was a reduction in the numbers of visits to a physician due to economic difficulties (Yes/No), whether the respondent took any medication (Yes/No), and whether the respondent stopped taking any medication due to economic difficulties (Yes/No) were also recorded. Body mass index (BMI, body weight in kilograms divided by the square of the height in meters) was calculated using the values for self-reported weight and height. The BMI values were assigned to categories according to World Health Organization criteria (26).

Food insecurity was assessed using a psychometric scale adapted from the Brazilian Food Insecurity Scale; this scale was adapted from the US Household Food Security Survey Module (27–29). This tool was used to assess the quantitative and qualitative components of food insecurity within the 3 months before the respondent answered the survey. A score ranging from 0 to 14 was obtained as an outcome of the total number of affirmative answers. Each score was used to assign the respondent to one of four categories of food insecurity (i.e., "food security," "low food insecurity," "moderate food insecurity," and "severe food insecurity"; **Table 1**).

Statistical Analysis

The statistical analysis was performed using the Statistical Package for the Social Sciences - IBM-SPSS for Windows 24.0®. To assure the representativeness of the sample for the 65 years and older Portuguese population, weighting coefficients were computed and used for the additional statistical analyses. The EpiDoC 3 study participants and non-participants were first compared regarding sociodemographic, socioeconomic, and health status characteristics. We then adjusted the weights based on the corresponding population stratification groups (gender, age group, and health region). Weighted proportions of food insecurity according to age group, gender, health region, years of education, income, and household income perception were calculated. Prevalence estimates for food insecurity were calculated as weighted proportions, consistent with the sample design. After the descriptive analyses were performed, each participant was assigned to the "Food Security" or "Food Insecurity" (including mild, moderate and severe food

TABLE 1 | Definitions of Food Security levels.

Food Security Level	Cut-offs	Definition
Food Security	If the household includes minors (<18 years old): 0 Household without minors (≥18 years): 0	Households show access at all times to enough food for an active and healthy life.
Low Food Insecurity	If the household includes minors (<18 years old): 1 - 5 Household without minors (≥18 years): 1 – 3	Households reports at least anxiety about lack of food to meet dietary needs. At this level, coping strategies to deal with economic and food constraints can also have an important on the reduction of diet quality.
Moderate Food Insecurity	If the household includes minors (<18 years old): 6 - 9 Household without minors (≥ 18 years): 4 – 5	Adults in the household reported food intake reduction and changes in eating patterns due to economic difficulties in accessing food.
Severe Food Insecurity	If the household includes minors (<18 years old): 10 - 14 Household without minors (≥ 18 years): 6 – 8	At this level, households without children experienced the physical sensation of hunger and households with children reported a reduction of children's food intake.

Adapted from the Brazilian Institute of Geography and Statistics. National Household Sample Survey - Food Security 2004/2009. Rio de Janeiro; 2010 (30).

insecurity) categories to evaluate the relationships between food insecurity and the other study variables. The magnitudes of the associations between the variables were calculated using binary logistic regression models. The dependent variable was food security status ["food insecurity" (event) vs. "food security"]. Independent variables were sequentially added to the model based on existing knowledge about the variables that could affect the event. Crude and adjusted odds ratios (ORs; age group, gender, health region, and years of education) and the corresponding 95% confidence intervals (CIs) were computed. EQ5D-3L and self-perception of general health status data were analyzed as continuous variables. We interpreted these variables considering that the EQ5D-3L values ranged from 0 to 1 and that the self-perception of general health status values ranged from 0 to 100. A significance level of $\alpha = 0.05$ (two-tailed) was used for all analyses.

Ethical Issues

The EpiDoC 3 study was performed according to the criteria established by the Declaration of Helsinki and revised in 2013 in Fortaleza (31). The study was reviewed and approved by the National (Portuguese) Committee for Data Protection and by the NOVA Medical School Ethics Committee. The participants gave informed signed consent to be included in all phases of the study.

RESULTS

The data were collected using telephone interviews of 1,885 Portuguese people ≥ 65 years of age living in communities in the mainland, or the Madeira or Azores islands, between July 2015 and September 2016. The sample consisted of 55.5% women and 44.5% men (mean ± standard deviation (SD), 74.3 ± 6.8 years (range, 65–104 years). The results for the sociodemographic and socioeconomic characteristics of this older population are presented in **Table 2**.

Prevalence of Food Insecurity

A Cronbach's α coefficient of 0.949 was found when we analyzed only the adult household-related items of the scale. The first validation of the Household Food Insecurity Scale used a sample from the Portuguese population. It was performed by Gregorio et al. in 2015. They found a Cronbach's α coefficient of 0.865 (27).

Twenty-three percent (n = 500) of 65 years and older households reported being food-insecure. Of this food-insecure group, 16.3% were in the low food insecurity, 4.8% were in the moderate, and 2% were in the severe food insecurity, group (**Table 3**). There were apparent differences between genders and age groups (**Table 4**). Older females were more likely to report living in a food-insecure household (26.5%) compared with older males (18.9%) (OR = 1.545, 95% CI 1.534–1.556). A higher proportion (25.9%) of food insecurity was found in the households of the individuals in the 70–74 years age group (OR = 1.405, 95% CI 1.392–1.417). The highest proportion of severe food insecurity was also found among the individuals in the 70–74 years age group (2.9%) (**Table 3**).

TABLE 2 | Sociodemographic and socioeconomic characteristics of older adults.

Variables	Total n (%)
AGE (n = 1885)	
65-69 years	563 (29.4)
70-74 years	475 (27)
75-79 years	393 (19.9)
≥80 years	454 (23.7)
GENDER (n = 1885)	
Female	1243 (55.5)
Male	642 (44.5)
EDUCATION LEVEL (n = 1877)	
0 years of education	174 (9.7)
1 - 4 years of education	1205 (63.8)
5 – 9 years of education	267 (13.9)
10- 12 years of education	117 (6.3)
>12 years of education	114 (6.4)
HEALTH REGION (n = 1885)	
North	501 (32.2)
Centre	414 (27.1)
Lisbon	371 (23.1)
Alentejo	136 (9.6)
Algarve	78 (4.1)
Azores	183 (1.8)
Madeira	202 (2)
INCOME (n = 1384)	
≤ 500€	950 (64.4)
501€ until 750€	208 (15.5)
751€ until 1000€	89 (9.6)
1001€ until 1500€	84 (6.4)
≥1501€	53 (4.1)
INCOME PERCEPTION (n = 1869)	
I live comfortably with my current income	223 (12.4)
I can live with my current income	777 (41.9)
It is difficult to live with the current income	585 (30.7)
It is very difficult to live with the current income	284 (14.9)

All percentages were weighted for correcting to population representativeness.

VARIABLES ASSOCIATED WITH FOOD INSECURITY

Sociodemographic Characteristics

The results for the analysis of the sociodemographic characteristics of the sample and for the application of a binary logistic regression model for the event (food insecurity, binary variable) are presented in **Table 4**. The results indicated that for the sociodemographic factors related to food insecurity, females (OR = 1.545, 95% CI 1.534–1.556), the oldest ages (70–74 years vs. 65–69 years: OR = 1.405, 95% CI 1.392–1.417; 75–79 years vs. 65–69 years: OR = 1.246, 95% CI 1.233–1.258; ≥80 years vs. 65–69 years: OR = 1.234, 95% CI 1.222–1.246), lower levels of education (0 years of school vs. 5–9 years: OR = 3.355,

TABLE 3 | Food Insecurity status by age group and gender.

Variables	Total *n* (%)	Food Security *n* (%)	Low Food Insecurity *n* (%)	Moderate Food Insecurity *n* (%)	Severe Food Insecurity *n* (%)
AGE (*n* = 1885)					
65-69 years	563 (29.4)	418 (80.1)	94 (14.1)	33 (4.0)	18 (1.8)
70-74 years	475 (27)	347 (74.1)	85 (19.4)	26 (2.6)	17 (2.9)
75-79	393 (19.9)	288 (76.4)	68 (16.6)	32 (6.1)	5 (0.9)
≥80 years	454 (23.7)	332 (76.5)	80 (15.1)	30 (6.1)	12 (2.2)
GENDER (*n* = 1885)					
Female	1243 (55.5)	865 (73.5)	241 (17.1)	93 (6.2)	44 (3.1)
Male	642 (44.5)	520 (81.1)	86 (15.1)	28 (3.1)	8 (0.7)

All percentages were weighted for correcting to population representativeness.

TABLE 4 | Food Insecurity status: Associations with Sociodemographic Characteristics.

Variables	Total *n* (%)	Food Security *n* (%)	Food Insecurity *n* (%)	Crude OR (95% CI)
AGE (*n* = 1885)				
65-69 years	563 (29.4)	418 (80.1)	155 (19.9)	1
70-74 years	475 (27)	347 (74.1)	128 (25.9)	1.405(1.392-1.417)
75-79 years	393 (19.9)	288 (76.4)	105 (23.6)	1.246 (1.233-1.258)
≥80 years	454 (23.7)	332 (76.5)	122 (23.5)	1.234 (1.222-1.246)
GENDER (*n* = 1885)				
Female	1243 (55.5)	865 (73.5)	378 (26.5)	1.545 (1.534-1.556)
Male	642 (44.5)	520 (81.1)	122 (18.9)	1
EDUCATION LEVEL (*n* = 1877)				
0 years of education	174 (9.7)	91 (65.6)	83 (34.4)	3.355 (3.306-3.404)
1 - 4 years of education	1205 (63.8)	852 (73.8)	436 (26.2)	2.269 (2.242-2.296)
5 – 9 years of education	267 (13.9)	223 (86.5)	44 (13.5)	1
10- 12 years of education	117 (6.3)	105 (89.2)	12 (10.2)	0.776 (0.760-0.793)
>12 years of education	114 (6.4)	108 (91.8)	6 (8.2)	0.572 (0.559-0.585)
HEALTH REGION (*n* = 1885)				
North	501 (32.2)	359 (75.6)	142 (24.4)	1
Centre	414 (27.1)	312 (76.1)	102 (23.9)	0.972 (0.964-0.980)
Lisboa	371 (23.1)	312 (81.2)	59 (18.8)	0.717 (0.710-0.724)
Alentejo	136 (9.6)	104 (78.4)	32 (21.6)	0.853 (0.842-0.864)
Algarve	78 (4.1)	57(77.8)	21 (22.2)	0.881 (0.866-0.897)
Azores	183 (1.8)	123 (68.1)	60 (31.9)	1.451 (1.417-1.485)
Madeira	202 (2)	118 (58.8)	84 (41.2)	2.161 (2.116-2.207)

All percentages were weighted for correcting to population representativeness.

95% CI 3.306–3.404; 1–4 years vs. 5–9 years: OR = 2.269, 95% CI 2.242–2.296), living in the Azores (Azores vs. North: OR = 1.451, 95% CI 1.417–1.485) and Madeira (Madeira vs. North: OR = 2.161, 95% CI 2.116–2.207) were associated with increased odds of living in a food-insecure household.

Socioeconomic Characteristics

The results for the application of a binary logistic regression model for the event food insecurity are presented in **Table 5**. The socioeconomic characteristics were included in the model and the results were presented as crude and adjusted ORs (i.e., adjusted by age group, gender, education level, and health region). The analysis of socioeconomic characteristics revealed that having an monthly income ≤500€ (i.e., ≤ 500€ vs. 501€ to 750€: OR = 3.125, 95% CI 4.091–4.210) and reporting having financial difficulties (*It is difficult to live with the current income* vs. *I can live with my current income*: OR = 6.366, 95% CI 6.304–6.429) or reporting that it was very difficult to live with the current income (*It is very difficult to live with the current income* vs. *I can live with my current income*: OR = 16.665, 95% CI 16.482–16.851) were associated with increased odds of living in a food-insecure household.

TABLE 5 | Food Insecurity status: Associations with Socioeconomic Characteristics.

Variables	Total *n* (%)	Food Security *n* (%)	Food Insecurity *n* (%)	Crude OR (95% CI)	Adjusted OR* (95% CI)
INCOME (*n* =1384)					
≤ 500€	950 (64.4)	614 (67.2)	336 (32.8)	4.150 (4.091-4.210)	4.442 (4.377-4.508)
501€ until 750€	208 (15.5)	177 (89.5)	31 (10.5)	1	1
751€ until 1000€	89 (9.6)	81 (94.9)	8 (5.1)	0.457 (0.444-0.470)	0.510 (0.496-0.525)
1001€ until 1500€	84 (6.4)	78 (92.4)	6 (7.6)	0.701 (0.681-0.721)	0.978 (0.950-1.008)
≥1501€	53 (4.1)	51 (89.5)	2 (10.5)	1.000 (0.971-1.031)	1.267 (1.226-1.310)
INCOME PERCEPTION (*n* = 1869)					
I live comfortably with my current income	223 (12.4)	217 (94.6)	6 (5.4)	0.688 (0.675-0.702)	0.774 (0.759-0.790)
I can live with my current income	777 (41.9)	703 (92.4)	74 (7.6)	1	1
It is difficult to live with the current income	585 (30.7)	359 (65.5)	226 (34.5)	6.366 (6.304-6.429)	6.228 (6.166-6.291)
It is very difficult to live with the current income	284 (14.9)	92 (42.0)	192 (58.0)	16.665 (16.482-16.851)	15.817 (15.637-15.998)

**Adjusted Odds Ratio to gender, age, education level, and health region.*
All percentages were weighted for correcting to population representativeness.

Chronic Diseases

The results for the crude and adjusted ORs (i.e., adjusted for age group, gender, education level, and health region) for the presence of household food insecurity and chronic disease are presented in **Table 6**. The results indicated that older adults living in food-insecure households had greater odds of having one or more chronic diseases (OR = 1.161, 95% CI 1.158–1.164). The chronic conditions were diabetes (OR = 1.832, 95% CI 1.818–1.846), hypercholesterolemia (OR = 1.138, 95% CI 1.129–1.146), pulmonary disease (OR = 1.628, 95% CI 1.606–1.651), cardiac disease (OR = 1.329, 95% CI 1.319–1.340), digestive disease (OR = 1.259, 95% CI 1.247–1.271), mental disease (OR = 1.334, 95% CI 1.322–1.347), and urinary disease (OR = 1.566, 95% CI 1.550–1.582). Except for the variable hypercholesterolemia (ORa = 0.992, 95% CI 0.988–1.004), these associations were present before and after adjusting the model. For the variable BMI, older adults from food-insecure households had greater odds of pre-obesity (pre-obesity vs. normal weight: OR = 1.364, 95% CI 1.353–1.376) and obesity (obesity vs. normal weight: OR = 1.493, 95% CI 1.477–1.508), and lower odds of being underweight (underweight vs. normal weight: OR = 0.572, 95% CI 0.543–0.603), before and after adjusting for age group, gender, education level, and health region.

Management of Chronic Diseases

The results for the application of a binary logistic regression model for the event food insecurity are presented in **Table 7**. The variables related to management of chronic disease were included in the model, and the results were presented as crude and adjusted ORs (i.e., adjusted for age group, gender, education level, and health region). The results of the analysis of the difficulties experienced by older adults in the management of these chronic diseases indicated that those who reported a decrease in medical visits or who stopped taking medication due to economic reasons had a higher odds (OR = 4.381, 95% CI 4.334–4.428, and OR = 5.477, 95% CI 5.422–5.532, respectively) of living in a food-insecure household, before and after adjustment of the model.

Health Related Quality of Life

The results for the crude ORs and adjusted ORs (i.e., adjusted for age group, gender, education level, and health region) for the presence of household food insecurity and HRQoL are presented in **Table 8**. The results indicated that before and after adjustment of the model, older adults from food-insecure households had higher odds of a lower HRQoL (EQ5D-3L score: OR = 0.212, 95% CI 0.210–0.214). The analysis of the self-perception of general health status (thermometer scale from the EQ5D-3L questionnaire adapted to one question) revealed that older adults who reported a better health status had lower odds of living in a food-insecure household, before and after adjusting the model (OR = 0.976, 95% CI 0.976–0.976).

DISCUSSION

This study aimed to estimate the prevalence of food insecurity and its association with chronic diseases and HRQoL in individuals ≥65 years of age living in households in the community. To our knowledge, a study with these objectives has not been published.

We found a food insecurity prevalence of 23%. Few studies of food insecurity in Portugal have been performed, and none have specifically examined the older adult population. A national study of the EpiDoc cohort revealed a food insecurity prevalence of 19.3% in the adult population (≥18 years) (23). The results of this current study indicated that this problem is more prevalent in the older population compared with the adult population. Other analyses adult populations found values for prevalence of food insecurity between 8.1% and 50.7% (32–34). However, comparing the results of our study and published studies should be done carefully because the methodological approaches, sources of collected data, and the times of data collection were different.

TABLE 6 | Food Insecurity status: Associations with Chronic Diseases.

Variables	Food Security *n* (%)	Food Insecurity *n* (%)	Crude OR (95% CI)	Adjusted OR* (95% CI)
CHRONIC DISEASES				
Number of Chronic Diseases	Mean±SD: 1.98±1.41	Mean±SD: 2.31±1.66	1.161 (1.158-1.164)	1.128 (1.125-.130)
DIABETES MELLITUS (*n* = 1626)				
No	910 (79.9)	294 (20.1)	1	1
Yes	286 (68.4)	136 (31.6)	1.832 (1.818-1.846)	1.764 (1.750-1.778)
HYPERCHOLESTEROLEMIA (*n* = 1568)				
No	518 (77.8)	162 (22.2)	1	1
Yes	631 (75.5)	257 (24.5)	1.138 (1.129-1.146)	1.992 (0.988-1.004)
PULMONARY DISEASES (*n* = 1644)				
No	1130 (77.3)	405 (22.7)	1	1
Yes	76 (67.6)	33 (32.4)	1.628 (1.606-1.651)	1.611 (1.588-1.634)
CARDIAC DISEASES (*n* = 1619)				
No	887 (78.4)	286 (21.6)	1	1
Yes	306 (73.2)	140 (26.8)	1.329 (1.319-1.340)	1.298 (1.287-1.308)
DIGESTIVE DISEASES (*n* = 1640)				
No	1029 (77.6)	358 (22.4)	1	1
Yes	178 (73.4)	75 (26.6)	1.259 (1.247-1.271)	1.296 (1.283-1.309)
MENTAL DISEASES (*n* = 1653)				
No	967 (77.8)	343 (22.2)	1	1
Yes	246 (72.4)	97 (27.6)	1.334 (1.322-1.347)	1.245 (1.233-1.257)
ONCOLOGIC DISEASES (*n* = 1654)				
No	1089 (76.8)	393 (23.2)	1	1
Yes	124 (77.0)	48 (23.0)	0.988 (0.977-1.000)	1.040 (1.028-1.052)
URINARY DISEASES (*n* = 1621)				
No	1065 (77.9)	396 (22.1)	1	1
Yes	126 (69.2)	34 (30.8)	1.566 (1.550-1.582)	1.994 (1.972-2.016)
BODY MASS INDEX CLASSIFICATION BMI CLASSES (*n* = 1634)**				
Underweight	15 (88.7)	2 (11.3)	0.572 (0,543-0,603)	0.421 (0.400-0.443)
Normal weight	375 (81.7)	110 (18.3)	1	1
Pre-obesity	579 (76.6)	180 (23.4)	1.364 (1.353-1.376)	1.388 (1.376-1.401)
Obesity	271 (75.0)	102 (25.0)	1.493 (1.477-1.508)	1.314 (1.300-1.328)

**Adjusted Odds Ratio to gender, age, education level, and health region.*
All percentages and means were weighted for correcting to population representativeness.
***BMI Classes: Underweight <18,5kg/m^2; Normal weight 18,5-24,9kg/m^2; Pré-obesity 25-29,9kg/m^2; Obesity ≥30kg/m^2*

Similarly, direct comparison of the values for prevalence found in our study with estimates from other countries is not always feasible because the methods of data collection differ. However, some studies used similar methodological approaches to our study. The results of a study performed by Goldberg et al. of a sample of 2,045 older adults ≥60 years of age who were included in the National Health and Nutrition Examination Survey (NHANES, USA) 2007–2008 indicated that >9% of older adult households were food-insecure (35). Russell et al. found that of a sample of 3,509 older adults in Australia, 13% reported food insecurity (5). Other studies performed in United States and Australian populations revealed a higher prevalence of food insecurity in disadvantaged urban areas (6, 8, 36). Compared with our study, these two studies found lower values for prevalence of food insecurity. However, the differences might be due to differences in the participants' ages (i.e., the other studies included participants <65 years of age). The differences could also be due to differences in the sources of collected data (i.e., national vs. regional samples), the socioeconomic disparities between each location (37–39), the socio-economic characteristics of the population (40) or because our sample was collected after a period of economic crisis (41). The data used for other studies were collected before the period of global economic recession (42).

Consistent with the results of previous studies, our study revealed that older adults in food-insecure households were more likely to be women, have less education, and live in households with a lower per capita income (5, 11, 12, 34, 37, 43–45). The income perception is the factor with the most robust association with food insecurity in older adults; it clearly

TABLE 7 | Food Insecurity status: Associations with Management of Chronic Diseases.

Variables	Food Security *n* (%)	Food Insecurity *n* (%)	Crude OR (95% CI)	Adjusted OR* (95% CI)
REDUCTION OF MEDICAL VISITS DUE TO ECONOMIC DIFFICULTIES (*n* = 1883)				
No	1305 (79.4)	393 (20.6)	1	1
Yes	78 (46.9)	107 (53.1)	4.381 (4.334-4.428)	4.350 (4.301-4.398)
TAKE MEDICATION (*n* = 1882)				
No	103 (76.2)	36 (23.8)	-	-
Yes	1280 (77.0)	463 (23.0)		
STOP TAKING MEDICATION DUE TO ECONOMIC DIFFICULTIES (*n* = 1875)				
No	1297 (80.4)	372 (19.6)	1	1
Yes	80 (42.8)	126 (57.2)	5.477 (5.422-5.532)	5.152 (5.099-5.207)

**Adjusted Odds Ratio to gender, age, health region, and level of education.*
All percentages were weighted for correcting to population representativeness.

TABLE 8 | Food Insecurity status: Associations with Health-related Quality of Life.

Variables	Food Security	Food Insecurity	Crude OR (95% CI)	Adjusted OR* (95% CI)
Health-Related Quality of Life - EQ5D-3L score (*n* = 1715)	Mean ± SD: 0.683 ± 0.318 Medium: 0.693 Minimum: −0.438 Maximum: 1	Mean ± SD: 0.511 ± 0.336 Medium: 0.536 Minimum: −0.344 Maximum: 1	0.212 (0.210–0.214)	0.251 (0.248–0.254)
Self-perception of general health status (*n* = 1715)	Mean ± SD: 70.06 ± 19.79 Medium: 70 Minimum: 0 Maximum: 100	Mean ± SD: 59.33 ± 22.02 Medium: 60 Minimum: 0 Maximum: 100	0.976 (0.976–0.976)	0.979 (0.978–0.979)

**Adjusted Odds Ratio to gender, age, education level, and health region.*
All means were weighted for correcting to population representativeness.

represents the relationship between economic factors and food insecurity (5, 13, 46).

Our findings for the self-reported noncommunicable diseases suggested that older adults with chronic diseases (i.e., diabetes, pulmonary disease, cardiac disease, digestive disease, mental disease, and urinary disease) had increased odds of living in a food-insecure household. Other studies have also found associations between food insecurity and higher values for prevalence of diabetes (34, 47–51), pulmonary disease (51), mental disease (12, 18, 48, 52, 53), cardiac disease (48, 54, 55) and poor health outcomes (56). The higher prevalence can be explained by the results of a study that found that food insecurity requires changes in the household food supply that reduce diet quality (57). Disturbance of the nutrient and dietary patterns linked with food insecurity may clarify the higher rates of chronic illness experienced by food-insecure individuals (55, 57).

There are other putative reasons for the higher prevalence of chronic diseases in older adults from food-insecure households. For example, a review performed by Gucciardi et al. revealed that due to the cost of out-of-pocket health care expenditures such as purchase of prescribed medications and supplies, food insecurity affects compliance with the self-management recommendations given to individuals with diabetes (50). Seligman et al. found that persons in food-insecure households may replace the consumption of healthy foods with less expensive foods that have poor nutritional value and a higher energy density. These individuals will then consume in excess of their energy needs and these intakes can be associated with the development of diabetes (49). This finding is consistent with the finding of another study of older adults (58).

The significant association between food insecurity and pulmonary disease revealed by our study is consistent with the results of studies performed in other countries that indicate that being a smoker is a predictor for reporting characteristics associated with food insecurity (5, 51).

Our study also revealed that a higher proportion of older adults from food-insecure households reported lower rates of being underweight and higher rates of pre-obesity and obesity (**Table 6**). The results of previous studies have been inconsistent in this area, especially in the older adult populations where this association is weak (12, 45, 55, 59–61). Consistent with our findings, some studies found that food insecurity is associated with greater BMI values (pre-obesity and obesity) in older adults (18, 62). However, other studies have not found this association

(12) or it has only been found in populations of older females but not in populations of older males (45, 61). These conflicting results may be related to the evidence that compared with direct assessment, self-reported measures of weight and height in older adults could give biased results (18, 45, 63). The aging process is accompanied by modifications in body composition (e.g., reductions in height resulting from compression of the vertebrae, loss of muscle tone, and variations in body weight). Older adults tend to report the values they maintained in adulthood (18, 45, 60, 64). Therefore, these findings suggest that the food-insecurity association with obesity reported among adults may have different characteristics in older adults.

Some studies have found that food-insecure older adults report lower investment in their health (8). Food insecurity, cost-related medication nonadherence, and a decrease in medical visits are three related problems with negative consequences and public health implications (65). Our study found that older adults who reported a decrease in medical visits or who stopped taking medication for economic reasons had 4.5 and 5.5 higher odds, respectively, of living in a food-insecure household.

Our findings suggested that those who reported that they stopped taking medication due to economic reasons had higher odds of living in a food-insecure household. In Portugal, the acquisition of medication is associated with different levels of reimbursement by the state (range, 15% to 95%). There is typically some expenditure by the elderly for medication. Elderly people who must purchase several medications may not be able to do so, especially if they have a low income. Afulani et al. assessed the association between food security and cost-related medication under use in a sample of 10,401 American older adults (National Health Interview Survey 2011–2012). Consistent with our findings, they found that older adults from food-insecure households were more likely to report cost-related medication under use than the adults living in food-secure households (66). Bengle et al. examined the relationship between cost-related medication nonadherence and food insecurity in a sample of 1,000 low-income Georgian older adult participants of the Older Americans Act Nutrition Program. They found that food-insecure participants were three times more likely to practice cost-related medication nonadherence than their counterparts (65). In a 2008 study of older Georgians, Bhargava et al. found that food-insecure individuals were more likely to report a poorer health status, had more chronic disease, and tended to have lower health care expenditures compared with their counterparts with similar health status. Taken together, these findings suggest that food-insecure older adults may be unable to meet healthcare needs and practice healthy food consumption behaviors (6). Other studies have found similar relationships between food insecurity and lack of adherence to medical treatments and drug therapies (8, 13, 34, 50).

In older adults, food insecurity and higher prevalence of chronic diseases contribute to declines in functionality and corresponding decreases in quality of life (9, 19). The relationships between nutrition and morbidity and mortality in aging are well-established, but more research on HRQoL and food insecurity in older adults is needed. Our findings indicated that older adults from food-insecure households reported a poor HRQoL (**Table 8**). These findings are consistent with those of a study of an older Australian cohort of community-living persons ≥49 years of age; this study revealed associations between food insecurity and poor HRQoL characteristics (19). Older adults living in food-insecure households report at least some inability to obtain enough food due to economic limitations and that consequently they reduced their diet quality or variety (28, 67). Diet quality and variety are significant determinants of HRQoL in the aging population (68, 69).

Our study also found that older adults from food-insecure households self-reported a lower health status value (**Table 8**). This finding is consistent with studies that found that than compared with food-secure older adults, food-insecure older adults self-report a poor health status (5, 8, 13, 65).

Our study had some limitations. First, it was based on a cross-sectional analysis that limited the ability to explore casual relationships and establish the temporal sequence of associations. Second, the method used to control the potential effects of sociodemographic variables was based on self-reported conditions, which might contributed to underestimates of the diagnosis of chronic conditions and BMI values (12, 18, 45, 63). Third, the food insecurity scale *"evaluates the food security situation of the household members as a set and not necessarily the condition of any specific household member"* (28, 29). Thus, it was not possible to define the food insecurity status of each older adult living in the household. Despite these limitations, our findings are a valuable resource in understanding key health-related factors associated with food insecurity in older adults. They can be used during development of preventive public health strategies and policies. To our knowledge, this study is one of the first to examine the prevalence of household food insecurity and its associations with chronic diseases and HRQoL of older adults living in the community. The strengths of our study include the use of a randomly selected sample that represented the population of Portugal. The instrument used to record information on food insecurity had high internal consistency measures for this sample. Our study also examined a relationship that has been overlooked in older populations: the association between management of chronic diseases and food insecurity. The results of this study contribute to understanding the inter-related issues that affect health status and disease evolution.

CONCLUSIONS

In conclusion, our results have implications for clinical practice and public policy development. For an increasingly aging population, the greater odds of food insecurity among households of older adults and the associated factors indicates the importance of considering this problem as one of the main public health challenges.

Ensuring that older adults have enough food to meet their needs may be an important way to help them enjoy good health and remain active while aging. Food insecurity in older adults is an undesirable problem that requires additional attention. Food insecurity is associated with higher odds of chronic disease, poor self-management of chronic disease, and lower HRQoL. Because it is determined by economic factors, food insecurity is socially and ethically unacceptable. Therefore, during a period marked by significant financial stress, implementation of strategies aimed at ensuring the food security of the aging population is needed. We suggest that other evaluation and monitoring studies should be performed and further investigation using longitudinal data are needed to determine the health consequences of food insecurity among older adults. These results would assist health professionals and policymakers to better understand the barriers to achieve improved health in this population.

ETHICS STATEMENT

EpiDoC 3 study was performed according to the principles established by the Declaration of Helsinki and revised in 2013 in Fortaleza. The study was reviewed and approved by the National Committee for Data Protection and by the NOVA Medical School Ethics Committee. Participants provided informed consent to contribute in all phases of the study.

AUTHOR CONTRIBUTIONS

All authors contributed to this work. HC, AR, and MG performed the initial study. SF and CN analyzed the data. SF, CN, and OS interpreted the data. SF wrote the manuscript. HC, AR, and MG provided scientific support and revised the manuscript. All authors contributed to the further discussion of the manuscript. All authors read and approved the final manuscript.

FUNDING

This project was supported by a grant from the Public Health Initiatives Programme (PT06), financed by the EEA Grants Financial Mechanism 2009–2014.

REFERENCES

1. United Nations. *World Population Ageing. Department of Economic and Social Affairs*. Population Division (2015).
2. Direção Geral da Saúde. *Portugal Idade Maior Em Números – 2014*. Lisboa (2014).
3. Kamp B. Position of the American Dietetic Association, American Society for Nutrition, and Society for Nutrition Education: food and nutrition programs for community-residing older adults. *J Am Diet Assoc.* (2010) 110:463–72. doi: 10.1016/j.jada.2009.12.009
4. Food and Agriculture Organization of the United Nations. *An Introduction to the Basic Concepts of Food Security Food Security Information for Action.* (2008).
5. Russell J, Flood VM, Yeatman H, Mitchell P. Prevalence and risk factors of food insecurity among a cohort of older Australians. *J Nutr Heal Aging* (2014) 18:3–8. doi: 10.1007/s12603-013-0339-6
6. Bhargava V, Lee JS, Jain R, Johnson MA, Brown A. Food insecurity is negatively associated with home health and out-of-pocket expenditures in older adults. *J Nutr.* (2012) 142:1888–95. doi: 10.3945/jn.112.163220
7. Wolfe WS, Olson CM, Kendall A, Frongillo EA. Understanding food insecurity in the elderly: a conceptual framework. *J Nutr Educ.* (1996) 28:92–100.
8. Lee JS, Frongillo EA. Nutritional and health consequences are associated with food insecurity. *J Nutr Community Int Nutr.* (2001) 1503–9. doi: 10.1093/jn/131.5.1503
9. Bernstein M, Munoz N. Position of the academy of nutrition and dietetics: food and nutrition for older adults: promoting health and wellness. *J Acad Nutr Diet.* (2012) 112:1255–77. doi: 10.1016/j.jand.2012.06.015
10. Lee JS, Johnson MA, Brown A, Nord M. Food security of older adults requesting older americans act nutrition program in georgia can be validly measured using a short form of the U.S. Household Food Security Survey Module 1 - 3. *J Nutr.* (2011) 141:1362–8. doi: 10.3945/jn.111.139378
11. Lee JS, Frongillo EA. Factors associated with food insecurity among U.S. elderly persons: importance of functional impairments. *J Gerontol B Psychol Sci Soc Sci.* (2001) 56:S94–9. doi: 10.1093/geronb/56.2.S94
12. Escamilla RP. functional limitations, depression, and cash assistance are associated with food insecurity among older urban adults in Mexico City. *J Heal Care Poor Underserved.* (2016) 27:1537–54. doi: 10.1353/hpu.2016.0130
13. Quine S, Morrell S. Food insecurity in community-dwelling older Australians. *Public Health Nutr.* (2006) 9:219–24. doi: 10.1079/PHN2005834
14. Wolfe WS, Frongillo EA, Valois P. Understanding the experience of food insecurity by elders suggests ways to improve its measurement 1. *J Nutr.* (2003) 133:2762–9. doi: 10.1093/jn/133.9.2762
15. United Nations. *World Population Prospects: The 2015 Revision.* New York, NY (2015).
16. World Health Organization. *Active Ageing: A Policy Framework.* Madrid (2002).
17. Vilar-Compte M, Gaitán-rossi P, Pérez-Escamilla R. Food insecurity measurement among older adults : implications for policy and food security governance. *Glob Food Sec.* (2017) 14:87–95. doi: 10.1016/j.gfs.2017.05.003
18. Kim K, Frongillo EA. Participation in food assistance programs modifies the relation of food insecurity with weight and depression in elders. *J Nutr.* (2007) 137:1005–10. doi: 10.1093/jn/137.4.1005
19. Russell JC, Flood VM, Yeatman H Wang JJ, Mitchell P. Food insecurity and poor diet quality are associated with reduced quality of life in older adults. *Nutr Diet.* (2016) 73:50–8. doi: 10.1111/1747-0080.12263
20. World Health Organization. *Draft 1: Global Strategy and Action Plan on Ageing and Health.* (2015).
21. World Health Organization. *Action Plan for implementation of European Strategy for the Prevention and Control of Noncommunicable Diseases 2012-2016.* Copenhagen (2012).
22. Rodrigues AM, Gouveia N, Pereira L, Eusébio M, Ramiro S. EpiReumaPt – the study of Rheumatic and Musculoskeletal diseases in Portugal : a detailed view of the methodology. *Acta Reumatol Port.* (2015) 40:110–24. Available online at: http://europepmc.org/abstract/med/26219965
23. Gregório MJ, Rodrigues AM, Graça P, de Sousa RD, Dias SS, Branco JC, et al. Food insecurity is associated with low adherence to the mediterranean diet and adverse health conditions in Portuguese adults. *Front Public Health.* (2018) 6:38. doi: 10.3389/fpubh.2018 00038
24. Canhão H, Rodrigues, Ana Maria Andre B, Gregório MJ, Sousa RD, Santos MJ, Dias SS, et al. Challenges of ageing in Portugal – data from EpiDoC cohort. *Acta Med Port.* (2017) 31:80–93. doi: 10.20344/amp.9817
25. Ferreira PL, Ferreira LN, Pereira LN. Contributos para a validação da versão Portuguesa do EQ-5D. *Acta Med Port.* (2013) 26:664–75.
26. World Health Organization. *Obesity: Preventing and Managing the Global Epidemic. Vol. 894,* WHO technical report series. Geneva (2000).
27. Gregório MJ, Nogueira PJ GP. *The First Validation of the Household Food Insecurity Scale in a Sample of Portuguese Population. Desigual Sociais no acesso a Uma Aliment Saudável um Estud na Popul Portgueasa.* Tese doutoramento, Fac Ciências da Nutr e Aliment da Univ do Porto (2015).
28. Pérez-Escamilla R, Segall-Corrêa AM, Kurdian Maranha L, Sampaio Md MDFA, Marín-León L, Panigassi G. An adapted version of the U.S. Department of Agriculture Food Insecurity module is a valid tool for assessing

household food insecurity in Campinas, *Brazil. J Nutr.* (2004) 134:1923–8. doi: 10.1093/jn/134.8.1923
29. Bickel G, Nord M, Price C, Hamilton W, Cook J. *Guide to Measuring Household Food Security Revised 2000. United States Department of Agriculture.* (2000). p. 1–76.
30. Instituto Brasileiro de Geografia e Estatística - IBGE. *Segurança Alimentar - Pesquisa Nacional Por Amostra de Domicílios 2004-2009. ISBN 978-8.* Rio de Janeiro (2010).
31. World Health Organization. *Vienna Vienna Declaration on Nutrition and Noncommunicable Diseases in the Context of Health 2020. In: WHO Ministerial Conference on Nutrition and Noncommunicable Diseases in the Context of Health 2020.* (2013).p. 1–3.
32. Branco MJ, Nunes B CT. *Uma Observação sobre "Insegurança Alimentar."* Lisboa (2003).
33. Direção Geral da Saúde. *RELATÓRIO INFOFAMÍLIA 2011-2014 - Quatro anos de monitorização da Segurança Alimentar e outras questões de saúde relacionadas com condições socioeconómicas, em agregados familiares portugueses utentes dos cuidados de saúde primários do Serviço Nacional de.* Lisboa (2017).
34. Alvares L, Amaral TF. Food insecurity and associated factors in the Portuguese population. *Food Nutr Bull.* (2014) 35:395–402. doi: 10.1177/156482651403500401
35. Goldberg SL, Mawn BE. Predictors of Food Insecurity among Older Adults in the United States. *Public Health Nurs.* (2014) 32:397–407. doi: 10.1111/phn.12173
36. Nolan M, Rikard-Bell G, Mohsin M, Williams M. Food insecurity in three socially disadvantaged localities in Sydney, Australia. *Heal Promot J Aust.* (2006) 17:247–54. doi: 10.1071/HE 06247
37. Smith MD, Rabbitt MP, Coleman- Jensen A. Who are the World's food insecure? new evidence from the food and agriculture organization's food insecurity experience scale. *World Dev.* (2017) 93:402–12. doi: 10.1016/j.worlddev.2017.01.006
38. Carter MA, Dubois L, Tremblay MS. Place and food insecurity : a critical review and synthesis of the literature. *Public Health Nutr.* (2017) 17:94–112. doi: 10.1017/S1368980013000633
39. Pérez-zepeda MU, Castrejón-pérez RC, Wynne-bannister E, García-peña C. Frailty and food insecurity in older adults. *Public Health Nutr.* (2016) 19:2844–9. doi: 10.1017/S1368980016000987
40. Bocquier A, Vieux F, Lioret S, Dubuisson C, Caillavet F, Darmon N. Socio-economic characteristics , living conditions and diet quality are associated with food insecurity in France. *Public Health Nutr.* (2015) 18:2952–61. doi: 10.1017/S1368980014002912
41. Instituto Nacional de Estatística. *Rendimento e Condições de Vida 2014.* Lisboa (2015).
42. Banco de Portugal. Boletim Económico. *Departamento de Estudos Económicos.* Lisboa (2016).
43. Dhurandhar EJ. The food-insecurity obesity paradox : a resource scarcity hypothesis. *Physiol Behav.* (2016) 162:88–92. doi: 10.1016/j.physbeh.2016.04.025
44. Stuff JE, Casey PH, Szeto KL, Gossett JM, Robbins JM, Simpson PM, et al. Household food insecurity is associated with adult health status. *J Nutr Commun Int Nutition.* (2004) 2330–5. doi: 10.1093/jn/134.9.2330
45. Hernandez DC, Reesor L, Murillo R. gender disparities in the food insecurity-overweight and food insecurity-obesity paradox among low-income older adults. *J Acad Nutr Diet.* (2017) 117:1087–96. doi: 10.1016/j.jand.2017.01.014
46. Radermacher H, Feldman S, Bird S. Food Security in Older Australians from Different Cultural Backgrounds. *J Nutr Educ Behav.* (2010) 42:328–36. doi: 10.1016/j.jneb.2009.10.004
47. Leung CW, Epel ES, Ritchie LD, Crawford PB, Laraia BA. Food insecurity is inversely associated with diet quality of lower-income adults. *J Acad Nutr Diet.* (2014) 14:1943–53.e2. doi: 10.1016/j.jand.2014.06.353
48. Vozoris NT, Tarasuk VS. Household food insufficiency is associated with poorer health. *J Nutr Community Int Nutition.* (2003) 133:120–6. doi: 10.1093/jn/133.1.120
49. Seligman HK, Bindman AB, Vittinghoff E, Kanaya AM, Kushel MB. Food insecurity is associated with diabetes mellitus : results from the national health examination and nutrition examination survey (NHANES) 1999 – 2002. *J Gen Intern Med.* (2007) 22:1018–23. doi: 10.1007/s11606-007-0192-6
50. Gucciardi E, Vahabi M, Norris N, Paul J, Monte D, Farnum C. The Intersection between Food Insecurity and Diabetes : a Review. *Curr Nutr Rep.* (2014) 3:324–32. doi: 10.1007/s13668-014-0104-4
51. Vaccaro JA, Huffman FG. Sex and Race / Ethnic Disparities in Food Security and Chronic Diseases in U . S . Older Adults. *Gerontol Geriatr Med.* (2017) 3:1–9. doi: 10.1177/2333721417718344
52. Leung CW, Epel ES, Willett WC, Rimm EB, Laraia BA. Household food insecurity is positively associated with depression among low-income supplemental nutrition assistance program participants and income-eligible nonparticipants. *J Nutr.* (2015) 145:622–7. doi: 10.3945/jn.114.199414
53. Jones AD. Food insecurity and mental health status: a global analysis of 149 countries. *Am J Prev Med.* (2017) 53:264–273. doi: 10.1016/j.amepre.2017.04.008
54. Saiz AM, Aul AM, Malecki KM, Bersch AJ, Bergmans RS, LeCaire TJ, et al. Food insecurity and cardiovascular health: Findings from a statewide population health survey in Wisconsin. *Prev Med.* (2016) 93:1–6. doi: 10.1016/j.ypmed.2016.09.002
55. Stuff JE, Casey PH, Connell CL, Catherine M, Ms JMG, Harsha D, et al. Household food insecurity and obesity, chronic disease, and chronic disease risk factors. *J Hunger Environ Nutr.* (2006) 2:43–62. doi: 10.1300/J477v01n02_04
56. Brucker DL. The association of food insecurity with health outcomes for adults with disabilities. *Disabil Health J.* (2016) 10:286–93. doi: 10.1016/j.dhjo.2016.12.006
57. Champagne CM, Casey PH, Connell CL, Stuff JE, Gossett JM, Harsha DW, et al. Poverty and food intake in rural america: diet quality is lower in food insecure adults in the mississippi Delta. *J Am Diet Assoc.* (2007) 107:1886–94. doi: 10.1016/j.jada.2007.08.003
58. Wang E, McGinnis K, Bryante K, Goulet J, Gibert C. Food insecurity and health : data from the veterans aging cohort study. *Public Health Rep.* (2015) 130:261–8. doi: 10.1177/003335491513000313
59. Martin-Fernandez J, Caillavet F, Lhuissier A, Chauvin P. Food insecurity, a determinant of obesity? - an analysis from a population-based survey in the paris metropolitan area, 2010. *Obes Facts* (2014) 7:120–9. doi: 10.1159/000362343
60. Dinour LM, Bergen D, Yeh MC. The food insecurity-obesity paradox: a review of the literature and the role food stamps may play. *J Am Diet Assoc.* (2007) 107:1952–61. doi: 10.1016/j.jada.2007.08.006
61. Ahn S, Smith ML, Hendricks M, Ory MG. Associations of food insecurity with body mass index among baby boomers and older adults. *Food Sec.* (2014) 6:423–33. doi: 10.1007/s12571-014-0344-6
62. Brewer DP, Ms CSC, Porter KN, Lee JS, Hausman DB. Physical limitations contribute to food insecurity and the food insecurity – obesity paradox in older adults at senior centers in georgia. *J Nutr Elder.* (2010) 29:150–69. doi: 10.1080/01639361003772343
63. J F, Stewart E, Stewart JM. Validity of self-report screening for overweight and obesity : evidence from the canadian community health survey. *Can J Public Heal.* (2008) 99:423–7.
64. Kuczmarski MF, Kuczmarski RJ, Najjar M. Effects of age on validity of self-reported height, weight, and body mass index: Findings from the third National Health and Nutrition Examination Survey, 1988-1994. *J Am Diet Assoc.* (2001) 28–34. doi: 10.1016/S0002-8223(01)00008-6
65. Bengle R, Sinnett S, Johnson T, Johnson MA, Brown A, Lee JS. Food insecurity is associated with cost- related medication non-adherence in community-dwelling , low-income older adults in Georgia. *J Nutr Elder.* (2010) 2:170–91. doi: 10.1080/01639361003772400
66. Afulani P, Herman D, Jensen A, Harrison G. Food insecurity and health outcomes among older adults : the role of cost-related medication underuse. *J Nutr Gerontol Geriatr.* (2015) 34:319–42. doi: 10.1080/21551197.2015.1054575

67. Graça P, Jorge Nogueira P, Gomes S, Abreu Santos C, Boavida J. Proposta Metodológica para a Avaliação da Insegurança Alimentar em Portugal. *Nutrícias* (2014) 21:4–11. Available online at: http://hdl.handle.net/10400.26/10175
68. McNaughton SA, Crawford D, Ball K, Salmon J. Understanding determinants of nutrition, physical activity and quality of life among older adults: the Wellbeing, Eating and Exercise for a Long Life (WELL) study. *Health Qual Life Outcomes* (2012) 10:109. doi: 10.1186/1477-7525-10-109
69. Amarantos E, Martinez A, Dwyer J. Nutrition and quality of life in older adults. *J Gerontol.* (2001) 56:54–64. doi: 10.1093/gerona/56.suppl_2.54

15

Mitophaging: Mitophagy in Aging and Disease

Daniela Bakula and Morten Scheibye-Knudsen**

Department of Cellular and Molecular Medicine, Center for Healthy Aging, University of Copenhagen, Copenhagen, Denmark

Edited by:
Konstantinos Palikaras, Foundation for Research and Technology Hellas, Greece

Reviewed by:
Nabil Eid, United Arab Emirates University, United Arab Emirates
Carsten Culmsee, University of Marburg, Germany

***Correspondence:**
Daniela Bakula
bakula@sund.ku.dk
Morten Scheibye-Knudsen
mscheibye@sund.ku.dk;
morten@forsoegsperson.dk

Maintaining mitochondrial health is emerging as a keystone in aging and associated diseases. The selective degradation of mitochondria by mitophagy is of particular importance in keeping a pristine mitochondrial pool. Indeed, inherited monogenic diseases with defects in mitophagy display complex multisystem pathologies but particularly progressive neurodegeneration. Fortunately, therapies are being developed that target mitophagy allowing new hope for treatments for previously incurable diseases. Herein, we describe mitophagy and associated diseases, coin the term mitophaging and describe new small molecule interventions that target different steps in the mitophagic pathway. Consequently, several age-associated diseases may be treated by targeting mitophagy.

Keywords: autophagy, mitophagy, aging, mitophaging, monogenic disorders, interventions

MITOCHONDRIAL INTEGRITY DEFINES ORGANISMAL HEALTH

Mitochondria, the powerhouses of eukaryotic cells, are the key organelles for energy production allowing organismal growth and survival. Besides serving as adenosine triphosphate generators, mitochondria act as signaling hubs for programmed cell death, regulate calcium homeostasis and are required for cholesterol, nucleotide and amino acid synthesis (Sun et al., 2016). To fulfil their broad range of biological roles, mitochondria contain more than 1,000 proteins that localize and function in four specialized compartments, the outer membrane, the inner membrane, the intermembrane space and the matrix. The minority of mitochondrial proteins are encoded by the circular mitochondrial genome, whereas the vast majority is encoded in the nuclear genome. However, mutations in both genomes can cause a heterogeneous group of disorders, known as mitochondrial diseases, which are characterized by severe metabolic and neurological defects. Due to their highly variable clinical features, the prevalence of mitochondrial diseases has likely been underestimated (Haas et al., 2007; Wallace, 2018). Nevertheless, advances in next generation sequencing technologies have simplified the clinical diagnosis and enabled molecular characterization of so far undescribed mitochondrial diseases (Calvo et al., 2012; Cui et al., 2013; Legati et al., 2016). Notably, computational approaches relying on phenotypic description of mitochondrial diseases can help to characterize new mitochondrial diseases of previously unknown pathogenesis (Scheibye-Knudsen et al., 2013).

Increased evidence indicates that mitochondrial integrity is disrupted during the aging process and contributes to the pathogenesis of age-related disorders in humans (Kauppila et al., 2017; Youle, 2019). In line with this, mice that carry a defective proof-reading mitochondrial DNA polymerase gamma show an accelerated aging phenotype that may be driven by the accumulation of mutations in the mitochondrial DNA (mtDNA) (Trifunovic et al., 2004). The described correlation between levels of mtDNA deletions in human brain and aging as well as the association between mtDNA haplogroups and diseases, further supports the direct influence of mitochondria on health- and lifespan in organisms (Cortopassi and Arnheim, 1990; Corral-Debrinski et al., 1992; Hudson et al., 2014; Wallace, 2015). Indeed, dysfunctional degradation of mitochondria through the process of mitophagy is increasingly associated with degenerative diseases and aging, a phenomenon we call mitophaging. Evidently, the maintenance of functional mitochondria is necessary to sustain cellular homeostasis and organismal health.

MITOCHONDRIAL QUALITY CONTROL MECHANISMS

Mitochondria have evolved multiple mechanisms ensuring mitochondrial quality. For instance, mitochondrial chaperones and proteases are constantly preventing the accumulation of misfolded and aggregated proteins by monitoring proteostasis through the mitochondrial unfolded protein stress response (UPR^{mt}) (Melber and Haynes, 2018), a mechanism that has been shown to be critical for longevity in mammals (Houtkooper et al., 2013; Mouchiroud et al., 2013). Further, mitochondria are dynamic organelles existing in large tubular and highly dynamic networks that constantly undergo fission and fusion processes, thereby leading to the dilution of non-functional mitochondria (Youle and van der Bliek, 2012).

Nevertheless, autophagy is the only known pathway that mediates the turnover of whole mitochondria to avoid cellular damage and apoptosis. The degradation process is mediated by a double-membrane vesicle, known as the autophagosome, and it was first observed in mammalian cells by electron microscopy (De Duve and Wattiaux, 1966). For a long time, autophagy was considered a non-selective bulk degradation pathway, however, when the yeast mitochondrial protein Uth1p was found to be involved in the selective degradation of mitochondria (Kissová et al., 2004), the term "mitophagy" was subsequently introduced (Lemasters, 2005).

Herein, we discuss the role of mitophagy in impacting human disease development and the aging process itself. Further, interventions that target mitophagy will be discussed that may provide a promising strategy for the treatment of a broad spectrum of diseases.

WHAT IS MITOPHAGY?

The process of mitophagy can act either as a response to various stress stimuli including nutrient starvation and oxidative stress or as a programmed removal of mitochondria (Palikaras et al., 2018; Pickles et al., 2018). Different pathways are known to regulate mitophagy, the best-studied pathway is mediated by the phosphatase and tensin homologue (PTEN)-induced putative kinase 1 (PINK1) and the E3-ubiquitin ligase Parkin (**Figure 1A**). Mutations in both genes encoding PINK1 and Parkin (PARK2), have been reported to cause autosomal recessive forms of Parkinson's Disease (PD) (Kitada et al., 1998; Valente et al., 2004). Under un-stressed conditions, PINK1 is imported via the translocase of the outer membrane and translocase of the inner membrane (TOM/TIM) complex in a membrane potential dependent manner into mitochondria, leading to proteolytic cleavage of PINK1 (Jin et al., 2010; Deas et al., 2011; Meissner et al., 2011). The N-terminal truncated PINK1 is subsequently released to the cytosol, and degraded by the proteasome (Yamano and Youle, 2013). Loss of mitochondrial membrane potential disrupts the transport of PINK1 across the mitochondrial membrane leading to the accumulation of uncleaved PINK1 at the outer mitochondrial membrane. Subsequently, PINK1 regulates the recruitment and activation of the cytosolic Parkin via direct phosphorylation of the Parkin Ub-like (UBL) domain or via the phosphorylation of ubiquitin (Kondapalli et al., 2012; Shiba-Fukushima et al., 2012; Iguchi et al., 2013; Kane et al., 2014; Kazlauskaite et al., 2014; Koyano et al., 2014; Ordureau et al., 2014; Wauer et al., 2015). Once activated, Parkin drives the ubiquitination of multiple substrates, which leads to a positive feed forward mechanism through the generation of additional substrates for Pink1 (Ordureau et al., 2014).

In recent years, several substrates, in particular mitochondrial outer membrane proteins and autophagy receptors, have been identified to be ubiquitinated by the PINK1/Parkin-mediated signaling pathway (Sarraf et al., 2013). For instance, the mitochondrial fusion proteins mitofusin 1 and 2 (Mfn1 and Mfn2) are degraded in a PINK1/parkin dependent manner to make mitochondria accessible for degradation and to prevent fusion of damaged mitochondria with the healthy network (Gegg et al., 2010; Tanaka et al., 2010). However, conditional double-knockout of Mfn1 and Mfn2 in mice leads to mitochondrial dysfunction and, in line with this, Mfn2-depleted cardiomyocytes are deficient in Parkin recruitment to the mitochondrial outer membrane (Chen et al., 2011; Chen and Dorn, 2013). A similar priming function of mitochondria has been described for other mitochondrial proteins such as Miro1 and VDAC1 (Geisler et al., 2010; Wang et al., 2011; Sun et al., 2012; Safiulina et al., 2019). Recently, the apoptotic protein BAK has been identified as a Parkin target, further connecting Parkin-mediated mitophagy to the regulation of cellular apoptosis (Bernardini et al., 2019). The ubiquitination events driven by PINK1 and Parkin enable the recruitment of autophagy substrate receptors to the mitochondrial membrane including p62, Optineurin and NDP52, thereby promoting the engulfment of mitochondria by autophagosomes (Geisler et al., 2010; Wong and Holzbaur, 2014; Lazarou et al., 2015).

Notably, transcriptional regulation is a crucial process for functional PINK1-Parkin-mediated mitophagy. For instance, PINK1-Parkin-mediated mitophagy induction upon cellular stress such as through reactive oxygen species or ethanol exposure leads to the nuclear translocation of several transcription factors, including the transcription factor EB (TFEB) and the nuclear respiratory factors (NRFs), controlling the expression of mitochondrial, autophagy and lysosomal genes (Nezich et al., 2015; Ivankovic et al., 2016; Eid et al., 2019). Parkin expression itself has also been shown to be tightly controlled by stress pathways such as the unfolded protein response pathway and its activating transcription factor 4 (ATF4) (Bouman et al., 2011). Altogether, this highlights the great number of potential therapeutic avenues to target the PINK1-Parkin signaling pathway.

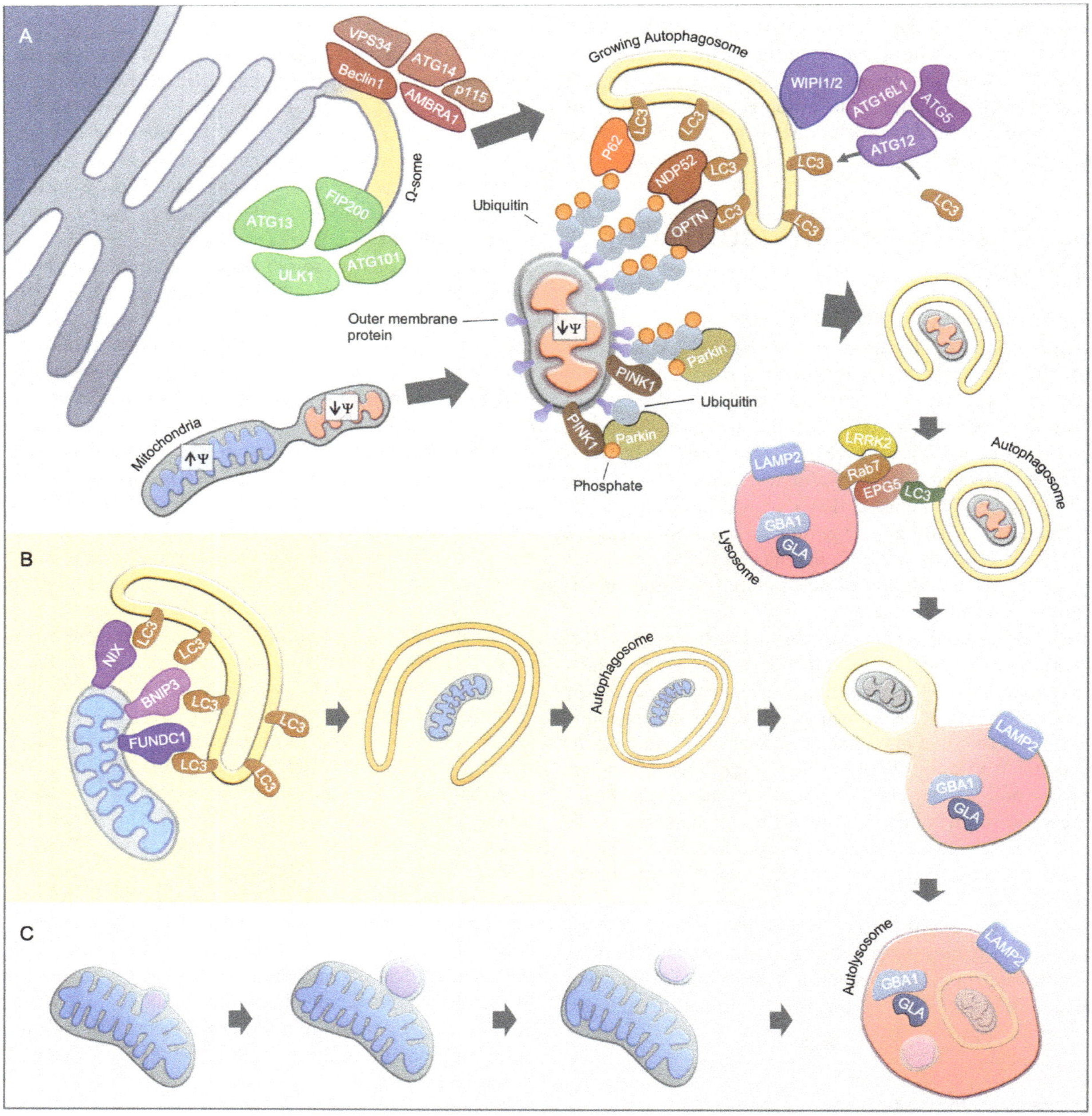

FIGURE 1 | Mitophagy pathways. **(A)** Ubiquitin-dependent PINK1/Parkin-mediated mitophagy. Upon mitochondrial damage, PINK1 is stabilized at the outer mitochondrial membrane, leading to Parkin activation and subsequent ubiquitination of mitochondrial proteins. Finally, autophagy receptors such as NDP52, OPTN, and p62 are recruited to mediate the engulfment of mitochondria by the autophagosomal membrane through the interaction with LC3. A possible source of the autophagosomal membrane is provided by the endoplasmic reticulum, where the autophagy core complexes VPS34 and ULK1 initiate the membrane formation. The membrane formation is further mediated by WIPI1 and WIPI2, leading to the recruitment of the ATG16L1-complex and LC3, thereby facilitating the formation of autophagosomes. Finally, autophagosomes fuses with acidic lysosomes, a step that is regulated by concerted action of autophagosomal and lysosomal proteins. **(B)** Ubiquitin-independent receptor-mediated mitophagy. Ubiquitin-independent receptor mediated mitophagy is mediated by the recruitment of autophagy receptor proteins such as NIX, BNIP3, and FUNDC1 to the mitochondrial membrane. The receptor proteins recruit LC3, which enables the engulfment of mitochondria by autophagosomes. **(C)** Alternative degradation pathways. Piecemeal mitophagy and mitochondrial-derived vesicle degradation are cellular pathways that mediate localized degradation of mitochondria.

Pink1/Parkin-independent mitophagy pathways mainly rely on receptor proteins which mediate the recruitment of LC3/GABARAPs for the removal of mitochondria (**Figure 1B**). For instance, the BCL2-related protein NIX (also known as BNIP3L) mediates mitophagy in mammals during reticulocyte differentiation, a process that requires the elimination of mitochondria (Schweers et al., 2007; Sandoval et al., 2008; Novak et al., 2010). In line with this, *NIX* knockout mice develop anemia and reticulocytosis (Schweers et al., 2007; Sandoval et al., 2008). The interaction of NIX with LC3 protein members is mediated via the LC3-interacting (LIR) motif, however, re-expression of LIR-mutant NIX in NIX deficient reticulocytes partially rescued the observed phenotype, indicating LC3-independent or even autophagy-independent mechanisms for mitochondrial clearance in reticulocyte differentiation (Novak et al., 2010). Another LIR-motif containing protein, FUNDC1, regulates mitophagy under hypoxic conditions by promoting mitochondrial fission (Liu et al., 2012; Chen et al., 2016). During cardiac progenitor cell differentiation, FUNDC1 and NIX, but not Pink1 and Parkin, are upregulated to maintain a functional mitochondrial network (Lampert et al., 2019). Mitophagy is therefore also regulated in a lineage dependent fashion.

Localized removal of mitochondrial subdomains can be mediated by piecemeal mitophagy or mitochondrial-derived vesicles (**Figure 1C**). Mitochondrial-derived vesicle formation is thought to be dependent on PINK1/Parkin but independent of the canonical autophagy machinery (Soubannier et al., 2012; McLelland et al., 2014). Whereas, the accumulation of misfolded mitochondrial protein aggregates leads to localized recruitment of Parkin and autophagy proteins, thereby facilitating the degradation of mitochondrial subdomains (Burman et al., 2017). A PINK1/Parkin-independent piecemeal mitophagy has been recently reported that drives LC3C- and p62-mediated degradation of mitochondrial subregions (Le Guerroué et al., 2017). However, the protein machinery for these mitochondrial degradation pathways may overlap with the classic mitophagy pathways as well as their physiological relevance needs to be further investigated.

MITOPHAGING

A decline in mitochondrial function is a hallmark of the aging process and is connected to other aging hallmarks such as telomere dysfunction, genome instability and cellular senescence. However, it remains largely unclear how these processes are interconnected and finally provoke disruption of the cellular and tissue integrity (López-Otín et al., 2013). There is accumulating evidence that mitophagy impacts health- and lifespan in different model organisms. Using a transgenic mouse strain that expresses the fluorescent mitophagy reporter mt-Keima, a decreased mitophagy level was observed in the hippocampal dentate gyrus in 21-month old mice compared to 3-month old mice (Sun et al., 2015). A decline in mitophagy was also observed in aged mouse hearts, in line with this, altered mitophagy has been shown to influence different cardiac pathologies (Hoshino et al., 2013; Bravo-San Pedro et al., 2017). Other tissues that contribute to aging phenotypes are also characterized by defective mitophagy, as shown recently for aged skeletal muscle satellite cells isolated from humans or mice (García-Prat et al., 2016). Notably, decreased expression of mitophagy genes was observed in the skeletal muscle of physically inactive elderly women (Drummond et al., 2014).

The effect of changes in mitophagy on health- and lifespan has been particularly demonstrated by using the model organisms *C. elegans* and *D. melanogaster*. Several genetic studies in *D. melanogaster* revealed that the overexpression of mitochondrial and mitophagy genes leads to increased health- and/or lifespan. For instance, the overexpression of the mitochondrial fission protein dynamin-related protein 1 (DRP1) increased the lifespan along with a prolonged healthspan in flies (Rana et al., 2017). The importance of mitochondrial fission on drosophila lifespan was further demonstrated by the observation that lifespan extension caused by the overexpression of p62 was abrogated in DRP1 mutant flies (Aparicio et al., 2019). Lifespan extension in flies was also observed after overexpression of Parkin and Pink1, whereby, Parkin overexpression counteracted increased Mfn2 levels, which can be observed during aging (Todd and Staveley, 2012; Rana et al., 2013). These findings are consistent with studies in *C. elegans*, where mitophagy has been shown to contribute to lifespan regulation (Palikaras et al., 2015; Schiavi et al., 2015). Evidently, there is substantial data supporting a role of declining mitophagy, mitophaging, in aging.

WHAT HAPPENS WHEN MITOPHAGY GOES WRONG?

Impaired mitophagy contributes to the pathogenesis of several human diseases, in particular to age-related sporadic disorders, such as Parkinson's disease, Alzheimer's disease, cardiomyopathies and cancer (Bernardini et al., 2017; Fivenson et al., 2017; Levine and Kroemer, 2019). While these observations yield interesting correlations between certain disease states and alterations in mitophagy it is difficult to deduct causation. Here, monogenic diseases with specific defects in mitophagy may give us mechanistic understanding of pathogenesis and biology (**Table 1**). Thus, monogenic disorders may provide valuable tools for studying molecular pathomechanisms that are driven by defective mitophagy. To explore the clinical phenotype of autophagy diseases, we identified the clinical descriptions in the literature of all the diseases in **Table 1** and performed hierarchical clustering based on the prevalence of those features (**Figure 2A**; Scheibye-Knudsen et al., 2013; Andreassen et al., 2019). Although the clustering did connect clinically similar diseases (such as Charcot–Marie–Tooth 2A2 and 2B), it became immediately apparent that there is no good correlation between clinical outcome and the putative molecular function of the gene responsible for the disease. Indeed, principal component analysis also did not show any obvious separation of clinical groups based on proposed molecular functions (**Figure 2B**). This suggests that our knowledge of the pathogeneses of most of these disorders is quite limited. Nevertheless, when looking at the average prevalence of clinical features across all aging diseases there was a considerable overrepresentation of neurological features suggesting that defects in autophagy often leads to brain disease (**Figure 2C**). More specifically, the phenotype in the autophagy disorders show significant overlap with what is seen in mitochondrial diseases indicating that mitochondrial dysfunction may be driving diseases in many autophagy-related

TABLE 1 | Examples of autophagy/mitophagy-related monogenic disorders.

Disease	Gene	Protein function	Symptoms	References
Amyotrophic lateral sclerosis	OPTN (AD)	Autophagy receptor	Motor neuron degeneration	Weil et al., 2018
Alzheimer's disease	APP (AD)	Transmembrane protein	Dementia	Fang et al., 2019
Ataxia-telangiectasia	ATM (AR)	DNA-damage response	Cerebellar degeneration, Telangiectasia, Radiosensitivity	Fang et al., 2016
Autosomal dominant optic atrophy	OPA1 (AD)	Mitochondrial fusion protein	Optic atrophy	White et al., 2009; Liao et al., 2017
Barth syndrome	TAZ (XLR)	Mitochondrial protein	3-Methylglutaconic aciduria, Cardiomyopathy, Neutropenia; Muscle weakness	Hsu et al., 2015
Charcot–Marie–Tooth disease	MFN2, RAB7 (AD, AR)	Mitochondrial fusion protein, endolysosomal protein	Neuropathy, Muscle weakness	Yamano et al., 2014; Rizzo et al., 2016
Charlevoix-Saguenay spastic ataxia	SACS (AR)*	Co-chaperone	Cerebellar degeneration, Neuropathy, Spasticity	Bradshaw et al., 2016; Morani et al., 2019
Cockayne syndrome	ERCC6 (AR)	DNA damage repair	Cerebellar degeneration, Short stature, Sun sensitivity	Scheibye-Knudsen et al., 2012
Danon disease	LAMP2 (XLD)	Autolysosome formation	Cardiomyopathy, Developmental delay, Myopathy	Tanaka et al., 2000; Hashem et al., 2017
Fabry disease	GLA (XL)	Lysosomal enzyme	Nephropathy, Cardiomyopathy, Hearing loss, Neuorpathy	Chévrier et al., 2010; Ivanova et al., 2019
Fanconi anemia	FANCC (AR)	DNA damage repair	Short stature, Anemia, Skin pigmentation changes, Osteopenia	Sumpter et al., 2016
Frontotemporal dementia and/or amyotrophic lateral sclerosis	TBK1, SQSTM1 (AD)	Serine/threonine protein kinase, autophagy receptor	Dementia, Motor neuron degeneration,	Geisler et al., 2010; Richter et al., 2016
Gaucher disease	GBA1 (AR)	Lysosomal enzyme	Hepatosplenomegali, Pancytopenia, Gaucher cells	Osellame et al., 2013
Intellectual developmental disorder with short stature and variable skeletal anomalies	WIPI2 (AR)	Autophagosome formation	Mental retardation, Cerebral atrophy, Short stature	Zachari et al., 2019
Krabbe disease	GALC (AR)*	Lysosomal enzyme	Spasticity, Leukodystrophy, Myoclonus	Del Grosso et al., 2019
Lafora disease	EPM2A (AR)	Glycogen synthesis	Seizures, Mental retardation	Lahuerta et al., 2018
Microcephaly 18	WDFY3 (AD)	Selective autophagy, aggrephagy	Cognitive deficits, Microcephaly	Napoli et al., 2018
MRXST	HUWE1 (XL)	E3-ubiquitin protein ligase	Mental retardation, Macrocephaly, Macroorchidism, Seizures	Di Rita et al., 2018
Mucolipidosis II	GNPTAB (AR)*	Lysosomal enzyme	Developmental delay, Short stature, Cardiomegaly, Dysostosis multiplex	Otomo et al., 2009
Multiple sulfatase deficiency	SUMF1 (AR)*	ER-resident enzyme	Cerebellar degeneration, Mental retardation, Hepatosplenomegaly	Settembre et al., 2008
NADGP	SQSTM1 (AR)	Autophagy receptor	Cerebellar degeneration, Mental retardation, Vertical gaze palsy, Dystonia	Geisler et al., 2010
NBIA5	WDR45 (XLD)*	Autophagosome formation	Cerebellar degeneration, Developmental delay, Brain iron accumulation, Dystonia	Saitsu et al., 2013
NEDSBAS	WDR45B (AR)*	Autophagosome formation	Seizures, Developmental delay, Spasticity, Cerebral atrophy	Bakula et al., 2017; Suleiman et al., 2018

(Continued)

TABLE 1 | Continued

Disease	Gene	Protein function	Symptoms	References
Neuronal Ceroid Lipofuscinosis	PPT1 (AR)*	Lysosomal enzyme	Mental retardation, Seizures, Cerebellar degeneration	Mukherjee et al., 2019
Niemann-Pick disease	NPC1 (AR)*	Lysosomal protein	Seizures, Jaundice, Hepatosplenomegaly, Mental retardation	Pacheco et al., 2007
Parkinson's disease	LRRK2, PARK2, PARK6 (AD)	Mitochondrial proteins	Bradykinesia, Rigidity, Tremor, Dementia	Ryan et al., 2015
Pompe disease	GAA (AR)*	Lysosomal enzyme	Muscle weakness, Cardiomyopathy, Hypotonia	Raben et al., 2012
Spastic paraplegia 15	ZFYVE26 (AR)*	Autophagosome formation	Spasticity, Hyperactive reflexes, Mental retardation	Vantaggiato et al., 2013; Denton et al., 2018
Spastic paraplegia 49	TECPR2 (AR)*	LC3/GABARAP binding protein	Developmental delay, Spasticity, Dysmorphism, Microcephaly, Hypotonia, Short stature	Oz-Levi et al., 2012
Spinocerebellar ataxia 25	ATG5 (AR)	Autophagosome formation	Developmental delay, Cerebellar degeneration Mental retardation	Sun et al., 2015
Spinocerebellar ataxia 4	VPS13D (AR)	Lysosomal enzyme	Hyperactive reflexes, Muscle atrophy, Cerebeller degeneration	Anding et al., 2018
Vici syndrome	EPG5 (AR)*	Autolysosome formation	Cataracts, Cardiomyopathy, Developmental delay, Hypotonia, Immune deficiency, Corpus callosum agenesis	Cullup et al., 2013
Wolfram syndrome	WFS1 (AR)	Calcium homeostasis	Diabetes mellitus type 1 Optic atrophy, Hearing loss, Diabetes insipidus	Cagalinec et al., 2016
Xeroderma pigmentosum group A	XPA (AR)	DNA damage repair	Sun sensitivity, Cerebellar degeneration, Cancer, Neuropathy	Fang et al., 2014
Zellweger syndrome	PEX13 (AR)	Peroxisome biogenesis	Developmental delay, Dysmorphism, Hepatosplenomegaly, Seizures	Lee et al., 2017

For genes that are marked with an asterisk the function in mitophagy remains largely unknown, however, defects in autophagy and mitochondrial dysfunction have been reported. Abbreviations: AD, autosomal dominant; AR, autosomal-recessive; XLR, X-linked recessive; XLD, X-linked dominant.

disorders ranging from lysosomal diseases to bonafide mitophagy deficiencies (**Figures 2C,D**). In the following we will examine a few key examples of these disorders.

Defects in the Autophagic Machinery

To date, only a few monogenic diseases caused by single mutations in the autophagy core machinery have been reported. One of them, spinocerebellar ataxia-25 (SCAR25), is caused by a mutation in the *autophagy-related 5* gene (*ATG5*), encoding a protein that is part of the ATG12-ATG5-ATG16L1 complex, which facilitates LC3/GABARAP conjugation (Mizushima, 2020). So far, two siblings have been identified with SCAR25, presenting with clinical symptoms such as truncal ataxia and intellectual disability (Kim et al., 2016). In line with the neurological phenotypes, a neuron-specific knockout of *ATG5* in mice causes neuronal degeneration, by contrast, a complete *ATG5* knockout is neonatal lethal (Kuma et al., 2004; Hara et al., 2006). Ataxia is a common feature of many mitochondrial disorders (Scheibye-Knudsen et al., 2013), however, mitochondrial viability in SCAR25 has not been investigated so far. Thus, the contribution of mitochondrial defects to the reported clinical features in SCAR25 remains speculative, since ATG5-independent mitophagy pathways have been reported (Honda et al., 2014; Hirota et al., 2015).

Mutations in members of the human WD-repeat protein interacting with phosphoinositides (WIPI) family are known to cause neurological deficits. The WIPI protein family consists of four members, WIPI1–WIPI4, that contribute to the early steps of autophagosome formation (Proikas-Cezanne et al., 2004). The family member WIPI2 localizes in a phosphatidylinositol 3-phosphate-dependent manner to the autophagosomal membrane, where it facilitates ATG16L1 recruitment and LC3 lipidation (Dooley et al., 2014; Bakula et al., 2017). Recently, patients with mutations in the *WIPI2* gene have been described with multisystemic clinical features, primarily, neurological and skeletal deficiencies that are characterized by severe mental retardation and short stature (Jelani et al., 2019). Notably, WIPI2 overexpression prevents age-related autophagy

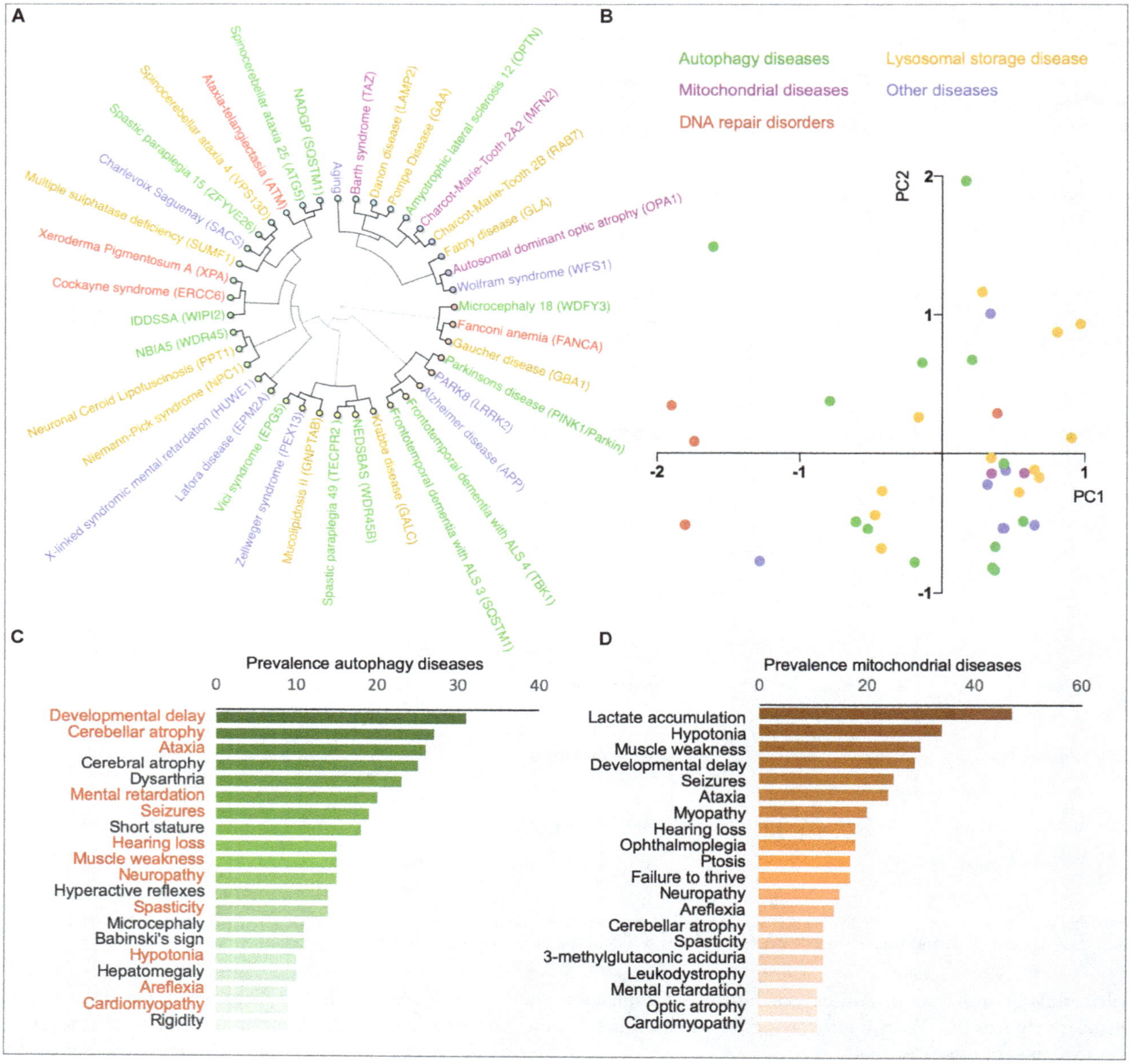

FIGURE 2 | Phenotype clustering of autophagy diseases. **(A)** Hierarchical clustering of diseases based on the published prevalence of clinical features in the diseases (for data and references see www.mitodb.com). **(B)** Principal component analysis of diseases based on the prevalence of clinical features. **(C)** The average prevalence of top-20 clinical features in all autophagy-related disorders (Red, shared with the top-20 features in mitochondrial disorders). **(D)** The average prevalence of clinical features in mitochondrial diseases.

decline in dorsal root ganglion neurons (Stavoe et al., 2019). Patients with mutations in the genes *WIPI3* (*WDR45B*) or *WIPI4* (*WDR45*) show severe and progressive neurodegenerative phenotypes (Haack et al., 2012; Hayflick et al., 2013; Saitsu et al., 2013; Suleiman et al., 2018). Notably, *WIPI4* mutations result in degeneration of the substantia nigra, a target area of the brain affected in Parkinson's disease (Mann et al., 1992). In line with these observations, *WIPI3* or *WIPI4* knockout mice show neurological defects, possibly caused by defective neuronal autophagy (Zhao et al., 2015; Ji et al., 2019). WIPI3 and −4 knockout mice display mitochondrial dysmorphology, which was also evident in WIPI4 mutant human fibroblast cells (Zhao et al., 2015; Seibler et al., 2018; Ji et al., 2019). The patient phenotypes caused by mutations in the *WIPI* genes highlight the importance of the WIPI protein members for neuronal function, however, the contribution of WIPI-mediated clearance of mitochondria in neurodegeneration remains unclear.

Deficiency in the late stage of autophagy is observed in the autosomal recessive neurological disorder, Vici syndrome. The disease is caused by mutations in the *ectopic P-granules autophagy protein 5* gene (*EPG5*), encoding for a Rab7 effector protein that is required for the fusion of late autophagosomes with lysosomes (Cullup et al., 2013; Wang et al., 2016). The disease is characterized by multisystemic defects that show some overlap with mitochondrial diseases, such as agenesis of corpus callosum, cardiomyopathy, immunodeficiency, cataracts and hypopigmentation (Cullup et al., 2013). Mitochondria with abnormal shape and distribution were observed in muscle tissue biopsies from patients with Vici syndrome or *EPG5* knockout mice (Cullup et al., 2013; Zhao et al., 2013). The importance of EPG5 in mitochondrial homeostasis was further highlighted by a study showing deficient mitochondrial clearance during spermatogenesis in an *EPG5*-deficient medaka fish line (Herpin et al., 2015).

Cargo recognition and degradation in selective autophagy is mediated by autophagy receptor proteins, such as optineurin and p62. Both proteins are associated with the progressive neurological disorder amyotrophic lateral sclerosis (ALS), which is primarily caused by loss of motor neurons (Maruyama et al., 2010; Fecto et al., 2011). Around 10% of ALS cases are caused by inherited single gene mutations and frequently show comorbidity with frontotemporal dementia (FTD). Interestingly, optineurin and p62 are phosphorylated by tank-binding kinase 1 (TBK1), a serine/threonine kinase that has also been implicated in ALS-FTD disease development (Cirulli et al., 2015; Freischmidt et al., 2015; Pottier et al., 2015). Thus, there is a striking correlation with mutations in multiple mitophagy players leading to ALS.

Defects in Mitochondrial Quality Control

Proteins involved in the regulation of mitochondrial quality control are essential modulators of mitophagy, consequently, understanding their molecular mechanisms may give important insights into the consequences of impaired mitophagy. In recent years, mitochondrial dysfunction has been extensively discussed as an important contributor to neurodegeneration in familial Parkinson's disease, as well as in idiopathic forms (Bose and Beal, 2016). Early onset recessive familial Parkinson's disease can be caused by mutations in the genes *Park2* (*Parkin*), *Park6* (*Pink1*), or *Park7* (*DJ-1*). All three proteins localize to mitochondria and loss of each of them leads to increased sensitivity toward oxidative stress along with mitochondrial and energetic dysfunction (Dodson and Guo, 2007). Pink1 and Parkin are directly involved in the mitophagy pathway, whereas, the precise function of DJ-1 remains under discussion. Interestingly, overexpression of Pink1 and Parkin rescues the observed phenotype caused by DJ-1 deficiency, suggesting partial redundancies in the mitophagic apparatus (Irrcher et al., 2010).

Mitochondrial fission and fusion are critical events for controlled degradation of damaged mitochondria. Optic atrophy 1 (OPA1) is an inner mitochondrial membrane protein that regulates the fusion of mitochondria, together with MFN1 and MFN2. Mutation in the *OPA1* gene has been observed to cause autosomal dominant optic atrophy (ADOA) often accompanied by myopathy and progressive ataxia (Yu-Wai-Man et al., 2010). Myopathy and neurodegeneration is also observed in patients with Charcot–Marie–Tooth syndrome caused by loss of the *MFN2* gene (Calvo et al., 2009), underscoring the importance of mitochondrial function in muscle and brain tissues. For both diseases impaired mitophagy has been reported, suggesting that dysfunctional mitophagy may contribute to the described disease pathology (White et al., 2009; Rizzo et al., 2016; Liao et al., 2017).

Defects in Lysosomal Function

Another group of diseases that may be partial driven by deficient mitophagy, are lysosomal storage disorders, a heterogenous group of more than 60 rare monogenic diseases that are caused by defects in lysosomal function (Platt et al., 2018). Some of the most well described are Gaucher disease and Niemann–Pick type C. Gaucher disease is caused by mutations in the *glucocerebrosidase* (*GBA*) gene, encoding a lysosomal enzyme required to hydrolyze the glycolipid glucosylceramide. Patients with Gaucher disease display features in multiple organs caused by lysosomal accumulation of glucosylceramide with a subset of patients display progressive neurodegeneration. Notably, the *GBA* gene represents a major risk locus for inherited Parkinson's disease supporting the idea that mitophagy is important in this disease (Goker-Alpan et al., 2004; Lwin et al., 2004). Reduced mitochondrial respiration, increased ROS production and increased alpha-synuclein accumulation can be observed in various GBA deficiency models, cellular changes that are also described to be central drivers of neuronal loss in Parkinson's disease (Osellame et al., 2013; Chen et al., 2019). Nieman Pick type C is caused by mutations in the *NPC1* gene and is characterized by developmental delay, progressive neurodegeneration, dysphagia and vertical gaze palsy, a combination of phenotypes that can also be observed in mitochondrial disorders. In patient-derived fibroblast cells and NPC1-deficient neuronal cells impaired autophagy and an accumulation of mitochondrial fragments have been observed upon lysosomal cholesterol accumulation (Pacheco et al., 2007; Elrick et al., 2012; Ordonez et al., 2012).

Secondary Defects in Mitophagy

In addition to diseases with primary defects in mitophagy, several diseases have been described with secondary mitophagic dysfunction. In the context of monogenic diseases displaying premature aging, loss of mitophagy was first described in Cockayne syndrome, a disease characterized by progressive neurodegeneration reminiscent of mitochondrial disorders (Scheibye-Knudsen et al., 2012). The pathogenesis likely involves dysregulation of uncoupling proteins (U) due to decreased activity of the PGC-1alpha transcription factor. UCPs regulate mitochondrial membrane potential and consequently a reduction in UCPs lead to increased mitochondrial membrane potential and loss of PINK1 mediated mitophagy. Accordingly, overexpression of UCP2 can rescue mitochondrial and mitophagic defects in Cockayne syndrome. Notably, the same pathogenesis is found in related DNA repair disorders xeroderma pigmentosum group A and ataxia-telangiectasia (Fang et al., 2014, 2016).

Another disease that is characterized by mitochondrial deficiency is Zellweger syndrome, which belongs to a subgroup of peroxisome biogenesis disorders (Salpietro et al., 2015). Zellweger syndrome is caused by mutations in one of 14 human

PEX genes, encoding for peroxin proteins that are required for the maintenance of peroxisomes (Waterham and Ebberink, 2012). Zellweger syndrome patients show dysmorphic features and suffer from severe neurological symptoms. Recently, PEX13 was shown to be required for mitophagy, but interestingly, dispensable for starvation-induced autophagy (Lee et al., 2017). Similarly, PEX5, an interaction partner of PEX13, has been shown to modulate autophagy via regulation of the mTOR signaling pathway (Eun et al., 2018), in line with this, mitochondrial defects can be observed in *PEX5* knockout models (Baumgart et al., 2001). However, it is still unclear, to what extent the clinical features of Zellweger syndrome are driven by mitophagic defects.

IS MITOPHAGY A THERAPEUTIC TARGET?

An increasing number of human diseases have been associated with impaired mitophagy, thus, interventions that modulate mitophagy may provide the possibility of counteracting disease development or progression (**Figure 3**). In recent years, multiple small molecules as well as lifestyle interventions have been shown to modulate autophagy, thereby causing health- and lifespan benefits in different organisms (Galluzzi et al., 2017). Due to the dependency on core autophagy regulators, mitophagy is modulated by most of the classic autophagy inducers such as the mTOR inhibitor rapamycin, the AMP-activated protein kinase (AMPK) activator AICAR as well as caloric restriction and exercise. In particular, the effectiveness of rapamycin and rapalogs has been intensively studied in the context of lifespan regulation and human disease development and rapamycin remain the most well documented compound for life- and healthspan extension in laboratory animals (Saxton and Sabatini, 2017). Further connections between longevity and mitophagy comes from work on the metabolite NAD^+ and the NAD^+-dependent acetylase Sirtuin 1 (SIRT1). Here, it has been shown that stimulation of SIRT1 through NAD^+ augmentation or small molecules leads to activation of the energy responsive kinase AMPK that in turns regulates a central autophagy regulator, Unc-51-like kinase 1 (ULK1) (Egan et al., 2011; Price et al., 2012). Further, SIRT1 and AMPK also regulate the transcription factor PGC-1alpha, a key regulator of mitochondrial function that was initially found to control UCP levels and thereby mitochondrial membrane potential (Puigserver et al., 1998; Cantó et al., 2009). Indeed, SIRT1 activation leads to UCP-2 upregulation, stimulation of mitophagy and rescue of aging features in models of premature aging (Fang et al., 2014; Scheibye-Knudsen et al., 2014). Notably, direct stimulation of AMPK through the AMP-mimetic compound AICAR regulates mitochondrial dynamics via the induction of mitochondrial fission, further highlighting the broad effect of AMPK on mitochondrial function (Toyama et al., 2016).

Due to their great diversity, natural compounds are a tremendous source for novel mitophagy modulators. Urolithin A, a gut metabolite of ellagic acid, extends health- and lifespan in *C. elegans* as well as improving muscle function in rodent models via the induction of mitophagy (Ryu et al., 2016). The effectiveness of urolithin A was further highlighted in animal models of Alzheimer's disease, where the disease pathology was ameliorated in the group of urolithin A-treated mice (Fang et al., 2019). In a human clinical trial study, the safety of urolithin A was evaluated, and signatures of improved mitochondrial function were demonstrated (Andreux et al., 2019). Similar to Urolithin A, the potency of antibacterial compound actinonin was demonstrated in Alzheimer's disease models (Fang et al., 2019). Actinonin inhibits mitochondrial translation, thereby inducing mitophagy via the activation of the PINK1/Parkin-regulated signaling pathway (Richter et al., 2013; Sun et al., 2015; Burman et al., 2017). Another natural compound that has been suggested as a potential intervention for aging and diseases is the polyamine spermidine (Eisenberg et al., 2009; Madeo et al., 2018; Schwarz et al., 2018). The administration of spermidine leads to an induction of mitophagy in cardiomyocytes, along with cardio protection in mice (Eisenberg et al., 2016). The induction of autophagy via spermidine has been associated, among others, with the inhibition of the acetyltransferase EP300 and the ATM-driven activation of the PINK1/Parkin-regulated mitophagy pathway (Pietrocola et al., 2015; Qi et al., 2016).

Transcriptional regulation of mitophagy has also been shown as a viable pathway for increased mitochondrial health. An example is the synthetic compound PMI that stimulates mitophagy via the activation of the transcription factor Nrf2, which controls the expression of mitophagy genes including p62 (East et al., 2014; Bertrand et al., 2015). PMI treatment facilitates LC3 recruitment and mitochondrial ubiquitination in a PINK1/Parkin-independent manner, notably without disrupting the mitochondrial membrane potential (East et al., 2014).

Besides targeting mitophagy core proteins, intervention strategies targeting mitochondrial proteins may present a useful approach for disorders that are characterized by abnormal mitochondrial dynamic. Mdivi-1, has been identified in a yeast screen for mitochondrial fission inhibitors and several studies indicate its therapeutic potential for the treatment of neurological disorders (Cassidy-Stone et al., 2008; Cui et al., 2010; Solesio et al., 2012). However, the specificity of Mdivi-1 toward its putative target Drp1 has recently been questioned and needs to be further clarified (Bordt et al., 2017). USP30, a deubiquitinase that targets mitochondrial proteins, may present another promising target to facilitate mitophagy, since improved mitochondrial function was obtained upon USP30 depletion in different Parkinson's disease models (Bingol et al., 2014). Notably, MF-094 has been recently identified as a selective inhibitor of USP30 that may thereby facilitate mitophagy through increased ubiquitination of outer membrane proteins (Kluge et al., 2018). Thus, a number of mitophagy modulators have been identified, yet the main goal will be the precise and specific targeting of damaged mitochondria. One possible way is to apply chimeric molecules such as the recently generated autophagy-targeting chimeric molecule (AUTAC4) that selectively targets the mitochondrial membrane for ubiquitination and subsequent degradation (Takahashi et al., 2019). These approaches may be particularly efficacious in conditions of mitophaging where the mitophagy apparatus is likely intact but mitophagy occurs at suboptimal levels.

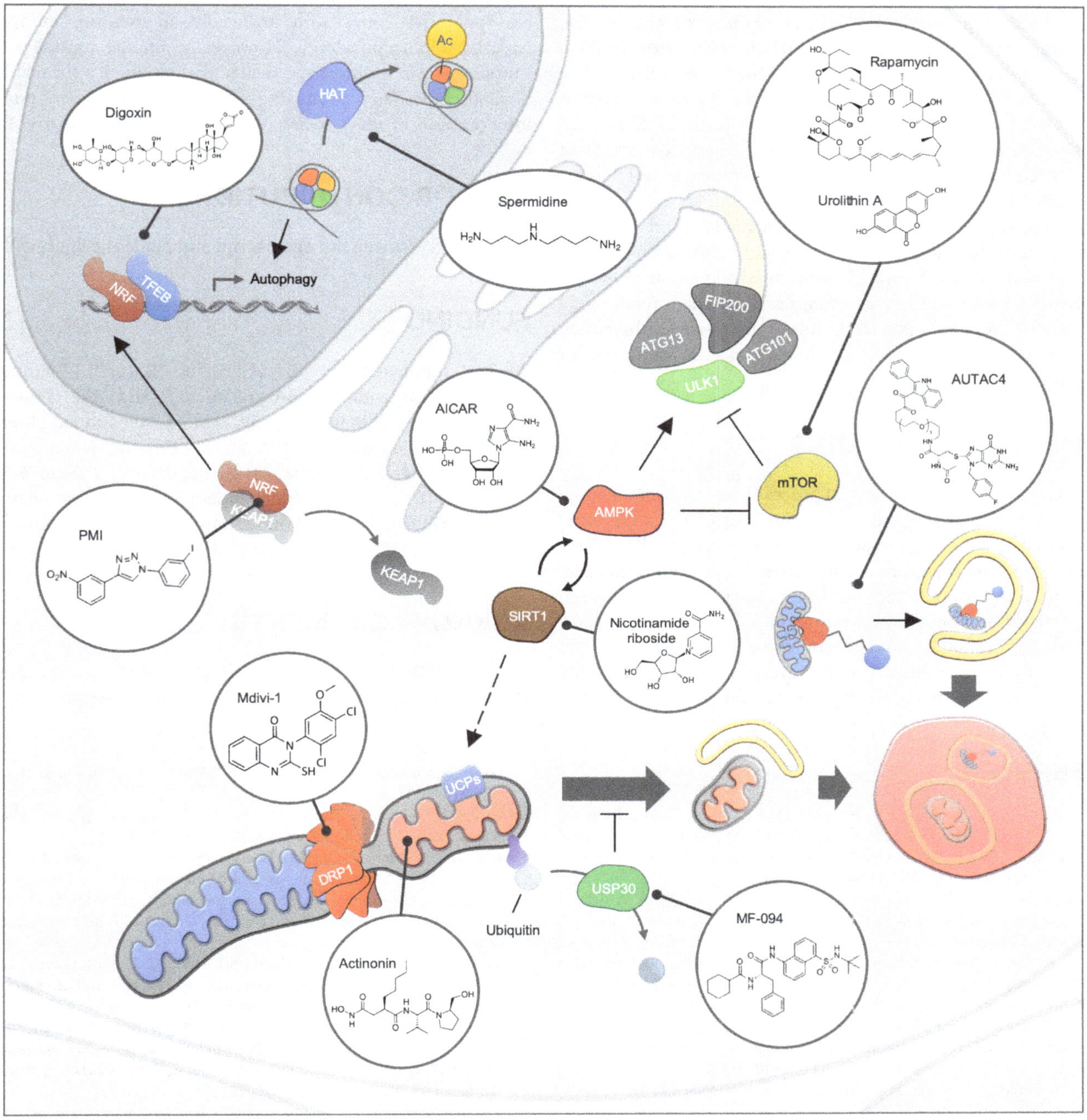

FIGURE 3 | Mitophagy interventions. An overview of different mitophagy modulating compounds and their targets. Abbreviations: Ac, Acetylation; HAT, Histone acetyltransferase.

In diseases characterized by dysfunctional lysosomes, stimulation of mitophagy may be detrimental due to an accumulation of undigested cargo material. In this regard, the inhibition of mitophagy is considered as a therapeutic strategy. In a mouse model of Pompe disease autophagy inhibition next to an enzyme replacement therapy has been proposed as a potential intervention (Raben et al., 2010). In line with this, knockdown of the mTOR pathway inhibitor TSC2 in muscle of Pompe disease mice reduced accumulation of autophagy markers and a decline in muscle atrophy was osberved (Lim et al., 2017). However, strategies to facilitate the fusion of autophagosomes and lysosomes in lysosomal storage disorders are also proposed for the treatment of several lysosomal storage disorders (Spampanato et al., 2013; Bartolomeo et al., 2017). TFEB, which controls the expression of autophagy as well as lysosomal genes and longevity (Napolitano and Ballabio, 2016), may provide a promising target since its agonists, such as the clinically approved cardiac drug digoxin or the natural compound ikarugamycin, improve metabolic function in mice and extend lifespan in *C. elegans* (Wang et al., 2017). The therapeutic potential of TFEB in Parkinson's disease was further highlighted by a recent study that showed restored TFEB and improved neurological function upon rapamycin treatment in Q311X mutant parkin mice independently of the parkin E3 ligase (Siddiqui et al., 2015).

In summary, great progress has been made in recent years, however, the clinical safety of mitophagy modulating drugs needs to be further clarified. More refined tools that allow the distinction between mitophagy and general macroautophagy may be beneficial and could accelerate future discoveries. Altogether, this will enable us to step closer toward clinical validation of mitophagy modulators.

CONCLUDING REMARKS

Mitophagy is emerging as a central process preserving organismal and, especially, neurological health. Since most trials targeting age-associated neurodegeneration in the last decades have been disappointing, new pharmaceutical avenues are direly needed. Here, mitophagy stimulators could play a key role. Indeed, several clinical trials are underway testing the efficacy of mitophagy modulating compounds and the outcome of these studies will undoubtedly prove critical for the future translatability of the field. Nonetheless, the regulatory mechanism of mitophagy and its contribution to age-associated diseases still remains elusive and potential issues with artificially augmenting mitophagy have not been considered. However, given the central role of mitophaging in multiple age-related pathologies it appears highly likely that these new promising approaches may present possible interventions in age-associated diseases. The future is bright!

AUTHOR CONTRIBUTIONS

DB and MS-K wrote the manuscript and made the figures.

FUNDING

DB is supported by the German Research Foundation (Forschungsstipendium; BA 6276/1-1) and the Lundbeck foundation (# R303-2018-3159). MS-K is funded through the Nordea Foundation (#02-2017-1749), the Novo Nordisk Foundation (#NNF17OC0027812), the Danish Cancer Society (#R167-A11015_001), the Independent Research Fund Denmark (#7016-00230B), the Neye Foundation, the Lundbeck Foundation (#R324-2019-1492) and *Insilico* Medicine.

ACKNOWLEDGMENTS

We would like to express our deep gratitude to Dr. Brenna Osborne for her critical comments to our manuscript.

REFERENCES

Anding, A. L., Wang, C., Chang, T.-K., Sliter, D. A., Powers, C. M., Hofmann, K., et al. (2018). Vps13D encodes a ubiquitin-binding protein that is required for the regulation of mitochondrial size and clearance. *Curr. Biol. CB* 28:287-295.e6. doi: 10.1016/j.cub.2017.11.064

Andreassen, S. N., Ben Ezra, M., and Scheibye-Knudsen, M. (2019). A defined human aging phenome. *Aging* 11, 5786–5806. doi: 10.18632/aging.102166

Andreux, P. A., Blanco-Bose, W., Ryu, D., Burdet, F., Ibberson, M., Aebischer, P., et al. (2019). The mitophagy activator urolithin A is safe and induces a molecular signature of improved mitochondrial and cellular health in humans. *Nat. Metab.* 1, 595–603. doi: 10.1038/s42255-019-0073-4

Aparicio, R., Rana, A., and Walker, D. W. (2019). Upregulation of the autophagy adaptor p62/SQSTM1 prolongs health and lifespan in middle-aged drosophila. *Cell Rep.* 28:1029–1040.e5. doi: 10.1016/j.celrep.2019.06.070

Bakula, D., Müller, A. J., Zuleger, T., Takacs, Z., Franz-Wachtel, M., Thost, A.-K., et al. (2017). WIPI3 and WIPI4 β-propellers are scaffolds for LKB1-AMPK-TSC signalling circuits in the control of autophagy. *Nat. Commun.* 8:15637. doi: 10.1038/ncomms15637

Bartolomeo, R., Cinque, L., De Leonibus, C., Forrester, A., Salzano, A. C., Monfregola, J., et al. (2017). mTORC1 hyperactivation arrests bone growth in lysosomal storage disorders by suppressing autophagy. *J. Clin. Invest.* 127, 3717–3729. doi: 10.1172/JCI94130

Baumgart, E., Vanhorebeek, I., Grabenbauer, M., Borgers, M., Declercq, P. E., Fahimi, H. D., et al. (2001). Mitochondrial alterations caused by defective peroxisomal biogenesis in a mouse model for Zellweger syndrome (PEX5 knockout mouse). *Am. J. Pathol.* 159, 1477–1494. doi: 10.1016/S0002-9440(10)62534-5

Bernardini, J. P., Brouwer, J. M., Tan, I. K., Sandow, J. J., Huang, S., Stafford, C. A., et al. (2019). Parkin inhibits BAK and BAX apoptotic function by distinct mechanisms during mitophagy. *EMBO J.* 38:e99916. doi: 10.15252/embj.201899916

Bernardini, J. P., Lazarou, M., and Dewson, G. (2017). Parkin and mitophagy in cancer. *Oncogene* 36, 1315–1327. doi: 10.1038/onc.2016.302

Bertrand, H. C., Schaap, M., Baird, L., Georgakopoulos, N. D., Fowkes, A., Thiollier, C., et al. (2015). Design, synthesis, and evaluation of triazole derivatives that induce Nrf2 dependent gene products and inhibit the Keap1-Nrf2 protein-protein interaction. *J. Med. Chem.* 58, 7186–7194. doi: 10.1021/acs.jmedchem.5b00602

Bingol, B., Tea, J. S., Phu, L., Reichelt, M., Bakalarski, C. E., Song, Q., et al. (2014). The mitochondrial deubiquitinase USP30 opposes parkin-mediated mitophagy. *Nature* 510, 370–375. doi: 10.1038/nature13418

Bordt, E. A., Clerc, P., Roelofs, B. A., Saladino, A. J., Tretter, L., Adam-Vizi, V., et al. (2017). The putative Drp1 inhibitor mdivi-1 is a reversible mitochondrial complex I inhibitor that modulates reactive oxygen species. *Dev. Cell* 40:583-594.e6. doi: 10.1016/j.devcel.2017.02.020

Bose, A., and Beal, M. F. (2016). Mitochondrial dysfunction in Parkinson's disease. *J. Neurochem.* 139(Suppl. 1), 216–231. doi: 10.1111/jnc.13731

Bouman, L., Schlierf, A., Lutz, A. K., Shan, J., Deinlein, A., Kast, J., et al. (2011). Parkin is transcriptionally regulated by ATF4: evidence for an interconnection between mitochondrial stress and ER stress. *Cell Death. Differ* 18, 769–782. doi: 10.1038/cdd.2010.142

Bradshaw, T. Y., Romano, L. E. L., Duncan, E. J., Nethisinghe, S., Abeti, R., Michael, G. J., et al. (2016). A reduction in Drp1-mediated fission compromises mitochondrial health in autosomal recessive spastic ataxia of Charlevoix Saguenay. *Hum. Mol. Genet.* 25, 3232–3244. doi: 10.1093/hmg/ddw173

Bravo-San Pedro, J. M., Kroemer, G., and Galluzzi, L. (2017). Autophagy and mitophagy in cardiovascular disease. *Circ. Res.* 120, 1812–1824. doi: 10.1161/CIRCRESAHA.117.311082

Burman, J. L., Pickles, S., Wang, C., Sekine, S., Vargas, J. N. S., Zhang, Z., et al. (2017). Mitochondrial fission facilitates the selective mitophagy of protein aggregates. *J. Cell Biol.* 216, 3231–3247. doi: 10.1083/jcb.201612106

Cagalinec, M., Liiv, M., Hodurova, Z., Hickey, M. A., Vaarmann, A., Mandel, M., et al. (2016). Role of mitochondrial dynamics in neuronal development: mechanism for wolfram syndrome. *PLoS Biol.* 14:e1002511. doi: 10.1371/journal.pbio.1002511

Calvo, J., Funalot, B., Ouvrier, R. A., Lazaro, L., Toutain, A., De Mas, P., et al. (2009). Genotype-phenotype correlations in Charcot-Marie-Tooth disease type 2 caused by mitofusin 2 mutations. *Arch. Neurol.* 66, 1511–1516. doi: 10.1001/archneurol.2009.284

Calvo, S. E., Compton, A. G., Hershman, S. G., Lim, S. C., Lieber, D. S., Tucker, E. J., et al. (2012). Molecular diagnosis of infantile mitochondrial disease with targeted next-generation sequencing. *Sci. Transl. Med.* 4:118ra10. doi: 10.1126/scitranslmed.3003310

Cantó, C., Gerhart-Hines, Z., Feige, J. N., Lagouge, M., Noriega, L., Milne, J. C., et al. (2009). AMPK regulates energy expenditure by modulating NAD+ metabolism and SIRT1 activity. *Nature* 458, 1056–1060. doi: 10.1038/nature07813

Cassidy-Stone, A., Chipuk, J. E., Ingerman, E., Song, C., Yoo, C., Kuwana, T., et al. (2008). Chemical inhibition of the mitochondrial division dynamin reveals its role in Bax/Bak-dependent mitochondrial outer membrane permeabilization. *Dev. Cell* 14, 193–204. doi: 10.1016/j.devcel.2007.11.019

Chen, C., Turnbull, D. M., and Reeve, A. K. (2019). Mitochondrial dysfunction in Parkinson's disease-cause or consequence? *Biology* 8:20038. doi: 10.3390/biology8020038

Chen, M., Chen, Z., Wang, Y., Tan, Z., Zhu, C., Li, Y., et al. (2016). Mitophagy receptor FUNDC1 regulates mitochondrial dynamics and mitophagy. *Autophagy* 12, 689–702. doi: 10.1080/15548627.2016.1151580

Chen, Y., and Dorn, G. W. (2013). PINK1-phosphorylated mitofusin 2 is a Parkin receptor for culling damaged mitochondria. *Science* 340, 471–475. doi: 10.1126/science.1231031

Chen, Y., Liu, Y., and Dorn, G. W. (2011). Mitochondrial fusion is essential for organelle function and cardiac homeostasis. *Circ. Res.* 109, 1327–1331. doi: 10.1161/CIRCRESAHA.111.258723

Chévrier, M., Brakch, N., Céline, L., Genty, D., Ramdani, Y., Moll, S., et al. (2010). Autophagosome maturation is impaired in Fabry disease. *Autophagy* 6, 589–599. doi: 10.4161/auto.6.5.11943

Cirulli, E. T., Lasseigne, B. N., Petrovski, S., Sapp, P. C., Dion, P. A., Leblond, C. S., et al. (2015). Exome sequencing in amyotrophic lateral sclerosis identifies risk genes and pathways. *Science* 347, 1436–1441. doi: 10.1126/science.aaa3650

Corral-Debrinski, M., Horton, T., Lott, M. T., Shoffner, J. M., Flint Beal, M., and Wallace, D. C. (1992). Mitochondrial DNA deletions in human brain: regional variability and increase with advanced age. *Nat. Genet.* 2, 324–329. doi: 10.1038/ng1292-324

Cortopassi, G. A., and Arnheim, N. (1990). Detection of a specific mitochondrial DNA deletion in tissues of older humans. *Nucleic Acids Res.* 18, 6927–6933. doi: 10.1093/nar/18.23.6927

Cui, H., Li, F., Chen, D., Wang, G., Truong, C. K., Enns, G. M., et al. (2013). Comprehensive next-generation sequence analyses of the entire mitochondrial genome reveal new insights into the molecular diagnosis of mitochondrial DNA disorders. *Genet. Med. Off. J. Am. Coll. Med. Genet.* 15, 388–394. doi: 10.1038/gim.2012.144

Cui, M., Tang, X., Christian, W. V., Yoon, Y., and Tieu, K. (2010). Perturbations in mitochondrial dynamics induced by human mutant PINK1 can be rescued by the mitochondrial division inhibitor mdivi-1. *J. Biol. Chem.* 285, 11740–11752. doi: 10.1074/jbc.M109.066662

Cullup, T., Kho, A. L., Dionisi-Vici, C., Brandmeier, B., Smith, F., Urry, Z., et al. (2013). Recessive mutations in EPG5 cause Vici syndrome, a multisystem disorder with defective autophagy. *Nat. Genet.* 45, 83–87. doi: 10.1038/ng.2497

De Duve, C., and Wattiaux, R. (1966). Functions of lysosomes. *Annu. Rev. Physiol.* 28, 435–492. doi: 10.1146/annurev.ph.28.030166.002251

Deas, E., Plun-Favreau, H., Gandhi, S., Desmond, H., Kjaer, S., Loh, S. H. Y., et al. (2011). PINK1 cleavage at position A103 by the mitochondrial protease PARL. *Hum. Mol. Genet.* 20, 867–879. doi: 10.1093/hmg/ddq526

Del Grosso, A., Angella, L., Tonazzini, I., Moscardini, A., Giordano, N., Caleo, M., et al. (2019). Dysregulated autophagy as a new aspect of the molecular pathogenesis of Krabbe disease. *Neurobiol. Dis.* 129, 195–207. doi: 10.1016/j.nbd.2019.05.011

Denton, K., Mou, Y., Xu, C.-C., Shah, D., Chang, J., Blackstone, C., et al. (2018). Impaired mitochondrial dynamics underlie axonal defects in hereditary spastic paraplegias. *Hum. Mol. Genet.* 27, 2517–2530. doi: 10.1093/hmg/ddy156

Di Rita, A., Peschiaroli, A., Acunzo, P. D., Strobbe, D., Hu, Z., Gruber, J., et al. (2018). HUWE1 E3 ligase promotes PINK1/PARKIN-independent mitophagy by regulating AMBRA1 activation via IKKα. *Nat. Commun.* 9:3755. doi: 10.1038/s41467-018-05722-3

Dodson, M. W., and Guo, M. (2007). Pink1, Parkin, DJ-1 and mitochondrial dysfunction in Parkinson's disease. *Curr. Opin. Neurobiol.* 17, 331–337. doi: 10.1016/j.conb.2007.04.010

Dooley, H. C., Razi, M., Polson, H. E. J., Girardin, S. E., Wilson, M. I., and Tooze, S. A. (2014). WIPI2 links LC3 conjugation with PI3P, autophagosome formation, and pathogen clearance by recruiting Atg12-5-16L1. *Mol. Cell* 55, 238–252. doi: 10.1016/j.molcel.2014.05.021

Drummond, M. J., Addison, O., Brunker, L., Hopkins, P. N., McClain, D. A., LaStayo, P. C., et al. (2014). Downregulation of E3 ubiquitin ligases and mitophagy-related genes in skeletal muscle of physically inactive, frail older women: a cross-sectional comparison. *J. Gerontol. A. Biol. Sci. Med. Sci.* 69, 1040–1048. doi: 10.1093/gerona/glu004

East, D. A., Fagiani, F., Crosby, J., Georgakopoulos, N. D., Bertrand, H., Schaap, M., et al. (2014). PMI: a $\Delta\Psi$m independent pharmacological regulator of mitophagy. *Chem. Biol.* 21, 1585–1596. doi: 10.1016/j.chembiol.2014.09.019

Egan, D. F., Shackelford, D. B., Mihaylova, M. M., Gelino, S., Kohnz, R. A., Mair, W., et al. (2011). Phosphorylation of ULK1 (hATG1) by AMP-activated protein kinase connects energy sensing to mitophagy. *Science* 331, 456–461. doi: 10.1126/science.1196371

Eid, N., Ito, Y., Horibe, A., Otsuki, Y., and Kondo, Y. (2019). Ethanol-induced mitochondrial damage in sertoli cells is associated with parkin overexpression and activation of mitophagy. *Cells* 8:30283. doi: 10.3390/cells8030283

Eisenberg, T., Abdellatif, M., Schroeder, S., Primessnig, U., Stekovic, S., Pendl, T., et al. (2016). Cardioprotection and lifespan extension by the natural polyamine spermidine. *Nat. Med.* 22, 1428–1438. doi: 10.1038/nm.4222

Eisenberg, T., Knauer, H., Schauer, A., Büttner, S., Ruckenstuhl, C., Carmona-Gutierrez, D., et al. (2009). Induction of autophagy by spermidine promotes longevity. *Nat. Cell Biol.* 11, 1305–1314. doi: 10.1038/ncb1975

Elrick, M. J., Yu, T., Chung, C., and Lieberman, A. P. (2012). Impaired proteolysis underlies autophagic dysfunction in Niemann–Pick type C disease. *Hum. Mol. Genet.* 21, 4876–4887. doi: 10.1093/hmg/dds324

Eun, S. Y., Lee, J. N., Nam, I.-K., Liu, Z.-Q., So, H.-S., Choe, S.-K., et al. (2018). PEX5 regulates autophagy via the mTORC1-TFEB axis during starvation. *Exp. Mol. Med.* 50:4. doi: 10.1038/s12276-017-0007-8

Fang, E. F., Hou, Y., Palikaras, K., Adriaanse, B. A., Kerr, J. S., Yang, B., et al. (2019). Mitophagy inhibits amyloid-β and tau pathology and reverses cognitive deficits in models of Alzheimer's disease. *Nat. Neurosci.* 22, 401–412. doi: 10.1038/s41593-018-0332-9

Fang, E. F., Kassahun, H., Croteau, D. L., Scheibye-Knudsen, M., Marosi, K., Lu, H., et al. (2016). NAD+ replenishment improves lifespan and healthspan in ataxia telangiectasia models via mitophagy and DNA repair. *Cell Metab.* 24, 566–581. doi: 10.1016/j.cmet.2016.09.004

Fang, E. F., Scheibye-Knudsen, M., Brace, L. E., Kassahun, H., SenGupta, T., Nilsen, H., et al. (2014). Defective mitophagy in XPA via PARP-1 hyperactivation and NAD(+)/SIRT1 reduction. *Cell* 157, 882–896. doi: 10.1016/j.cell.2014.03.026

Fecto, F., Yan, J., Vemula, S. P., Liu, E., Yang, Y., Chen, W., et al. (2011). SQSTM1 mutations in familial and sporadic amyotrophic lateral sclerosis. *Arch. Neurol.* 68, 1440–1446. doi: 10.1001/archneurol.2011.250

Fivenson, E. M., Lautrup, S., Sun, N., Scheibye-Knudsen, M., Stevnsner, T., Nilsen, H., et al. (2017). Mitophagy in neurodegeneration and aging. *Neurochem. Int.* 109, 202–209. doi: 10.1016/j.neuint.2017.02.007

Freischmidt, A., Wieland, T., Richter, B., Ruf, W., Schaeffer, V., Müller, K., et al. (2015). Haploinsufficiency of TBK1 causes familial ALS and fronto-temporal dementia. *Nat. Neurosci.* 18, 631–636. doi: 10.1038/nn.4000

Galluzzi, L., Pedro, J. M. B.-S., Levine, B., Green, D. R., and Kroemer, G. (2017). Pharmacological modulation of autophagy: therapeutic potential and persisting obstacles. *Nat. Rev. Drug Discov.* 16, 487–511. doi: 10.1038/nrd.2017.22

García-Prat, L., Martínez-Vicente, M., Perdiguero, E., Ortet, L., Rodríguez-Ubreva, J., Rebollo, E., et al. (2016). Autophagy maintains stemness by preventing senescence. *Nature* 529, 37–42. doi: 10.1038/nature16187

Gegg, M. E., Cooper, J. M., Chau, K.-Y., Rojo, M., Schapira, A. H. V., and Taanman, J.-W. (2010). Mitofusin 1 and mitofusin 2 are ubiquitinated in a PINK1/parkin-dependent manner upon induction of mitophagy. *Hum. Mol. Genet.* 19, 4861–4870. doi: 10.1093/hmg/ddq419

Geisler, S., Holmström, K. M., Skujat, D., Fiesel, F. C., Rothfuss, O. C., Kahle, P. J., et al. (2010). PINK1/Parkin-mediated mitophagy is dependent on VDAC1 and p62/SQSTM1. *Nat. Cell Biol.* 12, 119–131. doi: 10.1038/ncb2012

Goker-Alpan, O., Schiffmann, R., LaMarca, M. E., Nussbaum, R. L., McInerney-Leo, A., and Sidransky, E. (2004). Parkinsonism among Gaucher disease carriers. *J. Med. Genet.* 41, 937–940. doi: 10.1136/jmg.2004.024455

Haack, T. B., Hogarth, P., Kruer, M. C., Gregory, A., Wieland, T., Schwarzmayr, T., et al. (2012). Exome sequencing reveals de novo WDR45 mutations causing a phenotypically distinct, X-linked dominant form of NBIA. *Am. J. Hum. Genet.* 91, 1144–1149. doi: 10.1016/j.ajhg.2012.10.019

Haas, R. H., Parikh, S., Falk, M. J., Saneto, R. P., Wolf, N. I., Darin, N., et al. (2007). Mitochondrial disease: a practical approach for primary care physicians. *Pediatrics* 120, 1326–1333. doi: 10.1542/peds.2007-0391

Hara, T., Nakamura, K., Matsui, M., Yamamoto, A., Nakahara, Y., Suzuki-Migishima, R., et al. (2006). Suppression of basal autophagy in neural cells causes neurodegenerative disease in mice. *Nature* 441, 885–889. doi: 10.1038/nature04724

Hashem, S. I., Murphy, A. N., Divakaruni, A. S., Klos, M. L., Nelson, B. C., Gault, E. C., et al. (2017). Impaired mitophagy facilitates mitochondrial damage in Danon disease. *J. Mol. Cell. Cardiol.* 108, 86–94. doi: 10.1016/j.yjmcc.2017.05.007

Hayflick, S. J., Kruer, M. C., Gregory, A., Haack, T. B., Kurian, M. A., Houlden, H. H., et al. (2013). β-Propeller protein-associated neurodegeneration: a new X-linked dominant disorder with brain iron accumulation. *Brain J. Neurol.* 136, 1708–1717. doi: 10.1093/brain/awt095

Herpin, A., Englberger, E., Zehner, M., Wacker, R., Gessler, M., and Schartl, M. (2015). Defective autophagy through epg5 mutation results in failure to reduce germ plasm and mitochondria. *FASEB J.* 29, 4145–4161. doi: 10.1096/fj.14-265462

Hirota, Y., Yamashita, S., Kurihara, Y., Jin, X., Aihara, M., Saigusa, T., et al. (2015). Mitophagy is primarily due to alternative autophagy and requires the MAPK1 and MAPK14 signaling pathways. *Autophagy* 11, 332–343. doi: 10.1080/15548627.2015.1023047

Honda, S., Arakawa, S., Nishida, Y., Yamaguchi, H., Ishii, E., and Shimizu, S. (2014). Ulk1-mediated Atg5-independent macroautophagy mediates elimination of mitochondria from embryonic reticulocytes. *Nat. Commun.* 5:4004. doi: 10.1038/ncomms5004

Hoshino, A., Mita, Y., Okawa, Y., Ariyoshi, M., Iwai-Kanai, E., Ueyama, T., et al. (2013). Cytosolic p53 inhibits Parkin-mediated mitophagy and promotes mitochondrial dysfunction in the mouse heart. *Nat. Commun.* 4:2308. doi: 10.1038/ncomms3308

Houtkooper, R. H., Mouchiroud, L., Ryu, D., Moullan, N., Katsyuba, E., Knott, G., et al. (2013). Mitonuclear protein imbalance as a conserved longevity mechanism. *Nature* 497, 451–457. doi: 10.1038/nature12188

Hsu, P., Liu, X., Zhang, J., Wang, H.-G., Ye, J.-M., and Shi, Y. (2015). Cardiolipin remodeling by TAZ/tafazzin is selectively required for the initiation of mitophagy. *Autophagy* 11, 643–652. doi: 10.1080/15548627.2015.1023984

Hudson, G., Gomez-Duran, A., Wilson, I. J., and Chinnery, P. F. (2014). Recent Mitochondrial DNA mutations increase the risk of developing common late-onset human diseases. *PLoS Genet.* 10:e1004369. doi: 10.1371/journal.pgen.1004369

Iguchi, M., Kujuro, Y., Okatsu, K., Koyano, F., Kosako, H., Kimura, M., et al. (2013). Parkin-catalyzed ubiquitin-ester transfer is triggered by PINK1-dependent phosphorylation. *J. Biol. Chem.* 288, 22019–22032. doi: 10.1074/jbc.M113.467530

Irrcher, I., Aleyasin, H., Seifert, E. L., Hewitt, S. J., Chhabra, S., Phillips, M., et al. (2010). Loss of the Parkinson's disease-linked gene DJ-1 perturbs mitochondrial dynamics. *Hum. Mol. Genet.* 19, 3734–3746. doi: 10.1093/hmg/ddq288

Ivankovic, D., Chau, K.-Y., Schapira, A. H. V., and Gegg, M. E. (2016). Mitochondrial and lysosomal biogenesis are activated following PINK1/parkin-mediated mitophagy. *J. Neurochem.* 136, 388–402. doi: 10.1111/jnc.13412

Ivanova, M. M., Changsila, E., Iaonou, C., and Goker-Alpan, O. (2019). Impaired autophagic and mitochondrial functions are partially restored by ERT in Gaucher and Fabry diseases. *PLoS One* 14:e0210617. doi: 10.1371/journal.pone.0210617

Jelani, M., Dooley, H. C., Gubas, A., Mohamoud, H. S. A., Khan, M. T. M., Ali, Z., et al. (2019). A mutation in the major autophagy gene. WIPI2, associated with global developmental abnormalities. *Brain J. Neurol.* 142, 1242–1254. doi: 10.1093/brain/awz075

Ji, C., Zhao, H., Li, D., Sun, H., Hao, J., Chen, R., et al. (2019). Role of Wdr45b in maintaining neural autophagy and cognitive function. *Autophagy* 0, 1–11. doi: 10.1080/15548627.2019.1632621

Jin, S. M., Lazarou, M., Wang, C., Kane, L. A., Narendra, D. P., and Youle, R. J. (2010). Mitochondrial membrane potential regulates PINK1 import and proteolytic destabilization by PARL. *J. Cell Biol.* 191, 933–942. doi: 10.1083/jcb.201008084

Kane, L. A., Lazarou, M., Fogel, A. I., Li, Y., Yamano, K., Sarraf, S. A., et al. (2014). PINK1 phosphorylates ubiquitin to activate Parkin E3 ubiquitin ligase activity. *J. Cell Biol.* 205, 143–153. doi: 10.1083/jcb.201402104

Kauppila, T. E. S., Kauppila, J. H. K., and Larsson, N.-G. (2017). Mammalian mitochondria and aging: an update. *Cell Metab.* 25, 57–71. doi: 10.1016/j.cmet.2016.09.017

Kazlauskaite, A., Kondapalli, C., Gourlay, R., Campbell, D. G., Ritorto, M. S., Hofmann, K., et al. (2014). Parkin is activated by PINK1-dependent phosphorylation of ubiquitin at Ser65. *Biochem. J.* 460, 127–139. doi: 10.1042/BJ20140334

Kim, M., Sandford, E., Gatica, D., Qiu, Y., Liu, X., Zheng, Y., et al. (2016). Mutation in ATG5 reduces autophagy and leads to ataxia with developmental delay. *eLife* 5:e12245. doi: 10.7554/eLife.12245

Kissová, I., Deffieu, M., Manon, S., and Camougrand, N. (2004). Uth1p is involved in the autophagic degradation of mitochondria. *J. Biol. Chem.* 279, 39068–39074. doi: 10.1074/jbc.M406960200

Kitada, T., Asakawa, S., Hattori, N., Matsumine, H., Yamamura, Y., Minoshima, S., et al. (1998). Mutations in the parkin gene cause autosomal recessive juvenile parkinsonism. *Nature* 392, 605–608. doi: 10.1038/33416

Kluge, A. F., Lagu, B. R., Maiti, P., Jaleel, M., Webb, M., Malhotra, J., et al. (2018). Novel highly selective inhibitors of ubiquitin specific protease 30 (USP30) accelerate mitophagy. *Bioorg. Med. Chem. Lett.* 28, 2655–2659. doi: 10.1016/j.bmcl.2018.05.013

Kondapalli, C., Kazlauskaite, A., Zhang, N., Woodroof, H. I., Campbell, D. G., Gourlay, R., et al. (2012). PINK1 is activated by mitochondrial membrane potential depolarization and stimulates Parkin E3 ligase activity by phosphorylating Serine 65. *Open Biol.* 2:120080. doi: 10.1098/rsob.120080

Koyano, F., Okatsu, K., Kosako, H., Tamura, Y., Go, E., Kimura, M., et al. (2014). Ubiquitin is phosphorylated by PINK1 to activate parkin. *Nature* 510, 162–166. doi: 10.1038/nature13392

Kuma, A., Hatano, M., Matsui, M., Yamamoto, A., Nakaya, H., Yoshimori, T., et al. (2004). The role of autophagy during the early neonatal starvation period. *Nature* 432, 1032–1036. doi: 10.1038/nature03029

Lahuerta, M., Aguado, C., Sánchez-Martín, P., Sanz, P., and Knecht, E. (2018). Degradation of altered mitochondria by autophagy is impaired in Lafora disease. *FEBS J.* 285, 2071–2090. doi: 10.1111/febs.14468

Lampert, M. A., Orogo, A. M., Najor, R. H., Hammerling, B. C., Leon, L. J., Wang, B. J., et al. (2019). BNIP3L/NIX and FUNDC1-mediated mitophagy is required for mitochondrial network remodeling during cardiac progenitor cell differentiation. *Autophagy* 15, 1182–1198. doi: 10.1080/15548627.2019.1580095

Lazarou, M., Sliter, D. A., Kane, L. A., Sarraf, S. A., Wang, C., Burman, J. L., et al. (2015). The ubiquitin kinase PINK1 recruits autophagy receptors to induce mitophagy. *Nature* 524, 309–314. doi: 10.1038/nature14893

Le Guerroué, F., Eck, F., Jung, J., Starzetz, T., Mittelbronn, M., Kaulich, M., et al. (2017). Autophagosomal content profiling reveals an LC3C-dependent piecemeal mitophagy pathway. *Mol. Cell* 68:786–796.e6. doi: 10.1016/j.molcel.2017.10.029

Lee, M. Y., Sumpter, R., Zou, Z., Sirasanagandla, S., Wei, Y., Mishra, P., et al. (2017). Peroxisomal protein PEX13 functions in selective autophagy. *EMBO Rep* 18, 48–60. doi: 10.15252/embr.201642443

Legati, A., Reyes, A., Nasca, A., Invernizzi, F., Lamantea, E., Tiranti, V., et al. (2016). New genes and pathomechanisms in mitochondrial disorders unraveled by NGS technologies. *Biochim. Biophys. Acta* 1857, 1326–1335. doi: 10.1016/j.bbabio.2016.02.022

Lemasters, J. J. (2005). Selective mitochondrial autophagy, or mitophagy, as a targeted defense against oxidative stress, mitochondrial dysfunction, and aging. *Rejuvenation Res.* 8, 3–5. doi: 10.1089/rej.2005.8.3

Levine, B., and Kroemer, G. (2019). Biological functions of autophagy genes: a disease perspective. *Cell* 176, 11–42. doi: 10.1016/j.cell.2018.09.048

Liao, C., Ashley, N., Diot, A., Morten, K., Phadwal, K., Williams, A., et al. (2017). Dysregulated mitophagy and mitochondrial organization in optic atrophy due to OPA1 mutations. *Neurology* 88, 131–142. doi: 10.1212/WNL.0000000000003491

Lim, J.-A., Li, L., Shirihai, O. S., Trudeau, K. M., Puertollano, R., and Raben, N. (2017). Modulation of mTOR signaling as a strategy for the treatment of Pompe disease. *EMBO Mol. Med.* 9, 353–370. doi: 10.15252/emmm.201606547

Liu, L., Feng, D., Chen, G., Chen, M., Zheng, Q., Song, P., et al. (2012). Mitochondrial outer-membrane protein FUNDC1 mediates hypoxia-induced mitophagy in mammalian cells. *Nat. Cell Biol.* 14, 177–185. doi: 10.1038/ncb2422

López-Otín, C., Blasco, M. A., Partridge, L., Serrano, M., and Kroemer, G. (2013). The hallmarks of aging. *Cell* 153, 1194–1217. doi: 10.1016/j.cell.2013.05.039

Lwin, A., Orvisky, E., Goker-Alpan, O., LaMarca, M. E., and Sidransky, E. (2004). Glucocerebrosidase mutations in subjects with parkinsonism. *Mol. Genet. Metab.* 81, 70–73. doi: 10.1016/j.ymgme.2003.11.004

Madeo, F., Eisenberg, T., Pietrocola, F., and Kroemer, G. (2018). Spermidine in health and disease. *Science* 359:aan2788. doi: 10.1126/science.aan2788

Mann, V. M., Cooper, J. M., Krige, D., Daniel, S. E., Schapira, A. H., and Marsden, C. D. (1992). Brain, skeletal muscle and platelet homogenate mitochondrial function in Parkinson's disease. *Brain J. Neurol.* 115(Pt 2), 333–342. doi: 10.1093/brain/115.2.333

Maruyama, H., Morino, H., Ito, H., Izumi, Y., Kato, H., Watanabe, Y., et al. (2010). Mutations of optineurin in amyotrophic lateral sclerosis. *Nature* 465, 223–226. doi: 10.1038/nature08971

McLelland, G.-L., Soubannier, V., Chen, C. X., McBride, H. M., and Fon, E. A. (2014). Parkin and PINK1 function in a vesicular trafficking pathway regulating mitochondrial quality control. *EMBO J.* 33, 282–295. doi: 10.1002/embj.201385902

Meissner, C., Lorenz, H., Weihofen, A., Selkoe, D. J., and Lemberg, M. K. (2011). The mitochondrial intramembrane protease PARL cleaves human Pink1 to regulate Pink1 trafficking. *J. Neurochem.* 117, 856–867. doi: 10.1111/j.1471-4159.2011.07253.x

Melber, A., and Haynes, C. M. (2018). UPRmt regulation and output: a stress response mediated by mitochondrial-nuclear communication. *Cell Res* 28, 281–295. doi: 10.1038/cr.2018.16

Mizushima, N. (2020). The ATG conjugation systems in autophagy. *Curr. Opin. Cell Biol.* 63, 1–10. doi: 10.1016/j.ceb.2019.12.001

Morani, F., Doccini, S., Sirica, R., Paterno, M., Pezzini, F., Ricca, I., et al. (2019). Functional transcriptome analysis in ARSACS KO cell model reveals a role of sacsin in autophagy. *Sci. Rep.* 9:11878. doi: 10.1038/s41598-019-48047-x

Mouchiroud, L., Houtkooper, R. H., Moullan, N., Katsyuba, E., Ryu, D., Cantó, C., et al. (2013). The NAD(+)/sirtuin pathway modulates longevity through activation of mitochondrial UPR and FOXO signaling. *Cell* 154, 430–441. doi: 10.1016/j.cell.2013.06.016

Mukherjee, A. B., Appu, A. P., Sadhukhan, T., Casey, S., Mondal, A., Zhang, Z., et al. (2019). Emerging new roles of the lysosome and neuronal ceroid lipofuscinoses. *Mol. Neurodegener.* 14:4. doi: 10.1186/s13024-018-0300-6

Napoli, E., Song, G., Panoutsopoulos, A., Riyadh, M. A., Kaushik, G., Halmai, J., et al. (2018). Beyond autophagy: a novel role for autism-linked Wdfy3 in brain mitophagy. *Sci. Rep.* 8:11348. doi: 10.1038/s41598-018-29421-7

Napolitano, G., and Ballabio, A. (2016). TFEB at a glance. *J. Cell Sci.* 129, 2475–2481. doi: 10.1242/jcs.146365

Nezich, C. L., Wang, C., Fogel, A. I., and Youle, R. J. (2015). MiT/TFE transcription factors are activated during mitophagy downstream of Parkin and Atg5. *J. Cell Biol.* 210, 435–450. doi: 10.1083/jcb.201501002

Novak, I., Kirkin, V., McEwan, D. G., Zhang, J., Wild, P., Rozenknop, A., et al. (2010). Nix is a selective autophagy receptor for mitochondrial clearance. *EMBO Rep.* 11, 45–51. doi: 10.1038/embor.2009.256

Ordonez, M. P., Roberts, E. A., Kidwell, C. U., Yuan, S. H., Plaisted, W. C., and Goldstein, L. S. B. (2012). Disruption and therapeutic rescue of autophagy in a human neuronal model of Niemann Pick type C1. *Hum. Mol. Genet.* 21, 2651–2662. doi: 10.1093/hmg/dds090

Ordureau, A., Sarraf, S. A., Duda, D. M., Heo, J.-M., Jedrychowski, M. P., Sviderskiy, V. O., et al. (2014). Quantitative proteomics reveal a feedforward mechanism for mitochondrial PARKIN translocation and ubiquitin chain synthesis. *Mol. Cell* 56, 360–375. doi: 10.1016/j.molcel.2014.09.007

Osellame, L. D., Rahim, A. A., Hargreaves, I. P., Gegg, M. E., Richard-Londt, A., Brandner, S., et al. (2013). Mitochondria and quality control defects in a mouse model of Gaucher disease–links to Parkinson's disease. *Cell Metab.* 17, 941–953. doi: 10.1016/j.cmet.2013.04.014

Otomo, T., Higaki, K., Nanba, E., Ozono K., and Sakai, N. (2009). Inhibition of autophagosome formation restores mitochondrial function in mucolipidosis II and III skin fibroblasts. *Mol. Genet. Metab.* 98, 393–399. doi: 10.1016/j.ymgme.2009.07.002

Oz-Levi, D., Ben-Zeev, B., Ruzzo, E. K., Hitomi, Y., Gelman, A., Pelak, K., et al. (2012). Mutation in TECPR2 reveals a role for autophagy in hereditary spastic paraparesis. *Am. J. Hum. Genet.* 91, 1065–1072. doi: 10.1016/j.ajhg.2012.09.015

Pacheco, C. D., Kunkel, R., and Lieberman, A. P. (2007). Autophagy in Niemann-Pick C disease is dependent upon Beclin-1 and responsive to lipid trafficking defects. *Hum. Mol. Genet.* 16, 1495–1503. doi: 10.1093/hmg/ddm100

Palikaras, K., Lionaki, E., and Tavernarakis, N. (2015). Coordination of mitophagy and mitochondrial biogenesis during ageing in *C. elegans*. *Nature* 521, 525–528. doi: 10.1038/nature14300

Palikaras, K., Lionaki, E., and Tavernarakis, N. (2018). Mechanisms of mitophagy in cellular homeostasis, physiology and pathology. *Nat. Cell Biol.* 20, 1013–1022. doi: 10.1038/s41556-018-0176-2

Pickles, S., Vigié, P., and Youle, R. J. (2018). Mitophagy and Quality Control Mechanisms in Mitochondrial Maintenance. *Curr. Biol. CB* 28, R170–R185. doi: 10.1016/j.cub.2018.01.004

Pietrocola, F., Lachkar, S., Enot, D. P., Niso-Santano, M., Bravo-San Pedro, J. M., Sica, V., et al. (2015). Spermidine induces autophagy by inhibiting the acetyltransferase EP300. *Cell Death. Differ.* 22, 509–516. doi: 10.1038/cdd.2014.215

Platt, F. M., d'Azzo, A., Davidson, B. L., Neufeld, E. F., and Tifft, C. J. (2018). Lysosomal storage diseases. *Nat. Rev. Dis. Primer* 4:27. doi: 10.1038/s41572-018-0025-4

Pottier, C., Bieniek, K. F., Finch, N., van de Vorst, M., Baker, M., Perkersen, R., et al. (2015). Whole-genome sequencing reveals important role for TBK1 and OPTN mutations in frontotemporal lobar degeneration without motor neuron disease. *Acta Neuropathol.* 130, 77–92. doi: 10.1007/s00401-015-1436-x

Price, N. L., Gomes, A. P., Ling, A. J. Y., Duarte, F. V., Martin-Montalvo, A., North, B. J., et al. (2012). SIRT1 is required for AMPK activation and the beneficial effects of resveratrol on mitochondrial function. *Cell Metab.* 15, 675–690. doi: 10.1016/j.cmet.2012.04.003

Proikas-Cezanne, T., Waddell, S., Gaugel, A., Frickey, T., Lupas, A., and Nordheim, A. (2004). WIPI-1alpha (WIPI49), a member of the novel 7-bladed WIPI protein family, is aberrantly expressed in human cancer and is linked to starvation-induced autophagy. *Oncogene* 23, 9314–9325. doi: 10.1038/sj.onc.1208331

Puigserver, P., Wu, Z., Park, C. W., Graves, R., Wright, M., and Spiegelman, B. M. (1998). A cold-inducible coactivator of nuclear receptors linked to adaptive thermogenesis. *Cell* 92, 829–839. doi: 10.1016/s0092-8674(00)81410-5

Qi, Y., Qiu, Q., Gu, X., Tian, Y., and Zhang, Y. (2016). ATM mediates spermidine-induced mitophagy via PINK1 and Parkin regulation in human fibroblasts. *Sci. Rep.* 6:24700. doi: 10.1038/srep24700

Raben, N., Schreiner, C., Baum, R., Takikita, S., Xu, S., Xie, T., et al. (2010). Suppression of autophagy permits successful enzyme replacement therapy in a lysosomal storage disorder–murine Pompe disease. *Autophagy* 6, 1078–1089. doi: 10.4161/auto.6.8.13378

Raben, N., Wong, A., Ralston, E., and Myerowitz, R. (2012). Autophagy and mitochondria in Pompe disease: nothing is so new as what has long been forgotten. *Am. J. Med. Genet. C Semin. Med. Genet.* 160C, 13–21. doi: 10.1002/ajmg.c.31317

Rana, A., Oliveira, M. P., Khamoui, A. V., Aparicio, R., Rera, M., Rossiter, H. B., et al. (2017). Promoting Drp1-mediated mitochondrial fission in midlife prolongs healthy lifespan of Drosophila melanogaster. *Nat. Commun.* 8:448. doi: 10.1038/s41467-017-00525-4

Rana, A., Rera, M., and Walker, D. W. (2013). Parkin overexpression during aging reduces proteotoxicity, alters mitochondrial dynamics, and extends lifespan. *Proc. Natl. Acad. Sci. U.S.A.* 110, 8638–8643. doi: 10.1073/pnas.1216197110

Richter, B., Sliter, D. A., Herhaus, L., Stolz, A., Wang, C., Beli, P., et al. (2016). Phosphorylation of OPTN by TBK1 enhances its binding to Ub chains and promotes selective autophagy of damaged mitochondria. *Proc. Natl. Acad. Sci. U.S.A.* 113, 4039–4044. doi: 10.1073/pnas.1523926113

Richter, U., Lahtinen, T., Marttinen, P., Myöhänen, M., Greco, D., Cannino, G., et al. (2013). A mitochondrial ribosomal and RNA decay pathway blocks cell proliferation. *Curr. Biol.* 23, 535–541. doi: 10.1016/j.cub.2013.02.019

Rizzo, F., Ronchi, D., Salani, S., Nizzardo, M., Fortunato, F., Bordoni, A., et al. (2016). Selective mitochondrial depletion, apoptosis resistance, and increased mitophagy in human Charcot-Marie-Tooth 2A motor neurons. *Hum. Mol. Genet.* 25, 4266–4281. doi: 10.1093/hmg/ddw258

Ryan, B. J., Hoek, S., Fon, E. A., and Wade-Martins, R. (2015). Mitochondrial dysfunction and mitophagy in Parkinson's: from familial to sporadic disease. *Trends Biochem. Sci.* 40, 200–210. doi: 10.1016/j.tibs.2015.02.003

Ryu, D., Mouchiroud, L., Andreux, P. A., Katsyuba, E., Moullan, N., Nicolet-Dit-Félix, A. A., et al. (2016). Urolithin A induces mitophagy and prolongs lifespan in *C. elegans* and increases muscle function in rodents. *Nat. Med.* 22, 879–888. doi: 10.1038/nm.4132

Safiulina, D., Kuum, M., Choubey, V., Gogichaishvili, N., Liiv, J., Hickey, M. A., et al. (2019). Miro proteins prime mitochondria for Parkin translocation and mitophagy. *EMBO J.* 38:e99384. doi: 10.15252/embj.201899384

Saitsu, H., Nishimura, T., Muramatsu, K., Kodera, H., Kumada, S., Sugai, K., et al. (2013). De novo mutations in the autophagy gene WDR45 cause static encephalopathy of childhood with neurodegeneration in adulthood. *Nat. Genet.* 45, 445–449. doi: 10.1038/ng.2562

Salpietro, V., Phadke, R., Saggar, A., Hargreaves, I. P., Yates, R., Fokoloros, C., et al. (2015). Zellweger syndrome and secondary mitochondrial myopathy. *Eur. J. Pediatr.* 174, 557–563. doi: 10.1007/s00431-014-2431-2

Sandoval, H., Thiagarajan, P., Dasgupta, S. K., Schumacher, A., Prchal, J. T., Chen, M., et al. (2008). Essential role for Nix in autophagic maturation of erythroid cells. *Nature* 454, 232–235. doi: 10.1038/nature07006

Sarraf, S. A., Raman, M., Guarani-Pereira, V., Sowa, M. E., Huttlin, E. L., Gygi, S. P., et al. (2013). Landscape of the PARKIN-dependent ubiquitylome in response to mitochondrial depolarization. *Nature* 496, 372–376. doi: 10.1038/nature12043

Saxton, R. A., and Sabatini, D. M. (2017). mTOR Signaling in Growth. *Metabolism, and Disease. Cell* 168, 960–976. doi: 10.1016/j.cell.2017.02.004

Scheibye-Knudsen, M., Mitchell, S. J., Fang, E. F., Iyama, T., Ward, T., Wang, J., et al. (2014). A high-fat diet and NAD(+) activate Sirt1 to rescue premature aging in cockayne syndrome. *Cell Metab.* 20, 840–855. doi: 10.1016/j.cmet.2014.10.005

Scheibye-Knudsen, M., Ramamoorthy, M., Sykora, P., Maynard, S., Lin, P.-C., Minor, R. K., et al. (2012). Cockayne syndrome group B protein prevents the accumulation of damaged mitochondria by promoting mitochondrial autophagy. *J. Exp. Med.* 209, 855–869. doi: 10.1084/jem.20111721

Scheibye-Knudsen, M., Scheibye-Alsing, K., Canugovi, C., Croteau, D. L., and Bohr, V. A. (2013). A novel diagnostic tool reveals mitochondrial pathology in human diseases and aging. *Aging* 5, 192–208. doi: 10.18632/aging.100546

Schiavi, A., Maglioni, S., Palikaras, K., Shaik, A., Strappazzon, F., Brinkmann, V., et al. (2015). Iron-starvation-induced mitophagy mediates lifespan extension upon mitochondrial stress in *C. elegans*. *Curr. Biol. CB* 25, 1810–1822. doi: 10.1016/j.cub.2015.05.059

Schwarz, C., Stekovic, S., Wirth, M., Benson, G., Royer, P., Sigrist, S. J., et al. (2018). Safety and tolerability of spermidine supplementation in mice and older adults with subjective cognitive decline. *Aging* 10, 19–33. doi: 10.18632/aging.101354

Schweers, R. L., Zhang, J., Randall, M. S., Loyd, M. R., Li, W., Dorsey, F. C., et al. (2007). NIX is required for programmed mitochondrial clearance during reticulocyte maturation. *Proc. Natl. Acad. Sci. U.S.A.* 104, 19500–19505. doi: 10.1073/pnas.0708818104

Seibler, P., Burbulla, L. F., Dulovic, M., Zittel, S., Heine, J., Schmidt, T., et al. (2018). Iron overload is accompanied by mitochondrial and lysosomal dysfunction in WDR45 mutant cells. *Brain* 141, 3052–3064. doi: 10.1093/brain/awy230

Settembre, C., Fraldi, A., Jahreiss, L., Spampanato, C., Venturi, C., Medina, D., et al. (2008). A block of autophagy in lysosomal storage disorders. *Hum. Mol. Genet.* 17, 119–129. doi: 10.1093/hmg/ddm289

Shiba-Fukushima, K., Imai, Y., Yoshida, S., Ishihama, Y., Kanao, T., Sato, S., et al. (2012). PINK1-mediated phosphorylation of the Parkin ubiquitin-like domain primes mitochondrial translocation of Parkin and regulates mitophagy. *Sci. Rep.* 2:1002. doi: 10.1038/srep01002

Siddiqui, A., Bhaumik, D., Chinta, S. J., Rane, A., Rajagopalan, S., Lieu, C. A., et al. (2015). Mitochondrial quality control via the PGC1α-TFEB signaling pathway is compromised by parkin Q311X mutation but independently restored by rapamycin. *J. Neurosci. Off. J. Soc. Neurosci.* 35, 12833–12844. doi: 10.1523/JNEUROSCI.0109-15.2015

Solesio, M. E., Saez-Atienzar, S., Jordán, J., and Galindo, M. F. (2012). Characterization of mitophagy in the 6-hydoxydopamine Parkinson's disease model. *Toxicol. Sci. Off. J. Soc. Toxicol.* 129, 411–420. doi: 10.1093/toxsci/kfs218

Soubannier, V., McLelland, G.-L., Zunino, R., Braschi, E., Rippstein, P., Fon, E. A., et al. (2012). A vesicular transport pathway shuttles cargo from mitochondria to lysosomes. *Curr. Biol. CB* 22, 135–141. doi: 10.1016/j.cub.2011.11.057

Spampanato, C., Feeney, E., Li, L., Cardone, M., Lim, J.-A., Annunziata, F., et al. (2013). Transcription factor EB (TFEB) is a new therapeutic target for Pompe disease. *EMBO Mol. Med.* 5, 691–706. doi: 10.1002/emmm.201202176

Stavoe, A. K., Gopal, P. P., Gubas, A., Tooze, S. A., and Holzbaur, E. L. (2019). Expression of WIPI2B counteracts age-related decline in autophagosome biogenesis in neurons. *eLife* 8:e44219. doi: 10.7554/eLife.44219

Suleiman, J., Allingham-Hawkins, D., Hashem, M., Shamseldin, H. E., Alkuraya, F. S., and El-Hattab, A. W. (2018). WDR45B-related intellectual disability, spastic quadriplegia, epilepsy, and cerebral hypoplasia: a consistent neurodevelopmental syndrome. *Clin. Genet.* 93, 360–364. doi: 10.1111/cge.13054

Sumpter, R., Sirasanagandla, S., Fernández, ÁF., Wei, Y., Dong, X., Franco, L., et al. (2016). Fanconi Anemia Proteins Function in Mitophagy and Immunity. *Cell* 165, 867–881. doi: 10.1016/j.cell.2016.04.006

Sun, N., Youle, R. J., and Finkel, T. (2016). The mitochondrial basis of aging. *Mol. Cell* 61, 654–666. doi: 10.1016/j.molcel.2016.01.028

Sun, N., Yun, J., Liu, J., Malide, D., Liu, C., Rovira, I. I., et al. (2015). Measuring In Vivo Mitophagy. *Mol. Cell* 60, 685–696. doi: 10.1016/j.molcel.2015.10.009

Sun, Y., Vashisht, A. A., Tchieu, J., Wohlschlegel, J. A., and Dreier, L. (2012). Voltage-dependent anion channels (VDACs) recruit Parkin to defective mitochondria to promote mitochondrial autophagy. *J. Biol. Chem.* 287, 40652–40660. doi: 10.1074/jbc.M112.419721

Takahashi, D., Moriyama, J., Nakamura, T., Miki, E., Takahashi, E., Sato, A., et al. (2019). AUTACs: cargo-specific degraders using selective autophagy. *Mol. Cell* 76:797–810.e10. doi: 10.1016/j.molcel.2019.09.009

Tanaka, A., Cleland, M. M., Xu, S., Narendra, D. P., Suen, D.-F., Karbowski, M., et al. (2010). Proteasome and p97 mediate mitophagy and degradation of mitofusins induced by Parkin. *J. Cell Biol.* 191, 1367–1380. doi: 10.1083/jcb.201007013

Tanaka, Y., Guhde, G., Suter, A., Eskelinen, E. L., Hartmann, D., Lüllmann-Rauch, R., et al. (2000). Accumulation of autophagic vacuoles and cardiomyopathy in LAMP-2-deficient mice. *Nature* 406, 902–906. doi: 10.1038/35022595

Todd, A. M., and Staveley, B. E. (2012). Expression of Pink1 with α-synuclein in the dopaminergic neurons of Drosophila leads to increases in both lifespan and healthspan. *Genet. Mol. Res. GMR* 11, 1497–1502. doi: 10.4238/2012.May.21.6

Toyama, E. Q., Herzig, S., Courchet, J., Lewis, T. L., Losón, O. C., Hellberg, K., et al. (2016). AMP-activated protein kinase mediates mitochondrial fission in response to energy stress. *Science* 351, 275–281. doi: 10.1126/science.aab4138

Trifunovic, A., Wredenberg, A., Falkenberg, M., Spelbrink, J. N., Rovio, A. T., Bruder, C. E., et al. (2004). Premature ageing in mice expressing defective mitochondrial DNA polymerase. *Nature* 429, 417–423. doi: 10.1038/nature02517

Valente, E. M., Abou-Sleiman, P. M., Caputo, V., Muqit, M. M. K., Harvey, K., Gispert, S., et al. (2004). Hereditary early-onset Parkinson's disease caused by mutations in PINK1. *Science* 304, 1158–1160. doi: 10.1126/science.1096284

Vantaggiato, C., Crimella, C., Airoldi, G., Polishchuk, R., Bonato, S., Brighina, E., et al. (2013). Defective autophagy in spastizin mutated patients with hereditary spastic paraparesis type 15. *Brain J. Neurol.* 136, 3119–3139. doi: 10.1093/brain/awt227

Wallace, D. C. (2015). Mitochondrial DNA variation in human radiation and disease. *Cell* 163, 33–38. doi: 10.1016/j.cell.2015.08.067

Wallace, D. C. (2018). Mitochondrial genetic medicine. *Nat. Genet.* 50, 1642–1649. doi: 10.1038/s41588-018-0264-z

Wang, C., Niederstrasser, H., Douglas, P. M., Lin, R., Jaramillo, J., Li, Y., et al. (2017). Small-molecule TFEB pathway agonists that ameliorate metabolic syndrome in mice and extend *C. elegans* lifespan. *Nat. Commun.* 8, 1–14. doi: 10.1038/s41467-017-02332-3

Wang, X., Winter, D., Ashrafi, G., Schlehe, J., Wong, Y. L., Selkoe, D., et al. (2011). PINK1 and Parkin target Miro for phosphorylation and degradation to arrest mitochondrial motility. *Cell* 147, 893–906. doi: 10.1016/j.cell.2011.10.018

Wang, Z., Miao, G., Xue, X., Guo, X., Yuan, C., Wang, Z., et al. (2016). The Vici Syndrome Protein EPG5 Is a Rab7 Effector that Determines the Fusion Specificity of Autophagosomes with Late Endosomes/Lysosomes. *Mol. Cell* 63, 781–795. doi: 10.1016/j.molcel.2016.08.021

Waterham, H. R., and Ebberink, M. S. (2012). Genetics and molecular basis of human peroxisome biogenesis disorders. *Biochim. Biophys. Acta BBA Mol. Basis Dis.* 1822, 1430–1441. doi: 10.1016/j.bbadis.2012.04.006

Wauer, T., Swatek, K. N., Wagstaff, J. L., Gladkova, C., Pruneda, J. N., Michel, M. A., et al. (2015). Ubiquitin Ser65 phosphorylation affects ubiquitin structure, chain assembly and hydrolysis. *EMBO J.* 34, 307–325. doi: 10.15252/embj.201489847

Weil, R., Laplantine, E., Curic, S., and Génin, P. (2018). Role of optineurin in the mitochondrial dysfunction: potential implications in neurodegenerative diseases and Cancer. *Front. Immunol.* 9:1243. doi: 10.3389/fimmu.2018.01243

White, K. E., Davies, V. J., Hogan, V. E., Piechota, M. J., Nichols, P. P., Turnbull, D. M., et al. (2009). OPA1 deficiency associated with increased autophagy in retinal ganglion cells in a murine model of dominant optic atrophy. *Invest. Ophthalmol. Vis. Sci.* 50, 2567–2571. doi: 10.1167/iovs.08-2913

Wong, Y. C., and Holzbaur, E. L. F. (2014). Optineurin is an autophagy receptor for damaged mitochondria in parkin-mediated mitophagy that is disrupted by an ALS-linked mutation. *Proc. Natl. Acad. Sci. U.S.A.* 111, E4439–E4448. doi: 10.1073/pnas.1405752111

Yamano, K., Fogel, A. I., Wang, C., van der Bliek, A. M., and Youle, R. J. (2014). Mitochondrial Rab GAPs govern autophagosome biogenesis during mitophagy. *eLife* 3:e01612. doi: 10.7554/eLife.01612

Yamano, K., and Youle, R. J. (2013). PINK1 is degraded through the N-end rule pathway. *Autophagy* 9, 1758–1769. doi: 10.4161/auto.24633

Youle, R. J. (2019). Mitochondria-Striking a balance between host and endosymbiont. *Science* 365:aaw9855. doi: 10.1126/science.aaw9855

Youle, R. J., and van der Bliek, A. M. (2012). Mitochondrial fission, fusion, and stress. *Science* 337, 1062–1065. doi: 10.1126/science.1219855

Yu-Wai-Man, P., Griffiths, P. G., Gorman, G. S., Lourenco, C. M., Wright, A. F., Auer-Grumbach, M., et al. (2010). Multi-system neurological disease is common in patients with OPA1 mutations. *Brain J. Neurol.* 133, 771–786. doi: 10.1093/brain/awq007

Zachari, M., Gudmundsson, S. R., Li, Z., Manifava, M., Shah, R., Smith, M., et al. (2019). Selective Autophagy of Mitochondria on a Ubiquitin-Endoplasmic-Reticulum Platform. *Dev. Cell* 50:627–643.e5. doi: 10.1016/j.devcel.2019.06.016

Zhao, H., Zhao, Y. G., Wang, X., Xu, L., Miao, L., Feng, D., et al. (2013). Mice deficient in Epg5 exhibit selective neuronal vulnerability to degeneration. *J. Cell Biol.* 200, 731–741. doi: 10.1083/jcb.201211014

Zhao, Y. G., Sun, L., Miao, G., Ji, C., Zhao, H., Sun, H., et al. (2015). The autophagy gene Wdr45/Wipi4 regulates learning and memory function and axonal homeostasis. *Autophagy* 11, 881–890. doi: 10.1080/15548627.2015.1047127

16

Chronic Sustained Hypoxia-induced Redox Remodeling Causes Contractile Dysfunction in Mouse Sternohyoid Muscle

Philip Lewis[1], *David Sheehan*[2], *Renata Soares*[3], *Ana Varela Coelho*[3] and *Ken D. O'Halloran*[1]*

[1] Department of Physiology, School of Medicine, University College Cork, Cork, Ireland, [2] School of Biochemistry and Cell Biology, University College Cork, Cork, Ireland, [3] Instituto de Tecnologia Química e Biológica António Xavier, New University of Lisbon, Lisbon, Portugal

Edited by:
Brian McDonagh,
University of Liverpool, UK

Reviewed by:
Leonardo F. Ferreira,
University of Florida, USA
Esther Barreiro,
Institut Hospital del Mar d'Investigacions Mèdiques, Spain

***Correspondence:**
Ken D. O'Halloran,
Department of Physiology, School of Medicine, University College Cork, 3-079, Western Gateway Building, Western Road, Cork, Ireland
k.ohalloran@ucc.ie

Chronic sustained hypoxia (CH) induces structural and functional adaptations in respiratory muscles of animal models, however the underlying molecular mechanisms are unclear. This study explores the putative role of CH-induced redox remodeling in a translational mouse model, with a focus on the sternohyoid—a representative upper airway dilator muscle involved in the control of pharyngeal airway caliber. We hypothesized that exposure to CH induces redox disturbance in mouse sternohyoid muscle in a time-dependent manner affecting metabolic capacity and contractile performance. C57Bl6/J mice were exposed to normoxia or normobaric CH (FiO_2 = 0.1) for 1, 3, or 6 weeks. A second cohort of animals was exposed to CH for 6 weeks with and without antioxidant supplementation (tempol or N-acetyl cysteine in the drinking water). Following CH exposure, we performed 2D redox proteomics with mass spectrometry, metabolic enzyme activity assays, and cell-signaling assays. Additionally, we assessed isotonic contractile and endurance properties *ex vivo*. Temporal changes in protein oxidation and glycolytic enzyme activities were observed. Redox modulation of sternohyoid muscle proteins key to contraction, metabolism and cellular homeostasis was identified. There was no change in redox-sensitive proteasome activity or HIF-1α content, but CH decreased phospho-JNK content independent of antioxidant supplementation. CH was detrimental to sternohyoid force- and power-generating capacity and this was prevented by chronic antioxidant supplementation. We conclude that CH causes upper airway dilator muscle dysfunction due to redox modulation of proteins key to function and homeostasis. Such changes could serve to further disrupt respiratory homeostasis in diseases characterized by CH such as chronic obstructive pulmonary disease. Antioxidants may have potential use as an adjunctive therapy in hypoxic respiratory disease.

Keywords: hypoxia, oxidative stress, antioxidants, respiratory muscle, COPD

Introduction

The striated muscles of breathing are the final common effectors of the respiratory control system, critical in the maintenance of respiratory homeostasis. Pharyngeal dilator muscles are an important subset of the respiratory muscles serving to control the patency of the upper airway. Pharyngeal dilator muscle damage or dysfunction increases the risk of obstructive airway events. Upper airway muscle dysfunction is implicated in human obstructive sleep apnea (OSA), a common respiratory disorder characterized by repeated occlusions of the pharyngeal airway during sleep. Of note, OSA is prevalent in patients with chronic obstructive pulmonary disease (COPD), presenting as the "overlap syndrome" (Owens et al., 2008; McNicholas, 2009; Owens and Malhotra, 2010), but the reasons for the emergence of this co-morbidity are unclear.

Chronic sustained hypoxia (CH) is a dominant feature of respiratory diseases including COPD, but the putative role of CH in respiratory muscle remodeling and dysfunction is generally under-explored. Little is known about the effects of CH exposure on the respiratory muscles and there exists a general paucity of information concerning the pharyngeal dilator muscles despite the potential clinical relevance. Respiratory and limb muscle remodeling are features of COPD (Orozco-Levi, 2003; Doucet et al., 2004, 2010; Levine et al., 2013) and interestingly, exposure to CH elicits differential structural and functional adaptations in respiratory and limb muscles (El-Khoury et al., 2003, 2012; Faucher et al., 2005; McMorrow et al., 2011; Gamboa and Andrade, 2012; Carberry et al., 2014). We speculate that hypoxic remodeling of respiratory muscle has relevance to respiratory muscle plasticity in respiratory disease. Hypoxia-related remodeling of upper airway muscles may underpin poor upper airway control in COPD.

Pharyngeal dilator muscles are phasically active during inspiration and muscle activity is increased during hypoxic exposure (O'Halloran et al., 2002; Edge et al., 2014). Contractile activity increases reactive oxygen species (ROS) production which are pivotal for muscle adaptation to high altitude and respiratory diseases characterized by hypoxia (Zuo and Clanton, 2005; Marin-Corral et al., 2009; Murray, 2009; Chaudhary et al., 2012; El-Khoury et al., 2012; Levine et al., 2013; Puig-Vilanova et al., 2015). Thus, CH likely challenges respiratory muscles, including the pharyngeal dilator muscles, with enhanced ROS on two fronts—increased contractile activity during reflex hyperventilation and hypoxia *per se*. We postulated a role for ROS in eliciting CH-induced redox remodeling of key muscle proteins with resultant functional changes in the sternohyoid muscle—a representative pharyngeal dilator muscle. The supra- and infra-hyoid muscles of the upper airway control the position of the hyoid bone, displacing it anteriorly during inspiration to enlarge the caliber of the pharynx. Sternohyoid muscle length correlates to airway volume (Van Lunteren et al., 1987) and the muscle is recruited during increased respiratory drive (O'Halloran et al., 2002) and obstructive airway events (Edge et al., 2012). Sternohyoid muscle damage is reported in the English bulldog, an animal model of OSA (Petrof et al., 1994). We have extensively characterized sternohyoid muscle physiology (O'Halloran, 2006; Skelly et al., 2010; Shortt and O'Halloran, 2014; McDonald et al., 2015), including several studies in animal models of chronic hypoxia (Bradford et al., 2005; McMorrow et al., 2011; Skelly et al., 2011, 2012a,b, 2013; O'Connell et al., 2013; Carberry et al., 2014; McDonald et al., 2014). The sternohyoid muscle is suited to *ex vivo* study of contractile function due to ease of access, longitudinal arrangement of its fibers and the opportunity, employed in the present study, to keep bony origin and insertions intact in isolated preparations.

Given that ventilation, muscle contractile behavior, and the level of hypoxia experienced by the respiratory muscles, are likely temporally modified during the process of acclimatization to CH, we characterized protein carbonyl and free thiol content (the most common and most specific form of protein oxidation respectively (Dalle-Donne et al., 2006; El-Shafey et al., 2011) in the sternohyoid after 1, 3, or 6 weeks of CH exposure. In addition, we sought to identify redox-modified proteins in the sternohyoid muscle after 6 weeks of CH using 2D redox proteomics combined with mass spectrometry (Cole et al., 2014; Hu et al., 2014; Rainville et al., 2014) having reasoned that this information will aid the determination of how and where ROS exert their effects in muscle cells following CH exposure. We postulated that chymotrypsin-like activity of the 20S proteasome is increased in the sternohyoid after 6 weeks of CH given that proteasomal activity is highly sensitive to ROS (McClung et al., 2008; Aiken et al., 2011). Hypoxia through the hypoxia-inducible factor (HIF)-1α transcription factor promotes a more glycolytic phenotype in tissues to reduce the reliance on oxygen in ATP production (Howald et al., 1990; Murray, 2009; Wheaton and Chandel, 2011). HIF expression correlates with muscle fiber type and activity and is also modulated by ROS. Therefore, we reasoned that glyceraldehyde-3-phosphate dehydrogenase (GAPDH) and lactate dehydrogenase (LDH) activities would be temporally modified in the sternohyoid in response to CH exposure. We also assessed HIF-1α content, phospho-MAPK content (p38, JNK, ERK1/2), and sternohyoid isotonic contractile and endurance properties *ex vivo* after 6 weeks of CH in the presence or absence of chronic antioxidant supplementation with tempol or N-acetyl cysteine (NAC). We tested the hypothesis that CH causes aberrant redox modulation of sternohyoid muscle function which is reversible by antioxidant supplementation.

Materials and Methods

Ethical Approval

All protocols involving animals described in this study were approved by local ethics committee and were performed under license from the Irish Government Department of Health and Children in accordance with EU legislation.

Animal Model

In the first series of experiments, 48 adult male C576Bl/J mice (Charles River Laboratories, UK) were exposed to 1, 3, or 6 weeks of CH ($FiO_2 = 0.1$) or normoxia (6 groups: $n = 8$ per group, matched for age and weight) in environmental chambers (OxyCycler Model A84, BioSpherix Ltd, USA) with precise control of ambient oxygen concentration. All mice were housed at room temperature on a 12:12-h light–dark cycle. Food and water were available *ad libitum*, and the chambers were opened briefly once a week for cleaning. In a second series, 32 adult male C576Bl/J mice were exposed to normoxia or CH with or without antioxidant supplementation with tempol or NAC for 6 weeks (4 groups: $n = 8$ per group, matched for age and weight). At the end of the gas treatment periods, animals were anesthetized by 5% isoflurane inhalation in oxygen and euthanized by cervical dislocation. Blood samples were taken in capillary tubes for hematocrit determination.

Molecular Studies

Tissue Preparation for Molecular Studies

Sternohyoid muscles were excised, snap frozen in liquid nitrogen and stored at −80°C. Frozen muscle samples were homogenized in 10% w/v modified radioimmunoprecipitation (RIPA) assay buffer (1X RIPA, 200 mM sodium fluoride, 1 mM phenylmethylsulfonyl fluoride, protease inhibitor cocktail, phosphatase inhibitor cocktail (Fisher Scientific, Ireland) and centrifuged at 13,000 *g* for 15 min to separate the insoluble fraction from crude protein homogenate. Protein concentrations were evaluated using a bicinchoninic assay (Pierce Biotechnology (Fisher Scientific), Ireland) against bovine serum albumin standards. Two additional muscles, the soleus and extensor digitorum longus (EDL), slow and fast fiber type limb muscles respectively, were also prepared in this manner for determination of total protein carbonyl and free thiol content for comparison to sternohyoid.

Total Protein Carbonyl and Free Thiol Content

As previously described (Cole et al., 2014; Hu et al., 2014; Rainville et al., 2014), muscle homogenates were incubated with either 2 mM fluorescein-thiosemicarbazide (FTSC) or 2 mM iodoacetamidofluorescein (IAF) (Sigma-Aldrich Co., Ireland) for 2 h in the dark on ice for detection of free protein carbonyl and thiol groups respectively. Samples were then precipitated with 20% trichloroacetic acid (TCA) in acetone, followed by centrifugation at 11,000 *g* for 3 min. Protein pellets were then washed with ice-cold excess 1:1 ethylacetate/ethanol or acetone (for FTSC and IAF respectively) to remove excess TCA, interfering salts and non-protein contaminants. Samples were dried, re-suspended in sample buffer containing 5% beta-mercaptoethanol and heated at 95°C for 5 min before electrophoretic separation on a 12% polyacrylamide gel (1D). Fluorescent images of the gels were captured on a Typhoon Trio+ Variable-Mode Imager (GE Healthcare, UK). Protein bands were visualized by colloidal coomassie staining (Dyballa and Metzger, 2009) and images were captured on a calibrating image densitometer (GS-800, Bio-Rad, USA).

2D Redox Proteomics

As previously described (Cole et al., 2014; Hu et al., 2014; Rainville et al., 2014), this method separates proteins according to their isoelectric point and molecular mass such that they appear as spots when stained on polyacrylamide gels; protein spots can be analyzed independently. Briefly, sternohyoid muscle samples were treated as described above for 1D preparation until re-suspension in sample buffer. Samples were instead re-suspended in rehydration buffer (7 M urea, 2 M thiourea, 2% (w/v) 3-[(3-Cholamidopropyl)dimethylammonio]-1-propanesulfonate, 4% (v/v) ampholytes (Pharmalyte 3–10, Amersham, UK), 1% (v/v) destreak reagent (Amersham) and a trace amount of bromophenol blue) and loaded onto 70 mm pH 3–10 non-linear immobilized pH gradient (IPG) strips (GE Healthcare) overnight. IPG strips were focused on a Protean isoelectric focusing (IEF) cell (BioRad) with linear voltage increases: 250 V for 15min; 4000 V for 2 h; then up to 20,000 V. Following IEF, strips were equilibrated (20 min) in equilibration buffer (6 M urea, 0.375 M Tris, pH 8.8, 2% (w/v) sodium-dodecyl sulfate, and 20% (v/v) glycerol) containing 2% (w/v) dithiothreitol, and then for 20 min in equilibration buffer containing 2.5% (w/v) iodoacetamide. Equilibrated strips were then subjected to gel electrophoresis. Fluorescent and colloidal coomassie stained gel images were captured as described above.

Image Analysis

Quantity One image analysis software (Bio-Rad) was used to subtract background and quantify optical density for total protein carbonyl and free thiol content. For each sample, intensity of fluorescence was normalized to intensity of coomassie staining. For 2D separations, alignment of gels, spot matching, and quantification of spot volumes was carried out using Progenesis SameSpots image analysis software (Version 4.5; Non-linear Dynamics, USA).

Protein Digestion and Identification

Gel spots were used for in-gel protein digestion with trypsin. The extracted peptides were loaded onto a R2 micro column (RP-C18 equivalent) where they were desalted, concentrated and eluted directly onto a MALDI plate using α-cyano-4-hydroxycinnamic acid (5 mg/ml) as matrix solution in 50% (v/v) acetonitrile and 5% (v/v) formic acid. Mass spectra of the peptides were acquired with positive reflectron mass spectrometry (MS) and MS/MS modes using MALDI-TOF/TOF MS instrument (4800 *plus* MALDI TOF/TOF analyzer). The collected MS and MS/MS spectra were analyzed in combined mode using Mascot (version 2.2; Matrix Science, Boston, MA) search engine and SwissProt (release 02_2013, 539,165 entries) database restricted to 50 ppm peptide mass tolerance for the parent ions, an error of 0.3 Da for the fragments, one missed cleavage in peptide masses, and carbamidomethylation of Cys and oxidation of Met as fixed and variable amino acid modifications, respectively. No taxonomy restrictions were applied. The identified proteins were only considered if a MASCOT score above 95% confidence was obtained ($p < 0.05$) and at least one peptide was identified with a score above 95% confidence ($p < 0.05$). This analysis was conducted by the Analytical Services Unit, Instituto de Tecnologia Química e Biológica (ITQB), New University of Lisbon, Lisbon, Portugal.

Chymotrypsin-like Proteasome Activity

Chymotrypsin-like activity of the 20S proteasome was measured fluorometrically in accordance with the manufacturer's instructions (Abcam, UK).

Glycolytic Enzyme Activities

For GAPDH activity measurement, samples were added to 13.5 mM sodium pyrophosphate buffer (pH 8.5) containing 30 mM sodium arsenate, 0.25 mM NAD with 3.325 mM DTT. Samples were incubated at 25°C for 10 min to achieve temperature equilibration and to establish a blank rate, if any. 0.5 mM DL-glyceraldehdye-3-phosphate was added and absorbance was recorded for 10 min at 339 nm. Measured rates were corrected by measuring the blank rate of the reaction. One unit is defined as 1 μmol NADH generated/minute/mg protein. Similarly, total LDH activity was calculated as rate of absorbance at 339 nm produced by oxidation of NADH at 25°C and pH 7.3 in 0.2 M Tris-HCL buffer containing 1 mM sodium pyruvate and 0.22 mM NADH.

HIF-1α and Phospho-MAPK Content

HIF-1α content and phospho-(p)-p38, p-JNK, p-ERK1/2 content were assayed by an immuno-linked luminescence assay in accordance with manufacturer's instructions (Mesoscale Discovery, Gaithersburg, USA). HeLa cells treated with and without cobalt chloride for 16 h provided positive and negative controls respectively for the HIF-1α assay. Lysate from Jurkat cells treated with 1 mol rapamycin for 3 h to activate MAPK phosphatase 1 was used as negative control for the MAPK assay. Lysate from Jurkat cells treated with 50 nM calyculin A and 200 nM PMA for 15 min to stimulate phosphorylation of MAPK proteins was used as a positive control (Mesoscale Discovery).

Isotonic Muscle Function

Ex Vivo Muscle Preparation

Animals were anesthetized by 5% isoflurane inhalation in air and euthanized by cervical dislocation. Sternohyoid muscles were excised and placed in a bath of Krebs solution (NaCl 120 mM, KCl 5 mM, Ca^{2+} gluconate 2.5 mM, $MgSO_4$ 1.2 mM, NaH_2PO_4 1.2 mM, $NaHCO_3$ 25 mM, glucose 11.5 mM, and 25 μM d-tubocurarine) at room temperature and gassed with carbogen (95% O_2/5% CO_2) before mounting in the test bath for assessment of muscle contractile and endurance performance. Whole intact mouse sternohyoid muscle bundles were arranged between the electrodes with the sternum anchored at a fixed base and hyoid bone connected by a non-elastic string to a dual-mode lever force transducer (Aurora Scientific, Canada) such that fibers were orientated vertically. Upon placement in the test bath, bundles were incubated at 35°C in Krebs solution gassed with carbogen (95% O_2/5% CO_2). Muscle performance has previously been shown (Skelly et al., 2010) to be optimal under hyperoxic conditions (95% O_2) compared to normoxic conditions (21% O_2). Bundles were equilibrated for 5 min in gassed Krebs solution prior to initiating the experimental protocol.

Protocol

Bundles were set to optimum length (Lo—length at which peak twitch force occurs) by adjusting the position of the force transducer with a micro-positioner and stimulating with repeated single pulses whilst adjusting muscle length until peak twitch force was reached. Contractile kinetics [time to peak (TTP) and half-relaxation time (T50)] were measured from the peak twitch force recordings. After 5 min of equilibration, the lever of the force transducer was set to maximum rigidity (~500 mN; >100% load) and a tetanic contraction was elicited by stimulating the bundle with supra-maximal voltage at 100 Hz for 300 ms. The peak isometric force ($Fmax$) was established allowing determination of 100% load for isotonic assessments. Shortening contractions were elicited in incremental steps ranging from 0 to 100% load with 1 min rest between each step. Peak shortening velocity ($Vmax$) was determined during the initial 30 ms of shortening (see **Figure 1**) as this is when velocity is greatest (Watchko et al., 1997; Van Lunteren et al., 2007; Van Lunteren and Pollarine, 2010). Power was determined at each step as the product of force/cross-sectional area (CSA) x shortening velocity/Lo. Peak specific work ($Wmax$) was calculated as force/CSA x shortening (L/Lo) at the load where the product of these variables was greatest.

Isotonic Function Data Analysis

Muscle cross-sectional area (CSA) was calculated as the blotted dry muscle bundle weight divided by the product of Lo and the specific density which was assumed to be 1.056 g/cm^3. Specific force was calculated as N/cm^2. Specific shortening velocity was calculated as Lo/s. Specific power was calculated as Watts/cm^2. $Wmax$ was calculated as Joules/cm^3.

Statistical Analyses

Statistical comparisons of the total mean fluorescence intensity for 1D preparations and FTSC/IAF- and coomassie-labeled spot volumes (2D) were measured using Student t-tests, Mann-Whitney U-tests, or One-Way ANOVA as appropriate after testing for normality and equal variance in the data sets. Student t-test or Mann-Whitney U-test was used as appropriate to compare control and CH groups for chymotrypsin-like activity of the 20S proteasome, and GAPDH and LDH activities. Tissue limitations restricted the measurement of all molecular components at all three time points of CH exposure. HIF-1α content and p-MAPK contents were compared between groups by One-Way

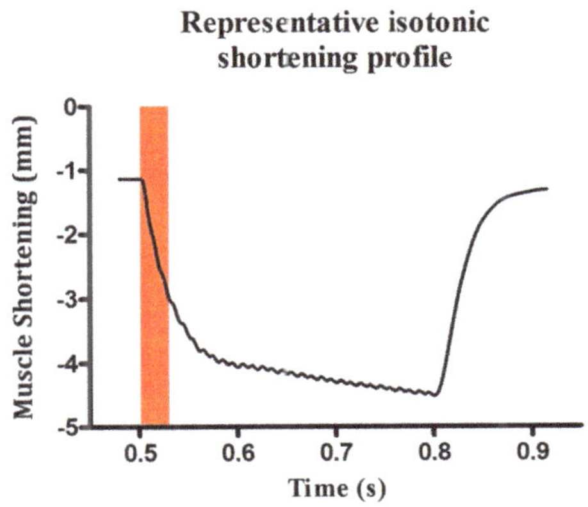

FIGURE 1 | Representative profile of sternohyoid peak shortening velocity. An original record illustrating a representative contraction at 0% load. Maximum velocity of shortening was calculated during the first 30 ms of the contraction.

ANOVA followed by Tukey's multiple comparison *post-hoc* test, or the Kruskal-Wallis test followed by Dunn's multiple comparison *post-hoc* test as appropriate, after testing for normality and equal variance in the data sets. Statistical comparisons were performed between groups for sternohyoid contractile and endurance performance using One-Way ANOVA followed by Tukey's multiple comparison *post-hoc* tests. Power-load relationship was assessed by Two-Way ANOVA followed by Bonferroni's *post-hoc* multiple comparison tests. Linear regression analysis was performed to assess the relationship between oxidative stress markers (protein free thiol and carbonyl groups) and sternohyoid muscle power. $P < 0.05$ was the criterion for statistical significance in all tests.

Results

Animal Model

Hematocrit was significantly ($p < 0.001$) increased by CH exposure (**Table 1**). Antioxidant supplementation in animals exposed to 6 weeks of CH had no effect on hematocrit compared to CH alone. Animals drank equivalent volumes of water (with or without antioxidant) per day. Body mass decreased after 1 week of CH exposure but all hypoxic animals returned to a growth curve equivalent to the control animals for weeks two through to six of the gas treatments (data not shown).

Total Protein Carbonyl and Free Thiol Content

Significant increases in sternohyoid carbonyl content were observed after 3 ($p < 0.001$) and 6 ($p < 0.001$) weeks of CH (**Figure 2A**)—indicative of increased sternohyoid protein oxidation. Sternohyoid protein free thiol content changes were bi-phasic (**Figure 2B**). There was a significant increase in sternohyoid protein free thiol content after 1 ($p < 0.05$) and 3 ($p < 0.01$) weeks of CH; however free thiol content was significantly lower than control after 6 weeks of CH ($p < 0.001$). For comparison, two limb muscles, namely soleus, and extensor digitorum longus (EDL) were also studied. Unlike the sternohyoid, there were no significant changes to the carbonyl content of the EDL proteome after CH exposure (**Figure 3A**). There was, however, significant increases in EDL free thiol content after 1 ($p < 0.01$), 3 ($p < 0.001$), and 6 ($p < 0.001$) weeks of CH—though the magnitude of the increase is seen to decrease over time (**Figure 3B**). Similar to the sternohyoid muscle, but unlike the EDL, significant increases in soleus protein carbonyl content were observed after 3 ($p < 0.05$), and 6 ($p < 0.01$) weeks of CH (**Figure 4A**). Soleus protein free thiol content was significantly increased after 1 ($p < 0.001$), 3 ($p < 0.01$), and 6 ($p < 0.001$) weeks of CH compared to controls (**Figure 4B**). Consistent with EDL, there was a decline in increased free thiol content in the soleus with progressive CH.

TABLE 1 | Hematocrit values after 1, 3, or 6 weeks of normoxia or chronic sustained hypoxia (CH).

	Normoxia	CH	*P*-value[a]
HEMATOCRIT (%)			
One Week	34 ± 2	52 ± 2	$P < 0.001$
Three Weeks	38 ± 1	65 ± 1	$P < 0.001$
Six Weeks	32 ± 1	62 ± 1	$P < 0.001$

Data are presented as mean ± SEM; n = 8 per group. [a]Student unpaired t-test.

2D Redox Proteomics

In the sternohyoid, 498, 264, and 996 resolved spots were matched in FTSC-, IAF-labeled and coomassie-stained separations respectively. A significant relative volume difference was observed in 87 FTSC, 51 IAF, and 156 coomassie spots comparing control and CH groups ($p < 0.05$). Proteins were selected for mass spectrometry analysis based on separation, resolution, abundance, and overlap in fluorescence-stain and muscle separations. Protein smears and gel defects were excluded. Results for protein remodeling are presented in **Table 2** with proteins grouped according to cellular location and/or function. Selected spots can be visualized on the representative coomassie stained gel shown in **Figure 5**. A change in FTSC and IAF fluorescence

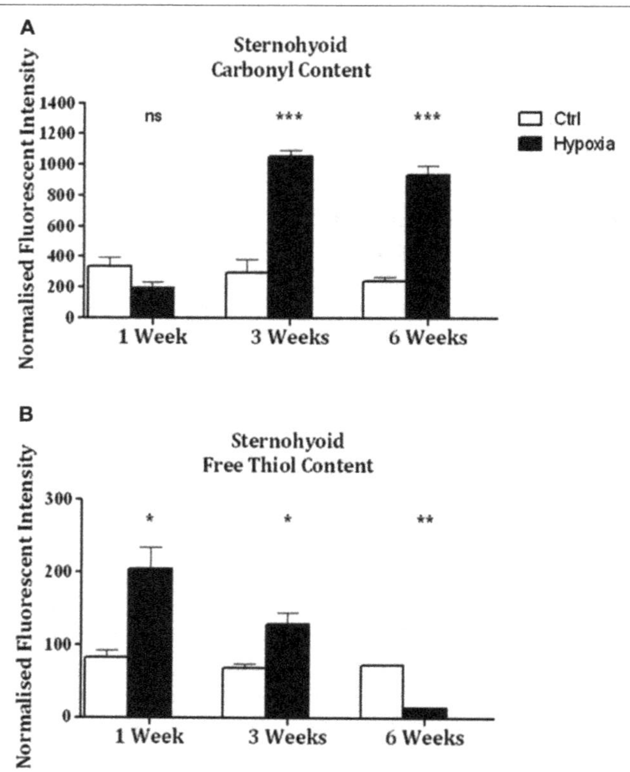

FIGURE 2 | Sternohyoid protein carbonyl and free thiol content after 1, 3, and 6 weeks of sustained hypoxia compared to normoxic controls. **(A)** Sternohyoid protein carbonyl content (mean ± SEM) after 1, 3, and 6 weeks of normoxia or sustained hypoxia expressed as normalized fluorescence intensity; $n = 5$–8 per group; **(B)** Sternohyoid protein free thiol content (mean ± SEM) after 1, 3, and 6 weeks of normoxia or sustained hypoxia expressed as normalized fluorescence intensity; $n = 7$–8 per group; *$p < 0.05$, **$p < 0.01$, ***$p < 0.001$, ns, not significant; Student *t*-test or Mann-Whitney test as appropriate. Ctrl, normoxic control; Hypoxia, sustained hypoxia ($FiO_2 = 0.1$).

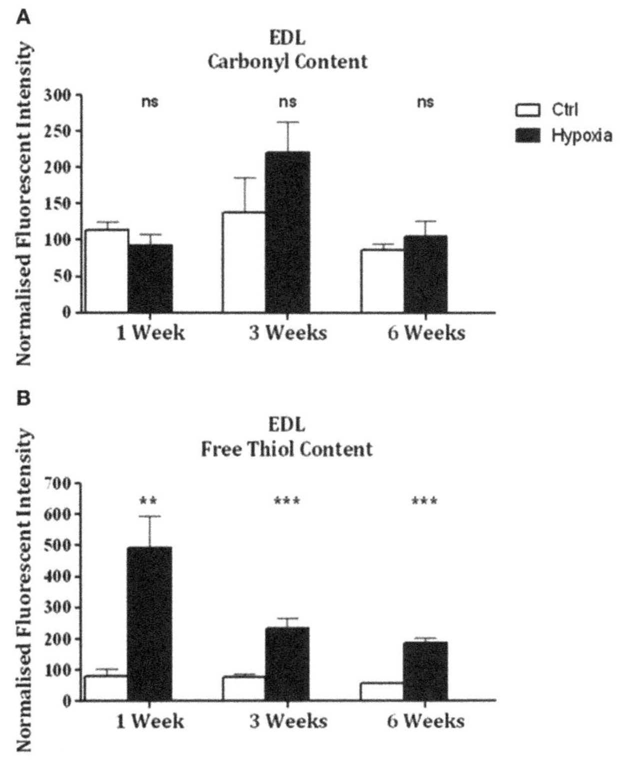

FIGURE 3 | EDL protein carbonyl and free thiol content after 1, 3, and 6 weeks of sustained hypoxia compared to normoxic controls. (A) EDL protein carbonyl content (mean ± SEM) after 1, 3, and 6 weeks of sustained hypoxia expressed as normalized fluorescence intensity; $n = 4$–8 per group; **(B)** EDL protein free thiol content (mean ± SEM) after 1, 3, and 6 weeks of sustained hypoxia expressed as normalized fluorescence intensity; $n = 6$–8 per group; $^{**}p < 0.01$, $^{***}p < 0.001$, ns, not significant; Student *t*-test or Mann-Whitney test as appropriate; Ctrl, normoxic control; Hypoxia, sustained hypoxia ($FiO_2 = 0.1$).

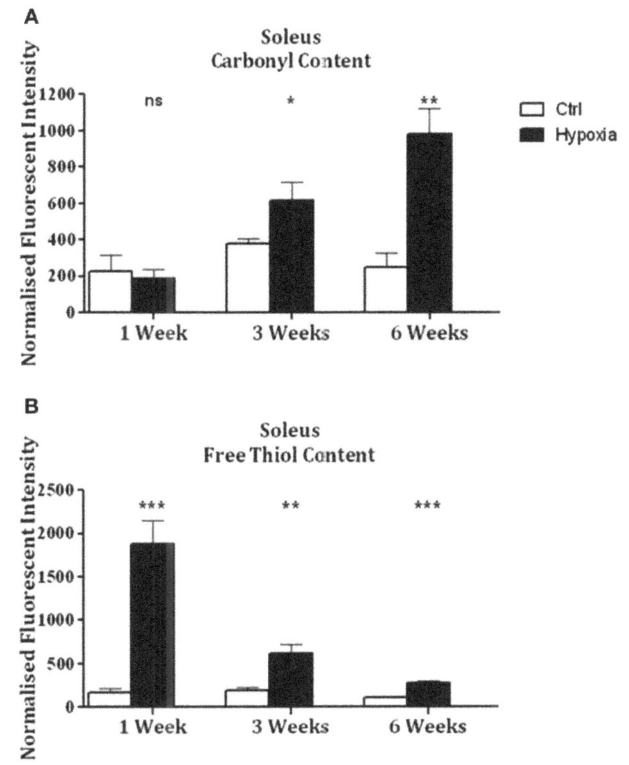

FIGURE 4 | Soleus protein carbonyl and free thiol content after 1, 3, and 6 weeks of sustained hypoxia compared to normoxic controls. (A) Soleus protein carbonyl content (mean ± SEM) after 1, 3, and 6 weeks of sustained hypoxia expressed as normalized fluorescence intensity; $n = 4$–8 per group; **(B)** Soleus protein free thiol content (mean ± SEM) after 1, 3, and 6 weeks of sustained hypoxia expressed as normalized fluorescence intensity; $n = 8$ per group; $^{*}p < 0.05$, $^{**}p < 0.01$, $^{***}p < 0.001$, ns, not significant; Student *t*-test or Mann-Whitney test as appropriate; Ctrl, normoxic control; Hypoxia, sustained hypoxia ($FiO_2 = 0.1$).

intensity signal independent of, or differential to, coomassie signal is indicative of protein redox remodeling.

Sternohyoid Glycolytic Enzyme Activities

Sternohyoid GAPDH activity was significantly increased after 1 week of CH ($p < 0.05$) but significantly decreased after 3 weeks of CH ($p < 0.01$) (data not shown). LDH activity in the sternohyoid (data not shown) was significantly increased after 1 week of CH ($p < 0.05$).

Sternohyoid Chymotrypsin-like Proteasome Activity

Chymotrypsin-like proteasome activity was unchanged in the sternohyoid after 6 weeks of CH (data not shown).

Sternohyoid HIF-1α Content

There was no change in sternohyoid HIF-1α content following 6 weeks of CH with or without antioxidant supplementation (data not shown).

Sternohyoid Phospho-MAPK Content

There was no change in sternohyoid p-p38 content following 6 weeks of CH with or without antioxidant supplementation (**Figure 6A**). However, 6 weeks of CH significantly decreased sternohyoid p-JNK content compared to control (One-Way ANOVA ($p < 0.01$) followed by Tukey's multiple comparison test ($p < 0.05$); chronic antioxidant supplementation with either tempol or NAC did not prevent this (**Figure 6B**). A similar effect was observed for sternohyoid p-ERK1/2 content. A Kruskal-Wallis test revealed a significant difference in the mean values of the groups. However, Dunn's multiple comparisons test revealed no significant differences between pairs (**Figure 6C**).

Sternohyoid Protein Carbonyl and Free Thiol Content after Antioxidant Treatment

In the second cohort of animals, significant increases in sternohyoid protein carbonyl content were again observed after 6 weeks of CH ($p < 0.001$). Chronic antioxidant supplementation with either Tempol ($p < 0.001$) or NAC ($p < 0.001$) significantly ameliorated the CH-induced increase in protein carbonyl content

TABLE 2 | Identifications by mass spectrometry of proteins undergoing significant redox remodeling in the sternohyoid muscle after 6 weeks of sustained hypoxia.

Spot #	Protein	Mw (Da)	GI number	Mascot score	Matched peptides	Sequence coverage	Carbonyl *p*-value, fold	Free thiol *p*-value, fold	Expression *p*-value, fold
ELECTRON TRANSPORT CHAIN									
1	Cytochrome bc - 1 complex subunit 1	52,819	341941780	430	6	26%	-	<0.01, −1.4	<0.001, −2
2	ATP Synthase subunit α	59,716	416677	997	6	53%	-	-	<0.01, +1.5
TCA CYCLE									
3	Aconitase hydratase	85,410	60391212	1210	11	41%	<0.01, +1.4	<0.001, −2	<0.01, −2.6
4	2-oxo-glutarate dehydrogenase, mt	116,375	146345472	477	4	22%	-	<0.01, −2.4	<0.01, +2.8
GLYCOLYSIS									
5	Fructose bis-phosphate aldolase A	39,331	113607	588	3	70%	-	<0.01, −2.9	-
6	Glyceraldehyde-3-phosphate dehydrogenase	35,787	120702	531	4	48%	-	<0.01, −1.6	<0.001, −2
7	Phosphoglycerate kinase 1	44,534	1730519	534	4	45%	-	-	<0.01,+1.7
8	Phosphoglycerate mutase 2	28,809	6093745	1010	9	57%	-	-	<0.01, +1.7
9	Pyruvate kinase isozymes M1/M2	57,305	146345448	837	6	53%	<0.01, −1.2	-	<0.01, +1.3
PHOSPHAGEN AND LIPID METABOLISM									
10	Glycerol-3-phosphate dehydrogenase [NAD(+)]	37,548	121557	412	3	48%	-	<0.01, −2	<0.01, −2.6
11	Creatine kinase m-type	43,014	124056470	784	7	42%	<0.01, +1.2	-	<0.01, −1.2
STRESS RESPONSE AND IRON HOMEOSTASIS									
12	Glycogen phosphorylase	97,225	14916635	1450	13	47%	<0.01, −1.3	-	<0.01, +4.1
13	90kDa heat shock protein	83,229	341941065	742	6	31%	-	-	<0.01, −1.3
14	Alpha crystallin B chain	20,056	6166129	761	7	65%	<0.01, +1.2	-	-
15	Myoglobin	17,059	127676	923	7	43%	-	-	<0.01, −1.7
16	Serotransferrin	76,674	21363012	121	1	17%	<0.01, −1.4	<0.01, +1.8	-
17	Carbonic anhydrase III	29,348	30581036	966	8	71%	<0.01, +1.2	<0.01, -2.7	<0.01, +1.9
18	Albumin	68,648	5915682	1340	11	53%	-	-	<0.01, −1.8
CROSS-BRIDGE AND SARCOPLASMIC RETICULUM									
19	Calsequestrin	46,420	341940315	543	4	19%	<0.01, −1.5	-	<0.01, −2.3

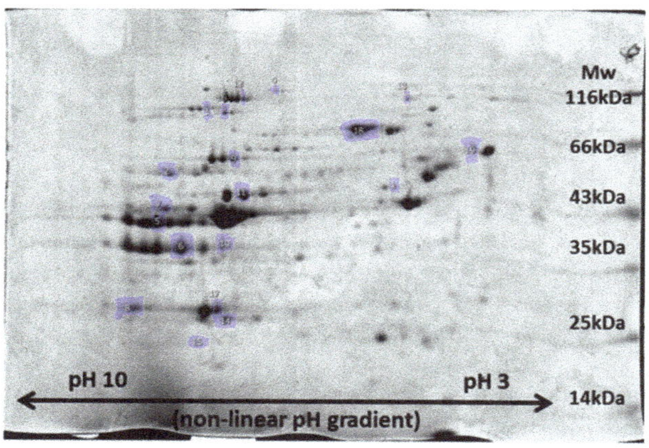

FIGURE 5 | Representative image of 2D-PAGE sternohyoid muscle protein profile after coomassie staining of proteins. A molecular mass marker ranging from 14 to 116 kDa is shown for size reference and isoelectric point is indicated along the range pH 10-3. Spot numbers match those presented in **Table 2**.

(**Figure 7A**). Similarly, sternohyoid protein free thiol content was significantly lower than control after 6 weeks of CH ($p < 0.01$) and antioxidant treatment with Tempol ($p < 0.001$) and NAC ($p < 0.05$) ameliorated this effect (**Figure 7B**).

Sternohyoid Muscle Function

There are no significant differences observed across groups for contractile kinetics, twitch force, V*max*, W*max*, or isotonic fatigue index (**Table 3**) as determined by One-Way ANOVA or Kruskal-Wallis test; however, CH exposure increased the contraction time, and decreased endurance (**Table 3**). NAC supplementation in CH increased peak twitch force, V*max*, W*max*, and endurance (**Table 3**). Fmax is significantly different across groups; decreased in CH compared to control and significantly increased by NAC supplementation in CH compared to CH alone as revealed by Tukey's multiple comparison *post-hoc* test (**Table 3**).

Sternohyoid muscle isotonic contractile function (power) was significantly depressed by CH exposure (**Figure 8**; Two-Way ANOVA: gas treatment: $p < 0.001$). Significant correlations were observed for oxidative stress markers and sternohyoid muscle function (**Figure 9**). The deleterious effects of CH exposure on sternohyoid function were prevented with antioxidant supplementation in CH using either tempol or NAC (**Figure 8**).

Discussion

This is the first study to identify proteins in an upper airway muscle undergoing redox remodeling following exposure to CH. CH decreased sternohyoid force- and power-generating

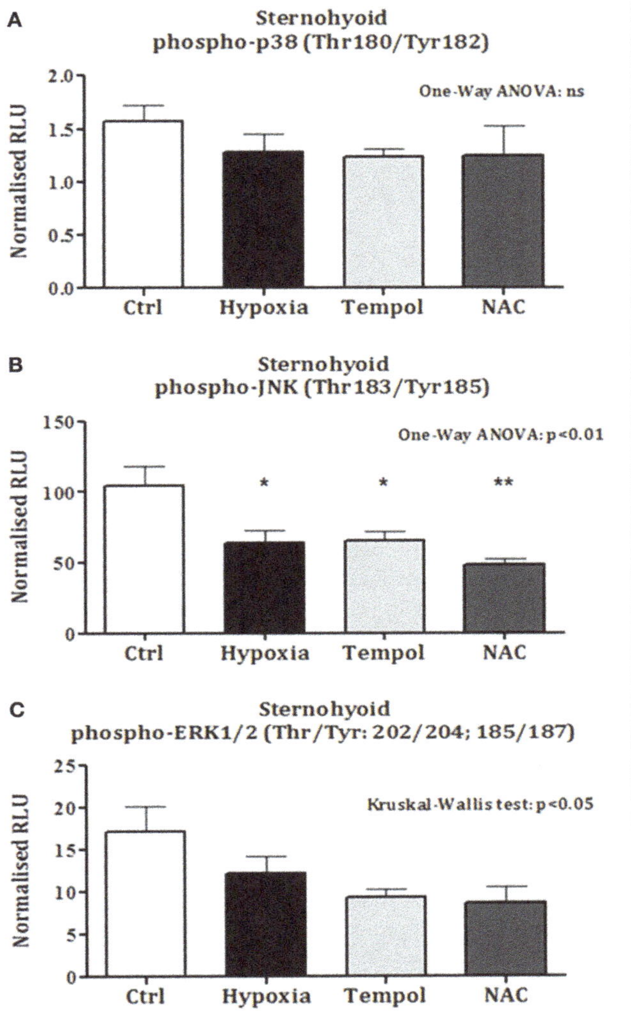

FIGURE 6 | Sternohyoid phospho-MAPK contents after 6 weeks of normoxia and sustained hypoxia ± chronic antioxidant supplementation. (A) Sternohyoid phospho-p38 content (mean ± SEM) expressed as normalized relative luminescence units; $n = 5$–7 per group; **(B)** Sternohyoid phospho-JNK content (mean ± SEM expressed as normalized relative luminescence units; $n = 5$–7 per group; **(C)** Sternohyoid phospho-ERK 1/2 content (mean ± SEM) expressed as normalized relative luminescence units; $n = 5$–7 per group; $^*p < 0.05$ and $^{**}p < 0.01$ vs. control, Tukey's multiple comparison test; Ctrl, normoxic control; Hypoxia, sustained hypoxia ($FiO_2 = 0.1$); Tempol, tempol + sustained hypoxia; NAC, NAC + sustained hypoxia; RLU, relative luminescence units.

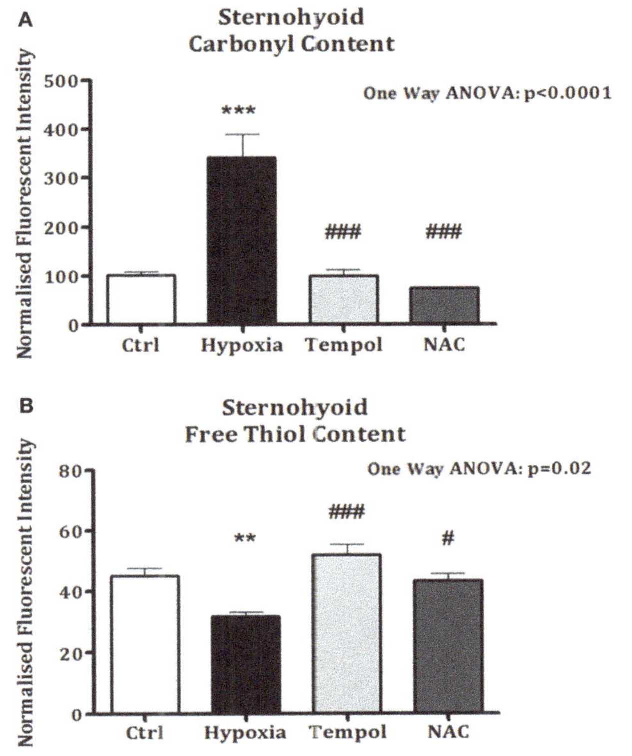

FIGURE 7 | Sternohyoid protein carbonyl and free thiol content following 6 weeks of normoxia and sustained hypoxia ± chronic antioxidant supplementation. (A) Sternohyoid protein carbonyl content (mean ± SEM) expressed as normalized fluorescence intensity; $n = 5$–7 per group; **(B)** Sternohyoid protein free thiol content (mean ± SEM) expressed as normalized fluorescence intensity; $n = 5$–7 per group; $^{**}p < 0.05$ and $^{***}p < 0.001$ vs. control, $^{\#}p < 0.05$ and $^{\#\#\#}p < 0.001$ vs. hypoxia, Tukey's multiple comparison test; Ctrl, normoxic control; Hypoxia, sustained hypoxia ($FiO_2 = 0.1$); Tempol, tempol + sustained hypoxia; NAC, NAC + sustained hypoxia.

capacity. Antioxidant supplementation prevented CH-induced sternohyoid dysfunction. The main findings of this study are: (1) CH induces temporal changes in protein carbonylation and free thiol oxidation in the sternohyoid, responses different to that seen in limb muscles; (2) Proteins key to muscle contraction, metabolism, and homeostasis are redox-modified in the sternohyoid following 6 weeks of CH; (3) Glycolytic enzyme activities are temporally affected in the sternohyoid following progressive CH exposure; (4) CH has no effect on sternohyoid HIF-1α content; (5) CH decreases p-JNK in sternohyoid independent of antioxidant status; (6) CH causes sternohyoid muscle dysfunction; (7) Oxidative stress markers and muscle function were significantly correlated; (8) Both protein oxidation and contractile impairment following CH are fully reversed by chronic antioxidant supplementation.

Muscle Redox Status

In skeletal muscle adaptation to high altitude and respiratory diseases featuring hypoxia, ROS have been shown to cause protein redox remodeling and to modify protein function with resultant changes in metabolic processes, homeostasis and contractile performance (Zuo and Clanton, 2005; Marin-Corral et al., 2009; Murray, 2009; Chaudhary et al., 2012; Levine et al., 2013; Puig-Vilanova et al., 2015). However, the cause and motive for increased ROS production is unclear and may differ in skeletal muscles given their varied functional roles. In the present study, we observed time-dependent increases in protein oxidation (both increased carbonyl content and decreased free thiol content) in CH-exposed sternohyoid muscle (differential to responses in limb muscles, which is likely pivotal for time-dependent and

TABLE 3 | Sternohyoid muscle contractile properties after 6 weeks of normoxia and sustained hypoxia ± chronic antioxidant supplementation.

	Normoxia	Hypoxia	Tempol	NAC	*P*-Value[a]
TTP (ms)	9 ± 0	10 ± 0	11 ± 1	10 ± 0	ns
T50 (ms)	11 ± 1	11 ± 1	14 ± 3	12 ± 2	ns
Pt (N/cm^2)	2.5 ± 0.4	1.6 ± 0.2	1.9 ± 0.2	3.0 ± 0.9	ns
Fmax (N/cm^2)	12.3 ± 1.5	8.0 ± 0.6*	11.0 ± 0.3	16.0 ± 2.3##	<0.01
Vmax (Lo/s)	5.4 ± 0.7	5.2 ± 0.9	6.1 ± 0.7	6.1 ± 0.4	ns
Wmax (J/cm^3)	0.6 ± 0.1	0.6 ± 0.1	0.8 ± 0.1	0.9 ± 0.1	ns
Fatigue Index (% of initial power)	63 ± 14	36 ± 7	33 ± 11	46 ± 12	ns

*Data are presented as mean ± SEM; n = 5–8 per group; [a]One Way ANOVA, *p < 0.05 vs. Normoxia and ##p 0.01 vs. Hypoxia, Tukey's post-hoc multiple comparison test; ns, not significant; Hypoxia, 6 weeks of sustained hypoxia (FiO_2 = 0.1); Tempol, tempol + hypoxia; NAC, NAC + hypoxia.*

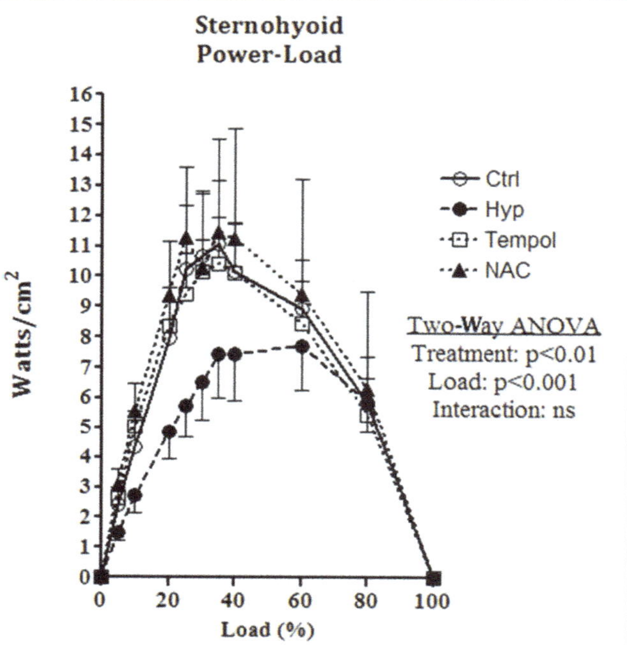

FIGURE 8 | Sternohyoid power-load relationship following 6 weeks of normoxia and sustained hypoxia ± chronic antioxidant supplementation. Sternohyoid specific power (mean ± SEM) expressed as Watts/CSA (cm^2) as a function of load expressed as a percentage of peak force (force/peak force*100); *n* = 5–7 per group; Ctrl, normoxic control; Hyp, sustained hypoxia (FiO_2 = 0.1); Tempol, tempol + sustained hypoxia; NAC, NAC + sustained hypoxia. *P*-values shown for two factor (treatment × load) analysis of variance highlighting a significant effect of 6 weeks of sustained hypoxia on sternohyoid power-load relationship. Antioxidant supplementation reversed the effects of hypoxia.

differential structural and functional remodeling reported in previous studies (El-Khoury et al., 2003, 2012; Faucher et al., 2005; Gamboa and Andrade, 2010, 2012; McMorrow et al., 2011; Carberry et al., 2014). This, in turn, may be of clinical significance given that CH is potentially implicated in the progression of respiratory diseases.

Clearly there is differential muscle protein redox remodeling which appears unrelated to fiber type *per se* given the similarities between the EDL and sternohyoid muscles, and unrelated to respiratory vs. limb muscle differences *per se* given the differences observed in the EDL compared with the soleus. As the soleus is a postural muscle, it exhibits greater contractile activity than the EDL which is used for more powerful movements of the limbs. The combination of activity and hypoxic exposure is potentially synergistic in driving protein oxidation, with reflex hyperventilation and hypoxia combining to drive protein oxidation in the sternohyoid. Furthermore, a comparison of basal carbonyl signals from sternohyoid and limb muscle proteomes suggests that basal workload of a given muscle is more important in determining carbonylation of proteins than fiber type *per se*.

2D redox proteomic profiling of the sternohyoid muscle after 6 weeks of CH exposure reveals key proteins in muscle that are targeted by ROS, many of which are redox modified in COPD muscle (Marin-Corral et al., 2009). It is clear from **Table 2** that extensive remodeling occurs to mitochondrial, metabolic, and associated proteins, suggesting that the mitochondria are the primary source of remodeling stress. Reflex hyperventilation increases metabolic demand and subsequent metabolic substrate flux to the respiratory chain. With hypoxia, stockpiling of electrons occurs, increasing electron leak and subsequent ROS formation. This is supported by the findings of decreased muscle mitochondrial density and mitochondrial remodeling in hypoxia, high altitude, and respiratory-related diseases (Hoppeler et al., 1990, 2003; Gosker et al., 2000; Wijnhoven et al., 2006; Viganò et al., 2008; Gamboa and Andrade, 2010, 2012). The fold change in free thiol content following 1 week of CH is greatest in soleus>EDL>sternohyoid suggesting that fiber type, more so than contractile activity, is key to this change.

EDL free thiol content remains elevated above control whereas carbonyl content was unchanged after 6 weeks of CH; however the pattern of change is similar to the sternohyoid and soleus muscles. It is likely to be a combination of hypoxia, muscle fiber composition, and workload in hypoxia that accounts for the differential changes in respiratory and limb muscle protein oxidation and functional changes. In keeping with the notion of muscle specific effects of CH, other studies have reported differential effects of oxidation, based on carbonyl and thiol measurements as well as other indicators of altered cellular oxidative/reductive state which are proposed to depend on the activity and/or local cellular environment of the relevant protein (Haycock et al., 1998; Kadiiska et al., 2005; El-Shafey et al., 2011). See additional discussion in the supplementary file.

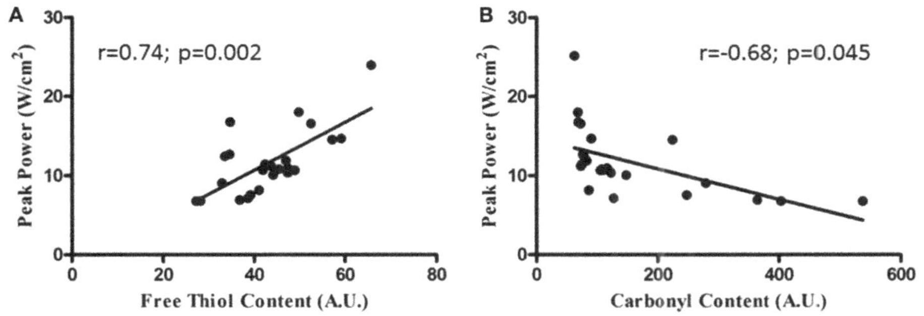

FIGURE 9 | Relationship between sternohyoid power and oxidative stress markers. Relationship between sternohyoid specific peak power and muscle oxidative stress markers [protein free thiol content **(A)** and carbonyl content **(B)**] plotting data from all animals in the second cohort of studies; $n = 24$. Note the correlation coefficients and statistically significant relationships.

Muscle Redox Signaling

Decreased sternohyoid GAPDH activity with progressive hypoxia is consistent with the decreased expression measured by proteomic profiling after 6 weeks of CH. CH-induced changes in LDH activity in the sternohyoid follow a similar pattern to GAPDH. As muscle function and metabolism are intrinsically interlinked through HIF signaling (Semenza et al., 1994; Vogt et al., 2001; Kim et al., 2006), one might have expected a CH-induced increase in HIF-1α content. However, decreased GAPDH expression and decreased GAPDH and LDH activities observed in the sternohyoid muscle of our mouse model are suggestive of decreased HIF-1α content. Interestingly, after 6 weeks of CH exposure we observed that there was no change in sternohyoid HIF-1α content. It is plausible that the degree of hypoxia experienced by the sternohyoid may change temporally with acclimatization to hypoxia such that HIF-1α may have been activated earlier in the exposure. Of note, for example, GAPDH activity is increased in sternohyoid muscle after 1 but not 3 weeks of CH. Protein carbonylation is elevated in CH sternohyoid after 6 weeks suggesting that although ROS are presumably elevated in the muscle there is no ROS-dependent HIF-1α activation. Moreover, antioxidant supplementation did not affect HIF-1α content in CH sternohyoid. Thus, our results suggest that redox modulation of sternohyoid metabolism and function is HIF-1α independent.

The MAPK proteins are involved in a diverse array of cellular signaling events and are vital to muscle growth and homeostasis. p38 activity in muscle is strongly associated with promoting atrophy in COPD limb muscle (Lemire et al., 2012) and is potentially required for hypoxia signaling of HIF via mitochondrial ROS production (Emerling et al., 2005). However, neither HIF-1α content nor chymotrypsin-like 20S proteasome activity changed in the sternohyoid muscle following CH. Indeed, hypertrophy of fast fibers in the sternohyoid is reported following CH exposure in the rat (McMorrow et al., 2011) suggesting enhanced protein synthesis. This is especially interesting, as the present study has established for the first time, that the CH sternohyoid has decreased (not increased) power-generating capacity, highlighting a potent redox-dependent inhibitory effect of CH on the contractile machinery of the airway dilator muscle, rather than CH-induced muscle atrophy.

p-JNK content is decreased in the sternohyoid following CH exposure. Differential regulation of p38 and JNK occurs at the MAP2K level and is potentially influenced by contractile activity and mechanical stress (Sawada et al., 2001). The combination of hypoxic/redox stress, muscle fiber type combination, and mechanical activity of the sternohyoid is likely important in determining the stress kinase response to CH exposure. A ROS/p-JNK-dependent mechanism is implicated in CH-induced sternohyoid dysfunction but it is important to note that antioxidant supplementation did not prevent the CH-induced decrease in p-JNK (or p-ERK1/2), whereas antioxidants prevented sternohyoid redox stress and contractile dysfunction following CH exposure.

Sternohyoid Isotonic Performance

The sternohyoid force- and power-generating capacity was significantly depressed by CH exposure. Muscle oxidative stress markers and contractile power were significantly correlated; moreover, antioxidant supplementation during CH exposure prevented both protein redox stress and contractile dysfunction. Therefore, we posit that CH-induced redox remodeling of key proteins in metabolism and the contractile apparatus is central to CH-induced sternohyoid muscle dysfunction. Concerning the potential clinical relevance of our findings, sternohyoid dysfunction could serve to increase obstructive airway events *in vivo*—further disrupting respiratory homeostasis in diseases characterized by hypoxic stress. We speculate that CH-induced redox remodeling and functional deficit in pharyngeal dilator muscles potentially underpins the higher prevalence of OSA observed in COPD patients (the overlap syndrome) (Owens and Malhotra, 2010).

Summary and Conclusions

This study highlights the application of a redox proteomics approach to a translational animal model of hypoxia. CH exposure causes progressive redox remodeling in the sternohyoid (upper airway dilator) muscle with differential responses to limb muscles. CH results in metabolic protein structural remodeling with resultant changes in enzyme activity. Redox and expression changes were shown to occur to various protein chaperones including those important to cross-bridge maintenance. Ultimately, it appears that CH-induced redox changes result in functional deficit in the sternohyoid, given that antioxidant supplementation during CH exposure prevents both protein stress and functional impairment. We hypothesize a pivotal role for ROS in pharyngeal dilator muscle structural and functional (mal)adaptations to CH. The putative role of hypoxia in driving respiratory muscle remodeling in human respiratory disease warrants investigation.

Author Contributions

The study was conceived and designed by PL and KO. Experiments and data analyses were performed by PL in the laboratories of KO and DS. Mass spectrometry experiments were performed and analyzed by RS in the laboratory of AV. The manuscript was written by PL and KO with contributions from the other authors.

Acknowledgments

This project was funded by The Health Research Board (Ireland), and by the Strategic Research Fund, University College Cork, Ireland.

References

Aiken, C. T., Kaake, R. M., Wang, X., and Huang, L. (2011). Oxidative stress-mediated regulation of proteasome complexes. *Mol. Cell. Proteomics* 10, R110.006924. doi: 10.1074/mcp.R110.006924

Bradford, A., McGuire, M., and O'Halloran, K. D. (2005). Does episodic hypoxia affect upper airway dilator muscle function? Implications for the pathophysiology of obstructive sleep apnoea. *Respir. Physiol. Neurobiol.* 147, 223–234. doi: 10.1016/j.resp.2005.04.001

Carberry, J. C., McMorrow, C., Bradford, A., Jones, J. F. X., and O'Halloran, K. D. (2014). Effects of sustained hypoxia on sternohyoid and diaphragm muscle during development. *Eur. Respir. J.* 43, 1149–1158. doi: 10.1183/09031936.00139512

Chaudhary, P., Suryakumar, G., Prasad, R., Singh, S. N., Ali, S., and Ilavazhagan, G. (2012). Chronic hypobaric hypoxia mediated skeletal muscle atrophy: role of ubiquitin-proteasome pathway and calpains. *Mol. Cell. Biochem.* 364, 101–113. doi: 10.1007/s11010-011-1210-x

Cole, C., Coelho, A. V., James, R. H., Connelly, D., and Sheehan, D. (2014). Proteomic responses to metal-induced oxidative stress in hydrothermal vent-living mussels, Bathymodiolus sp., on the Southwest Indian Ridge. *Mar. Env. Res.* 96, 29–37. doi: 10.1016/j.marenvres.2013.09.003

Dalle-Donne, I., Aldini, G., Carini, M., Colombo, R., Rossi, R., and Milzani, A. (2006). Protein carbonylation, cellular dysfunction, and disease progression. *J. Cell. Mol. Med.* 10, 389–406. doi: 10.1111/j.1582-4934.2006.tb00407.x

Doucet, M., Debigaré, R., Joanisse, D. R., Côté, C., Leblanc, P., Grégoire, J., et al. (2004). Adaptation of the diaphragm and the vastus lateralis in mild-to-moderate COPD. *Eur. Respir. J.* 24, 971–979. doi: 10.1183/09031936.04.00020204

Doucet, M., Dubé, A., Joanisse, D. R., Debigaré, R., Michaud, A., Paré, M.-È., et al. (2010). Atrophy and hypertrophy signalling of the quadriceps and diaphragm in COPD. *Thorax* 65, 963–970. doi: 10.1136/thx.2009.133827

Dyballa, N., and Metzger, S. (2009). Fast and sensitive colloidal coomassie G-250 staining for proteins in polyacrylamide gels. *J. Vis. Exp.* 30:e1431. doi: 10.3791/1431

Edge, D., Jones, J. F. X., Bradford, A., and O'Halloran, K. D. (2012). Effect of chronic intermittent hypoxia on reflex recruitment of sternohyoid EMG during airway obstruction in the anaesthetised rat. *Proc Physiol Soc* 27, PC223.

Edge, D., McDonald, F. B., Jones, J. F. X., Bradford, A., and O'Halloran, K. D. (2014). Effect of chronic intermittent hypoxia on the reflex recruitment of the genioglossus during airway obstruction in the anesthetized rat. *Prog. Brain Res.* 209, 147–168. doi: 10.1016/B978-0-444-63274-6.00008-4

El-Khoury, R., Bradford, A., and O'Halloran, K. D. (2012). Chronic hypobaric hypoxia increases isolated rat fast-twitch and slow-twitch limb muscle force and fatigue. *Physiol. Res.* 61, 195–201.

El-Khoury, R., O'Halloran, K. D., and Bradford, A. (2003). Effects of chronic hypobaric hypoxia on contractile properties of rat sternohyoid and diaphragm muscles. *Clin. Exp. Pharmacol. Physiol.* 30, 551–554. doi: 10.1046/j.1440-1681.2003.03874.x

El-Shafey, A. F., Armstrong, A. E., Terrill, J. R., Grounds, M. D., and Arthur, P. G. (2011). Screening for increased protein thiol oxidation in oxidatively stressed muscle tissue. *Free Radic. Res.* 45, 991–999. doi: 10.3109/10715762.2011.590136

Emerling, B. M., Platanias, L. C., Black, E., Nebreda, A. R., Davis, R. J., and Chandel, N. S. (2005). Mitochondrial reactive oxygen species activation of p38 mitogen-activated protein kinase is required for hypoxia signaling. *Mol. Cell. Biol.* 25, 4853–4862. doi: 10.1128/MCB.25.12.4853-4862.2005

Faucher, M., Guillot, C., Marqueste, T., Kipson, N., Mayet-Sornay, M.-H., Desplanches, D., et al. (2005). Matched adaptations of electrophysiological, physiological, and histological properties of skeletal muscles in response to chronic hypoxia. *Pflügers Arch.* 450, 45–52. doi: 10.1007/s00424-004-1370-6

Gamboa, J. L., and Andrade, F. H. (2010). Mitochondrial content and distribution changes specific to mouse diaphragm after chronic normobaric hypoxia. *Am. J. Physiol. Regul. Integr. Comp. Physiol.* 298, R575–R583. doi: 10.1152/ajpregu.00320.2009

Gamboa, J. L., and Andrade, F. H. (2012). Muscle endurance and mitochondrial function after chronic normobaric hypoxia: contrast of respiratory and limb muscles. *Pflügers Arch.* 463, 327–338. doi: 10.1007/s00424-011-1057-8

Gosker, H. R., Wouters, E. F., van der Vusse, G. J., and Scholsa, M. (2000). Skeletal muscle dysfunction in chronic obstructive pulmonary disease and chronic heart failure: underlying mechanisms and therapy perspectives. *Am. J. Clin. Nutr.* 71, 1033–1047.

Haycock, J. W., Mac Neil, S., and Mantle, D. (1998). Differential protein oxidation in Duchenne and Becker muscular dystrophy. *Neuroreport* 9, 2201–2207. doi: 10.1097/00001756-199807130-00010

Hoppeler, H., Howald, H., and Cerretelli, P. (1990). Human muscle structure after exposure to extreme altitude. *Experientia* 46, 1185–1187. doi: 10.1007/BF01936933

Hoppeler, H., Vogt, M., Weibel, E. R., and Flück, M. (2003). Response of skeletal muscle mitochondria to hypoxia. *Exp. Physiol.* 88, 109–119. doi: 10.1113/eph8802513

Howald, H., Pette, D., Simoneau, J. A., Uber, A., Hoppeler, H., and Cerretelli, P. (1990). Effect of chronic hypoxia on muscle enzyme activities. *Int. J. Sport. Med.* 11(Suppl. 1), S10–S14. doi: 10.1055/s-2007-1024847

Hu, W., Culloty, S., Darmody, G., Lynch, S., Davenport, J., Ramirez-Garcia, S., et al. (2014). Toxicity of copper oxide nanoparticles in the blue mussel, Mytilus edulis: a redox proteomic investigation. *Chemosphere* 108, 289–299. doi: 10.1016/j.chemosphere.2014.01.054

Kadiiska, M. B., Gladen, B. C., Baird, D. D., Germolec, D., Graham, L. B., Parker, C. E., et al. (2005). Biomarkers of oxidative stress study II: are oxidation products of lipids, proteins, and DNA markers of CCl4 poisoning? *Free Radic. Biol. Med.* 38, 698–710. doi: 10.1016/j.freeradbiomed.2004.09.017

Kim, J., Tchernyshyov, I., Semenza, G. L., and Dang, C. V. (2006). HIF-1-mediated expression of pyruvate dehydrogenase kinase: a metabolic switch required for cellular adaptation to hypoxia. *Cell Metab.* 3, 177–185. doi: 10.1016/j.cmet.2006.02.002

Lemire, B. B., Debigaré, R., Dubé, A., Thériault, M.-E., Côté, C. H., and Maltais, F. (2012). MAPK signaling in the quadriceps of patients with chronic obstructive pulmonary disease. *J. Appl. Physiol.* 113, 159–166. doi: 10.1152/japplphysiol.01518.2011

Levine, S., Bashir, M. H., Clanton, T. L., Powers, S. K., and Singhal, S. (2013). COPD elicits remodeling of the diaphragm and vastus lateralis muscles in humans. *J. Appl. Physiol.* 114, 1235–1245. doi: 10.1152/japplphysiol.01121.2012

Marin-Corral, J., Minguella, J., Ramírez-Sarmiento, A. L., Hussain, S. N. A., Gea, J., and Barreiro, E. (2009). Oxidised proteins and superoxide anion production in the diaphragm of severe COPD patients. *Eur. Respir. J.* 33, 1309–1319. doi: 10.1183/09031936.00072008

McClung, J. M., Whidden, M. A., Kavazis, A. N., Falk, D. J., Deruisseau, K. C., and Powers, S. K. (2008). Redox regulation of diaphragm proteolysis during mechanical ventilation. *Am. J. Physiol. Regul. Integr. Comp. Physiol.* 294, R1608–R1617. doi: 10.1152/ajpregu.00044.2008

McDonald, F. B., Edge, D., and O'Halloran, K. D. (2014). Chronic nitric oxide synthase inhibition does not impair upper airway muscle adaptation to chronic intermittent hypoxia in the rat. *Prog. Brain Res.* 212, 237–251. doi: 10.1016/B978-0-444-63488-7.00012-4

McDonald, F. B., Skelly, J. R., and O'Halloran, K. D. (2015). The β_2-adrenoceptor agonist terbutaline recovers rat pharyngeal dilator muscle force decline during severe hypoxia. *Oral Dis.* 21, e121–e127. doi: 10.1111/odi.12247

McMorrow, C., Fredsted, A., Carberry, J., O'Connell, R. A., Bradford, A., Jones, J. F. X., et al. (2011). Chronic hypoxia increases rat diaphragm muscle endurance and sodium-potassium ATPase pump content. *Eur. Respir. J.* 37, 1474–1481. doi: 10.1183/09031936.00079810

McNicholas, W. T. (2009). Chronic obstructive pulmonary disease and obstructive sleep apnea: overlaps in pathophysiology, systemic inflammation, and cardiovascular disease. *Am. J. Respir. Crit. Care Med.* 180, 692–700. doi: 10.1164/rccm.200903-0347PP

Murray, A. J. (2009). Metabolic adaptation of skeletal muscle to high altitude hypoxia: how new technologies could resolve the controversies. *Genome Med.* 1:117. doi: 10.1186/gm117

O'Halloran, K. D., McGuire, M., O'Hare, T., and Bradford, A. (2002). Chronic intermittent asphyxia impairs rat upper airway muscle responses to acute hypoxia and asphyxia. *Chest* 122, 269–275. doi: 10.1378/chest.122.1.269

O'Connell, R. A., Carberry, J., and O'Halloran, K. D. (2013). Sternohyoid and diaphragm muscle form and function during postnatal development in the rat. *Exp. Physiol.* 98, 1386–1400. doi: 10.1113/expphysiol.2013.073346

O'Halloran, K. D. (2006). Effects of nicotine on rat sternohyoid muscle contractile properties. *Respir. Physiol. Neurobiol.* 150, 200–210. doi: 10.1016/j.resp.2005.05.018

Orozco-Levi, M. (2003). Structure and function of the respiratory muscles in patients with COPD: impairment or adaptation? *Eur. Respir. J. Suppl.* 46, 41s–51s. doi: 10.1183/09031936.03.00004607

Owens, R. L., Eckert, D. J., Yeh, S. Y., and Malhotra, A. (2008). Upper airway function in the pathogenesis of obstructive sleep apnea: a review of the current literature. *Curr. Opin. Pulm. Med.* 14, 519–524. doi: 10.1097/MCP.0b013e3283130f66

Owens, R. L., and Malhotra, A. (2010). Sleep-disordered breathing and COPD: the overlap syndrome. *Respir Care* 55, 1333–1344; discussion: 1344–1346.

Petrof, B. J., Pack, A. I., Kelly, A. M., Eby, J., and Hendricks, J. C. (1994). Pharyngeal myopathy of loaded upper airway in dogs with sleep apnea. *J. Appl. Physiol.* 76, 1746–1752.

Puig-Vilanova, E., Rodriguez, D. A., Lloreta, J., Ausin, P., Pascual-Guardia, S., Broquetas, J., et al. (2015). Oxidative stress, redox signaling pathways, and autophagy in cachectic muscles of male patients with advanced COPD and lung cancer. *Free Radic. Biol. Med.* 79, 91–108. doi: 10.1016/j.freeradbiomed.2014.11.006

Rainville, L.-C., Carolan, D., Varela, A. C., Doyle, H., and Sheehan, D. (2014). Proteomic evaluation of citrate-coated silver nanoparticles toxicity in Daphnia magna. *Analyst* 139, 1678–1686. doi: 10.1039/c3an02160b

Sawada, Y., Nakamura, K., Doi, K., Takeda, K., Tobiume, K., Saitoh, M., et al. (2001). Rap1 is involved in cell stretching modulation of p38 but not ERK or JNK MAP kinase. *J. Cell Sci.* 114, 1221–1227.

Semenza, G. L., Roth, P. H., Fang, H. M., and Wang, G. L. (1994). Transcriptional regulation of genes encoding glycolytic enzymes by hypoxia-inducible factor 1. *J. Biol. Chem.* 269, 23757–23763.

Shortt, C. M., and O'Halloran, K. D. (2014). Hydrogen peroxide alters sternohyoid muscle function. *Oral Dis.* 20, 162–170. doi: 10.1111/odi.12084

Skelly, J. R., Bradford, A., Jones, J. F., and O'Halloran, K. D. (2010). Superoxide scavengers improve rat pharyngeal dilator muscle performance. *Am. J. Respir. Cell Mol. Biol.* 42, 725–731. doi: 10.1165/rcmb.2009-0160OC

Skelly, J. R., Edge, D., Shortt, C. M., Jones, J. F., Bradford, A., and O'Halloran, K. D. (2012a). Respiratory control and sternohyoid muscle structure and function in aged male rats: decreased susceptibility to chronic intermittent hypoxia. *Respir. Physiol. Neurobiol.* 180, 175–182. doi: 10.1016/j.resp.2011.11.004

Skelly, J. R., Edge, D., Shortt, C. M., Jones, J. F., Bradford, A., and O'Halloran, K. D. (2012b). Tempol ameliorates pharyngeal dilator muscle dysfunction in a rodent model of chronic intermittent hypoxia. *Am. J. Respir. Cell Mol. Biol.* 46, 139–148. doi: 10.1165/rcmb.2011-0084OC

Skelly, J. R., O'Connell, R. A., Jones, J. F., and O'Halloran, K. D. (2011). Structural and functional properties of an upper airway dilator muscle in aged obese male rats. *Respiration* 82, 539–549. doi: 10.1159/000332348

Skelly, J. R., Rowan, S. C., Jones, J. F., and O'Halloran, K. D. (2013). Upper airway dilator muscle weakness following intermittent and sustained hypoxia in the rat: effects of a superoxide scavenger. *Physiol. Res.* 16, 187–196.

Van Lunteren, E., Haxhiu, M. A., and Cherniack, N. S. (1987). Relation between upper airway volume and hyoid muscle length. *J. Appl. Physiol.* 63, 1443–1449.

Van Lunteren, E., and Pollarine, J. (2010). Improvement of diaphragm and limb muscle isotonic contractile performance by K+ channel blockade. *J. Neuroeng. Rehabil.* 7:1. doi: 10.1186/1743-0003-7-1

Van Lunteren, E., Pollarine, J., and Moyer, M. (2007). Isotonic contractile impairment due to genetic CLC-1 chloride channel deficiency in myotonic mouse diaphragm muscle. *Exp. Physiol.* 92, 717–729. doi: 10.1113/expphysiol.2007.038190

Viganò, A., Ripamonti, M., De Palma, S., Capitanio, D., Vasso, M., Wait, R., et al. (2008). Proteins modulation in human skeletal muscle in the early phase of adaptation to hypobaric hypoxia. *Proteomics* 8, 4668–4679. doi: 10.1002/pmic.200800232

Vogt, M., Puntschart, A., Geiser, J., Zuleger, C., Billeter, R., and Hoppeler, H. (2001). Molecular adaptations in human skeletal muscle to endurance training under simulated hypoxic conditions. *J Appl. Physiol.* 91, 173–182.

Watchko, J. F., Daood, M. J., Sieck, G. C., LaBella, J. J., Ameredes, B. T., Koretsky, A. P. et al. (1997). Combined myofibrillar and mitochondrial creatine kinase deficiency impairs mouse diaphragm isotonic function. *J. Appl. Physiol.* 82, 1416–1423.

Wheaton, W. W., and Chandel, N. S. (2011). Hypoxia. 2. Hypoxia regulates cellular metabolism. *Am. J. Physiol. Cell Physiol.* 300, C385–C393. doi: 10.1152/ajpcell.00485.2010

Wijnhoven, J. H., Janssen, J. M., van Kuppevelt, T. H., Rodenburg, R. J. T., and Dekhuijzen, P. N. R. (2006). Metabolic capacity of the diaphragm in patients with COPD. *Respir. Med.* 100. 1064–1071. doi: 10.1016/j.rmed.2005.09.029

Zuo, L., and Clanton, T. L. (2005). Reactive oxygen species formation in the transition to hypoxia in skeletal muscle. *Am. J. Physiol. Cell Physiol.* 289, C207–C216. doi: 10.1152/ajpcell.00449.2004

17

Aging, Disability, and Informal Caregivers: A Cross-sectional Study in Portugal

*Maria Ana Pego[1] and Carla Nunes[2,3]**

[1] Unidade de Investigação e Desenvolvimento em Enfermagem, Escola Superior de Enfermagem de Lisboa, Lisbon, Portugal, [2] Centro de Investigação em Saúde Pública, Escola Nacional de Saúde Pública, Universidade Nova de Lisboa, Lisbon, Portugal, [3] Escola Nacional de Saúde Pública, Universidade Nova de Lisboa, Lisbon, Portugal

Edited by:
Giuseppe Liotta,
Università degli Studi di Roma Tor Vergata, Italy

Reviewed by:
William Keith Gray,
Northumbria Healthcare NHS Foundation Trust, United Kingdom
Marios Kyriazis,
ELPIs Foundation for Indefinite Lifespans, United Kingdom

****Correspondence:***
Carla Nunes
cnunes@ensp.unl.pt

Objectives: Aging is pushing states to rethink long-term care policies in several dimensions. This study aims to characterize the reality of dependent older people regarding their demographic and health characteristics, to describe their informal carers and understand the availability of informal care.

Methods: A cross-sectional study was developed in Portugal in 2013. Descriptive statistical analyses and binary logistic analysis were conducted.

Results: Results show that the informal long-term care sector is primarily aimed at older people with severe limitations in their activities of daily living and at the chronically ill, particularly older women. Additionally, 39.5% of dependent older persons do not have informal care and only receive informal aid in cases of extreme need.

Discussion: Results show a critical situation for both social groups (older persons and caregivers) and the prospect of an alarming situation in the near future (aging and reduced availability of informal caregivers) unless a new approach for long-term care is developed.

Keywords: informal care, dependent elderly, epidemiology, aging, Portugal

INTRODUCTION

Improvements in living conditions and the quality of health services have led to a significant increase in the proportion of older people in the population, a trend that is expected to continue over the next decades. Public health authorities face the challenge of promoting the reform of health policies that are aimed at older people, due to the progressive loss of functionality and the consequent increase in dependence for their activities of daily living (ADL), leading the older person to an increased need for long-term care. These personal care components are often provided in combination with basic medical services (medication, health monitoring, prevention, rehabilitation, or palliative care services) and, sometimes, with lower level help, namely those related with Instrumental Activities of Daily Living (IADL), such as meals, shopping, and housework (1).

At first glance, one realizes that demographic, social, and economic changes are "pushing" states to reassess long-term care policies, mainly due to the restructuring of the family leading to a reduction in the availability of informal caregivers. The atomization of families, the greater volatility of marital relations, the reduction in the average size of families, declining birth rates, and the increasing participation of women in the labor market have substantially altered family structures and functioning (2).

Informal care is generally defined as the unpaid care provided to older and dependent people by a person with whom they have a social relationship, such as a spouse, parent, child, other relative, neighbor, friend, or other non-kin (3). In Europe, there is a multiplicity of forms of organization for long-term care, in which the North tends to have a greater provision of public services and formal care and the South favors the informal care sector provided by the family, due to the limited availability of formal resources (namely, systems of social protection for older people) and a "familiar" culture (4–10). For example, a significant proportion of long-term care is provided in this way in Spain (in 2008, 78% of care was provided by informal caregivers) and in France (in 2008, this amounted to 37%), according to Costa-Font and Courbage (11). Portugal shares the main characteristics of other Southern European countries, i.e., the family (in particular women) is the main provider of care, but differs in one key aspect: it has a high female participation rate in the labor market (9, 10, 12–14).

In a context of global aging and significant changes in family structures, it is necessary to comprehend the reality of informal care in order to understand its relevance to the care of the aging population. This study specifically contributes to the knowledge of the informal sector of care and aims to (i) describe the national reality of the dependent older person in Portugal regarding demographic, residential, and health characteristics; (ii) describe the informal carers, in terms of kinship, frequency of care, and geographical proximity between carer and older person; (iii) understand the availability of informal care. This article focuses on long-term care for the elderly in Portugal, framed in a context of significant changes in family structures and shifts in social solidarity networks. Thus, we argue that the current model of long-term care, based mainly on the informal sector, has not been able to keep up with the actual demands of the elderly in Portugal. Hence, we expect to find a significant part of the geriatric population in need of care. We also expect to find a relationship between the severity of the limitations perceived by older persons and the availability of an informal carer, i.e., only the most dependent and elderly have access to an informal caregiver.

MATERIALS AND METHODS

Data Source

This study is cross-sectional, observational, and analytical. Data are obtained from the fourth wave of the Survey of Health, Aging and Retirement in Europe (SHARE) (15), the first one that included Portugal. SHARE is the first longitudinal and cross-national research project collecting data on aging and access to the informal care sector.

In each country, data collection is based on probability household samples (drawn either by simple random selection or multistage random selection) where all people aged above 50 years and their partners were interviewed using Computer Assisted Personal Interviews. Although the sampling frame includes people living in institutions, the SHARE base sample excludes these individuals. For the Portuguese SHARE sample, the target population was defined as all Portuguese-speaking residents, born before 1960 and their spouses/partners. For each country, the sample size originally defined was 2,000 individuals. In Portugal response rate of 60%, was expected, with an expected proportion of non-sampling units of 10%. Analysis of the width and magnitude of the 95% confidence interval (95% CI) were used in order to evaluate the uncertainty of estimates. The SHARE study (fourth wave) was subject to several ethics reviews: The Ethics Committee of the University of Mannheim, Germany, Ethics Council of the Max Planck Society and by national ethics committees or institutional review boards whenever this was required. This study was conducted in full accordance with the World Medical Association Declaration of Helsinki. Written consents from all participants involved in this study were obtained.

Study Sample

For the purpose of this study two additional restrictions were applied: (1) 65 years or older and (2) functional dependence [limited in at least one ADL or one Instrumental Activity of Daily Living (IADL)]. In order to restrict the samples according to the functional dependence of the older person, we used the Katz Index (16) to characterize the ADL, and the Lawton and Brody Scale (17) to characterize the IADL.

Table 1 presents the variables used in the analysis to characterize dependent older people and informal caregivers.

TABLE 1 | Variables used in the analysis to characterize dependent old person and informal caregivers.

Variables	Categories
Dependent old person	
Sex	Male; female
Age	65–69; 70–74; 75–79; 80–84; 85–99
No. of children	0; 1; 2; 3[a]; 4[a]; 5[a]; 6 or more[a]
Marital status	Married or registered partnership, living with spouse; married, separated from spouse[a]; never married[a]; divorced[a]; widowed[a]
Type of building	Farm house; 1 or 2 family house; building with three or more flats
Household area	Major city[a]; small city[a]; village[a]; rural area
Educational level	First level (4 years); second level[a] (6 years); third level[a] (9 years); secondary school; higher education; no education
Limitation[b]	Severely limited; limited, but not severely[a]; not limited
Chronic illness	[a]Yes; no
Informal caregivers	
Kinship	Daughters and sons (named as "children"); brother or sister; spouse; son-in-law or daughter-in-law; neighbor; other relative; housekeeper; grandchildren; friend
Gender	Male; female
Geo. proximity	Live in the same house; live in the same building; live less than 1 km away; between 1 and 5 km away; between 5 and 25 km away; between 25 and 100 km away; more than 100and away
Frequency of care	Daily care; weekly care; monthly care; less-frequent care

[a]Categories merged in multivariate analyses especially due to small frequencies.
[b]Perceived limitations on ADL—derives from the following question: "For the past six months at least, to what extent have you been limited because of a health problem in activities people usually do?"

Statistical Analysis

Descriptive statistical analyses were conducted to characterize the dependent elderly population and the informal caregivers, considering the variables presented in **Table 1**. Thereafter, binary and multivariate logistic analyses (using both methods: enter and forward LR: likelihood ratio) were used to characterize the availability of informal care (Model 1), being cared for by someone within the household, named here "inside care" (Model 2), being cared for by someone outside the household, named here "outside care" (Model 3). Considering the above variables (**Table 1**), crude, adjusted (by sex and age and by all significant variables), and corresponding confidence intervals were presented. We used SPSS statistical software with a 0.05% significance level. All models were tested and validated, namely through Hosmer and Lesmeshow's goodness-of-fit test and analyses of residuals.

RESULTS

The findings from the descriptive statistics are presented in **Table 2**, globally (276) and stratified by type of help: without informal care (109), with inside care (89), and with outside care (78). The categories that best define each profile are in bold.

Table 2 shows that women were a majority in all situations, which is as expected because the sample includes more women than men. Regarding age, it is also likely that the most elderly tend to have more informal inside care. Regarding marital status, the most striking aspect is the fact that, among those who receive outside care, the majority are widowed (56.4%). Regarding the number of children, it appears that those who receive outside care differ from the rest. Indeed, they are characterized by having three or more children. Regarding the type of accommodation there is a clear distinction between those who do not have an informal carer and live primarily in a family home (54.8%), and those who have an informal carer and live primarily in buildings with more than three flats. **Table 2** shows that among those who have no care and those who are less dependent in ADL form the majority (55.0%).

The percentage of chronically ill is considerably lower among those who do not have informal care. However, it should be noted that even those who do not receive informal care have a very high percentage of chronically ill (65.1%). Inside caregivers are mainly spouses (55.5%) and adult children (24.2%), and the remaining caregivers are neighbors, housekeepers, friends, and other relatives. Of the spouses 56.3% are male and 43.6% female, and 71.4% of the adult children caregivers are female and 62.5% of the remaining caregivers are female. **Table 3** shows that the primary outside care providers are adult children (38.6%), followed by neighbors (15.9%), friends (8.4%), housekeepers (7.5%), and other relatives (27.7%).

The majority of daily care is delivered by adult children (39.6%), other relatives (24.5%, including spouses, brothers or sisters, grandchildren, daughters or sons-in-law), neighbors (15.1%), and housekeepers (11.3%). These caregivers are predominantly female (64.8%) and live less than a mile away (78.13%).

TABLE 2 | Descriptive statistics.

Categories	All, *n* (%)	Without informal care, *n* (%)	Outside care, *n* (%)	Inside care, *n* (%)
Gender				
Male	91 (33.0)	43 (39.4)	28 (31.5)	20 (25.6)
Female	**185 (67.0)**	**66 (60.6)**	**61 (68.5)**	**58 (74.4)**
Total	276 (100)	109 (39.5)	89 (32.2)	78 (28.3)
Age				
65–69	**68 (25.9)**	**34 (31.2)**	19 (22.6)	15 (21.4)
70–74	48 (18.3)	32 (29.4)	8 (9.5)	8 (11.4)
75–79	67 (25.5)	28 (25.7)	17 (20.2)	**22 (31.4)**
80–84	53 (20.2)	12 (11.0)	**26 (30.9)**	15 (21.4)
85–99	27 (10.3)	3 (2.8)	14 (16.7)	10 (14.3)
Total	263 (100)	109 (41.4)	84 (31.9)	70 (26.6)
Number of children				
0	18 (7.7)	4 (3.7)	8 (16.7)	6 (7.8)
1	56 (23.9)	25 (22.9)	10 (20.8)	21 (27.3)
2	**80 (34.2)**	**42 (38.5)**	**16 (33.3)**	**22 (28.6)**
3	34 (14.5)	19 (17.4)	3 (6.3)	12 (15.6)
4	15 (6.4)	10 (9.2)	1 (2.1)	4 (5.2)
5	10 (4.3)	3 (2.8)	3 (6.3)	4 (5.2)
6 or more children	21 (9.0)	6 (5.5)	7 (14.6)	8 (10.4)
Total	234 (100)	109 (46.5)	48 (20.5)	77 (32.9)
Marital status				
Married[a]	**175 (63.4)**	**84 (77.1)**	**66 (74.2)**	25 (32.1)
Married, separated from spouse	2 (0.7)	0 (0)	0 (0)	2 (2.6)
Never married	8 (2.9)	2 (1.8)	2 (2.2)	4 (5.1)
Divorced	8 (2.9)	3 (2.8)	2 (2.2)	3 (3.8)
Widowed	83 (30.1)	20 (18.3)	19 (21.3)	**44 (56.4)**
Total	276 (100)	109 (39.5)	89 (32.2)	**78 (28.3)**
Type of building				
Farm house	12 (5.8)	6 (6.5)	1 (2.3)	5 (7)
1 or 2 family house	**104 (50.0)**	**51 (54.8)**	21 (47.7)	32 (45.1)
Building with 3 or more flats	92 (44.2)	36 (38.7)	**22 (50)**	**34 (47.9)**
Total	208 (100)	93 (44.7)	**44 (21.2)**	**71 (34.1)**
Household area				
Major city	**89 (42.8)**	**36 (38.7)**	**19 (43.2)**	**34 (47.9)**
Small city	33 (15.9)	16 (17.2)	8 (18.2)	9 (12.7)
Village	24 (11.5)	11 (11.8)	3 (6.8)	10 (14.1)
Rural area	62 (29.8)	30 (32.3)	14 (31.8)	18 (25.4)
Total	208 (100)	93 (44.7)	44 (21.2)	71 (34.1)
Educational level				
First level (4 years)	**147 (53.8)**	**62 (56.9)**	**47 (53.4)**	**38 (50)**
Second level[a] (2 years)	19 (7.0)	8 (7.3)	5 (5.7)	6 (7.9)
Third level[a] (3 years)	15 (5.5)	4 (3.7)	8 (9.1)	3 (3.9)
Secondary school	16 (5.9)	5 (4.6)	5 (5.7)	6 (7.9)
Higher education	14 (5.1)	8 (7.3)	4 (4.5)	2 (2.6)
No education	62 (22.7)	22 (20.2)	19 (21.6)	21 (27.6)
Total	273 (100)	109 (39.9)	88 (32.2)	76 (27.8)
Perceived limitations in ADL				
Severely limited	**144 (52.2)**	28 (25.7)	**67 (75.3)**	**49 (62.8)**
Limited, but not severely	98 (35.5)	**60 (55.0)**	17 (19.1)	21 (26.9)
Not limited	34 (12.3)	21 (19.3)	5 (5.6)	8 (10.3)
Total	276 (100)	109 (39.5)	89 (32.2)	78 (28.3)
Chronic illness				
Yes	**216 (78.3)**	**71 (65.1)**	**77 (86.5)**	**68 (87.2)**
No	60 (21.7)	38 (34.9)	12 (13.5)	10 (12.8)
Total	276 (100)	109 (39.5)	89 (32.2)	78 (28.3)

[a]*Or registered partnership, living with spouse.*

TABLE 3 | Characterization of the informal caregivers—outside care.

	Daily, *n* (%)	Weekly, *n* (%)	Monthly, *n* (%)	Less freq., *n* (%)	All, *n* (%)
Kinship					
Spouse	1 (1.89)	1 (2.70)	0 (0)	0 (0)	2 (1.68)
Children	21 (39.62)	18 (48.65)	1 (14.29)	6 (27.27)	46 (38.66)
Brother or sister	3 (5.66)	3 (8.11)	0 (0)	2 (9.09)	8 (6.72)
Daughter-in-law or son-in-law	3 (5.66)	3 (8.11)	2 (28.57)	1 (4.55)	9 (7.56)
Neighbor	8 (15.09)	5 (13.51)	1 (14.29)	5 (22.73)	19 (15.97)
Housekeepers	6 (11.32)	2 (5.41)	0 (0)	1 (4.55)	9 (7.56)
Grandchildren	4 (7.55)	2 (5.41)	0 (0)	1 (4.55)	7 (5.88)
Friend	5 (9.43)	0 (0)	2 (28.57)	3 (13.64)	10 (8.40)
Other relative	2 (3.77)	3 (8.11)	1 (14.29)	3 (13.64)	9 (7.56)
Total	53 (100)	37 (100)	7 (100)	22 (100)	119(100)
Gender					
Male	13 (35.14)	10 (34.48)	2 (33.33)	9 (56.25)	
Female	24 (64.86)	19 (65.52)	4 (66.67)	7 (43.75)	
Total	37 (100)	29 (100)	6 (100)	16 (100)	
Geographic proximity					
In the same household	12 (37.5)	4 (13.79)	0 (0)	1 (10)	
In the same building	2 (6.25)	0 (0)	0 (0)	1 (10)	
Less than 1 km away	11 (34.38)	10 (34.48)	1 (25)	4 (40)	
Between 1 and 5 km away	2 (6.25)	1 (3.45)	0 (0)	1 (10)	
Between 5 and 25 km away	5 (15.63)	9 (31.03)	1 (25)	1 (10)	
Between 25 and 100 km away	0 (0)	5 (17.24)	2 (50)	1 (10)	
More than 100 km away	0 (0)	0 (0)	0 (0)	1 (10)	
Total	32 (100)	29 (100)	4 (100)	10 (100)	

As for weekly care, this is performed mainly by adult children (48.6%), other relatives (32.4%), and neighbors (13.5%); the caregivers are predominantly female (65.5%) and most live less than a kilometer away (48.2%). As shown in **Table 3**, as the frequency of care decreases, the distance between the caregiver and the person cared for increases. To explain and model the availability of informal carers for older persons in need of care, binary logistic models were used (Model 1—all informal care, Model 2—inside care, and Model 3—outside care). OR and CI of statistically significant variables are presented in **Table 4**.

Model 1 ($G2 = 78{,}075$; $p < 0.001$) has an explanatory capacity of 76%, with a sensitivity of 75.6% and a specificity of 76.3%. The corresponding values for Model 2 are $G2 = 46{,}145$ ($p < 0.001$), 78.8%, 71.4%, and 81.6% and for Model 3 are $G2 = 41{,}008$ ($p < 0.001$), 63.3%, 92.4%, and 50.3%.

Model 1 presents age, marital status, and limitations perceived in ADL as significant variables. Thus, it is observed that people aged 85–99 years have a 13.1 times higher probability of being informally cared for than those aged 65–69 years old. On the other hand, an older person living without a spouse is 5.1 times more likely to be informally cared for than an older person living with a spouse. It was also shown that older persons that perceive severe restrictions in their ADL have a probability 8.8 times higher of being informally cared for than those that perceive no limitation or little limitation in their ADL.

Model 2 identifies age and limitations perceived in ADL as significant variables: people aged 85–99 years have an 8.7 times greater likelihood of being informally cared for by someone within the household than people 65–69 years old. People aged 80–84 are 5.1 times more likely to be informally cared for than those aged 65–69 years old. Those that are severely limited are 6.6 times more likely to be cared for by an inside carer than those with little or no limitations in ADL.

Model 3 identifies education, marital status, perceived limitations in ADL, and the presence of chronic disease as significant variables. An older person with a secondary level of education is 9.4 times more likely to be cared for by an outside carer than an older person with no education. An older person living without a spouse is 2.8 times more likely to have outside care than those who live with their spouse. The results also show that an older person that perceives severe limitation in ADL is 2.3 times more likely to have outside care than those who perceive little or no limitation. Finally, older people with chronic disease have a 4.8 times higher probability of having outside care than those who are not chronically ill.

DISCUSSION

The majority of the informally cared for dependent elderly live with their main caregiver (53.3%). This result is expected, because older age groups are probably more dependent and in need of more frequent care and supervision in their daily activities. Similar studies (10) have shown that in Southern Europe, the main caregivers live inside the household. On the other hand, informal care is predominantly provided by family members (79.3%) (6, 18). Originally, it is the absence of a spouse that seems to influence the use of outside care, i.e., not having the possibility of being cared for by a spouse increases the probability of having a carer from outside the household.

Regarding outside care, it is mostly provided by adult children (38.6%), something that is also mentioned in the literature (10, 19). The main caregivers living outside the household are

TABLE 4 | Model 1, 2, and 3—results from the logistic regression analyses.

Model 1—availability of informal care

Independent variables	Crude odds ratio (95% CI; *p*)	Adjusted odds ratio[a] (95% CI; *p*)	Forward LR model,[b] odds ratio (95% CI; *p*)
Age			
65–69 years[c]	–	–	–
70–74 years	0.498 (0.228:1.087; *p* = 0.08)	–	0.461 (0.149:1.433; *p* = *0.181*)
75–79 years	1.290 (0.644:2.585; *p* = *0.473*)	–	1.532 (0.576:4.078; *p* = *0.393*)
80–84 years	2.922 (1.289:6.623; *p* = *0.010*)	–	1.437 (0.475:4.345; *p* = *0.520*)
85–99 years	10.271 (2.847:37.050; *p* = 0.001)	–	13.173 (2.772:62.601; *p* = 0.001)
Perceived limitations in the ADL			
Little or no limitation[c]	–	–	–
Severely limited	6.429 (1.904:6.616; *p* = 0.001)	6.481 (3.555:11.813; *p* = 0.001)	8.840 (3.958:19.612; *p* = 0.001)
Marital status			
Married and living without a spouse[c]	–	–	–
Does not live with the spouse	2.581 (1.483:4.493; *p* = 0.001)	1.933 (1.025:3.646; *p* = 0.042)	5.100 (2.288:11.371; *p* = 0.001)

Model 2—availability of informal care from someone inside the household

Independent variables	Raw odds ratio (95% CI; *p*)	Adjusted odds ratio[a] (95% CI; *p*)	Forward LR model,[b] odds ratio (95% CI; *p*)
Age			
68–69 years[c]	–	–	–
70–74 years	0.466 (0.189:1.148; *p* = *0.097*)	–	0.593 (0.128:2.742; *p* = 0.504)
75–79 years	1.156 (0.543:2.459; *p* = *0.707*)	–	1.704 (0.490:5.921; *p* = 0.402)
80–84 years	3.263 (1.544:6.895; *p* = *0.002*)	–	5.136 (1.471:17.930; *p* = 0.010)
85–99 years	6.200 (2.465:15.592; *p* = 0.001)	–	8.743 (2.236:34.180; *p* = 0.002)
Perceived limitations in the ADL			
Little or no limitation[c]	–	–	–
Severely limited	6.768 (3.843:11.919; *p* = 0.001)	6.414 (3.512:11.714; *p* = 0.001)	6.652 (2.236:34.180; *p* = 0.001)

Model 3—availability of informal care from someone outside the household

Independent variables	Raw odds ratio (95% CI; *p*)	Adjusted odds ratio[a] (95% CI; *p*)	Forward LR model,[b] odds ratio (95% CI; *p*)
Educational level			
No education[c]	–	–	–
First level (4 years)	0.813 (0.424:1.559; *p* = 0.533)	0.896 (0.453:1.772; *p* = *0.752*)	0.945 (0.446:2.003; *p* = 0.883)
Second (2 years) and third level (3 years)	0.779 (0.305:1.991; *p* = 0.602)	0.810 (0.292:2.251; *p* = *0.687*)	1.224 (0.39:3.846; *p* = 0.729)
Secondary education	1.633 (0.486:5.484; *p* = *0.428*)	1.543 (0.412:5.781; *p* = *0.520*)	9.436 (1.665:53.472; *p* = 0.011)
Higher education	0.272 (0.056:1.312; *p* = *0.105*)	0.239 (0.046:1.232; *p* = *0.087*)	0.253 (0.048:1.324; *p* = 0.104)
Perceived limitations in the ADL			
No limitation or little limitation[c]	–	–	–
Severely limited	2.923 (1.680:5.088; *p* = 0.001)	2.937 (1.635:5.274; *p* = 0.001)	2.316 (1.155:4.644; *p* = 0.018)
Chronic illness			
No[c]	–	–	–
Yes	3.370 (1.615:7.035; *p* = 0.001)	1.424 (0.745:2.722; *p* = *0.285*)	4.779 (1.668:13.691; *p* = 0.004)
Marital status			
Lives with the spouse[c]	–	–	–
Does not live with the spouse	3.165 (1.799:5.567; *p* = 0.001)	2.940 (1.492:5.795; *p* = 0.002)	2.772 (1.424:5.396; *p* = 0.003)

[a]*Adjusted to gender and age.*
[b]*Forward model LR, embodying all the variables under analysis.*
[c]*Reference class.*

female. This is shown in several reports on Europe, especially Southern Europe (4, 9, 10, 20).

The results show that the main recipients are older women limited in their ADL, chronically ill, and of advanced age. The literature shows that women have a higher life expectancy; however, the quality of life after age 65 declines substantially due to limitations in ADL and chronic illness (21).

The main caregivers among coresident caregivers are spouses (55.5%). Furthermore, geographical distance is extremely relevant in determining the frequency of care. Caregivers that care occasionally live outside the household. This shows that there is a nuclearization of the family, supporting the argument made on changes in family structure (10, 22–24).

In addition to the characterization of informal caregivers, our study aims to highlight the limitations of the current model of care. A significant proportion (39.5%) of the dependent elderly do not receive any type of informal care. The literature highlights the limitations of the current model of long-term care imposed by changes in family structures (10, 22–24).

Regarding the availability of inside care (all care, inside or outside), one variable is consistently identified: the limitation perceived in ADL, and the higher the limitation is perceived, the greater the availability of informal carers.

People aged 80–99 years are more likely to have inside care, and older persons aged 85–89 years are more likely to have informal care. Other authors (4, 10, 19, 25) state that it is mainly the most elderly and therefore those who are more dependent who have more access to an informal caregiver. Thus, informal caregivers predominantly help the most vulnerable, dependent and older persons.

In the first and third models, the variable living without a spouse influences the availability of an informal caregiver; this means that in the absence of a spouse, older people are more likely to be informally cared for and cared for by an outside carer. Older persons residing without a spouse receive help from non-resident caregivers. Regarding the first model, it may be the fact that the spouses also have functional limitations which prevents them from providing care to their spouses. On the other hand, it turns out that being married and living with their spouse is not decisive for obtaining help from informal caregivers. This may be related to the similar percentage of married older persons and those living with a spouse among those without informal help. This does not mean that spouses do not provide care, but the marital status does not explain the availability of informal caregivers. Other studies (10, 23) reflect the same relationship between informal care and marital status, explaining that the care from a spouse is sometimes not regarded by the older person as care, and this influences the answers of the older person.

The third model has two explanatory variables that differ from the other two models: level of education and the presence of chronic disease. Older people with chronic illness are more likely to have informal care (4, 25). Older people with secondary and postsecondary education are more likely to be cared for by someone from outside, mainly by a housekeeper (7.56%). Similar data were found in a study on the Spanish situation in which users with secondary and postsecondary education are more likely to have paid care from paid domestic workers (26).

Finally, it appears that the number of children is not decisive for receiving help from informal caregivers. It is not the amount of available resources that determines whether or not there is access to long-term care. Daatland (27) states that it is the quality of the relationship between parents and children that favors the assumption of the caregiver role by the children and not the number of children.

In general the results of this study are aligned with the literature, reinforcing the internal and external validity of this study, and adding scientific evidence (namely through the magnitude of the results) to this study of this issue. Nevertheless, we would like to emphasize that these results should be carefully interpreted and generalized due to the fact that the sample under analysis is limited. The wide range of some confidence intervals reflects the uncertainty of these results. Additionally, data collection was based on self-report questionnaires (for instance, the perceived limitations in ADL and the presence of chronic illness variables) and participants may not have responded truthfully, either because they cannot remember (memory bias) or because they wish to present themselves in a more socially acceptable manner (social desirability bias). The absence of some relevant variables referred to in the literature (economic status, availability of formal care, health status of care giver, among others) also constitutes a limitation of this study.

CONCLUSION

Based on this study, it appears that the informal long-term care sector in Portugal is primarily aimed at older people with severe limitations in their ADL and at the chronically ill, particularly older women. The absence of a spouse tends to mean that someone from outside the household responds to the need for care. Our study also shows that there are a significant proportion of dependent older persons without any kind of informal care (39.5%), which supports the argument that the current limitations of the long-term care model are imposed by changes in family structures.

Additionally, the main informal caregivers are family members and mostly women. However, the gender gap is not as clear when the primary caregiver is the spouse. Nonetheless, women represent 68% of the dependent elderly. Regarding adult children caregivers, the majority are female (71.4%). Among the caregivers who live with the older person, spouses are the main caregivers, in contrast to caregivers who live outside the household, where the majority are adult children and other relatives. It seems that there is a marked nuclearization of the family, supporting the argument in terms of the changes in family structure. On the other hand, the solidarity networks are mainly composed of family members. Regarding geographical distance, this is extremely relevant to the frequency of care, i.e., the closer the caregiver lives, the higher the frequency of care provided.

Taken as a whole, the current model of care, based on the informal long-term care sector, leaves out a significant proportion of dependent older persons and it seems that it is only in cases of extreme need that aid arises, i.e., only the most dependent and dependent older persons are helped by the informal care sector.

The results of this study show a critical situation for both social groups (older persons and caregivers) and an alarming prospect in the near future (a continuously aging society, a scarcity of young informal caregivers, the reduced availability of informal caregivers to care for the older person), something that is a global challenge, since many countries have the same characteristics. A new approach for long-term care is urgently required, a greater provision of public services and formal care is needed, especially at community and household level rather than institutionalization, allowing the elderly to live in their own context as long as is possible and promoting and safeguarding relationships and responsibilities with (and of) informal caregivers. Complementary studies on formal care are needed to understand the full context and to carefully evaluate different possible approaches (including elderly, caregivers and social/health services).

ETHICS STATEMENT

The SHARE study (fourth wave) was subject to several ethics reviews: The Ethics Committee of the University of Mannheim, Germany, Ethics Council of the Max Planck Society and by national ethics committees or institutional review boards whenever this was required. This study was conducted in full accordance with the World Medical Association Declaration of Helsinki. Written consents from all participants involved in this study were obtained.

AUTHOR CONTRIBUTIONS

MP designed the research, conducted the data analyses, and wrote the first draft, and reviewed and approved the final manuscript. CN designed the research, supervised the data analyses, and reviewed and approved the final manuscript.

REFERENCES

1. Lipszyc B, Sail E, Xavier A. *Long-Term Care: Need, Use and Expenditure in the EU-27*. Brussels: European Commission (2012). p. 7–9. Economic Papers 469.
2. Carneiro R, Chau F, Soares C, Fialho J, Sacadura M. *O Envelhecimento da População: Dependência, Ativação e Qualidade*. Lisboa: Centro de Estudos dos Povos e Culturas de Expressão Portuguesa (2012). p. 31–52.
3. Triantafillou J, Naiditch M, Stiehr K, Carretero S, Di Santo T, Bednarik R, et al. *Informal Care in the Long-Term Care System*. Athens/Vienna: European Overview paper, Interlinks (2010). p. 11–7.
4. José J, Wall K, Correia S. *Working Paper: Trabalhar e cuidar de um idoso dependente: problemas e soluções*. Lisboa: Instituto de Ciências Sociais da Universidade de Lisboa (2002). p. 5–11.
5. Comas-Herrera A, Wittenberg R. *European Study of Long-Term Care Expenditure*. Brussels: European Commission, Employment and Social Affairs (2003). p. 19–23.
6. Daatland O, Lowenstein A. Intergenerational solidarity and the family-welfare state balance. *Eur J Ageing* (2005) 2:174–82. doi:10.1007/s10433-005-0001-1
7. Costa-Font J. Devolution, diversity and welfare reform: long-term care in the 'Latin Rim'. *Soc Policy Adm* (2010) 44:481–94. doi:10.1111/j.1467-9515.2010.00724.x
8. Daatland S, Herlofson K, Lima I. Balancing generations: on the strength and character of family norms in the West and East of Europe. *Ageing Soc* (2011) 31:1159–79. doi:10.1017/S0144686X10001315
9. Tavora I. The southern European social model: familialism and the high rates of female employment in Portugal. *J Eur Soc Policy* (2011) 22:63–76. doi:10.1177/0958928711425269
10. Solé-Auró A, Crimmins E. Who cares? A comparison of informal and formal care provision in Spain, England and the USA. *Ageing Soc* (2014) 34:495–517. doi:10.1017/S0144686X12001134
11. Costa-Font J, Courbage C. *Financing Long-Term Care in Europe*. Hampshire: Palgrave Macmillan (2012). p. 3–14.
12. Wall K, Cunha V, Vasconcelos P. Families and informal support networks in Portugal: the reproduction of inequality. *J Eur Soc Policy* (2001) 11:213–33. doi:10.1177/095892870101100302
13. Pimentel L. O Sexo dos Anjos: os cuidados às pessoas idosas dependentes como uma esfera de acção preferencialmente feminina. *Ex aequo* (2011) 23:23–37.
14. Santana S. Reforming long-term care in Portugal: dealing with the multidimensional character of quality. In: Costa-Font J, editor. *Reforming Long-Term Care in Europe*. West Sussex: Wiley-Blackwell (2011). p. 154–69.
15. Börsch-Supan A, Brandt M, Hunkler C, Kneip T, Korbmacher J, Malter F, et al. Data resource profile: the survey of health, ageing and retirement in Europe (SHARE). *Int J Epidemiol* (2013) 42:992–1001. doi:10.1093/ije/dyt088
16. Katz SD. Progress in the development of the index of ADL. *Gerontologist* (1970) 10:20–30. doi:10.1093/geront/10.1_Part_1.20
17. Lawton M, Brody E. Assessment of older people: self-maintaining and instrumental activities of daily living. *Gerontologist* (1969) 9:179–86. doi:10.1093/geront/9.3_Part_1.179
18. Bettio F, Simonazzi A, Villa P. Change in care regimes and female migration: the 'care drain' in the Mediterranean. *J Eur Soc Policy* (2006) 16:271–85. doi:10.1177/0958928706065598
19. Lafortune G, Balestat G. *Trends in Severe Disability among Elderly People: Assessing the Evidence in 12 OECD Countries and the Future Implications*. Paris: OECD Publishing (2007). p. 6–23.
20. Crompton R. *Employment and the Family. The Reconfiguration of Work and the Family Life in Contemporary Societies*. Cambridge: Cambridge University Press (2006). p. 31–62.
21. Artazcoz L, Rueda S. Social inequalities in health among the elderly: a challenge for public health research. *J Epidemiol Community Health* (2007) 61:466–7. doi:10.1136/jech.2006.058081
22. Pickard L, Wittenberg R, Comas-Herreras A, Davies B, Darton R. Relying on informal care in the new century? Informal care for elderly people in England to 2031. *Ageing Soc* (2000) 20:745–72. doi:10.1017/S0144686X01007978
23. Stuifbergen M, Van Delden J, Dykstra P. The implications of today's family structures for support giving to older parents. *Ageing Soc* (2008) 28:413–34. doi:10.1017/S0144686X07006666
24. Principi A, Lamura G, Sirolla C, Mestheneos L, Bien BM, Brown J, et al. Work restrictions experienced by midlife family care-givers of older people: evidence from six European countries. *Ageing Soc* (2014) 34:209–31. doi:10.1017/S0144686X12000967
25. Romão A, Pereira A, Gerardo F. *As Necessidades dos Cuidadores Informais. Estudo na área do envelhecimento*. Lisboa: Santa Casa da Misericórdia de Lisboa (2008). p. 10–33.
26. Rogero-García J, Rosenberg M. Paid and unpaid support received by co-resident informal caregivers attending to community-dwelling older adults in Spain. *Eur J Ageing* (2011) 8:95–107. doi:10.1007/s10433-011-0184-6
27. Daatland O. Ageing, families and welfare systems: comparative perspectives. *Z Gerontol Geriatr* (2001) 34:16–20. doi:10.1007/s003910170086

18

Can Endurance Exercise Preconditioning Prevention Disuse Muscle Atrophy?

Michael P. Wiggs *

Department of Applied Physiology and Kinesiology, Center for Exercise Science, University of Florida, Gainesville, FL, USA

Edited by:
Brian McDonagh,
University of Liverpool, UK

Reviewed by:
Nazareno Paolocci,
Johns Hopkins University, USA
Daniela Caporossi,
University of Rome Foro Italico, Italy

***Correspondence:**
Michael P. Wiggs,
Department of Applied Physiology and Kinesiology,
Center for Exercise Science,
University of Florida,
Room 25 Florida Gym, Gainesville,
FL 32611, USA
mwiggs@ufl.edu

Emerging evidence suggests that exercise training can provide a level of protection against disuse muscle atrophy. Endurance exercise training imposes oxidative, metabolic, and heat stress on skeletal muscle which activates a variety of cellular signaling pathways that ultimately leads to the increased expression of proteins that have been demonstrated to protect muscle from inactivity –induced atrophy. This review will highlight the effect of exercise-induced oxidative stress on endogenous enzymatic antioxidant capacity (i.e., superoxide dismutase, glutathione peroxidase, and catalase), the role of oxidative and metabolic stress on PGC1-α, and finally highlight the effect heat stress and HSP70 induction. Finally, this review will discuss the supporting scientific evidence that these proteins can attenuate muscle atrophy through exercise preconditioning.

Keywords: bed rest, unloading, immobilization, superoxide dismutase, HSP70, PGC1-α, mitophagy, oxidative stress

Introduction

Prolonged periods of inactivity results in a loss of muscle protein, fiber atrophy, and impaired muscle function. It is widely recognized that maintaining skeletal muscle structure and function is important in promoting health and quality of life (Wolfe, 2006). A loss of muscle mass can impair the ability to perform activities of daily living, prolong periods of rehabilitation and be a major risk factor for chronic disease. Therefore, it is important to find ways to attenuate rapid muscle atrophy during periods of prolonged disuse.

Common disuse atrophy conditions include prolonged bed rest, limb immobilization/casting, and prolonged exposure to microgravity. The rapid decrease in muscle size observed during disuse is due to both a reduction in muscle protein synthesis and an increase in protein degradation. Therefore, countermeasures to prevent muscle wasting generally target these pathways. In this regard, it is well established that exercise training is able to increase muscle protein synthesis and has been used as a counter-measure to disuse muscle atrophy in many of these conditions (reviewed in Glover and Phillips, 2010). Indeed, both resistance and endurance exercise have been shown to attenuate muscle disuse muscle atrophy in both human and animal models of muscle atrophy and this has been termed "exercise preconditioning."

However, not all disuse atrophy conditions allow for exercise training during the period of muscle inactivity. For example, during casting and limb immobilization, it is physically impossible to exercise the affected muscles. Another example is mechanical ventilation induced-diaphragm atrophy. This is caused by inactivity of the diaphragm during mechanical ventilation (MV), which causes rapid (e.g., within 12 h) atrophy of the diaphragm (Powers et al., 2013). Recently our lab demonstrated that endurance exercise training prior to MV protected the diaphragm from muscle atrophy (Smuder et al., 2012a). To date, this is one of the few studies to examine the protective effects of exercise preconditioning against disuse muscle atrophy. Therefore, this review will highlight several potential cytoprotective proteins that are altered with exercise training that may be critical in protecting against disuse muscle atrophy. The review will begin with a brief discussion the regulation of muscle size, followed by the pertinent adaptations related to mitochondria, since mitochondrial health plays a key role in maintaining muscle size and function, and finaly the potential cytoprotective proteins induced by exercise will be discussed.

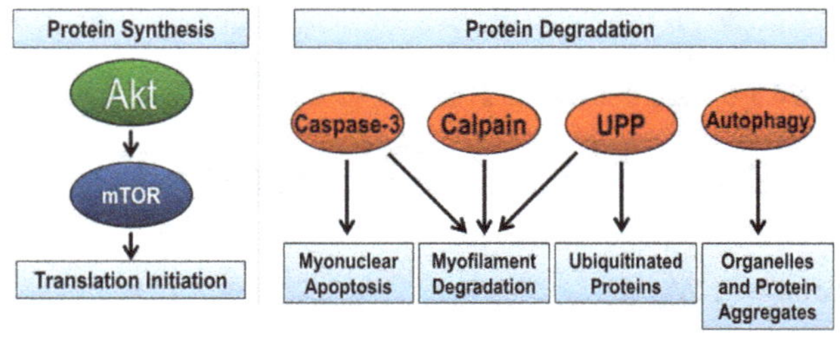

FIGURE 1 | Pathways regulating skeletal muscle size. The balance between protein synthesis and protein degradation determines muscle size. Muscle protein synthesis is regulated through the Akt/mTOR pathway. There are four pathways of protein degradation to degrade cellular components, caspase-3 removes nuclei (apoptosis) and along with the calpain family of proteins can breakdown the contractile proteins (myofilaments) in muscle into smaller polypeptides. The ubiquitin-proteasome pathway (UPP) breaks down the small peptides and any other protein targeted by ubiquitination for degradation. Finally, autophagy breaks down organelles, such as mitochondria and endoplasmic reticulum, and large protein aggregates.

Overview of the Regulation of Muscle Size

Muscle atrophy results from decrease in protein synthesis and an increase in protein degradation that ultimately leads to a decrease in myofiber size due to loss of contractile proteins, organelles, nuclei, and cytoplasm (Thomason and Booth, 1990). Indeed, animal studies have demonstrated that an increase in protein degradation and a decrease in protein synthesis contribute to disuse atrophy. This section will briefly describe the molecular basis for these processes (detailed review by Schiaffino et al., 2013).

Skeletal Muscle Proteolysis

In regards to proteolysis, skeletal muscle utilizes four complementary pathways to remove damaged, misfolded, or unnecessary proteins (**Figure 1**). These pathways include calpain, caspase-3, ubiquitin proteasome pathway, and autophagy (reviewed in Jackman and Kandarian, 2004). The calpain family of proteins is calcium dependent proteases that are important in the initiation of the breakdown of actin, myosin, and other structural proteins. Indeed, target pharmacological inhibition of calpain protects against disuse muscle atrophy (Tischler et al., 1990; Goll et al., 2003; Maes et al., 2007; Nelson et al., 2012; Talbert et al., 2013a). Caspase-3 is a member of the cysteine-aspartic acid protease family. Caspase-3 is most often defined by its central role in the removal of nuclei by myonuclear apoptosis; however, recent info also demonstrates the caspase-3 can work in concert with calpain in the cleavage of myofibrillar proteins (Du et al., 2004; Dupont-Versteegden, 2006; Smuder et al., 2010). Similar to calpain, inhibition or genetic knockdown of caspase-3 is sufficient to attenuate disuse muscle atrophy (McClung et al., 2007; Nelson et al., 2012; Talbert et al., 2013a; Zhu et al., 2013). Together, it is believed that calpain and caspase-3 are required for disuse atrophy because they begin the initial breakdown of the contractile apparatus of the muscle (Jackman and Kandarian, 2004). Further breakdown of these proteins is accomplished by the ubiquitin-proteasome pathway (Lecker et al., 1999). The proteasome pathway is also important in the degradation of misfolded, smaller polypeptides, and unnecessary proteins. Presently, the role of autophagy in disuse atrophy remains unclear. Early studies suggested that pharmacological inhibition of autophagy had minimal effects on muscle atrophy (Tischler et al., 1990); however, recent evidence suggests that autophagy may play an important role in disuse atrophy, specifically in the ability to selectively degrade organelles such as mitochondria (i.e., mitophagy) (Sandri, 2013). This will be discussed in greater detail in later sections.

Skeletal Muscle Protein Synthesis

Protein synthesis in cells is accomplished by a tightly controlled and structured scheme of signaling pathways, which culminate in the translation of messenger RNA (mRNA) into a specific protein. Within hours of disuse, muscle protein synthesis is rapidly depressed roughly 25–50% of control and reaches a new baseline level that persists throughout the period of inactivity (De Boer et al., 2007; Kortebein et al., 2008; Symons et al., 2009; Ferrando et al., 2010) The Akt/mTOR pathway is a crucial regulator of muscle mass by controlling formation of translation initiation machinery, the rate limiting step in protein synthesis (Bodine et al., 2001). Disuse atrophy results in decrease in this signaling pathway by decrease the phosphorylation of Akt and its downstream target mTOR. This ultimately leads to a decreased formation of the translation initiation complex and therefore, muscle protein synthesis.

In summary, it is believed that increased protein degradation and decreased protein synthesis contribute to disuse muscle atrophy. Of note, the increase in protein degradation persists only for a few days, while the decrease in protein synthesis happens within hours and remains depressed for the duration of disuse.

Endurance Exercise Training-Induced Adaptive Response in Skeletal Muscle

Classic studies elegantly demonstrate that prolonged endurance exercise training results in beneficial adaptations to skeletal muscle (Saltin et al., 1977; Holloszy and Coyle, 1984). Note that resistance exercise may also have positive effects in skeletal muscle. Unless otherwise stated, exercise training will specifically reference prolonged moderate to high intensity endurance exercise training. One of the fundamental principles of endurance training is a beneficial changes that with mitochondria in skeletal muscle. Given than exercise intensity and duration are sufficient to elicit a response, mitochondrial alterations are two-fold. First, there is an increase in mitochondrial turnover that is due to both an increase in new mitochondrion being made and slight increase in old mitochondria being removed. The end result is that exercise creates a larger population of mitochondria within skeletal muscle. In addition, increase in mitochondrial content improves the control of energy metabolism, and results in the oxidation of more fatty acids and less glycogen for ATP production. Indeed, these alterations are important because they are in contrast of many of the changes that occur with disuse atrophy, and will be discussed in detail later in this review.

Many of the adaptations that occur with exercise training occur due to an adaptive response. In other words, acute intense exercise training imposes a brief physiological stress on skeletal muscle. Examples of these stresses include oxidative, thermal, mechanical, metabolic, and cytokine production. In response to these stressors, signaling pathways are activated in order to increase the protein content of stress response proteins. This review will focus on several proteins that may play a role in cytoprotection, which are increased in response to acute exercise training due to oxidative, metabolic, and thermal stress.

The notion that exercise training can be cytoprotective against disuse muscle atrophy originates from the idea that repeated bouts of the exercise over a prolonged period of time results in an accumulation of these cytoprotective proteins, and therefore allows the skeletal muscle to be more resistant to the stress. It is important to note that many of the signaling pathways and proteins that are increased following endurance exercise are also found to be increased in disease states. Disuse muscle atrophy or disease states are associated with chronic exposure to stressors, and therefore the alterations in signaling pathways and protein expression are required for maintenance of cell homeostasis. In contrast, exercise-induced cellular stress is acute, lasting at most a few hours. Rest periods following exercise allows the skeletal muscle to handle the stressor and ultimately adapt. In theory exercise training may protect muscle from disuse atrophy by providing a "reserve" of cytoprotective proteins and increases the cell's ability to resist stress.

Role of Mitochondria and Oxidative Stress in Disuse Muscle Atrophy

Disuse muscle atrophy offers a different model of atrophy as opposed to many other models of atrophy because it is not associated with an increase in markers of inflammation. Therefore, the signals that promote atrophy are derived intracellularly. Evidence suggests that the major source of these intracellular signals arise in the mitochondria (Powers et al., 2012b).

Mitochondrial Morphology and Function are Altered During Disuse

The first studies to demonstrate that muscle inactivity was associated with alterations in mitochondria were completed in the early 1960s. These studies demonstrated that muscles subjected to denervation had mitochondria that were irregularly shaped and swollen (Aloisi et al., 1960; Carafoli et al., 1964; Muscatello and Patriarca, 1968) and had impaired mitochondrial coupling. Since these initial investigations, it has become well accepted that disuse muscle atrophy results in altered mitochondrial morphology and mitochondrial dysfunction (Powers et al., 2012b). Indeed, disuse atrophy disrupts the functioning of the oxidative phosphorylation system (i.e., electron transport chain), which results in the generation of superoxide (O_2^-). The O_2^- is dismutated to hydrogen peroxide and can then diffuse from the mitochondrion into the cytoplasm and negatively affect cell signaling pathways.

The Dual Role of Oxidative Stress in Disuse Muscle Atrophy and Exercise-Induced Adaptations in Skeletal Muscle

Several studies have demonstrated that disuse atrophy promotes an increase in reactive oxygen species (ROS) production in skeletal muscle (Adhihetty et al., 2007b; Muller et al., 2007; Kavazis et al., 2009). This increase is accompanied by a decreased expression of mitochondrial proteins and decreased mitochondrial respiration (i.e., ATP production). Increased ROS production alters redox signaling in muscle fibers that can increase proteolysis and decrease protein synthesis (reviewed in Powers, 2014). To further compound these effects, disuse muscle atrophy is associated with an overall decrease in antioxidant capacity in skeletal muscle (Lawler et al., 2003; Falk et al., 2006; Kavazis et al., 2009; Min et al., 2011). This decrease in antioxidant capacity is likely due to decreased antioxidant scavenging ability and not a decrease in antioxidant enzyme content (Kondo et al., 1993; Lawler et al., 2003).

Paradoxically, it is well established that endurance exercise increases oxidative stress in skeletal muscle. The first report of exercise-induced ROS in skeletal muscle was first reported over 30 years ago by Davies et al. (1982). Since that seminal report, many studies have confirmed that muscle contraction markedly increases the amount of ROS production compared to resting skeletal muscle (Powers and Jackson, 2008). An increase in ROS production has been demonstrated to be a powerful signaling molecule in activating signaling pathways. Importantly, increased ROS production acts as a powerful signal for the activation of transcription factors that increase endogenous antioxidant proteins (Powers et al., 2011). Indeed, evidence now suggests that the transient oxidative stress that occurs with exercise may be required for skeletal muscle adaptation to occur. Studies in animals (Gomez-Cabrera et al., 2005, 2008a) and humans (Ristow et al., 2009) have demonstrated that preventing exercise-induced oxidative stress blunted an increase in markers of mitochondrial biogenesis and endogenous antioxidants with training. Therefore, it appears that exercise-induced oxidative stress is required for the adaptive response of antioxidants.

The key difference between exercise-induced oxidative stress and oxidative stress associated with disuse atrophy is the duration of the exposure. Oxidative stress following exercise is transient in nature, while disuse atrophy results in chronic exposure to elevated ROS. Therefore the next section will briefly discuss endogenous antioxidants that are important in maintaining homeostasis in skeletal muscle and will discuss which of these antioxidants may confer protection due to exercise preconditioning.

The Role of Endogenous Antioxidants in Protection Against Disuse Atrophy

Skeletal muscle maintains a tightly controlled network of antioxidant defense mechanisms to reduce the potential for oxidative damage during periods of increased oxidative stress. Indeed, prolonged muscle inactivity is associated with a decrease in antioxidant capacity as well as an increase in ROS production and emission from mitochondria (Lawler et al., 2003; Falk et al., 2006; Kavazis et al., 2009; Min et al., 2011). In this section, we will provide a brief overview of three primary antioxidant enzymes in muscle: superoxide dismutase, glutathione peroxidase, and catalase and three accessory antioxidant enzymes: thioredoxin, glutaredoxin, and peroxiredoxin.

Superoxide Dismutase

Three isoforms of superoxide dismutase (SOD) are present in skeletal muscle. All three isoforms convert superoxide radicals into hydrogen peroxide and oxygen using a transition metal. SOD1 primarily is located within the cytosol and the mitochondrial intermembrane space and requires copper-zinc (Cu,-Zn-SOD) as a cofactor. SOD2 uses manganese (Mn-SOD) and is located only in the mitochondrial matrix. SOD3 also uses copper-zinc as a cofactor and is distributed in the extracellular space.

The general consensus in the literature is that chronic exercise training results in an overall increase in total SOD activity (reviewed in Powers et al., 2011). However, which specific isoform(s) are primarily responsible for the increase in activity is less clear. To further complicate matters, some studies have shown different responses in mRNA, protein content, and enzyme activity following exercise. For example, Strobel et al. demonstrated that 14 weeks of exercise training in mice resulted in no change in SOD2 mRNA, an increase in SOD2 protein content, and an unexplained decrease in SOD2 activity in skeletal muscle (Strobel et al., 2011). The variability in responses can likely be explained by experimental differences, such as differences in exercise protocols, muscle groups studied (i.e., fiber type), timing of tissue sampling, and under-powered studies. Nonetheless, generalizations can be made for each isoform.

SOD1 and SOD2 are the primary isoforms that have been studied to date. In regard to SOD1, numerous studies have shown an increase in either mRNA expression, protein content, or enzymatic activity (Oh-Ishi et al., 1996, 1997; Gore et al., 1998; Gomez-Cabrera et al., 2008a,b; Ristow et al., 2009; Meier et al., 2013). However, a similar number of studies can be found that have reported no change in at least one of these markers (Oh-Ishi et al., 1996; Lambertucci et al., 2007; Brooks et al., 2008). Therefore, since evidence exists both for and against, it is difficult to determine if an increase in SOD1 following exercise can be protective. There is a similar body of literature for SOD2; however, the majority of studies demonstrate at least one marker of SOD2 (i.e., mRNA expression, protein content, or enzymatic activity) is increased with exercise training (Oh-Ishi et al., 1997; Gore et al., 1998; Lambertucci et al., 2007; Gomez-Cabrera et al., 2008a; Ristow et al., 2009). To date, little is known about the response of SOD3 to exercise training.

Glutathione Peroxidase and Catalase

Hydrogen peroxide generated by the SOD family of antioxidants remains a reactive compound that can generate free radicals and is considered cytotoxic. Both glutathione peroxidase (GPX) and catalase are important antioxidants because they catalyze reactions that reduce hydrogen peroxide (reviewed in Powers and Jackson, 2008). In muscle cells, GPX expression is sensitive to oxidative stress (Zhou et al., 2001) and the majority of the literature suggests that GPX activity is increased following acute and chronic exercise (Laughlin et al., 1990; Criswell et al., 1993; Powers et al., 1994; Gore et al., 1998; Itoh et al., 2004; Lambertucci et al., 2007; Ristow et al., 2009; Smuder et al., 2011; Mangner et al., 2013). In contrast, changes in catalase expression following exercise is less clear, however the consensus is that catalase activity is not increased following training (Oh-Ishi et al., 1997; Smuder et al., 2011; Mangner et al., 2013).

Thioredoxin, Glutaredoxin, and Peroxiredoxin

In addition to the previously discussed antioxidant enzymes, skeletal muscle also contains several accessory enzymes that contribute directly or indirectly as antioxidants. The most important accessory antioxidant enzymes include thioredoxin, glutaredoxin, and peroxiredoxin.

The thioredoxin enzyme system is composed of both thioredoxin (Txn) and thioredoxin reductase (TxnRd). There are two isoforms of thioredoxin that are delineated from each other based on the cellular compartment in which they are found. Txn1 located in the cytosol and Txn2 found in the mitochondrial matrix (Arnér and Holmgren, 2000). Txn is an important disulfide reductase in the cell and therefore is important in maintaining proteins in their reduced state (Holmgren, 1989). Furthermore, it has recently been suggested that Txn2, in conjunction with glutathione (GSH), is an important regulator of hydrogen peroxide emission from mitochondria (Aon et al., 2012). Importantly, Txn protein content is decreased with hindlimb unloading (Matsushima et al., 2006). Unfortunately, there is a little evidence on the response of Txn1 or 2 following exercise training. However, recent reports suggest that TxnRd2, a necessary component in the system needed to catalyze the reduction (e.g., recycling) of Txn2, is increased in skeletal muscle following training (Fisher-Wellman et al., 2013).

Similar to Txn, glutaredoxin (Grx) is a thiodisulfide oxidoreductase that protects and repairs protein thiols during periods of oxidant stress (Holmgren, 1989). Grx protects protein thiols by the transfer of electrons from NADPH; this catalytic response is coupled with GSH and glutathione reductase. Three Grx isoforms are found in skeletal muscle. Grx1 is located in the cytosol and Grx2 and Grx5 are found in the mitochondria (Holmgren, 1989).

Peroxiredoxin (Prdx) is a peroxidase capable of reducing hydrogen peroxide and other hydroperoxides and peroxynitrate using electrons provided by thiol compounds (e.g., Txn) (Yin et al., 2012). There are six isoforms of Prdx; PrdxI, Prdx2, and Prdx6 are located in the cytosol whereas Prdx3 is located in the mitochondria (Yin et al., 2012). Prdx5 is located in both the cytosol and mitochondria whereas Prdx4 is found in the extracellular space (Yin et al., 2012).

The paucity of data on the response of accessory antioxidant enzymes to exercise training in skeletal muscle makes it difficult to make concrete statements on their role in the prevention of oxidative stress in skeletal muscle; however a few general conclusions can be reached. The Prdx isoforms are the most commonly studied group of enzymes following exercise training. Unfortunately, a clear pattern of expression following exercise or disuse does not exist. In general, Prdx expression is decreased with unloading in skeletal muscle; however exercise training does not consistently increase expression of any of the isoforms.

The Txn system is of interesting note because it has recently been reported that Txn2, in conjunction with glutathione (GSH), is an important regulator of hydrogen peroxide emission from mitochondria (Stanley et al., 2011; Aon et al., 2012). Importantly, Txn protein content is decreased with hindlimb unloading (Matsushima et al., 2006). Unfortunately, there is a little evidence on the response of Txn1 or 2 following exercise training. However, recent reports suggest that TxnRd2, a necessary component in the system needed to catalyze the reduction (e.g., recycling) of Txn2, is increased in skeletal muscle following training (Fisher-Wellman et al., 2013). Therefore, it stands to reason that exercise may prevent disuse atrophy-induced oxidative stress by increasing the buffering capacity of H_2O_2 in mitochondria.

In summary, endurance exercise training improves muscle antioxidant capacity as evidenced by several studies demonstrating less oxidative stress in trained muscles following a bout of intense exercise. The current body of literature suggests that the improvement in antioxidant capacity is due in part to increased activity of SOD2 and GPX, with the possibility that SOD1 may play a contributory role. Additional work is needed to clarify the importance and physiological roles that accessory antioxidant systems in regards to exercise training adaptations and disuse muscle atrophy, however promising new experiments suggest that these antioxidant systems may provide a novel approach to preventing disuse atrophy.

Can Increased Antioxidants Protect Against Disuse Muscle Atrophy?

It has been difficult to determine cause and effect for the hypothesis that increased antioxidant capacity can prevent disuse muscle atrophy. One reason for this is the lack of ability to use genetic knockout mice to determine gain or loss of function. SOD1 genetic knockout mice ($SOD1^{-/-}$) display increased markers of oxidative stress and marked muscle atrophy compared to wild type controls (Muller et al., 2006). Overexpression of SOD1 results in motor neuron disease and gross atrophy of skeletal muscle (Gurney et al., 1994; Rando et al., 1998; Zhang et al., 2013). It is believed that this sensitization of muscle to increased SOD1 activity is due to an imbalance between hydrogen peroxide generated by SOD1 without a concomitant increase in the enzymes that convert hydrogen peroxide to water and oxygen. Moreover, disruption of the SOD2 gene is lethal in mice due to neurodegeneration and cardiac dysfunction (Lebovitz et al., 1996). Therefore, it is difficult to conclude that increased expression of SOD1 or SOD2 can protect against oxidative stress during periods of disuse.

Without the ability to use transgenic animals, a common experimental design to determine the effect of antioxidant capacity on disuse muscle atrophy has been to provide exogenous antioxidant supplements. Examples of these supplements include vitamin C, vitamin E, trolox, N-acetylcysterine, and mitochondrial targeted antioxidants. Unfortunately, definitive proof that antioxidant supplementation protects against disuse atrophy does not exist because there is data for and against the idea that antioxidants can prevent disuse atrophy. For example, several studies using a variety of antioxidants in various disuse atrophy models suggest that antioxidant supplementation may provide protection against disuse atrophy (Kondo et al., 1991, 1992; Appell et al., 1997; Betters et al., 2004; Servais et al., 2007; Agten et al., 2011; Min et al., 2011; Talbert et al., 2013b), while several other papers provide evidence that antioxidant supplementation is not protective (Koesterer et al., 2002; Farid et al., 2005; Brocca et al., 2010; Desaphy et al., 2010). Indeed, these studies have spurred debates if oxidative stress is a cause of muscle atrophy or purely a consequence (Brocca et al., 2010; Powers et al., 2012a); compelling arguments for each side can be made. It is clear that more research is needed in this area, with a particular focus to address this issue in humans.

The Role of Mitochondria and PGC1-α in Disuse Muscle Atrophy

As previously mentioned, exercise training and disuse have opposite effects on skeletal muscle mitochondria. Prolonged exercise training results in an increase in mitochondrial turnover. However, because mitochondrial biogenesis is increased at a greater rate than removal of mitochondria, exercise training results in an increase in an overall increase in mitochondrial content. A potent activator of mitochondrial biogenesis is peroxisome proliferative activated receptor-γ coactivator 1α (PGC1-α) (**Figure 2**). Thus, the first part of this section will focus on PGC1-α's role

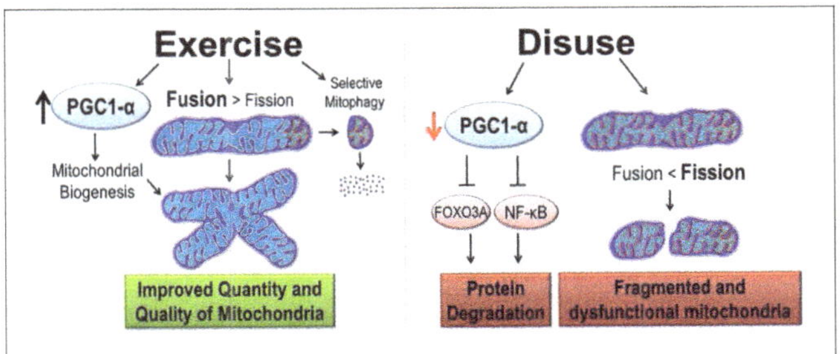

FIGURE 2 | Exercise and disuse effects on mitochondrial quality and quantity. Exercise training promotes cytoprotective effects by the induction of PGC1-α protein, considered the master regulator of mitochondrial biogenesis. Exercise improves quality in two ways. First, mitochondrial dynamics are shifted such that fusion is greater than fission resulting in larger mitochondrial network. Second, increased selective mitophagy removes old and dysfunctional mitochondria (denoted with red and orange organelles). In contrast, disuse decreases PGC1-α, removing its inhibition of protein degradation pathways. Furthermore, mitochondrial dynamics are shifted toward fission causing a small, fragmented, and dysfunctional mitochondria.

in mitochondrial turnover followed by a discussion on PGC1-α regulation of protein degradation.

PGC1–α Increases Mitochondrial Content is Skeletal Muscle

PGC1-α was first discovered in the lab of Bruce Spiegelman while studying adaptive thermogenesis in adipose tissue and skeletal muscle (Puigserver et al., 1998). This study speculated that increased expression of PGC1-α was an important modulator of mitochondrial biogenesis. Indeed, follow-up studies in skeletal muscle demonstrated that PGC1-α acts as co-activator by docking with transcription factors and aiding in the recruitment of regulatory protein complexes that increase gene transcription of proteins involved in mitochondrial biogenesis, rates of cellular respiration, and glucose uptake/utilization (Puigserver et al., 1998, 1999; Wu et al., 1999; St-Pierre et al., 2003).

In skeletal muscle, PGC1-α is frequently considered a "master regulator" of mitochondrial biogenesis because of its powerful role as a transcription co-factor. Indeed, PGC-1α interacts with and co-activates numerous transcription factors and nuclear receptors, including estrogen-related receptor-α (ERRα), nuclear respiratory factor-1 (NRF-1) and 2, myocyte enhancer factor 2 (MEF2), and mitochondrial transcription factor A (Tfam) (Spiegelman, 2007). All of these transcription factors directly regulate the expression of important nuclear-encoded mitochondrial genes necessary metabolic adaptations in skeletal muscle. Furthermore, overexpression of PGC1-α drives skeletal muscle fiber types to much more oxidative phenotype (Lin et al., 2002).

Mitochondrial and Metabolic Alteration with Disuse and Exercise

Prolonged disuse muscle atrophy is associated with impaired oxidative metabolism and an increase in glycolysis. This is due in part to a decrease in mitochondrial biogenesis, mitochondrial content, and electron transport chain components (Lecker et al., 2004; Kang and Ji, 2013). The onset of mitochondrial dysfunction is rapid and results in an increase in ROS production and metabolic stress due to increased reliance on glycolysis, decreased fat oxidation, and substrate accumulation, which ultimately leads to inefficient ATP production (Stein and Wade, 2005). The opposite is true for exercise trained muscle, which demonstrates an increase in oxidative metabolism, increased utilization of fat, and increased mitochondrial biogenesis (Holloszy and Coyle, 1984). It is becoming increasingly apparent that PGC1-α is an important mediator of these exercise-induced effects and may be an important mediator of exercise induced-cytoprotection. Because PGC1- α is such a power inducer of fuel intake and β-oxidation, it follows that the metabolic changes that occur with exercise-induced PGC1- α expression can protect against metabolic deficits seen with disuse atrophy.

PGC1- α Activity Regulates Protein Degradation Pathways

Although it is well established that the decrease in protein synthesis contributes to disuse atrophy; to date, there has been no data suggesting that PGC1-α signaling is directly mediates the protein synthesis pathways (Brault et al., 2010). However, PGC1-α transcriptional activity has been shown to prevent muscle protein degradation. This was first demonstrated by Sandri et al., who showed that over-expression of PGC1-α in mice prevented denervation-induced muscle atrophy by preventing the expression of key genes in the ubiquitin proteasome pathway and autophagy (Sandri et al., 2006). Furthermore, this study demonstrated that elevated PGC1-α content prevented transcriptional activity of FoxO3a. Upon activation, FoxO3a moves from the sarcoplasm into the nucleus where it acts as a potent translational activator of proteins in the ubiquitin-proteasome (i.e., atrogin-1 and MAFbx), autophagy, and apoptosis pathways. Additionally, a recent study suggests that PGC1-α can inhibit the NF-κB signaling pathway (Eisele et al., 2013), which is another important pathway in muscle protein degradation (reviewed in Jackman and Kandarian, 2004). Therefore, we conclude that PGC1-α is an important modulator of protein degradation pathways in disuse muscle atrophy and thus helps mediated the exercise preconditioning effect (**Figure 2**).

The rationale that PGC1-α mediates exercise-induced cytoprotection is two-fold. First, disuse muscle atrophy is associated with a decreased expression of PGC1-α content, as demonstrated in both animal and human models (Sandri et al., 2006; Sacheck et al., 2007; Kang and Ji, 2013). Therefore, it stands to reason, that preventing a decrease below basal levels of PGC1-α may prevent muscle atrophy. In this regard, PGC1-α expression is highly inducible with high intensity endurance exercise (Baar et al., 2002; Pilegaard et al., 2003; Smuder et al., 2012a) and importantly protein expression accumulates in skeletal muscle after training (Russell et al., 2003; Taylor et al., 2005). Thus, it follows that exercise training, prior to disuse muscle atrophy, can increase PGC1-α protein content such that the inactivity-induced decrease is mitigated or it only reaches the level of the basal untrained state. Indeed, expression of PGC1-α in fast-twitch muscles of mice, to levels commonly seen with exercise training, were able to attenuate disuse muscle atrophy (Sandri et al., 2006); thus, making PGC1-α a potentially important mediator of disuse atrophy protein degradation.

Endurance Exercise Improves Mitochondrial Quality

As previously mentioned, exercise training is a potent stimulus for mitochondrial biogenesis; however, recent evidence suggests that endurance training may also improve mitochondrial quality through two mutually exclusive pathways: alterations in mitochondrial dynamics and selective autophagic degradation of mitochondria (i.e., mitophagy).

Mitochondrial Dynamics

Isolated mitochondria are often represented as spherical shaped individual organelles, however, *in vitro* they form a complex interconnected network. The shape of the mitochondrial network is said to be dynamic because segments of mitochondria frequently divide (i.e., fission) and join (i.e., fusion). Mitochondrial dynamics are controlled by a family of mitochondrial shaping proteins (Dimmer and Scorrano, 2006; Iqbal and Hood, 2014). Key proteins that promote mitochondrial fission include

Dynamin-related protein-1 (Drp1) and Fission 1 (Fis1), whereas proteins regulating mitochondrial fusion include optic atrophy 1 (Opa1) and mitofusion 1 and 2 (Mfn1/2) (reviewed in Westermann, 2010; Chan, 2012). The role of fusion and fission in cells is complex, but it is believed that increased fusion of mitochondria is associated with improved function, while fission is a mechanism by which damaged portions of mitochondria are sectioned off the reticulum and targeted for degradation by autophagy (i.e., mitophagy).

Mitophagy

As previously discussed, autophagy is the degradation pathway that allows cells to degrade organelles and macromolecules. There are two classifications of autophagy, selective or non-selective (i.e., macroautophagy). Selective autophagy is defined by the autophagasome directly targeting an organelle that has been selected by the cell to be degraded. Often, selective autophagy refers to degradation of mitochondria or endoplasmic reticulum. Non-selective autophagy indiscriminately degrades organells and macromolecules. The process of autophagy consists of cytosolic components to be degraded that are sequestered into double membrane vesicles called autophagosomes. These autophagosomes fuse with lysosomes containing hydrolytic enzymes that break down cellular components (He and Klionsky, 2009). Although autophagy plays a prominent role in protein degradation during disuse, it also appears to have a housekeeping role by turning over organelles and degrading protein aggregates. Mice with genetic ablation of rate limiting proteins in the autophagic machinery display marked muscle atrophy and weakness (Masiero et al., 2009; Chang et al., 2012).

Mitophagy denotes the degradation of mitochondria through autophagy and is regulated independently of macroautophagy (Kanki and Klionsky, 2008). Following damage, the mitochondrial phosphatase and tensin homolog-induced kinase-1 (PINK1) becomes stabilized on the outer mitochondrial membrane (Vincow et al., 2013). PINK1 then recruits the protein Parkin, an e3 ubiquitin ligase, which tags several outer mitochondrial membrane proteins with ubiquitin and results in the fragmentation and isolation of impaired mitochondria (Narendra et al., 2010). Currently, little is known about the proteins that interact between the autophagasome and PINK1 and Parkin on the mitochondria. Briefly, several candidate proteins have been identified. For example BCL-2, a key anti-apoptotic factor, binds to proteins related to phagasome development (Liang et al., 1999). BNIP3 (Bcl-2 and 19 kD interacting protein-37) and BNIP3-like protein (BNIP3L) have also been identified as proteins than can pair autophagasomes with uqiquintated mitochondrial protein (Zhang and Ney, 2009). Finally, autophagy related gene 32 (Atg32) is another protein recently to confers selectivity of the autophagosome to mitochodnria (Kanki et al., 2009). The field of mitophagy is an active area of research that is rapidly evolving and complex field of study, and therefore the specifics are beyond the scope of this review. Please see the following references for in depth review (Twig and Shirihai, 2011; Youle and Narendra, 2011; Feng et al., 2013).

Mitochondrial Dynamics and Mitophagy in Exercise and Disuse

Mitochondrial dynamics and mitophagy are both altered with exercise training (**Figure 2**). In regard to mitochondrial dynamics, George Brooks' lab in the late 1980s was the first to demonstrate that the mitochondria reticulum became more expansive following chronic exercise training (Kirkwood et al., 1987). This suggested exercise training shifted the expression of fission and fusion machinery toward that of enhanced fusion. Improvements in biochemical and imaging techniques have provided evidence to support this theory. Exercise training is sufficient to increase expression of MFN1/2 and increases interactions between mitochondria (Ding et al., 2010; Picard et al., 2013; Iqbal and Hood, 2014). A primary pathway that drives the expression following exercise is PGC1 (Cartoni et al., 2005; Zechner et al., 2010) Concomitantly, fission protein expression is reduced with training (Perry et al., 2010; Iqbal and Hood, 2014). So what is the role of increased fusion of mitochondria? It is believed that the physiological relevance of increased fusion is mixing of mitochondrial content such as metabolic substrates, mitochondrial DNA, and proteins. Therefore, content mixing allows for a homogenous population of mitochondria, which in theory allows healthy mitochondria to positively affect damaged mitochondria.

Disuse atrophy is associated with a fragmented mitochondrial reticulum that is remodeled through autophagy (Romanello et al., 2010) (**Figure 2**). Note, mitochondria often appear enlarged in skeletal muscle atrophy (Powers et al., 2012b). This is not to be confused with a smaller, disorganized network. Instead, these mitochondria are enlarged due to swelling. Disuse atrophy results in an imbalance between fission and fusion events with an overall shift in the direction of fusion. Based on protein expression levels, disuse atrophy results in a down regulation of fusion machinery while fission events remain relatively constant (Iqbal and Hood, 2014; Cannavino et al., 2015). However, it is prudent to not exclude an increase in fission proteins with only a few data points. Indeed, expression of fission machinery is sufficient to cause muscle atrophy in mice (Romanello et al., 2010). Nonetheless, it is clear that disuse atrophy shifts the balance between fusion and fission results in small, fragmented mitochondria with a reduced capacity of ATP re-synthesis and increase in ROS emission (Twig et al., 2008).

It has recently been demonstrated that exercise training induces mitophagy, which is required for some of the exercise induced adaptations of skeletal muscle (Grumati et al., 2011; Lira et al., 2013). Although slightly counter intuitive, increased mitophagy following exercise is beneficial by improving overall mitochondrial quality through the selective removal of damaged or dysfunctional mitochondria (Safdar et al., 2011). Combined with evidence that exercise training or chronic stimulation of muscle results in a mitochondrial phenotype that resists oxidative stress and mitochondrial mediated apoptosis (Adhihetty et al., 2007a; O'leary and Hood, 2008), these data suggest that exercise training induced global changes in mitochondria may be cytoprotective by increasing quantity and improving quality of skeletal muscle mitochondria (**Figure 2**).

As previously discussed, disuse atrophy causes a decrease in mitochondrial number through targeted degradation.

Mitochondria are segregated by fission and then selectively targeted for degradation via mitophagy. This process is to remove damaged mitochondria and decrease mitochondrial number to match metabolic demands. Therefore, mitophagy, *per se*, is not a direct contributor to disuse atrophy.

In summary, it appears that a basal level of mitophagy is necessary to maintain cellular homeostasis. The function of mitophagy is to remove damaged and/or old organelles so that these can be replaced by newer, healthier organelles. Exercise training is the excellent example of mitophagy improving overall mitochondrial quality by increasing following exercise training and remodeling of the mitochondrial phenotype.

The Role of Heat Shock Protein 70 in Prevention of Muscle Atrophy

The heat shock family of proteins is known as molecular chaperone proteins that have been demonstrated to increase following exercise. In general, their role is three-fold: (1) facilitate folding of de novo synthesized proteins; (2) assist in the re-folding of misfolded proteins and denatured proteins, and (3) aid in the transport of those proteins to their correct cellular compartments (Feder and Hofmann, 1999). Heat shock proteins (HSPs) can be classified into a number of families that are traditionally named for their molecular mass. These include small HSPs (between 8 and 27 kDa), HSP60 (i.e., 60 kDa), HSP 70, and HSP90. Of these, HSP70 is the most studied and will be the focus of the following section.

HSP70 is Induced by Cell Stress and Exercise

HSP70, also commonly referred to as HSP72, is a highly conserved protein whose expression is increased following stress, hence why HSP70 is termed a stress-inducible member of the HSP family of proteins. Its expression is responsive to thermal stress, oxidative stress, mechanical stress, metabolic stress, and cytokines. Importantly, exercise training promotes these stressors and it is clear that exercise is a powerful inducer of HSP70 protein content.

The first evidence that exercise increased HSP70 protein content was generated in 1990 when Locke et al. postulated that exercising skeletal muscle from mice increased protein synthesis of stress protein similar to that of a protein produced during heat stress (Locke et al., 1990). Shortly thereafter, it was confirmed that exercise training increased HSP70 mRNA in both rodent (Salo et al., 1991) and human skeletal muscle (Puntschart et al., 1996). Since these original studies, it is now well accepted that a single bout of exercise is sufficient to increase HSP70 mRNA and protein expression in animals and humans in an intensity dependent manner (Milne and Noble, 2002; Morton et al., 2009). Importantly, prolonged exercise training increases baseline levels of HSP70 (Liu et al., 1999; Ecochard et al., 2000; González et al., 2000; Atalay et al., 2004; Kayani et al., 2008; Smuder et al., 2012b). It is important to note that mechanical unloading has the opposite effect of exercise on HSP70 content in muscle. Disuse atrophy is associated with a rapid decrease in HSP70 protein content (Lawler et al., 2006; Senf et al., 2008; Moriggi et al., 2010; Lomonosova et al., 2012).

Increased HSP70 Content Protects Against Disuse Muscle Atrophy

Early studies demonstrated that exposing mice to a non-lethal heat stress provides the animal with protection against a subsequent typically lethal heat exposure. These protective findings were attributed to a family of proteins that were induced by heat stress and these findings were soon translated to skeletal muscle (Garramone et al., 1994).In the study by Garramone et al., prior exposure to heat stress (i.e., greater than 41°C) conferred protection against ischemic injury in rat skeletal muscle (Garramone et al., 1994).

In regards to disuse muscle atrophy, there are several lines of evidence that induction of HSP70 content can protect against the negative biochemical and structural changes associated with muscle atrophy. First, prior exposure to heat stress demonstrates protection against atrophy in hind limb unloading, immobilization, and mechanical ventilation (Naito et al., 2000; Selsby and Dodd, 2005; Ichinoseki-Sekine et al., 2014). However, because heat stress may cause other adaptive responses independent of HSP70, these studies do not prove cause and effect. Direct evidence in support of this hypothesis comes from muscle-specific overexpression of HSP70. For example, Senf et al., demonstrated that HSP70 overexpression attenuated 4 days of immobilization-induced muscle atrophy (Senf et al., 2008). However, conversely, another study using whole body overexpression was unable to prevent 7 days of unloading-induced atrophy (Miyabara et al., 2012). Several possibilities exist for this discrepancy including species differences (rat/mice), duration of immobilization (4 day/7 days), and method of overexpression (single muscle electroporation/whole body overexpression). It important to note that the global (i.e., whole body) HSP70 overexpressing mice had significantly smaller muscles compared to their wild type littermates, suggesting altered physiology in these animals (Miyabara et al., 2012). Nonetheless, it appears that HSP70 is an important stress response protein that has the potential to protect against disuse muscle atrophy.

Mechanisms by which HSP70 Protects Against Muscle Atrophy

HSP70 is localized in many different subcellular locations including mitochondria, nucleus, ribosomes, and in the cytoplasm. Therefore, it is no surprise that HSP70 may protect against muscle atrophy through a multitude of different mechanisms (**Figure 3**). First, HSP70 is most well-known for its ability to serve as a chaperone and prevent dysfunction and/or targeted proteolysis of oxidized proteins by binding to and assisting in their re-folding. An important example of this mechanism is demonstrated by the ability of HSP70 to protect against damaging increases in intracellular calcium during muscle atrophy by binding to oxidized sarcoplasmic/endoplasmic reticulum Ca^{2+}-ATPase (SERCA) to preserve its function (Gehrig et al., 2012). Second, the chaperone function of HSP70 can maintain mitochondrial integrity by protecting mitochondria against apoptotic stimuli and contribute to the repair of damaged proteins (Kang et al., 1990; Mosser et al., 2000). Third, HSP72 can prevent disuse atrophy induced-proteolysis by inhibiting activation of FoxO3a

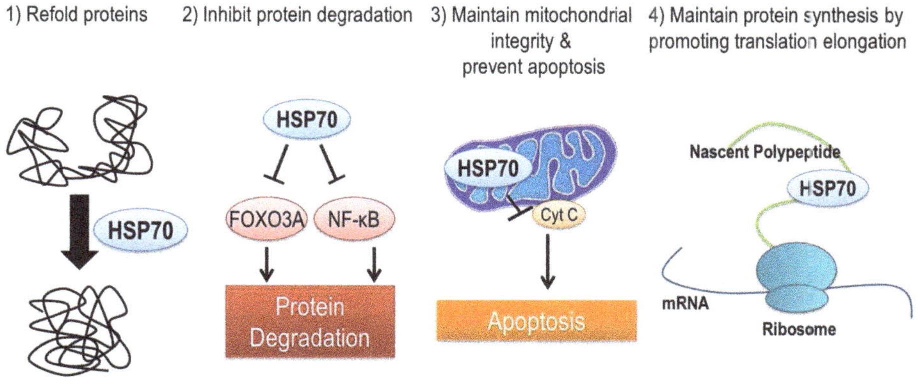

FIGURE 3 | HSP70 is an inducible chaperone protein that can be provide protection against muscle atrophy in several ways. (1) Refolding of misfolded or unfolded proteins, (2) inhibiting select pathways of protein degradation, (3) maintaining mitochondrial integrity and reducing apoptosis by preventing the release of cytochrome C from mitochondria, and (4) improving translation elongation and promoting protein synthesis.

and NF-κB signaling pathways (Senf et al., 2008, 2010). And finally, expression of HSP72 may prevent an atrophy induced decrease in muscle protein synthesis by maintaining the rate of translation elongation of nascent polypeptides (Nelson et al., 1992; Ku et al., 1995).

Conclusions

The idea that lifelong endurance training can be protective against disuse muscle atrophy has yet to be definitively proven in scientific literature, however the theory remains valid. An acute bout of exercise training results in a small stimulus that brings about an adaptive response. Prolonged exercise training results in an accumulation of these adaptive responses. Therefore, it follows that when skeletal muscle has adapted to small repeated stresses, it is much better suited to handle the stress brought on by disuse muscle atrophy. These adaptations include, but are not limited to, limiting oxidative stress during disuse atrophy by increased antioxidant systems to buffer increased ROS production or by having newer, healthier mitochondria that produce less ROS when inactive. There is also the possibility of increased proteins such as PGC1-α and HSP70 that can prevent activation of key protein degradation pathways, protect against mitochondrial dysfunction, maintain muscle protein synthesis, and assist in the refolding of damaged proteins. Furthermore, there are likely numerous other proteins that could be cytoprotective and therefore more work in this area needs to be done.

Acknowledgments

I would like to thank Dr. Scott Powers for his mentorship, encouragement and countless discussions that facilitated the scientific evidence and rationale behind this review.

References

Adhihetty, P. J., Ljubicic, V., and Hood, D. A. (2007a). Effect of chronic contractile activity on SS and IMF mitochondrial apoptotic susceptibility in skeletal muscle. *Am. J. Physiol. Endocrinol. Metab.* 292, E748–E755. doi: 10.1152/ajpendo.00311.2006

Adhihetty, P. J., O'leary, M. F., Chabi, B., Wicks, K. L., and Hood, D. A. (2007b). Effect of denervation on mitochondrially mediated apoptosis in skeletal muscle. *J. Appl. Physiol.* 102, 1143–1151. doi: 10.1152/japplphysiol.00768.2006

Agten, A., Maes, K., Smuder, A., Powers, S. K., Decramer, M., and Gayan-Ramirez, G. (2011). N-Acetylcysteine protects the rat diaphragm from the decreased contractility associated with controlled mechanical ventilation. *Crit. Care Med.* 39, 777–782. doi: 10.1097/CCM.0b013e318206cca9

Aloisi, M., Azzone, G., and Carafoli, E. (1960). Lesions of pigeon muscle mitochondria in avitaminosis B1 and denervation atrophy. *Arch. De Vecchi Anat. Patol.* 32:33.

Aon, M. A., Stanley, B. A., Sivakumaran, V., Kembro, J. M., O'Rourke, B., Paolocci, N., et al. (2012). Glutathione/thioredoxin systems modulate mitochondrial H2O2 emission: an experimental-computational study. *J. Gen. Physiol.* 139, 479–491. doi: 10.1085/jgp.201210772

Appell, H.-J., Duarte, J., and Soares, J. (1997). Supplementation of vitamin E may attenuate skeletal muscle immobilization atrophy. *Int. J. Sports Med.* 18, 157–160. doi: 10.1055/s-2007-972612

Arnér, E. S., and Holmgren, A. (2000). Physiological functions of thioredoxin and thioredoxin reductase. *Eur. J. Biochem.* 267, 6102–6109. doi: 10.1046/j.1432-1327.2000.01701.x

Atalay, M., Oksala, N. K., Laaksonen, D. E., Khanna, S., Nakao, C., Lappalainen, J., et al. (2004). Exercise training modulates heat shock protein response in diabetic rats. *J. Appl. Physiol.* 97, 605–611. doi: 10.1152/japplphysiol.01183.2003

Baar, K., Wende, A. R., Jones, T. E., Marison, M., Nolte, L. A., Chen, M., et al. (2002). Adaptations of skeletal muscle to exercise: rapid increase in the transcriptional coactivator PGC-1. *FASEB J.* 16, 1879–1886. doi: 10.1096/fj.02-0367com

Betters, J. L., Criswell, D. S., Shanely, R. A., Van Gammeren, D., Falk, D., Deruisseau, K. C., et al. (2004). Trolox attenuates mechanical ventilation–induced diaphragmatic dysfunction and proteolysis. *Am. J. Respir. Crit. Care Med.* 170, 1179–1184. doi: 10.1164/rccm.200407-939OC

Bodine, S. C., Stitt, T. N., Gonzalez, M., Kline, W. O., Stover, G. L., Bauerlein, R., et al. (2001). Akt/mTOR pathway is a crucial regulator of skeletal muscle hypertrophy and can prevent muscle atrophy in vivo. *Nat. Cell Biol.* 3, 1014–1019. doi: 10.1038/ncb1101-1014

Brault, J. J., Jespersen, J. G., and Goldberg, A. L. (2010). Peroxisome proliferator-activated receptor γ coactivator 1α or 1β overexpression inhibits muscle protein degradation, induction of ubiquitin ligases, and disuse atrophy. *J. Biol. Chem.* 285, 19460–19471. doi: 10.1074/jbc.M110.113092

Brocca, L., Pellegrino, M. A., Desaphy, J.-F., Pierno, S., Camerino, D. C., and Bottinelli, R. (2010). Is oxidative stress a cause or consequence of disuse muscle atrophy in mice? A proteomic approach in hindlimb-unloaded mice. *Exp. Physiol.* 95, 331–350. doi: 10.1113/expphysiol.2009.050245

Brooks, S. V., Vasilaki, A., Larkin, L. M., Mcardle, A., and Jackson, M. J. (2008). Repeated bouts of aerobic exercise lead to reductions in skeletal muscle free radical generation and nuclear factor κB activation. *J. Physiol.* 586, 3979–3990. doi: 10.1113/jphysiol.2008.155382

Cannavino, J., Brocca, L., Sandri, M., Grassi, B., Bottinelli, R., and Pellegrino, M. A. (2015). The role of alterations in mitochondrial dynamics and PGC-1alpha over-expression in fast muscle atrophy following hindlimb unloading. *J. Physiol.* doi: 10.1113/jphysiol.2014.286740. [Epub ahead of print].

Carafoli, E., Margreth, A., and Buffa, P. (1964). Early biochemical changes in mitochondria from denervated muscle and their relation to the onset of atrophy. *Exp. Mol. Pathol.* 3, 171–181. doi: 10.1016/0014-4800(64)90050-4

Cartoni, R., Léger, B., Hock, M. B., Praz, M., Crettenand, A., Pich, S., et al. (2005). Mitofusins 1/2 and ERRα expression are increased in human skeletal muscle after physical exercise. *J. Physiol.* 567, 349–358. doi: 10.1113/jphysiol.2005.092031

Chan, D. C. (2012). Fusion and fission: interlinked processes critical for mitochondrial health. *Annu. Rev. Genet.* 46, 265–287. doi: 10.1146/annurev-genet-110410-132529

Chang, N. C., Nguyen, M., Bourdon, J., Risse, P.-A., Martin, J., Danialou, G., et al. (2012). Bcl-2-associated autophagy regulator Naf-1 required for maintenance of skeletal muscle. *Hum. Mol. Genet.* 21, 2277–2287. doi: 10.1093/hmg/dds048

Criswell, D., Powers, S., Dodd, S., Lawler, J., Edwards, W., Renshler, K., et al. (1993). High intensity training-induced changes in skeletal muscle antioxidant enzyme activity. *Med. Sci. Sports Exerc.* 25, 1135–1140. doi: 10.1249/00005768-199310000-00009

Davies, K. J., Quintanilha, A. T., Brooks, G. A., and Packer, L. (1982). Free radicals and tissue damage produced by exercise. *Biochem. Biophys. Res. Commun.* 107, 1198–1205. doi: 10.1016/S0006-291X(82)80124-1

De Boer, M. D., Selby, A., Atherton, P., Smith, K., Seynnes, O. R., Maganaris, C. N., et al. (2007). The temporal responses of protein synthesis, gene expression and cell signalling in human quadriceps muscle and patellar tendon to disuse. *J. Physiol.* 585, 241–251. doi: 10.1113/jphysiol.2007.142828

Desaphy, J.-F., Pierno, S., Liantonio, A., Giannuzzi, V., Digennaro, C., Dinardo, M. M., et al. (2010). Antioxidant treatment of hindlimb-unloaded mouse counteracts fiber type transition but not atrophy of disused muscles. *Pharmacol. Res.* 61, 553–563. doi: 10.1016/j.phrs.2010.01.012

Dimmer, K. S., and Scorrano, L. (2006). (De) constructing mitochondria: what for? *Physiology* 21, 233–241. doi: 10.1152/physiol.00010.2006

Ding, H., Jiang, N., Liu, H., Liu, X., Liu, D., Zhao, F., et al. (2010). Response of mitochondrial fusion and fission protein gene expression to exercise in rat skeletal muscle. *Biochim. Biophys. Acta* 1800, 250–256. doi: 10.1016/j.bbagen.2009.08.007

Du, J., Wang, X., Miereles, C., Bailey, J. L., Debigare, R., Zheng, B., et al. (2004). Activation of caspase-3 is an initial step triggering accelerated muscle proteolysis in catabolic conditions. *J. Clin. Invest.* 113, 115–123. doi: 10.1172/JCI18330

Dupont-Versteegden, E. E. (2006). Apoptosis in skeletal muscle and its relevance to atrophy. *World J. Gastroenterol.* 12, 7463. doi: 10.3748/wjg.v12.i46.7463

Ecochard, L., Lhenry, F., Sempore, B., and Favier, R. (2000). Skeletal muscle HSP72 level during endurance training: influence of peripheral arterial insufficiency. *Pflüg. Arch.* 440, 918–924. doi: 10.1007/s004240000362

Eisele, P. S., Salatino, S., Sobek, J., Hottiger, M. O., and Handschin, C. (2013). The peroxisome proliferator-activated receptor γ coactivator 1α/β (PGC-1) coactivators repress the transcriptional activity of NF-κB in skeletal muscle cells. *J. Biol. Chem.* 288, 2246–2260. doi: 10.1074/jbc.M112.375253

Falk, D. J., Deruisseau, K. C., Van Gammeren, D. L., Deering, M. A., Kavazis, A. N., and Powers, S. K. (2006). Mechanical ventilation promotes redox status alterations in the diaphragm. *J. Appl. Physiol.* 101, 1017–1024. doi: 10.1152/japplphysiol.00104.2006

Farid, M., Reid, M. B., Li, Y.-P., Gerken, E., and Durham, W. J. (2005). Effects of dietary curcumin or N-acetylcysteine on NF-κB activity and contractile performance in ambulatory and unloaded murine soleus. *Nutr. Metab.* 2:20. doi: 10.1186/1743-7075-2-20

Feder, M. E., and Hofmann, G. E. (1999). Heat-shock proteins, molecular chaperones, and the stress response: evolutionary and ecological physiology. *Annu. Rev. Physiol.* 61, 243–282. doi: 10.1146/annurev.physiol.61.1.243

Feng, D., Liu, L., Zhu, Y., and Chen, Q. (2013). Molecular signaling toward mitophagy and its physiological significance. *Exp. Cell Res.* 319, 1697–1705. doi: 10.1016/j.yexcr.2013.03.034

Ferrando, A. A., Paddon-Jones, D., Hays, N. P., Kortebein, P., Ronsen, O., Williams, R. H., et al. (2010). EAA supplementation to increase nitrogen intake improves muscle function during bed rest in the elderly. *Clin. Nutr.* 29, 18–23. doi: 10.1016/j.clnu.2009.03.009

Fisher-Wellman, K. H., Mattox, T. A., Thayne, K., Katunga, L. A., La Favor, J. D., Neufer, P. D., et al. (2013). Novel role for thioredoxin reductase−2 in mitochondrial redox adaptations to obesogenic diet and exercise in heart and skeletal muscle. *J. Physiol.* 591, 3471–3486. doi: 10.1113/jphysiol.2013.254193

Garramone, R. R. Jr., Winters, R. M., Das, D. K., and Deckers, P. J. (1994). Reduction of skeletal muscle injury through stress conditioning using the heat-shock response. *Plast. Reconstr. Surg.* 93, 1242–1247. doi: 10.1097/00006534-199405000-00021

Gehrig, S. M., Van Der Poel, C., Sayer, T. A., Schertzer, J. D., Henstridge, D. C., Church, J. E., et al. (2012). Hsp72 preserves muscle function and slows progression of severe muscular dystrophy. *Nature* 484, 394–398. doi: 10.1038/nature10980

Glover, E. I., and Phillips, S. M. (2010). Resistance exercise and appropriate nutrition to counteract muscle wasting and promote muscle hypertrophy. *Curr. Opin. Clin. Nutr. Metab. Care* 13, 630–634. doi: 10.1097/MCO.0b013e32833f1ae5

Goll, D. E., Thompson, V. F., Li, H., Wei, W., and Cong, J. (2003). The calpain system. *Physiol. Rev.* 83, 731–801. doi: 10.1152/physrev.00029.2002

Gomez-Cabrera, M.-C., Borrás, C., Pallardó, F. V., Sastre, J., Ji, L. L., and Viña, J. (2005). Decreasing xanthine oxidase-mediated oxidative stress prevents useful cellular adaptations to exercise in rats. *J. Physiol.* 567, 113–120. doi: 10.1113/jphysiol.2004.080564

Gomez-Cabrera, M.-C., Domenech, E., Romagnoli, M., Arduini, A., Borras, C., Pallardo, F. V., et al. (2008a). Oral administration of vitamin C decreases muscle mitochondrial biogenesis and hampers training-induced adaptations in endurance performance. *Am. J. Clin. Nutr.* 87, 142–149.

Gomez-Cabrera, M.-C., Domenech, E., and Viña, J. (2008b). Moderate exercise is an antioxidant: upregulation of antioxidant genes by training. *Free Radic. Biol. Med.* 44, 126–131. doi: 10.1016/j.freeradbiomed.2007.02.001

González, B., Hernando, R., and Manso, R. (2000). Stress proteins of 70 kDa in chronically exercised skeletal muscle. *Pflüg. Arch.* 440, 42–49. doi: 10.1007/s004240051020

Gore, M., Fiebig, R., Hollander, J., Leeuwenburgh, C., Ohno, H., and Ji, L. (1998). Endurance training alters antioxidant enzyme gene expression in rat skeletal muscle. *Can. J. Physiol. Pharmacol.* 76, 1139–1145. doi: 10.1139/y98-125

Grumati, P., Coletto, L., Schiavinato, A., Castagnaro, S., Bertaggia, E., Sandri, M., et al. (2011). Physical exercise stimulates autophagy in normal skeletal muscles but is detrimental for collagen VI-deficient muscles. *Autophagy* 7, 1415–1423. doi: 10.4161/auto.7.12.17877

Gurney, M. E., Pu, H., Chiu, A. Y., Dal Canto, M. C., Polchow, C. Y., Alexander, D. D., et al. (1994). Motor neuron degeneration in mice that express a human Cu, Zn superoxide dismutase mutation. *Science* 264, 1772–1775. doi: 10.1126/science.8209258

He, C., and Klionsky, D. J. (2009). Regulation mechanisms and signaling pathways of autophagy. *Annu. Rev. Genet.* 43, 67. doi: 10.1146/annurev-genet-102808-114910

Holloszy, J. O., and Coyle, E. F. (1984). Adaptations of skeletal muscle to endurance exercise and their metabolic consequences. *J. Appl. Physiol.* 56, 831–838.

Holmgren, A. (1989). Thioredoxin and glutaredoxin systems. *J. Biol. Chem.* 264, 13963–13966.

Ichinoseki-Sekine, N., Yoshihara, T., Kakigi, R., Sugiura, T., Powers, S. K., and Naito, H. (2014). Heat stress protects against mechanical ventilation-induced diaphragmatic atrophy. *J. Appl. Physiol.* 117, 518–524. doi: 10.1152/japplphysiol.00170.2014

Iqbal, S., and Hood, D. (2014). The role of mitochondrial fusion and fission in skeletal muscle function and dysfunction. *Front. Biosci.* 20, 157–172.

Itoh, M., Oh-Ishi, S., Hatao, H., Leeuwenburgh, C., Selman, C., Ohno, H., et al. (2004). Effects of dietary calcium restriction and acute exercise on the antioxidant enzyme system and oxidative stress in rat diaphragm. *Am. J. Physiol. Regul. Integr. Comp. Physiol.* 287, R33–R38. doi: 10.1152/ajpregu.00598.2003

Jackman, R. W., and Kandarian, S. C. (2004). The molecular basis of skeletal muscle atrophy. *Am. J. Physiol. Cell Physiol.* 287, C834–C843. doi: 10.1152/ajpcell.00579.2003

Kang, C., and Ji, L. L. (2013). Muscle immobilization and remobilization downregulates PGC-1α signaling and the mitochondrial biogenesis pathway. *J. Appl. Physiol.* 115, 1618–1625. doi: 10.1152/japplphysiol.01354.2012

Kang, P.-J., Ostermann, J., Shilling, J., Neupert, W., Craig, E. A., and Pfanner, N. (1990). Requirement for hsp70 in the mitochondrial matrix for translocation and folding of precursor proteins. *Nature* 348, 137–143. doi: 10.1038/348137a0

Kanki, T., and Klionsky, D. J. (2008). Mitophagy in yeast occurs through a selective mechanism. *J. Biol. Chem.* 283, 32386–32393. doi: 10.1074/jbc.M802403200

Kanki, T., Wang, K., Cao, Y., Baba, M., and Klionsky, D. J. (2009). Atg32 is a mitochondrial protein that confers selectivity during mitophagy. *Dev. Cell* 17, 98–109. doi: 10.1016/j.devcel.2009.06.014

Kavazis, A. N., Talbert, E. E., Smuder, A. J., Hudson, M. B., Nelson, W. B., and Powers, S. K. (2009). Mechanical ventilation induces diaphragmatic mitochondrial dysfunction and increased oxidant production. *Free Radic. Biol. Med.* 46, 842–850. doi: 10.1016/j.freeradbiomed.2009.01.002

Kayani, A. C., Close, G. L., Jackson, M. J., and Mcardle, A. (2008). Prolonged treadmill training increases HSP70 in skeletal muscle but does not affect age-related functional deficits. *Am. J. Physiol. Regul. Integr. Comp. Physiol.* 294, R568–R576. doi: 10.1152/ajpregu.00575.2007

Kirkwood, S., Packer, L., and Brooks, G. (1987). Effects of endurance training on a mitochondrial reticulum in limb skeletal muscle. *Arch. Biochem. Biophys.* 255, 80–88. doi: 10.1016/0003-9861(87)90296-7

Koesterer, T., Dodd, S. L., and Powers, S. (2002). Increased antioxidant capacity does not attenuate muscle atrophy caused by unweighting. *J. Appl. Physiol.* 93, 1959–1965. doi: 10.1152/japplphysiol.00511.2002

Kondo, H., Miura, M., and Itokawa, Y. (1991). Oxidative stress in skeletal muscle atrophied by immobilization. *Acta Physiol. Scand.* 142, 527–528. doi: 10.1111/j.1748-1716.1991.tb09191.x

Kondo, H., Miura, M., and Itokawa, Y. (1993). Antioxidant enzyme systems in skeletal muscle atrophied by immobilization. *Pflüg. Arch.* 422, 404–406. doi: 10.1007/BF00374299

Kondo, H., Miura, M., Kodama, J., Ahmed, S. M., and Itokawa, Y. (1992). Role of iron in oxidative stress in skeletal muscle atrophied by immobilization. *Pflüg. Arch.* 421, 295–297. doi: 10.1007/BF00374844

Kortebein, P., Symons, T. B., Ferrando, A., Paddon-Jones, D., Ronsen, O., Protas, E., et al. (2008). Functional impact of 10 days of bed rest in healthy older adults. *J. Gerontol. Ser. A* 63, 1076–1081. doi: 10.1093/gerona/63.10.1076

Ku, Z., Yang, J., Menon, V., and Thomason, D. (1995). Decreased polysomal HSP-70 may slow polypeptide elongation during skeletal muscle atrophy. *Am. J. Physiol. Cell Physiol.* 268, C1369–C1374.

Lambertucci, R. H., Levada-Pires, A. C., Rossoni, L. V., Curi, R., and Pithon-Curi, T. C. (2007). Effects of aerobic exercise training on antioxidant enzyme activities and mRNA levels in soleus muscle from young and aged rats. *Mech. Ageing Dev.* 128, 267–275. doi: 10.1016/j.mad.2006.12.006

Laughlin, M., Simpson, T., Sexton, W., Brown, O., Smith, J., and Korthuis, R. (1990). Skeletal muscle oxidative capacity, antioxidant enzymes, and exercise training. *J. Appl. Physiol.* 68, 2337–2343.

Lawler, J. M., Song, W., and Demaree, S. R. (2003). Hindlimb unloading increases oxidative stress and disrupts antioxidant capacity in skeletal muscle. *Free Radic. Biol. Med.* 35, 9–16. doi: 10.1016/S0891-5849(03)00186-2

Lawler, J. M., Song, W., and Kwak, H. B. (2006). Differential response of heat shock proteins to hindlimb unloading and reloading in the soleus. *Muscle Nerve* 33, 200–207. doi: 10.1002/mus.20454

Lebovitz, R. M., Zhang, H., Vogel, H., Cartwright, J., Dionne, L., Lu, N., et al. (1996). Neurodegeneration, myocardial injury, and perinatal death in mitochondrial superoxide dismutase-deficient mice. *Proc. Natl. Acad. Sci. U.S.A.* 93, 9782–9787. doi: 10.1073/pnas.93.18.9782

Lecker, S. H., Jagoe, R. T., Gilbert, A., Gomes, M., Baracos, V., Bailey, J., et al. (2004). Multiple types of skeletal muscle atrophy involve a common program of changes in gene expression. *FASEB J.* 18, 39–51. doi: 10.1096/fj.03-0610com

Lecker, S. H., Solomon, V., Mitch, W. E., and Goldberg, A. L. (1999). Muscle protein breakdown and the critical role of the ubiquitin-proteasome pathway in normal and disease states. *J. Nutr.* 129, 227S–237S.

Liang, X. H., Jackson, S., Seaman, M., Brown, K., Kempkes, B., Hibshoosh, H., et al. (1999). Induction of autophagy and inhibition of tumorigenesis by beclin 1. *Nature* 402, 672–676. doi: 10.1038/45257

Lin, J., Wu, H., Tarr, P. T., Zhang, C.-Y., Wu, Z., Boss, O., et al. (2002). Transcriptional co-activator PGC-1α drives the formation of slow-twitch muscle fibres. *Nature* 418, 797–801. doi: 10.1038/nature00904

Lira, V. A., Okutsu, M., Zhang, M., Greene, N. P., Laker, R. C., Breen, D. S., et al. (2013). Autophagy is required for exercise training-induced skeletal muscle adaptation and improvement of physical performance. *FASEB J.* 27, 4184–4193. doi: 10.1096/fj.13-228486

Liu, Y., Mayr, S., Opitz-Gress, A., Zeller, C., Lormes, W., Baur, S., et al. (1999). Human skeletal muscle HSP70 response to training in highly trained rowers. *J. Appl. Physiol.* 86, 101–104.

Locke, M., Noble, E. G., and Atkinson, B. G. (1990). Exercising mammals synthesize stress proteins. *Am. J. Physiol.* 258. C723–C729.

Lomonosova, Y. N., Shenkman, B. S., and Nemirovskaya, T. L. (2012). Attenuation of unloading-induced rat soleus atrophy with the heat-shock protein inducer 17-(allylamino)-17-demethoxygeldanamycin. *FASEB J.* 26, 4295–4301. doi: 10.1096/fj.12-204412

Maes, K., Testelmans, D., Powers, S., Decramer, M., and Gayan-Ramirez, G. (2007). Leupeptin inhibits ventilator-induced diaphragm dysfunction in rats. *Am. J. Respir. Crit. Care Med.* 175, 1134–1138. doi: 10.1164/rccm.200609-1342OC

Mangner, N., Linke, A., Oberbach, A., Kullnick, Y., Gielen, S., Sandri, M., et al. (2013). Exercise training prevents TNF-α induced loss of force in the diaphragm of mice. *PLoS ONE* 8:e52274. doi: 10.1371/journal.pone.0052274

Masiero, E., Agatea, L., Mammucari, C., Blaauw, B., Loro, E., Komatsu, M., et al. (2009). Autophagy is required to maintain muscle mass. *Cell Metab.* 10, 507–515. doi: 10.1016/j.cmet.2009.10.008

Matsushima, Y., Nanri, H., Nara, S., Okufuji, T., Ohta, M., Hachisuka, K., et al. (2006). Hindlimb unloading decreases thioredoxin-related antioxidant proteins and increases thioredoxin-binding protein-2 in rat skeletal muscle. *Free Radic. Res.* 40, 715–722. doi: 10.1080/10715760600580488

McClung, J. M., Kavazis, A. N., Deruisseau, K. C., Falk, D. J., Deering, M. A., Lee, Y., et al. (2007). Caspase-3 regulation of diaphragm myonuclear domain during mechanical ventilation-induced atrophy. *Am. J. Respir. Crit. Care Med.* 175, 150–159. doi: 10.1164/rccm.200601-142OC

Meier, P., Renga, M., Hoppeler, H., and Baum, O. (2013). The impact of antioxidant supplements and endurance exercise on genes of the carbohydrate and lipid metabolism in skeletal muscle of mice. *Cell Biochem. Funct.* 31, 51–59. doi: 10.1002/cbf.2859

Milne, K. J., and Noble, E. G. (2002). Exercise-induced elevation of HSP70 is intensity dependent. *J. Appl. Physiol.* 93, 561–568. doi: 10.1152/japplphysiol.00528.2001

Min, K., Smuder, A. J., Kwon, O. S., Kavazis, A. N., Szeto, H. H., and Powers, S. K. (2011). Mitochondrial-targeted antioxidants protect skeletal muscle against immobilization-induced muscle atrophy. *J. Appl. Physiol.* 111, 1459–1466. doi: 10.1152/japplphysiol.00591.2011

Miyabara, E. H., Nascimento, T. L., Rodrigues, D. C., Moriscot, A. S., Davila, W. F., Aitmou, Y., et al. (2012). Overexpression of inducible 70-kDa heat shock protein in mouse improves structural and functional recovery of skeletal muscles from atrophy. *Pflüg. Arch. Eur. J. Physiol.* 463, 733–741. doi: 10.1007/s00424-012-1087-x

Moriggi, M., Vasso, M., Fania, C., Capitanio, D., Bonifacio, G., Salanova, M., et al. (2010). Long term bed rest with and without vibration exercise countermeasures: effects on human muscle protein dysregulation. *Proteomics* 10, 3756–3774. doi: 10.1002/pmic.200900817

Morton, J. P., Kayani, A. C., Mcardle, A., and Drust, B. (2009). The exercise-induced stress response of skeletal muscle, with specific emphasis on humans. *Sports Med.* 39, 643–662. doi: 10.2165/00007256-200939080-00003

Mosser, D. D., Caron, A. W., Bourget, L., Meriin, A. B., Sherman, M. Y., Morimoto, R. I., et al. (2000). The chaperone function of hsp70 is required for protection against stress-induced apoptosis. *Mol. Cell. Biol.* 20, 7146–7159. doi: 10.1128/MCB.20.19.7146-7159.2000

Muller, F. L., Song, W., Jang, Y. C., Liu, Y., Sabia, M., Richardson, A., et al. (2007). Denervation-induced skeletal muscle atrophy is associated with increased mitochondrial ROS production. *Am. J. Physiol. Reg. Integr. Comp. Physiol.* 293, R1159–R1168. doi: 10.1152/ajpregu.00767.2006

Muller, F. L., Song, W., Liu, Y., Chaudhuri, A., Pieke-Dahl, S., Strong, R., et al. (2006). Absence of CuZn superoxide dismutase leads to elevated oxidative stress and acceleration of age-dependent skeletal muscle atrophy. *Free Radic. Biol. Med.* 40, 1993–2004. doi: 10.1016/j.freeradbiomed.2006.01.036

Muscatello, U., and Patriarca, P. L. (1968). Denervation and disuse atrophy in pigeon breast muscle. An electron microscopic and biochemical study. *Am. J. Pathol.* 52, 1169.

Naito, H., Powers, S. K., Demirel, H. A., Sugiura, T., Dodd, S. L., and Aoki, J. (2000). Heat stress attenuates skeletal muscle atrophy in hindlimb-unweighted rats. *J. Appl. Physiol.* 88, 359–363.

Narendra, D. P., Jin, S. M., Tanaka, A., Suen, D.-F., Gautier, C. A., Shen, J., et al. (2010). PINK1 is selectively stabilized on impaired mitochondria to activate Parkin. *PLoS Biol.* 8:e1000298. doi: 10.1371/journal.pbio.1000298

Nelson, R. J., Ziegelhoffer, T., Nicolet, C., Werner-Washburne, M., and Craig, E. A. (1992). The translation machinery and 70 kd heat shock protein cooperate in protein synthesis. *Cell* 71, 97–105. doi: 10.1016/0092-8674(92)90269-I

Nelson, W. B., Smuder, A. J., Hudson, M. B., Talbert, E. E., and Powers, S. K. (2012). Cross-talk between the calpain and caspase-3 proteolytic systems in the diaphragm during prolonged mechanical ventilation. *Crit. Care Med.* 40, 1857–1863. doi: 10.1097/CCM.0b013e318246bb5d

Oh-Ishi, S., Kizaki, T., Nagasawa, J., Izawa, T., Komabayashi, T., Nagata, N., et al. (1997). Effects of endurance training on superoxide dismutase activiy, content and mRNA expression in rat muscle. *Clin. Exp. Pharmacol. Physiol.* 24, 326–332. doi: 10.1111/j.1440-1681.1997.tb01196.x

Oh-Ishi, S., Toshinai, K., Kizaki, T., Haga, S., Fukuda, K., Nagata, N., et al. (1996). Effects of aging and/or training on antioxidant enzyme system in diaphragm of mice. *Respir. Physiol.* 105, 195–202. doi: 10.1016/0034-5687(96)00057-6

O'leary, M. F., and Hood, D. A. (2008). Effect of prior chronic contractile activity on mitochondrial function and apoptotic protein expression in denervated muscle. *J. Appl. Physiol.* 105, 114–120. doi: 10.1152/japplphysiol.00724.2007

Perry, C. G., Lally, J., Holloway, G. P., Heigenhauser, G. J., Bonen, A., and Spriet, L. L. (2010). Repeated transient mRNA bursts precede increases in transcriptional and mitochondrial proteins during training in human skeletal muscle. *J. Physiol.* 588, 4795–4810. doi: 10.1113/jphysiol.2010.199448

Picard, M., Gentil, B. J., McManus, M. J., White, K., Louis, K. S., Gartside, S. E., et al. (2013). Acute exercise remodels mitochondrial membrane interactions in mouse skeletal muscle. *J. Appl. Physiol.* 115, 1562–1571. doi: 10.1152/japplphysiol.00819.2013

Pilegaard, H., Saltin, B., and Neufer, P. D. (2003). Exercise induces transient transcriptional activation of the PGC-1α gene in human skeletal muscle. *J. Physiol.* 546, 851–858. doi: 10.1113/jphysiol.2002.034850

Powers, S. K. (2014). Can antioxidants protect against disuse muscle atrophy? *Sports Med.* 44, 155–165. doi: 10.1007/s40279-014-0255-x

Powers, S. K., Criswell, D., Lawler, J., Martin, D., Ji, L. L., Herb, R. A., et al. (1994). Regional training-induced alterations in diaphragmatic oxidative and antioxidant enzymes. *Respir. Physiol.* 95, 227–237. doi: 10.1016/0034-5687(94)90118-X

Powers, S. K., and Jackson, M. J. (2008). Exercise-induced oxidative stress: cellular mechanisms and impact on muscle force production. *Physiol. Rev.* 88, 1243–1276. doi: 10.1152/physrev.00031.2007

Powers, S. K., Smuder, A., and Judge, A. (2012a). Oxidative stress and disuse muscle atrophy: cause or consequence? *Curr. Opin. Clin. Nutr. Metab. Care* 15, 240. doi: 10.1097/MCO.0b013e328352b4c2

Powers, S. K., Talbert, E. E., and Adhihetty, P. J. (2011). Reactive oxygen and nitrogen species as intracellular signals in skeletal muscle. *J. Physiol.* 589, 2129–2138. doi: 10.1113/jphysiol.2010.201327

Powers, S. K., Wiggs, M. P., Duarte, J. A., Zergeroglu, A. M., and Demirel, H. A. (2012b). Mitochondrial signaling contributes to disuse muscle atrophy. *Am. J. Physiol. Endocrinol. Metab.* 303, E31–E39. doi: 10.1152/ajpendo.00609.2011

Powers, S. K., Wiggs, M. P., Sollanek, K. J., and Smuder, A. J. (2013). Ventilator-induced diaphragm dysfunction: cause and effect. *Am. J. Physiol. Regul. Integr. Comp. Physiol.* 305, R464–R477. doi: 10.1152/ajpregu.00231.2013

Puigserver, P., Adelmant, G., Wu, Z., Fan, M., Xu, J., O'Malley, B., et al. (1999). Activation of PPARγ coactivator-1 through transcription factor docking. *Science* 286, 1368–1371. doi: 10.1126/science.286.5443.1368

Puigserver, P., Wu, Z., Park, C. W., Graves, R., Wright, M., and Spiegelman, B. M. (1998). A cold-inducible coactivator of nuclear receptors linked to adaptive thermogenesis. *Cell* 92, 829–839. doi: 10.1016/S0092-8674(00)81410-5

Puntschart, A., Vogt, M., Widmer, H., Hoppeler, H., and Billeter, R. (1996). Hsp70 expression in human skeletal muscle after exercise. *Acta Physiol. Scand.* 157, 411–417. doi: 10.1046/j.1365-201X.1996.512270000.x

Rando, T. A., Crowley, R. S., Carlson, E. J., Epstein, C. J., and Mohapatra, P. K. (1998). Overexpression of copper/zinc superoxide dismutase: a novel cause of murine muscular dystrophy. *Ann. Neurol.* 44, 381–386. doi: 10.1002/ana.410440315

Ristow, M., Zarse, K., Oberbach, A., Klöting, N., Birringer, M., Kiehntopf, M., et al. (2009). Antioxidants prevent health-promoting effects of physical exercise in humans. *Proc. Natl. Acad. Sci. U.S.A.* 106, 8665–8670. doi: 10.1073/pnas.0903485106

Romanello, V., Guadagnin, E., Gomes, L., Roder, I., Sandri, C., Petersen, Y., et al. (2010). Mitochondrial fission and remodelling contributes to muscle atrophy. *EMBO J.* 29, 1774–1785. doi: 10.1038/emboj.2010.60

Russell, A. P., Feilchenfeldt, J., Schreiber, S., Praz, M., Crettenand, A., Gobelet, C., et al. (2003). Endurance training in humans leads to fiber type-specific increases in levels of peroxisome proliferator-activated receptor-γ coactivator-1 and peroxisome proliferator-activated receptor-α in skeletal muscle. *Diabetes* 52, 2874–2881. doi: 10.2337/diabetes.52.12.2874

Sacheck, J. M., Hyatt, J.-P. K., Raffaello, A., Jagoe, R. T., Roy, R. R., Edgerton, V. R., et al. (2007). Rapid disuse and denervation atrophy involve transcriptional changes similar to those of muscle wasting during systemic diseases. *FASEB J.* 21, 140–155. doi: 10.1096/fj.06-6604com

Safdar, A., Bourgeois, J. M., Ogborn, D. I., Little, J. P., Hettinga, B. P., Akhtar, M., et al. (2011). Endurance exercise rescues progeroid aging and induces systemic mitochondrial rejuvenation in mtDNA mutator mice. *Proc. Natl. Acad. Sci. U.S.A.* 108, 4135–4140. doi: 10.1073/pnas.1019581108

Salo, D. C., Donovan, C. M., and Davies, K. J. (1991). HSP70 and other possible heat shock or oxidative stress proteins are induced in skeletal muscle, heart, and liver during exercise. *Free Rad. Biol. Med.* 11, 239–246. doi: 10.1016/0891-5849(91)90119-N

Saltin, B., Henriksson, J., Nygaard, E., Andersen, P., and Jansson, E. (1977). Fiber types and metabolic potentials of skeletal muscles in sedentary man and endurance runners. *Ann. N.Y. Acad. Sci.* 301, 3–29. doi: 10.1111/j.1749-6632.1977.tb38182.x

Sandri, M. (2013). Protein breakdown in muscle wasting: role of autophagy-lysosome and ubiquitin-proteasome. *Int. J. Biochem. Cell Biol.* 45, 2121–2129. doi: 10.1016/j.biocel.2013.04.023

Sandri, M., Lin, J., Handschin, C., Yang, W., Arany, Z. P., Lecker, S. H., et al. (2006). PGC-1alpha protects skeletal muscle from atrophy by suppressing FoxO3 action and atrophy-specific gene transcription. *Proc. Natl. Acad. Sci. U.S.A.* 103, 16260–16265. doi: 10.1073/pnas.0607795103

Schiaffino, S., Dyar, K. A., Ciciliot, S., Blaauw, B., and Sandri, M. (2013). Mechanisms regulating skeletal muscle growth and atrophy. *FEBS J.* 280, 4294–4314. doi: 10.1111/febs.12253

Selsby, J. T., and Dodd, S. L. (2005). Heat treatment reduces oxidative stress and protects muscle mass during immobilization. *Am. J. Physiol. Regul. Integr. Comp. Physiol.* 289, R134–R139. doi: 10.1152/ajpregu.00497.2004

Senf, S. M., Dodd, S. L., and Judge, A. R. (2010). FOXO signaling is required for disuse muscle atrophy and is directly regulated by Hsp70. *Am. J. Physiol. Cell Physiol.* 298, C38–C45. doi: 10.1152/ajpcell.00315.2009

Senf, S. M., Dodd, S. L., McClung, J. M., and Judge, A. R. (2008). Hsp70 overexpression inhibits NF-κB and Foxo3a transcriptional activities and prevents skeletal muscle atrophy. *FASEB J.* 22, 3836–3845. doi: 10.1096/fj.08-110163

Servais, S., Letexier, D., Favier, R., Duchamp, C., and Desplanches, D. (2007). Prevention of unloading-induced atrophy by vitamin E supplementation: links between oxidative stress and soleus muscle proteolysis? *Free Radic. Biol. Med.* 42, 627–635. doi: 10.1016/j.freeradbiomed.2006.12.001

Smuder, A. J., Kavazis, A. N., Hudson, M. B., Nelson, W. B., and Powers, S. K. (2010). Oxidation enhances myofibrillar protein degradation via calpain and caspase-3. *Free Radic. Biol. Med.* 49, 1152–1160. doi: 10.1016/j.freeradbiomed.2010.06.025

Smuder, A. J., Kavazis, A. N., Min, K., and Powers, S. K. (2011). Exercise protects against doxorubicin-induced oxidative stress and proteolysis in skeletal muscle. *J. Appl. Physiol.* 110, 935–942. doi: 10.1152/japplphysiol.00677.2010

Smuder, A. J., Min, K., Hudson, M. B., Kavazis, A. N., Kwon, O. S., Nelson, W. B., et al. (2012b). Endurance exercise attenuates ventilator-induced diaphragm dysfunction. *J. Appl. Physiol.* 112, 501–510. doi: 10.1152/japplphysiol.01086.2011

Smuder, A. J., Min, K., Hudson, M. B., Kavazis, A. N., Kwon, O.-S., Nelson, W. B., et al. (2012a). Endurance exercise attenuates ventilator-induced diaphragm dysfunction. *J. Appl. Physiol.* 112, 501–510. doi: 10.1152/japplphysiol.01086.2011

Spiegelman, B. M. (2007). "Transcriptional control of mitochondrial energy metabolism through the PGC1 coactivators," in *Novartis Foundation Symposium: Chichester, 1999* (New York, NY: John Wiley), 60.

Stanley, B. A., Sivakumaran, V., Shi, S., McDonald, I., Lloyd, D., Watson, W. H., et al. (2011). Thioredoxin reductase-2 is essential for keeping low levels of H2O2 emission from isolated heart mitochondria. *J. Biol. Chem.* 286, 33669–33677. doi: 10.1074/jbc.M111.284612

Stein, T., and Wade, C. (2005). Metabolic consequences of muscle disuse atrophy. *J. Nutr.* 135, 1824S–1828S.

St-Pierre, J., Lin, J., Krauss, S., Tarr, P. T., Yang, R., Newgard, C. B., et al. (2003). Bioenergetic analysis of peroxisome proliferator-activated receptor γ coactivators 1α and 1β (PGC-1α and PGC-1β) in muscle cells. *J. Biol. Chem.* 278, 26597–26603. doi: 10.1074/jbc.M301850200

Strobel, N. A., Peake, J. M., Matsumoto, A., Marsh, S. A., Coombes, J. S., and Wadley, G. D. (2011). Antioxidant supplementation reduces skeletal muscle mitochondrial biogenesis. *Med. Sci. Sports Exerc.* 43, 1017–1024. doi: 10.1249/MSS.0b013e318203afa3

Symons, T. B., Sheffield-Moore, M., Chinkes, D. L., Ferrando, A. A., and Paddon-Jones, D. (2009). Artificial gravity maintains skeletal muscle protein synthesis during 21 days of simulated microgravity. *J. Appl. Physiol.* 107, 34–38. doi: 10.1152/japplphysiol.91137.2008

Talbert, E. E., Smuder, A. J., Min, K., Kwon, O. S., and Powers, S. K. (2013a). Calpain and caspase-3 play required roles in immobilization-induced limb muscle atrophy. *J. Appl. Physiol.* 114, 1482–1489. doi: 10.1152/japplphysiol.00925.2012

Talbert, E. E., Smuder, A. J., Min, K., Kwon, O. S., Szeto, H. H., and Powers, S. K. (2013b). Immobilization-induced activation of key proteolytic systems in skeletal muscles is prevented by a mitochondria-targeted antioxidant. *J. Appl. Physiol.* 115, 529–538. doi: 10.1152/japplphysiol.00471.2013

Taylor, E. B., Lamb, J. D., Hurst, R. W., Chesser, D. G., Ellingson, W. J., Greenwood, L. J., et al. (2005). Endurance training increases skeletal muscle LKB1 and PGC-1α protein abundance: effects of time and intensity. *Am. J. Physiol. Endocrinol. Metab.* 289, E960–E968. doi: 10.1152/ajpendo.00237.2005

Thomason, D. B., and Booth, F. W. (1990). Atrophy of the soleus muscle by hindlimb unweighting. *J. Appl. Physiol.* 68, 1–12.

Tischler, M. E., Rosenberg, S., Satarug, S., Henriksen, E. J., Kirby, C. R., Tome, M., et al. (1990). Different mechanisms of increased proteolysis in atrophy induced by denervation or unweighting of rat soleus muscle. *Metab. Clin. Exp.* 39, 756–763. doi: 10.1016/0026-0495(90)90113-Q

Twig, G., Elorza, A., Molina, A. J., Mohamed, H., Wikstrom, J. D., Walzer, G., et al. (2008). Fission and selective fusion govern mitochondrial segregation and elimination by autophagy. *EMBO J.* 27, 433–446. doi: 10.1038/sj.emboj.7601963

Twig, G., and Shirihai, O. S. (2011). The interplay between mitochondrial dynamics and mitophagy. *Antioxid. Redox Signal.* 14, 1939–1951. doi: 10.1089/ars.2010.3779

Vincow, E. S., Merrihew, G., Thomas, R. E., Shulman, N. J., Beyer, R. P., Maccoss, M. J., et al. (2013). The PINK1–Parkin pathway promotes both mitophagy and selective respiratory chain turnover in vivo. *Proc. Natl. Acad. Sci. U.S.A.* 110, 6400–6405. doi: 10.1073/pnas.1221132110

Westermann, B. (2010). Mitochondrial fusion and fission in cell life and death. *Nat. Rev. Mol. Cell Biol.* 11, 872–884. doi: 10.1038/nrm3013

Wolfe, R. R. (2006). The underappreciated role of muscle in health and disease. *Am. J. Clin. Nutr.* 84, 475–482.

Wu, Z., Puigserver, P., Andersson, U., Zhang, C., Adelmant, G., Mootha, V., et al. (1999). Mechanisms controlling mitochondrial biogenesis and respiration through the thermogenic coactivator PGC-1. *Cell* 98, 115–124. doi: 10.1016/S0092-8674(00)80611-X

Yin, F., Sancheti, H., and Cadenas, E. (2012). Mitochondrial thiols in the regulation of cell death pathways. *Antioxid. Redox Signal.* 17, 1714–1727. doi: 10.1089/ars.2012.4639

Youle, R. J., and Narendra, D. P. (2011). Mechanisms of mitophagy. *Nat. Rev. Mol. Cell Biol.* 12, 9–14. doi: 10.1038/nrm3028

Zechner, C., Lai, L., Zechner, J. F., Geng, T., Yan, Z., Rumsey, J. W., et al. (2010). Total skeletal muscle PGC-1 deficiency uncouples mitochondrial derangements from fiber type determination and insulin sensitivity. *Cell Metab.* 12, 633–642. doi: 10.1016/j.cmet.2010.11.008

Zhang, J., and Ney, P. A. (2009). Role of BNIP3 and NIX in cell death, autophagy, and mitophagy. *Cell Death Differ.* 16, 939–946. doi: 10.1038/cdd.2009.16

Zhang, Y., Davis, C., Sakellariou, G. K., Shi, Y., Kayani, A. C., Pulliam, D., et al. (2013). CuZnSOD gene deletion targeted to skeletal muscle leads to loss of contractile force but does not cause muscle atrophy in adult mice. *FASEB J.* 27, 3536–3548. doi: 10.1096/fj.13-228130

Zhou, L. Z.-H., Johnson, A. P., and Rando, T. A. (2001). NFκB and AP-1 mediate transcriptional responses to oxidative stress in skeletal muscle cells. *Free Radic. Biol. Med.* 31, 1405–1416. doi: 10.1016/S0891-5849(01)00719-5

Zhu, S., Nagashima, M., Khan, M. A., Yasuhara, S., Kaneki, M., and Martyn, J. (2013). Lack of caspase–3 attenuates immobilization–induced muscle atrophy and loss of tension generation along with mitigation of apoptosis and inflammation. *Muscle Nerve* 47, 711–721. doi: 10.1002/mus.23642

19

Anxiety and Depression in the Portuguese Older Adults: Prevalence and Associated Factors

Rute Dinis de Sousa[1,2]*, *Ana Maria Rodrigues*[1,2,3,4], *Maria João Gregório*[1,2,5], *Jaime Da Cunha Branco*[1,2,3,6], *Maria João Gouveia*[7], *Helena Canhão*[1,2,3,8] *and Sara Simões Dias*[1,2,9]

[1] *Chronic Diseases Research Center (CEDOC), EpiDoC Unit, NOVA Medical School, Universidade Nova de Lisboa (NMS/UNL), Lisbon, Portugal,* [2] *EpiSaúde – Associação Científica, Évora, Portugal,* [3] *Sociedade Portuguesa de Reumatologia, Lisbon, Portugal,* [4] *Rheumatology Research Unit, Instituto de Medicina Molecular, Lisbon, Portugal,* [5] *Faculdade de Ciências da Nutrição e Alimentação da Universidade do Porto, Porto, Portugal,* [6] *Serviço de Reumatologia do Hospital Egas Moniz – Centro Hospitalar Lisboa Ocidental (CHLO-E.P.E.), Lisbon, Portugal,* [7] *Promoting Human Potential Research Group, ISPA – Instituto Universitário, Lisbon, Portugal,* [8] *Escola Nacional de Saúde Publica, Universidade Nova de Lisboa, Lisbon, Portugal,* [9] *Escola Superior de Saúde do Instituto Politécnico de Leiria, Leiria, Portugal*

Edited by:
Jeremy M. Jacobs,
Hadassah Medical Center, Israel

Reviewed by:
Wee Shiong Lim,
Tan Tock Seng Hospital, Singapore
Klara Komici,
Università degli Studi di Napoli Federico II, Italy

***Correspondence:**
Rute Dinis de Sousa
rute.sousa@nms.unl.pt

Anxiety and depression in the elderly individuals have been studied around the world, and some authors consider them among the most serious problems faced by modern societies. With recent economic crisis—very important in Southern European countries—isolation, loneliness, and exclusion of the active society, mental problems are probably raising and associated with distinct factors. In this cross-sectional analysis, nested in a longitudinal population-based cohort study, we analyze anxiety and depression prevalence, and their related factors, in a representative cohort of Portuguese seniors. We used data retrieved from second wave of follow-up of EpiDoC Cohort—EpiDoC 2 study, which is composed by 10,661 adults, representative of adult Portuguese population. This study included all ≥65 years old EpiDoC 2 study participants, who responded to Hospital Anxiety and Depression Scale (HADS), $n = 1,680$. Sociodemographic, lifestyles, self-reported non-communicable diseases, health-related quality of life (EQ-5D-3D), physical function (HAQ), and health resources consumption data were collected. Anxiety and depression were assessed with HADS. Anxiety and depression prevalence were estimated. Multivariable logistic regression was used to assess anxiety and depression score determinants. The estimated prevalence of anxiety among Portuguese elderly is 9.6% and depression is 11.8%. Seniors with anxiety and seniors with depression have a higher probability to self-report higher levels of physical disability (OR = 3.10; 96% CI 2.12–4.52; OR = 3.08, 95% CI 2.29–4.14, respectively) and lower levels of quality of life (OR = 0.03, 95% CI 0.01–0.09; OR = 0.03, 95% CI 0.01–0.06, respectively). Female gender (OR = 2.77, 95% CI 1.53–5.00), low educational level (OR = 2.30, 95% CI 1.22–4.36), allergic (OR = 2.02, 95% CI 1.14–3.55), and rheumatic disease (OR = 2.92, 95% CI 1.74–4.90) were significantly and independently associated with the presence of anxiety symptoms. Physical inactivity (OR = 1.64, 95% CI 1.11–2.42) and low educational level (OR = 2.40, 95% CI 1.41–4.09) were significantly and independently associated with depression symptoms. Subjects that reported to drink alcohol daily or occasionally were negatively associated with depression symptoms. Anxiety and depression are frequent among Portuguese elderly. These prevalence rates suggest that preventing mental illness in senior population is a crucial need. A well-designed prevention strategy might have an effective action in raising the well-being of elderly.

Keywords: older, anxiety, depression, non-communicable chronic diseases, lifestyles, quality of life, function

INTRODUCTION

Our world is now old and aging. Aging population is a long-term trend in Portugal, Europe, and around the World. According to United Nations data from 2015, the number of people over 65 has increased considerably in the largest regions of the world, and this aging is expected to accelerate in the coming decades (1). The same data point out that, in 2015, 1 in 8 people in the world were 60 years or older, totaling 901 million elderly people. A 176 million of these elderly people live in Europe.

In Portugal, the number of people over 65 years of age doubled in relation to the 1970s and, by 2015, was already over two million, with the population over 80 years old increasing fivefold. In concrete terms, there were 836,058 people aged 65 and over in Portugal in 1971. In 1977, they surpassed one million and, in 2012, two million. In 2015, they were 2,122,996 (2).

Although the epidemiological investigation has begun to converge regarding the estimation of the prevalence of anxiety and depression in elderly populations, there are still quite a few discrepancies (3). The sampling procedures diverge greatly: some studies use representative samples from the respective country, and others use samples of convenience. In addition, there is considerable instability in age cutoffs considered for the definition of the elderly or older adult. On the other hand, there is much variation in the operationalization of anxiety and depression, partly due to the use of different evaluation instruments. In fact, some authors consider that anxiety and depression are among the most serious problems faced by modern societies is depression among the elderly (4). Although depression is fairly common in the last years of life (5), there is great variation in its prevalence in studies worldwide (9–33%) (6).

Factors associated with aging, such as social isolation, reduced autonomy, financial insecurity, and poor health, cause an increase in the prevalence of these disorders (7).

Some studies point to psychosocial risk factors for anxiety disorders and late-onset depression: female gender, cognitive dysfunction, chronic illness, poor health perception, functional limitations, personality traits such as neuroticism and weak coping strategies (8, 9). Specifically, for anxiety disorder: not having children, low income, and experiencing traumatic events (10).

Given the social and economic context of our country, generating relevant evidence on anxiety and depressive symptoms in the Portuguese elderly population, and understanding them from a point of view that goes beyond the mental illness itself, by approaching the possible associated factors, is crucial. Data on elderly mental health and associated factors could be useful to address therapeutic programs and better planning of health care.

Therefore, to comprehend models of anxiety and depression independently in the Portuguese senior population, this study aims to: (1) determine the prevalence of anxiety and depression symptoms and (2) identify relevant associations between the symptoms of anxiety and depression and chronic self-reported non-communicable diseases, lifestyles, and sociodemographic characteristics.

MATERIALS AND METHODS

Sample

To analyze the older adult Portuguese population in terms of symptoms of anxiety and depression, their association with non-communicable chronic diseases, function, lifestyles, and quality of life we used data from the second wave of follow-up for EpiDoC Cohort—EpiDoC 2 (CoReumaPt) study—done by computer-assisted telephone interviews (CATIs).

The EpiDoC 2 evaluation consisted on a structured questionnaire, applied through phone call interviews to 10,153 eligible participants of EpiDoC 1 (EpiReumaPt) (11–13), a large population-based sample, who consented to be contacted again for follow-up. The study population comprised adults (≥18 years old) living in the community, in Portugal Mainland and Islands (Azores and Madeira). Exclusion criteria were as follows: being resident in institutions and individuals unable to speak Portuguese or to complete the assessment protocol. Participants were selected through a process of multistage random sampling. The sample was stratified by region and population size.

EpiDoC 2 (CoReumaPt) included 7,591 participants, representative of the adult Portuguese population. This study included 1,680 seniors (65 and more years old) of the EpiDoC 2 study, who responded to Hospital Anxiety and Depression Scale (HADS) (**Figure 1**).

Data Collection

Data collection was performed from March 26th 2013 to July 27th 2015. A trained research assistants' team was responsible for collecting the follow-up data from these subjects, by randomly call all the individuals. When a contact was not available, they would hold more attempts in different moments (morning, afternoon, evening, and weekends) to perform six attempts. The last contact had to have at least 1 month of interval from the previous one. Only then the contact would be abandoned. Rescheduling of the telephonic interviews to a more convenient moment was also an option. The interview was telephonically performed with the assistance of a CATI system.

Data were collected in a standardized form, and database access was protected by unique username and password, for each research team member, according to Portuguese Law of data collection (14).

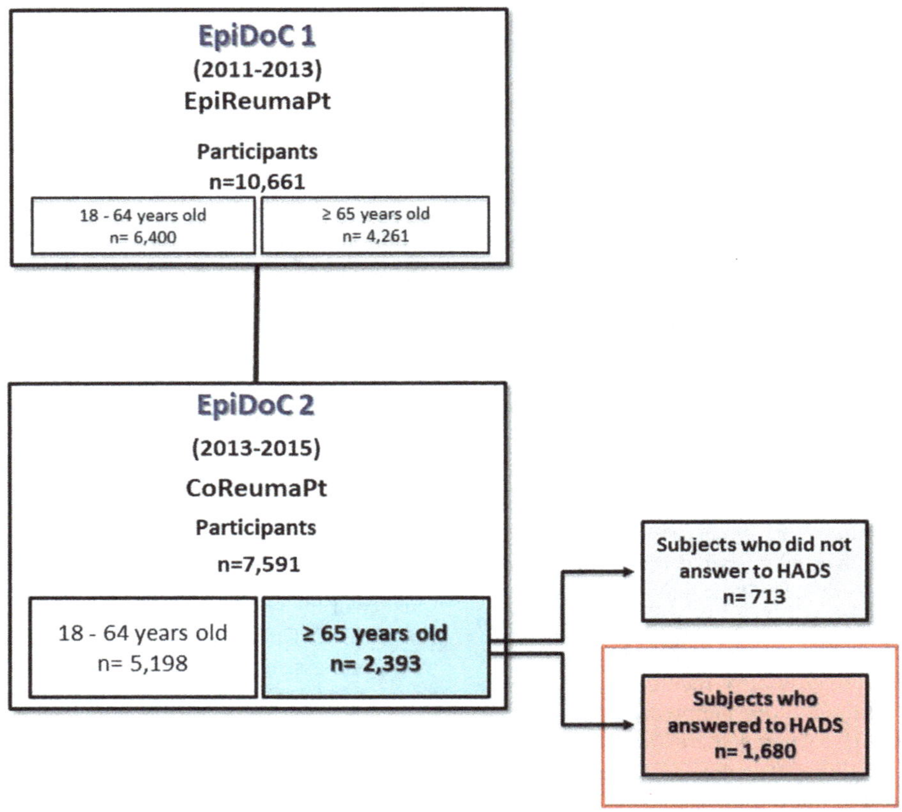

FIGURE 1 | Flowchart describing population eligible for this study.

Measurements, Assessment, and Instruments

Case Definition

To evaluate symptoms of anxiety and depression in EpiDoC 2 study, the HADS Portuguese validated version was applied (15). The HADS was originally developed by Zigmond and Snaith (16) as a screening tool to apprehend clinically significant states of anxiety and depression in a non-psychiatric hospital setting. Individual anxiety and depression scores were calculated by summation of the appropriate seven items and thus can range from 0 to 21, with higher scores indicating higher levels of anxiety or depression, respectively. In both subscales, a score between 0 and 7 is "normal," between 8 and 10 "mild," between 11 and 14 "moderate," and between 15 and 21 "severe" (idem). Presence of anxiety and depression symptoms was defined when HADS scale was ≥11, since Snaith suggested a score ≥11 was indicative of "caseness" to a mood disorder (17). We also used the HADS scale as a continuous outcome in the final analyses.

Sociodemographic and Socioeconomic Characteristics

Information on sociodemographic (sex, age, years of education, household composition, and NUT II), as well as socioeconomic variables (household income), was collected in the first wave—EpiDoC 1 study. Subjects were asked in the EpiDoC 2 study interview whether there have been changes.

Health Characteristics

In EpiDoC 1 study, individuals were asked if they had been previously diagnosed with some chronic disease (high cholesterol level, high blood pressure, rheumatic disease, allergy, gastrointestinal disease, cardiac disease, diabetes, thyroid and parathyroid disease, urolithiasis, pulmonary disease, hyperuricemia, cancer, neurologic disease, and hypogonadism), and this information was updated in the EpiDoC 2 study interview.

Self-reported height and weight were collected in EpiDoC 2. Based on these data, body mass index (BMI, weight/height^2, in kg/m^2) was calculated and categorized according to the World Health Organization classification in four categories: underweight (BMI < 18.5 kg/m^2), normal (BMI between 18.5 and 24.9 kg/m^2), overweight (BMI between 25 and 29.9 kg/m^2), and obesity (BMI ≥ 30 kg/m^2) (18).

Health-related quality of life was assessed using the Portuguese validated version of European Quality of Life questionnaire (EQ-5D-3L) (19, 20).

Function was evaluated based on the Portuguese version of Health Assessment Questionnaire (HAQ) (21, 22).

To assess health-care resources consumption, "number of medical appointments in the previous 12 months" and "hospitalization in the previous 12 months (yes/no)" was asked to participants.

Lifestyle Characteristics

In EpiDoC 2 study, questions concerning lifestyle habits included frequency of alcohol intake (daily, occasionally, and never), smoking habits (current smoker, past smoker, and never smoked), sleep habits (number of hours of sleep per day, categorized in <6 and ≥6 h/day). Physical activity level was classified based on the question related to the reported weekly frequency of physical activity. A frequency of once a week or more was considered "yes" to regular physical exercise.

Statistical Analysis

Sample Weights

EpiDoC was designed to obtain a representative sample of the Portuguese population (13). To guarantee its representativeness, weighted proportions have, for this matter, been computed and are described elsewhere (13).

To maintain the representativeness of the sample in relation to the Portuguese population (Mainland and Islands) in the second wave, extrapolation weights were again computed and used in further statistical analysis. These were obtained by calibrating the extrapolation weights originally designed for the EpiDoC 1 study sample. We first compared the participants and non-participants of EpiDoC 2 study, concerning their sociodemographic, socioeconomic and rheumatic disease screening, and health status characteristics. Then, we decided to adjust weights based on the stratification by seven NUTII regions [Norte, Centro, Lisboa, Alentejo, Algarve, and islands (Azores and Madeira)], gender (male and female), age categories (18–35, 36–55, 56–65, ≥8–35, 36–55 years old for NUTII Norte, Centro, and Lisboa; 18–65, 66+ for NUTII Alentejo, Algarve, and islands), and rheumatic disease screening (positive/negative).

Analysis and Statistical Software

Descriptive data for each categorical variable were presented as the absolute frequency and the correspondent proportion, weighted. The same adjustment has been done for the mean and SD for each continuous variable. Continuous variables were compared using Student's *t*-test or ANOVA, and nominal variables were compared using chi-square test.

To assess the determinants of anxiety and depression symptoms, we first performed univariate analysis to approach relations between independent variables (non-communicable chronic diseases, lifestyles, and sociodemographic characteristics) and outcomes (presence of anxiety and depression symptoms). When univariate analyses resulted in p-value < 0.1, those variables were included into the multivariable logistic regression models. Multivariable models were constructed using a forward selection method. The following independent variables were tested: age, gender, NUTS II, education level (0–4 vs ≥5 years), BMI (underweight, normal, overweight, and obese), alcohol intake (never, daily, and occasionally), current smoking, physical activity (yes/no), and chronic non-communicable diseases—high blood pressure, diabetes, high cholesterol level, pulmonary disease, cardiac disease, neurologic disease, allergies, neoplasic disease, thyroid disease, hyperuricemia, and rheumatic disease. Age, gender, and NUTS II were forced to stay in the model. The goodness of fit of the final multivariable regression model for the outcome anxiety has $p = 0.287$, and the goodness of fit of the final multivariable regression model for the outcome depression has $p = 0.4$.

Significance level was set at 0.05. All analyses were weighted and executed using STATA IC version 12 (StataCorp. 2011. Stata Statistical Software: Release 12. College Station, TX, USA: StataCorp LP).

Ethical Issues and Data Protection

EpiDoC 1 study was performed following the principles established by the Declaration of Helsinki (23) and revised in 2013 in Fortaleza. The study was reviewed and approved by the National Committee for Data Protection (Comissão Nacional de Proteção de Dados) and by the NOVA Medical School Ethics Committee. The participants provided informed consent to contribute in all phases of the study.

The EpiDoC 2 study was also approved by National Committee for Data Protection (in accordance with the Portuguese law number 67/98, October 26th, regarding protection of personal data) and was submitted to the same Ethics Committee. The study was conducted in accordance with the applicable laws and regulations including, but not limited to, the Guideline for Good Clinical Practice and the ethical principles stated in the Declaration of Helsinki (23).

Participants' confidentiality is safeguarded by the nonexistence of identifiers on the database (only unique ID participants' codes). Their names and contacts are stored separately from study data transmitted to the coordinating center. Thus, all data are kept anonymously and securely by the EpiDoC 2 study authorized staff. During EpiDoC 1 study, informed consent was also signed by those accepting to participate in the EpiDoC 2 study. There will be absolutely no disclosure of individual health information to the general public.

RESULTS

Our population of interest included 1,680 participants over 64 years old, 908 (54%) of those were females. Forty four percent were 75 years old or more. With respect to educational level, almost two-thirds of participants ($n = 1,259$; 76.03%) had less or equal to 4 years of education.

Most people with 65 years of age and more reported to live on a household income of less than 1,000€ per month; 35.8% reported the lowest income level of 500€/month. Moreover, elderlies tend to live in households are composed by only one (25.53%) or two persons (55.89%).

With respect to health-related characteristics, the observed mean number of non-communicable chronic diseases was 3.10 (±2.1). The most frequently reported chronic diseases were high blood pressure (57.3%), rheumatic diseases (50.53%), and high cholesterol level (49.7%).

People 65+ years old score EQ-5D-3L on average 0.61 (±0.77) for quality of life and 0.72 (±0.72) in HAQ for physical function.

The high consumption of health care resources by the older age group matches the health status. The average number of appointments was 7.74 (±8.40), and 24.16% was hospitalized in the last 12 months.

Regarding lifestyle habits, namely, in terms of alcohol intake and smoking habits, 36.43% of the individuals had reported a daily intake of alcohol beverages but only 5.39% were current smokers. Among the elderly, 43.65% of the subjects never consume alcohol and 66.35% of people aged 65 and above never smoked. Almost 60% of individuals above 65 years old do not engage in regular physical exercise, and around 70% of the Portuguese elderly sleep 6 or more hours per day.

Prevalence of Anxiety and Depression Symptoms in the Elderly

This study found 176 elderly out of 1,680 (10.48%) presenting anxiety symptoms (HADS-A ≥11), corresponding to a prevalence of 9.59% when weighted to Portuguese elderly population (**Table 1**). The mean score for HADS-A was 5.04 (±3.74).

In terms of depression symptoms, figures rise to 241 (14.34% in the present sample), equivalent to a prevalence of 11.77% of the Portuguese elderly population (**Table 1**). This population had a mean score for HADS-D of 5.27 (±4.07).

Sociodemographic, socioeconomic, lifestyle, and health-related characteristics of the Portuguese elderly population with and without anxiety symptoms are summarized in **Table 2**.

Table 3 summarizes sociodemographic, socioeconomic, lifestyle, and health-related seven characteristics of the Portuguese elderly population with and without depression symptoms.

Anxiety and Depression Symptoms and Physical Function in Seniors

Seniors with anxiety have a higher probability to have reported, even after the adjustment for sex, age, region, and number of non-communicable diseases, higher levels of physical disability (OR = 3.10; 96% CI 2.12–4.52).

Similar results were found for depression symptoms and seniors with depression have reported higher levels of physical disability (OR = 3.08, 95% CI 2.29–4.14).

TABLE 1 | Prevalence of anxiety and depression in the Portuguese senior population by age group.

	Elderly with anxiety symptoms (HADS-A ≥11)	Elderly with depression symptoms (HADS-D ≥11)
	n (%)	*n* (%)
Total	176 (9.59)	241 (11.77)
Age group		
65–69 y.o.	52 (12.38)	44 (7.29)
70–74 y.o.	45 (7.86)	65 (11.33)
75–79 y.o.	47 (8.99)	68 (15.16)
80–84 y.o.	20 (7.96)	42 (14.85)
≥85 y.o.	12 (9.56)	22 (1.68)

%, weighted percentage; HADS-A, Hospital Anxiety and Depression Scale—Anxiety subscale; HADS-D, Hospital Anxiety and Depression Scale-Depression subscale; y.o., year old.

Anxiety and Depression Symptoms and Quality of Life in the Elderly

In terms of quality of life (EQ-5D-3L score), seniors with anxiety have a higher probability to report lower levels of quality of life (OR = 0.03, 95% CI 0.01–0.09). These results were found after the adjustment for sex, age, region, and number of non-communicable diseases.

Multivariable analyses adjusting to sex, age, region, and number of non-communicable diseases also showed that seniors with depression symptoms have a higher probability to have reported lower levels of quality of life (OR = 0.03; 95% CI 0.01–0.06).

Anxiety and Depression Symptoms and Health-care Resources Consumption in the Elderly

Logistic regression adjusted to sex, age, region, and number of non-communicable diseases stressed that seniors with anxiety symptoms have a higher probability to have reported higher number of hospitalizations in the previous 12 months (OR = 2.53, 95% CI 1.37–4.67) and have reported a higher number of medical appointments in the previous 12 months.

Seniors with depression symptoms have also a higher probability to have reported higher number of hospitalizations in the previous 12 months (OR = 1.55, 95% CI 1.01–2.35). In terms of number of medical appointments in the previous 12 months, there is no significant difference between elderly with and without depressive symptoms.

Sociodemographic, Lifestyles, and Health Factors Independently Associated with Anxiety in Seniors

Multivariable logistic regression, including all previous significant independent variables, showed that being a woman (OR = 2.77, 95% CI 1.53–5.00) and have a low educational level (OR = 2.30, 95% CI 1.22–4.36) were significantly associated with anxiety symptoms. Regarding self-reported non-communicable chronic diseases, our results showed that only allergies (OR = 2.02, 95% CI 1.14–3.55) and rheumatic disease (OR = 2.92, 95% CI 1.74–4.90) were statistically significant associated with anxiety symptoms (**Table 4**).

Sociodemographic, Lifestyles, and Health Factors Independently Associated with Depression in Seniors

All previous significant independent variables were included in a multivariable logistic regression to depression symptoms. In this analysis, low educational level (OR = 2.40, 95% CI 1.41–4.09), physical inactivity (OR = 1.64, 95% CI 1.11–2.42), and alcohol intake on a daily (OR = 0.54, 95% CI 0.35–0.83) and occasionally basis (OR = 0.49, 95% CI 0.29–0.84) were protectors of depression (were associated with low risk of depression symptoms) (**Table 5**).

TABLE 2 | Sociodemographic, socioeconomic, lifestyle, and health-related characteristics of the Portuguese elderly population with and without anxiety symptoms.

Sociodemographic and socioeconomic characteristics		Elderly without anxiety symptoms (HADS-A <11)	Elderly with anxiety symptoms (HADS-A ≥11)	*p*-Value	Adjusted *p*-value
		Mean (SD) or *n* (%)	Mean (SD) or *n* (%)		
		n = 1,504 (90.41%)	*n* = 176 (9.59%)		
Age* (years)		74.24 (6.60)	73.96 (6.91)	0.059	0.131
Sex*	Female	768 (83.85)	140 (15.15)	<0.001†	<0.001†
	Male	736 (95.44)	36 (4.56)		
NUTS II*	Norte	476 (89.88)	67 (10.12)	0.906	0.977
	Centro	378 (89.93)	49 (10.07)		
	Lisboa e Vale do Tejo	291 (90.56)	23 (9.44)		
	Alentejo	95 (92.11)	11 (7.89)		
	Algarve	57 (93.14)	3 (6.86)		
	Região Autónoma dos Açores	80 (93.04)	7 (6.96)		
	Região Autónoma da Madeira	127 (91.03)	16 (8.97)		
Education level*	≤4 years of education	1,103 (88.55)	156 (11.45)	0.001†	0.002†
	>4 years of education	377 (95.98)	20 (4.02)		
Household income* (€)	≤500	384 (89.15)	58 (10.85)	0.430	0.411
	501–750	301 (91.75)	31 (8.25)		
	751–1,000	152 (88.38)	16 (11.62)		
	>1,000	275 (94.52)	16 (5.48)		
Household composition	1	374 (88.89)	55 (11.11)	0.388	0.900
	≥2	1,130 (90.90)	121 (9.10)		
Anthropometric data*					
BMI	Underweight	9 (84.23)	2 (15.77)	0.806	0.723
	Normal	397 (91.5)	47 (8.5)		
	Overweight	647 (90.2)	59 (9.8)		
	Obese	297 (91.32)	40 (8.68)		
Lifestyle characteristics					
Alcohol intake*	Never	630 (86.3)	102 (13.7)	0.002†	0.054
	Daily intake	571 (94.7)	40 (5.5)		
	Occasionally	300 (90.6)	34 (9.4)		
Smoke*	Never	969 (89.5)	145 (10.5)	0.480	0.344
	Past	449 (91.2)	25 (8.8)		
	Present	85 (95.5)	6 (4.5)		
No regular physical exercise*		873 (91.0)	109 (9.0)	0.590	0.482
Sleep habits (h)	<6	250 (87.7)	38 (12.3)	<0.001†	0.003†
	≥6	586 (95.9)	31 (4.1)		
Quality of life and physical function**					
EQ5D (0–1)		0.66 ± 0.01	0.31 ± 0.02	<0.001†	<0.001†
HAQ score (0–3)		0.63 ± 0.03	1.4 ± 0.06	<0.001†	<0.001†
Number of non-communicable diseases*		2.92 ± 1.95	4.76 ± 2.33	<0.001†	<0.001†
High blood pressure (Y/N)		825 (87.8)	128 (12.2)	0.011†	0.021†
Diabetes (Y/N)		341 (90.8)	47 (9.2)	0.808	0.874
High cholesterol level (Y/N)		712 (89.3)	105 (10.8)	0.489	0.908
Pulmonar disease (Y/N)		154 (82.6)	35 (17.4)	0.080	0.028†
Cardiac disease (Y/N)		370 (87.6)	67 (12.4)	0.127	0.104
Gastrointestinal diseases (Y/N)		380 (86.4)	72 (13.6)	0.037†	0.121
Neurologic diseases (Y/N)		106 (84.1)	22 (15.9)	0.080	0.256
Allergies (Y/N)		313 (83.0)	57 (17.0)	0.011†	0.015†
Neoplasic disease (Y/N)		128 (91.2)	15 (8.8)	0.732	0.600
Thyroid disease (Y/N)		156 (80.9)	41 (19.1)	<0.001†	0.085
Hyperuricemia (Y/N)		193 (89.1)	27 (10.9)	0.655	0.194
Rheumatic disease (Y/N)		685 (84.0)	125 (16.0)	<0.001†	<0.001†
Health resources consumption**					
Was hospitalizes since last contact		343 (85.0)	60 (15.1)	0.016†	0.003†
Went to medical appointments in hospitals since last contact		7.79 ± 0.36	13.9 ± 4.4	0.150	0.043†

%, weighted percentage; NUTS II, Nomenclatura das Unidades Territoriais, level II; BMI, body mass index (kg/m²); €, euro; HADS-A, Hospital Anxiety and Depression Scale—Anxiety subscale; HAQ, Health Assessment Questionnaire (0–3); EQ5D, European Quality of Life questionnaire five dimensions three levels (0–1).

†p-Value ≤ 0.05.

**p-Value was adjusted for age, sex, and region.*

***p-Value was adjusted for age, sex, region, and number of non-communicable diseases.*

TABLE 3 | Sociodemographic, socioeconomic, lifestyle, and health-related characteristics of the Portuguese elderly population with and without depression symptoms.

Sociodemographic and socioeconomic characteristics		Elderly without depression symptoms (HADS-D <11)	Elderly with depression symptoms (HADS-D ≥11)	*p*-Value	Adjusted *p*-value
		Mean (SD) or *n* (%)	Mean (SD) or *n* (%)		
		n = 1,439 (88.23%)	*n* = 241 (11.77%)		
Age* (years)		73.57 (6.51)	75.74 (7.23)	<0.001†	0.001†
Sex*	Female	747 (84.47)	161 (15.53)	<0.001†	<0.001†
	Male	692 (91.64)	80 (8.36)		
NUTS II*	Norte	463 (87.84)	80 (12.16)	0.020†	0.084
	Centro	360 (85.41)	67 (14.59)		
	Lisboa e Vale do Tejo	281 (93.63)	33 (6.37)		
	Alentejo	89 (87.2)	17 (12.8)		
	Algarve	50 (86.89)	10 (13.11)		
	Região Autónoma dos Açores	76 (87.77)	11 (12.23)		
	Região Autónoma da Madeira	120 (85.62)	23 (14.38)		
Education level*	≤4 years of education	1,046 (65.37)	213 (34.63)	<0.001†	<0.001†
	>4 years of education	373 (76.84)	24 (23.16)		
Household income* (€)	≤500	342 (80.53)	100 (19.47)	<0.001†	0.007†
	501–750	291 (88.06)	41 (11.94)		
	751–1,000	154 (96.26)	14 (3.74)		
	>1,000	271 (93.22)	20 (6.78)		
Household composition	1	347 (84.05)	82 (15.95)	0.009†	0.161
	≥2	1,092 (89.58)	159 (10.42)		
Anthropometric data*					
BMI	Underweight	9 (74.53)	2 (24.47)	0.293	0.245
	Normal	388 (89.99)	56 (10.01)		
	Overweight	620 (89.98)	86 (10.02)		
	Obese	284 (86.98)	53 (13.02)		
Lifestyle characteristics					
Alcohol intake*	Never	579 (83.2)	153 (16.8)	<0.001†	0.001†
	Daily intake	553 (91.7)	58 (8.3)		
	Occasionally	304 (92.1)	30 (7.9)		
Smoke*	Never	926 (85.8)	188 (14.2)	0.001†	0.154
	Past	434 (93.0)	40 (7.0)		
	Present	78 (90.2)	13 (9.8)		
No regular physical exercise*		807 (85.0)	175 (15.0)	<0.001†	0.001
Sleep habits (h)	<6	241 (86.1)	47 (13.9)	0.008†	0.048†
	≥6	528 (92.1)	59 (7.9)		
Quality of life and physical function**					
EQ5D (0–1)		0.67 ± 0.02	0.32 ± 0.02	<0.001†	<0.001†
HAQ score (0–3)		0.61 ± 0.03	1.38 ± 0.59	<0.001†	<0.001†
Number of non-communicable diseases		2.95 ± 1.93	4.36 ± 2.70	<0.001†	<0.001†
High blood pressure (Y/N)*		804 (87.2)	149 (12.76)	0.093	0.121
Diabetes (Y/N)*		315 (84.8)	73 (15.2)	0.039†	0.022†
High cholesterol level (Y/N)*		688 (86.0)	129 (14.0)	0.013†	0.056
Pulmonar disease (Y/N)*		150 (82.9)	39 (17.1)	0.023†	0.038†
Cardiac disease (Y/N)*		347 (83.6)	90 (16.5)	0.001†	0.015†
Gastrointestinal diseases (Y/N)*		367 (63.6)	85 (36.4)	0.019†	0.019†
Neurologic diseases (Y/N)*		102 (80.5)	26 (19.5)	0.028†	0.009†
Allergies (Y/N)		312 (87.9)	58 (12.1)	0.074	0.970
Neoplasic disease (Y/N)*		122 (87.3)	21 (12.7)	0.686	0.676
Thyroid disease (Y/N)*		157 (80.6)	40 (19.4)	0.001†	0.061
Hyperuricemia (Y/N)*		181 (83.2)	39 (16.8)	0.010†	0.009†
Rheumatic disease (Y/N)*		649 (82.9)	161 (17.1)	<0.001†	<0.001†
Health resources consumption**					
Was hospitalizes since last contact		334 (86.6)	69 (13.4)	0.226	0.043†
Went to medical appointments in hospitals since last contact		8.170 ± 0.634	8.961 ± 1.092	0.455	0.376

%, weighted percentage; NUTS II, Nomenclatura das Unidades Territoriais, level II; BMI, body mass index; €, euro; HADS-D, Hospital Anxiety and Depression Scale—Depression subscale; HAQ, Health Assessment Questionnaire (0–3); EQ5D, European Quality of Life questionnaire five dimensions three levels (0–1).

†p-Value ≤ 0.05.

**p-Value was adjusted for age, sex, and region.*

***p-Value was adjusted for age, sex, region, and number of non-communicable diseases.*

TABLE 4 | Factors associated with anxiety symptoms in seniors.

	Anxiety symptoms (yes/no)					
	Univariable logistic regression			Multivariable logistic regression		
	OR	95% CI	*p*-Value	OR	95% CI	*p*-Value
Gender						
Male	Ref.					
Female	3.74	2.12–6.62	0.000	2.77	1.53–5.00	0.001
Age (years)	0.98	0.94–1.02	0.371	0.96	0.92–1.00	0.078
NUTS II						
Norte	Ref.			Ref.		
Centro	0.99	0.63–1.57	0.982	0.98	0.60–1.60	0.939
Lisboa	0.92	0.29–3.00	0.897	0.97	0.37–2.54	0.949
Alentejo	0.76	0.37–1.57	0.462	0.79	0.36–1.73	0.553
Algarve	0.65	0.18–2.42	0.525	0.93	0.23–3.78	0.918
Azores	0.66	0.28–1.58	0.356	1.14	0.41–3.18	0.796
Madeira	0.87	0.46–1.66	0.683	0.91	0.48–1.75	0.785
Live alone (Y/N)	1.25	0.75–2.07	0.389			
Level of education						
≤4 years	3.09	1.72–5.54	0.000	2.30	1.22–4.36	0.010
>4 years	Ref.					
BMI						
Underweight	Ref.					
Normal	0.50	0.10–2.45	0.390			
Overweight	0.58	0.11–3.05	0.521			
Obese	0.51	0.10–2.52	0.407			
Alcohol intake						
Never	Ref.					
Daily intake	0.35	0.20–0.62	<0.001			
Occasionally	0.65	0.33–1.30	0.224			
Smoke						
Never	Ref.					
Past	0.82	0.33–2.06	0.680			
Present	0.40	0.15–1.06	0.066			
No regular physical exercise	0.85	0.48–1.53	0.590			
High blood pressure (Y/N)	2.03	1.18–3.50	0.011			
Diabetes (Y/N)	0.94	0.56–1.58	0.808			
High cholesterol level (Y/N)	1.23	0.69–2.20	0.489			
Pulmonar disease (Y/N)	1.64	0.94–2.85	0.080			
Cardiac disease (Y/N)	1.50	0.89–2.52	0.127			
Gastrointestinal diseases (Y/N)	1.80	1.03–3.13	0.039			
Neurologic diseases (Y/N)	1.85	0.93–3.67	0.080			
Allergies (Y/N)	2.43	1.23–4.79	0.011	2.02	1.14–3.55	0.015
Neoplasic disease (Y/N)	0.89	0.46–1.72	0.732			
Thyroid disease (Y/N)	2.51	1.50–4.20	<0.001			
Hyperuricemia (Y/N)	1.13	0.65–1.98	0.655			
Rheumatic disease (Y/N)	4.36	2.65–7.16	<0.001	2.92	1.74–4.90	<0.001

HADS-A, Hospital Anxiety and Depression Scale—Anxiety subscale; OR, odds ratio; CI, confidence interval; HAQ, Health Assessment Questionnaire (0–3); EQ5D, European Quality of Life questionnaire five dimensions three levels (0–1); BMI, body mass index.

[†]p-Value ≤ 0.05; GoF (p = 0.287).

DISCUSSION

This study showed a prevalence of 9.6% of anxiety symptoms among the Portuguese with 65 or more years old. This number is lower than the ones found in international studies over Australia, European, and American countries (24). These authors referred prevalence of significant anxiety symptoms between 15 and 52% in the elderly living in the community. Almost 10 years ago, an epidemiological study in Portugal, whose data were collected between 2008 and 2009, found the prevalence of generalized anxiety disorder in people over 65 years of age at 2.6% and the prevalence of any anxiety disorders 20% for the same age group (25).

Regarding depression, the estimated prevalence is of 11.8% for the Portuguese elderly living in the community, in line with the result of 12% for Major Depressive Disorder of the National Epidemiologic Study of Mental Health (25). In the Netherlands, however, depressive symptoms had a prevalence of 24% for older adults—55 years old and older (26), and Castro-Costa et al. exposed a prevalence of depressive symptoms ranging from 33% in France, Italy, and Spain, to 18–19%, in Sweden, Denmark, Netherlands, Germany, Austria, and Switzerland in adults over 50 years old (6).

Although the presented figures may suggest that Portuguese elderly are less anxious and depressed than other peoples

TABLE 5 | Factors associated with depression symptoms in seniors.

	Depression symptoms (yes/no)					
	Univariable logistic regression			Multivariable logistic regression		
	OR	95% CI	*p*-Value	OR	95% CI	*p*-Value
Gender						
Male	Ref.					
Female	2.02	1.42–2.85	<0.001	1.30	0.87–1.94	0.207
Age	1.05	1.02–1.07	<0.001	1.02	1.00–1.05	0.064
NUTS II						
Norte	Ref.					
Centro	1.23	0.84–1.82	0.289	1.11	0.73–1.70	0.607
Lisboa	0.49	0.29–0.84	0.009	0.51	0.28–0.96	0.037
Alentejo	1.06	0.58–1.94	0.849	1.18	0.64–2.18	0.603
Algarve	1.09	0.49–2.44	0.834	0.25	0.55–2.83	0.590
Azores	1.01	0.49–2.04	0.985	0.56	0.75–3.26	0.237
Madeira	1.21	0.70–2.11	0.492	1.20	0.66–2.18	0.547
Live alone (Y/N)	1.63	1.13–2.35	0.009			
Level of education (years)						
≤4	3.57	2.16–5.92	<0.001	2.40	1.41–4.09	0.001
>4	Ref.					
BMI						
Underweight	Ref.					
Normal	0.32	0.06–1.74	0.189			
Overweight	0.33	0.06–1.72	0.186			
Obese	0.44	0.08–2.30	0.334			
Alcohol intake						
Never	Ref.					
Daily intake	0.45	0.30–0.66	<0.001	0.54	0.35–0.83	0.005
Occasionally	0.42	0.26–0.70	0.001	0.49	0.29–0.84	0.009
Smoke						
Never	Ref.					
Past	0.46	0.30–0.70	<0.001			
Present	0.66	0.30–1.44	0.300			
No regular physical exercise	2.07	1.44–2.98	<0.001	1.64	1.11–2.42	0.013
High blood pressure (Y/N)	1.35	0.95–1.92	0.094			
Diabetes (Y/N)	1.50	1.02–2.21	0.040			
High cholesterol level (Y/N)	1.53	1.09–2.14	0.014			
Pulmonar disease (Y/N)	1.71	1.07–2.73	0.024			
Cardiac disease (Y/N)	1.83	1.27–2.64	0.001			
Gastrointestinal diseases (Y/N)	1.56	1.07–2.27	0.020			
Neurologic diseases (Y/N)	1.97	1.06–3.63	0.031			
Allergies (Y/N)	1.07	0.72–1.57	0.741			
Neoplasic disease (Y/N)	1.12	0.65–1.94	0.686			
Thyroid disease (Y/N)	2.01	1.31–3.08	0.001			
Hyperuricemia (Y/N)	1.74	1.14–2.65	0.011			
Rheumatic disease (Y/N)	2.94	2.04–4.23	<0.001	2.12	1.45–3.09	<0.001

HADS-D, Hospital Anxiety and Depression Scale-Depression subscale; OR, odds ratio; CI, confidence interval; HAQ, Health Assessment Questionnaire (0–3); EQ5D, European Quality of Life questionnaire five dimensions, three levels (0–1); BMI, body mass index.
Household composition: number of people that live in the house of the participant, including himself/herself.
†p-Value ≤ 0.05; GoF (p = 0.04056).

in Europe and around the globe, one should be very careful when comparing these numbers. There are core discrepancies regarding methods of data collection, different instruments of assessing depression and anxiety, different nosological entities considered (major depression disorder, minor depression disorder, generalized anxiety disorder vs symptoms of depression and anxiety), and finally different age groups cutoffs (≥50 and ≥55 vs ≥65).

As Byrne stressed differences in anxiety prevalence rates may be due to differences among populations, but also to differences in assessment tools and algorithms used for diagnosis such as State Trait Anxiety Inventory and Anxiety Disorder Scale (27). Some studies use the hierarchical approach to diagnosis, which may lead to lower prevalence by excluding individuals with diagnostic criteria that also have criteria for diagnosing other higher disorders in the hierarchy (3).

Our study demonstrates a close relationship between physical function and anxiety and depression showing that seniors with lower physical function are more likely to report anxiety and/or depression symptoms. Lenze and collaborators performed a literature review on the association of late life depression and anxiety with physical disability. Their findings indicated that depression was a risk factor for disability, but also in the other way, being disability a risk factor for depression (28). Brenes and colleagues studied the influence of anxiety on the progression of physical disability in a community-based observational work, concluding that, after adjusting for confounders, anxiety continued to predict the development of disability in activities of daily living (29).

In terms of quality of life, our results suggest that seniors with anxiety and/or depression are more likely to have reported lower levels of quality of life. Sivertsen and colleagues, in their review article of 74 studies, concluded the same, demonstrating that depressed older people had poor global quality of life than non-depressed individuals. They added that this association was stable over time and independently of how quality of life was measured (30). Brenes also considered anxiety in relation to quality of life, and her conclusions were similar: anxiety was significantly associated with all domains of quality of life, and as severity of anxiety symptoms increased, quality of life decreased (31). Having very low income was also related to higher depression. This is in line with what Valvanne and collaborators defended in their elderly population-based study in Finland (32). McCall and colleagues findings in USA also corroborated the conclusions that related low income to higher scores of depression (33).

To assess determinants for anxiety and depression, a multivariable logistic regression, using socioeconomic factors and chronic diseases was developed.

The results considering the outcome as a binary variable "Anxiety disorders (Yes/No)" showed that being a woman, having less than 5 years of education, having a rheumatic disease and allergies were factors highly associated to higher scores of the anxiety diagnosis in Portuguese elders. Beekman and colleagues had already pointed sex and education level out as relevant to understand anxiety in their study with LASA cohort data (34).

Although other studies found a significant higher rate of anxiety in women with 55 or more years old (35), this was not found in our population.

A global model using multivariable logistic regression was also used to capture the framework of factors related to depression in Portuguese elderly, level of education, physical inactivity, alcohol intake on a daily and occasionally basis, and rheumatic disease should be taken into account when considering depression in this population.

This is in line with the literature supporting that physical activity is associated with lower levels of depression (36) Also, several studies suggest that lower education is associated with depression (37–39).

Regarding alcohol intake, the results found denote that the daily or occasional consumption of alcoholic beverages decreases the probability of reporting depression among seniors. Although this result can be unsettling at first glance, it is important to retain that this study assessed consumption frequency, rather than type or quantity. In the literature, several studies associate alcohol misuse or alcoholism with higher levels of depression (40, 41). That is, however, a different matter.

Although literature often expresses a relationship between anxiety and/or depression and diabetes (42), pulmonary (43), and neoplasic diseases (44), these associations were not confirmed in Portuguese senior population. Our study confirms, however, conclusions of previous studies on rheumatic diseases (11, 45, 46) stressing their important association with both anxiety and depression, as well as the relationship between allergies and anxiety, patent in the literature (47).

Interestingly, the female sex is also described in literature as an important determinant of depression (46, 48). In our study, it was strongly significant even with multivariable analyses with single factors separately, such as non-communicable chronic diseases, quality of life, or function. But within a global model including all significant variables for depression, it loses its previous relevance.

Regarding age, Alameda County Study demonstrated a raise of depression prevalence with age (49). But multivariable analyses showed that the effect of age was related to physical health problems and disability associated with aging. Several studies concluded the same way, indicating that although depression prevalence increases with age, it should be due to age-related factors than age itself (50, 51).

Study limitations should be considered when interpreting results. Being cross-sectional, this analysis does not allow to draw conclusions about the effects of causality between the variables and the chronological order of the events.

Although Breeman defended HADS being used for clinical and non-clinical population (52), the use of a specific instrument to assess anxiety and depression in this particular age group is arguable.

Despite of what has been referred, several strengths related to both internal and external validity should be pointed out. Data come from large, nationally representative sample of the Portuguese elder population followed since 2011, allowing its generalization for the age group in our country. It should also be noted that data were collected by a team of 10 interviewers who were extensively and properly trained, whose proceedings were standardized, and regular and rigorously monitored to assess quality and reduce bias.

In conclusion, key findings of this study are as follows: (1) Portuguese elderly population have prevalence of anxiety and depression around 10 and 12%, respectively; (2) anxiety and depression are associated to different factors; (3) health-related quality of life and physical function play an important role in depression and anxiety; and (4) level of education distinguishes senior in terms of anxiety and depression.

ETHICS STATEMENT

This study was carried out in accordance with the recommendations of Guidelines for Good Clinical Practice and the ethical principles stated in the Declaration of Helsinki, National Committee for Data Protection (Comissão Nacional de Proteção de Dados) and by the NOVA Medical School Ethics Committee, with written informed consent from all subjects. All subjects gave written informed consent in accordance with the Declaration of Helsinki. The protocol was approved by the National Committee for Data Protection (Comissão Nacional de Proteção de Dados) and by the NOVA Medical School Ethics Committee.

AUTHOR CONTRIBUTIONS

RS conducted the study and wrote the paper. AR and MGr supported the development of the study design and methodology and reviewed the paper. JB is co-responsible for the EpiDoC Cohort and reviewed the paper. MGo and HC supported the whole development of the study and writing and reviewed the paper. SD supported the data analysis process.

REFERENCES

1. United Nations, Department of Economic and Social Affairs, Population Division. *World Population Prospects: The 2017 Revision, Key Findings and Advance Tables*. New York (2017). Working Paper No. ESA/P/WP/248.
2. PORDATA. *Indicadores de Envelhecimento – Portugal*. (2016). Available from: http://www.pordata.pt/Portugal/Indicadores+de+envelhecimento-526
3. Wolitzky-Taylor KB, Castriotta N, Lenze EJ, Stanley MA, Craske MG. Anxiety disorders in older adults: a comprehensive review. *Depress Anxiety* (2010) 27(2):190–211. doi:10.1002/da.20653
4. Chapman DP, Perry GS. Depression as a major component of public health for older adults. *Prev Chronic Dis* (2008) 5(1):A22.
5. Blazer DG II, Hybels CF. Origins of depression in later life. *Psychol Med* (2005) 35(9):1241–52. doi:10.1017/S0033291705004411
6. Castro-Costa E, Dewey M, Stewart R, Banerjee S, Huppert F, Mendonca-Lima C, et al. Prevalence of depressive symptoms and syndromes in later life in ten European countries: the SHARE study. *Br J Psychiatry* (2007) 191:393–401. doi:10.1192/bjp.bp.107.036772
7. Flint AJ. Epidemiology and comorbidity of anxiety disorders in the elderly. *Am J Psychiatry* (1994) 151(5):640–9. doi:10.1176/ajp.151.5.640
8. Schoevers RA, Beekman AT, Deeg DJ, Jonker C, van Tilburg W. Comorbidity and risk-patterns of depression, generalised anxiety disorder and mixed anxiety-depression in later life: results from the AMSTEL study. *Int J Geriatr Psychiatry* (2003) 18:994–1001. doi:10.1002/gps.1001
9. Vink D, Aartsen MJ, Schoevers RA. Risk factors for anxiety and depression in the elderly: a review. *J Affect Disord* (2008) 106(1–2):29–44. doi:10.1016/j.jad.2007.06.005
10. Lenze EJ, Wetherell JL. A lifespan view of anxiety disorders. *Dialogues Clin Neurosci* (2011) 13(4):381–99.
11. Branco JC, Rodrigues AM, Gouveia N, Eusebio M, Ramiro S, Machado PM, et al. Prevalence of rheumatic and musculoskeletal diseases and their impact on health-related quality of life, physical function and mental health in Portugal: results from EpiReumaPt – a national health survey. *RMD Open* (2016) 2(1):e000166. doi:10.1136/rmdopen-2015-000166
12. Gouveia N, Rodrigues AM, Ramiro S, Machado P, da Costa LP, Mourao AF, et al. EpiReumaPt: how to perform a national population based study – a practical guide. *Acta Reumatol Port* (2015) 40(2):128–36.
13. Rodrigues AM, Gouveia N, da Costa LP, Eusebio M, Ramiro S, Machado P, et al. EpiReumaPt – the study of rheumatic and musculoskeletal diseases in Portugal: a detailed view of the methodology. *Acta Reumatol Port* (2015) 40(2):110–24.
14. Lei n° 67/98 – Lei da Proteção de Dados Pessoais, 67 (1998).
15. Pais-Ribeiro J, Silva I, Ferreira T, Martins A, Meneses R, Baltar M. Validation study of a Portuguese version of the Hospital Anxiety and Depression Scale. *Psychol Health Med* (2007) 12(2):225–35; quiz 35–7. doi:10.1080/13548500500524088
16. Zigmond AS, Snaith RP. The Hospital Anxiety and Depression Scale. *Acta Psychiatr Scand* (1983) 67(6):361–70. doi:10.1111/j.1600-0447.1983.tb09716.x
17. Snaith RP. The Hospital Anxiety and Depression Scale. *Health Qual Life Outcomes* (2003) 1:29. doi:10.1186/1477-7525-1-29
18. WHO. *Physical Status: The Use and Interpretation of Anthropometry Report of a WHO Expert Committee*. Geneve: World Health Organization (1995).
19. Ferreira L, Ferreira P, Pereira L, Oppe M. EQ-5D Portuguese population norms. *Qual Life Res* (2014) 23(2):425–30. doi:10.1007/s11136-013-0488-4
20. Ferreira L, Ferreira P, Pereira L, Oppe M. The valuation of the EQ-5D in Portugal. *Qual Life Res* (2014) 23(2):413–23. doi:10.1007/s11136-013-0448-z
21. Benito-Garcia E, Santos M, Ramiro S, Medeiros S, Cordeiro R, Canas da Silva JA, et al. Propridades psicométricas da versão portuguesa do HAQ. *Acta Reumatol Port* (2006) 31:126–7.
22. Santos R, Reis P, Rebelo L, Costa Dias F, Miranda Rosa C, Viana de Queiroz M. "Health assessment questionnaire" (versão curta): adaptação para língua portuguesa e estudo da sua aplicabilidade. *Acta Reumatol Port* (1996) 76:15–20.
23. World Medical Association. World Medical Association Declaration of Helsinki: ethical principles for medical research involving human subjects. *JAMA* (2013) 310(20):2191–4. doi:10.1001/jama.2013.281053
24. Bryant C, Jackson H, Ames D. The prevalence of anxiety in older adults: methodological issues and a review of the literature. *J Affect Disord* (2008) 109(3):233–50. doi:10.1016/j.jad.2007.11.008
25. Almeida J, Xavier M, Cardoso G, Pereira M, Gusmão R, Corrêa B, et al. *Estudo epidemiológiológico nacional de saúde mental – 1° relatório*. Lisbon: Faculdade de Ciências Médicas, Universidade Nova de Lisboa (2013).
26. Hoogendijk EO, Deeg DJH, Poppelaars J, van der Horst M, Broese van Groenou MI, Comijs HC, et al. The Longitudinal Aging Study Amsterdam: cohort update 2016 and major findings. *Eur J Epidemiol* (2016) 31(9):927–45. doi:10.1007/s10654-016-0192-0
27. Byrne G. What happens to anxiety disorders in later life? *Rev Bras Psiquiatr* (2002) 24(Supl I):74–80. doi:10.1590/S1516-44462002000500014
28. Lenze EJ, Rogers JC, Martire LM, Mulsant BH, Rollman BL, Dew MA, et al. The association of late-life depression and anxiety with physical disability: a review of the literature and prospectus for future research. *Am J Geriatr Psychiatry* (2001) 9(2):113–35. doi:10.1097/00019442-200105000-00004
29. Brenes GA, Guralnik JM, Williamson JD, Fried LP, Simpson C, Simonsick EM, et al. The influence of anxiety on the progression of disability. *J Am Geriatr Soc* (2005) 53(1):34–9. doi:10.1111/j.1532-5415.2005.53007.x
30. Sivertsen H, Bjorklof GH, Engedal K, Selbaek G, Helvik AS. Depression and quality of life in older persons: a review. *Dement Geriatr Cogn Disord* (2015) 40(5–6):311–39. doi:10.1159/000437299
31. Brenes GA. Anxiety, depression, and quality of life in primary care patients. *Prim Care Companion J Clin Psychiatry* (2007) 9(6):437–43. doi:10.4088/PCC.v09n0606
32. Valvanne J, Juva K, Erkinjuntti T, Tilvis R. Major depression in the elderly: a Population Study in Helsinki. *Int Psychogeriatr* (1996) 8(3):437–43. doi:10.1017/S1041610296002797
33. McCall NT, Parks P, Smith K, Pope G, Griggs M. The prevalence of major depression or dysthymia among aged Medicare Fee-for-Service beneficiaries. *Int J Geriatr Psychiatry* (2002) 17(6):557–65. doi:10.1002/gps.642
34. Beekman AT, Bremmer MA, Deeg DJ, van Balkom AJ, Smit JH, de Beurs E, et al. Anxiety disorders in later life: a report from the Longitudinal Aging Study Amsterdam. *Int J Geriatr Psychiatry* (1998) 13(10):717–26. doi:10.1002/(SICI)1099-1166(1998100)13:10<717::AID-GPS857>3.0.CO;2-M
35. Himmelfarb S, Murrell SA. The prevalence and correlates of anxiety symptoms in older adults. *J Psychol* (1984) 116(2d Half):159–67. doi:10.1080/00223980.1984.9923632
36. Teixeira CM, Vasconcelos-Raposo J, Fernandes HM, Brustad RJ. Physical activity, depression and anxiety among the elderly. *Soc Indic Res* (2013) 113(1):307–18. doi:10.1007/s11205-012-0094-9
37. Forsell Y. Predictors for depression, anxiety and psychotic symptoms in a very elderly population: data from a 3-year follow-up study. *Soc Psychiatry Psychiatr Epidemiol* (2000) 35(6):259–63. doi:10.1007/s001270050237
38. Oh DH, Kim SA, Lee HY, Seo JY, Choi BY, Nam JH. Prevalence and correlates of depressive symptoms in Korean adults: results of a 2009 Korean Community Health Survey. *J Korean Med Sci* (2013) 28(1):128–35. doi:10.3346/jkms.2013.28.1.128
39. Cole M, Dendukuri N. Risk factors for depression among elderly community subjects: a systematic review and meta-analysis. *Am J Psychiatry* (2003) 160(6):1147–56. doi:10.1176/appi.ajp.160.6.1147
40. Boden JM, Fergusson DM. Alcohol and depression. *Addiction* (2011) 106(5):906–14. doi:10.1111/j.1360-0443.2010.03351.x
41. JS M. Alcohol and depression. *Br J Hosp Med* (1993) 50(5):261–4.

42. Barnard KD, Skinner TC, Peveler R. The prevalence of co-morbid depression in adults with Type 1 diabetes: systematic literature review. *Diabet Med* (2006) 23(4):445–8. doi:10.1111/j.1464-5491.2006.01814.x
43. Gudmundsson G, Gislason T, Janson C, Lindberg E, Suppli Ulrik C, Brondum E, et al. Depression, anxiety and health status after hospitalisation for COPD: a multicentre study in the Nordic countries. *Respir Med* (2006) 100(1):87–93. doi:10.1016/j.rmed.2005.04.003
44. Rodin G, Katz M, Lloyd N, Green E, Mackay JA, Wong RKS. Treatment of depression in cancer patients. *Curr Oncol* (2007) 14(5):180–8. doi:10.3747/co.2007.146
45. Margaretten M, Julian L, Katz P, Yelin E. Depression in patients with rheumatoid arthritis: description, causes and mechanisms. *Int J Clin Rheumtol* (2011) 6(6):617–23. doi:10.2217/ijr.11.62
46. Djernes JK. Prevalence and predictors of depression in populations of elderly: a review. *Acta Psychiatr Scand* (2006) 113(5):372–87. doi:10.1111/j.1600-0447.2006.00770.x
47. Tomoum MO, Klattcromwell C, DelSignore A, Ebert C, Senior BA. Depression and anxiety in chronic rhinosinusitis. *Allergy Rhinol* (2015) 5(8):674–81. doi:10.1002/alr.21528
48. Barefoot JC, Mortensen EL, Helms MJ, Avlund K, Schroll M. A longitudinal study of gender differences in depressive symptoms from age 50 to 80. *Psychol Aging* (2001) 16(2):342–5. doi:10.1037/0882-7974.16.2.342
49. Roberts RE, Kaplan GA, Shema SJ, Strawbridge WJ. Prevalence and correlates of depression in an aging cohort: the Alameda County Study. *J Gerontol B Psychol Sci Soc Sci* (1997) 52(5):S252–8. doi:10.1093/geronb/52B.5.S252
50. Steffens DC, Skoog I, Norton MC, Hart AD, Tschanz JT, Plassman BL, et al. Prevalence of depression and its treatment in an elderly population: the Cache County study. *Arch Gen Psychiatry* (2000) 57(6):601–7. doi:10.1001/archpsyc.57.6.601
51. van't Veer-Tazelaar PJ, van Marwijk HW, Jansen AP, Rijmen F, Kostense PJ, van Oppen P, et al. Depression in old age (75+), the PIKO study. *J Affect Disord* (2008) 106(3):295–9. doi:10.1016/j.jad.2007.07.004
52. Breeman S, Cotton S, Fielding S, Jones GT. Normative data for the Hospital Anxiety and Depression Scale. *Qual Life Res* (2015) 24(2):391–8. doi:10.1007/s11136-014-0763-z

20

Kinematic Changes during Prolonged Fast-walking in Old and Young Adults

Camila Fonseca Oliveira[1,2], Edgar Ramos Vieira[3], Filipa Manuel Machado Sousa[1,2] and João Paulo Vilas-Boas[1,2]*

[1] Center of Research, Education, Innovation and Intervention in Sport (CIFI²D), Faculty of Sport, University of Porto, Porto, Portugal, [2] Porto Biomechanics Laboratory (LABIOMEP), University of Porto, Porto, Portugal, [3] Department of Physical Therapy, Florida International University, Miami, FL, United States

Edited by:
Helena Canhao,
Unidade EpiDoC, Epidemiologia de doenças crônicas, Portugal

Reviewed by:
Lisa Robinson,
Newcastle upon Tyne Hospitals NHS Foundation Trust, United Kingdom
Vera Moniz-Pereira,
Universidade de Lisboa, Portugal

***Correspondence:**
Camila Fonseca Oliveira
fisiocamilafonseca@gmail.com

Walking biomechanics is known to be influenced by speed. However, most of the research examining the effects of walking speed and gait characteristics has been conducted after a fast-walking task, neglecting the changes that may occur during the task. The aim of the present study was to determine the impact of fast-walking over time on kinematics in young and old adults. Twenty-seven young adults (26.6 ± 6.0 years) and 23 old adults (71.0 ± 5.6 years) walked at 70% of their maximum heart rate for 20 min or until exhaustion, and the effects of fast-walking on temporospatial parameters and on angular kinematics were analyzed during the activity. During the protocol, both age-groups increased step-width variability. Significant effects of time were found for the ankle and hip at toe off for the older group. For the younger group, only the ankle angle at heel strike changed over time. For both groups, fast-walking induced changes in the coordination among the lower-limb angles that were more prominent during the swing phase of the gait. In conclusion, lower-limb kinematics changes in young adults were compatible with early signs of fatigue. The increased step-width variability in older adults may indicate an augmented risk of falling. Changes in the lower-limb walking kinematics of old adults suggest that the adjustments for weight acceptance and body propulsion were restricted to the hip and ankle joints. The kinematic changes among the lower-limb joint angles during the swing phase may compromise the quality of gait. These findings provide a foundation for future studies in the assessment of the risk of falls in older adults associated with walking at a faster pace.

Keywords: active-aging, fast-walking, kinematics, falls prevention, intra-limb coordination

INTRODUCTION

The world population is aging. Approximately 14% of the European population are over the age of 65 and it is expected that this proportion will double by 2050 (1). With more than a third of older adults experiencing at least one fall per year, the consequences of falls represent a major problem for the health systems of many countries and represent huge associated costs (1). Falls often occur during walking (2) and can be a result of aging-related changes on gait (3). Gait changes observed in older adults are primarily due to reduced muscle strength and lower-limb joint range of motion as a result of physiological and neuromuscular changes (4–6). Aging-related changes in gait may be of particular concern when walking faster than usual. Increased walking speed may magnify the effects and limitations that may occur over time, and such assessments may highlight other factors that may be associated with falls. Irrespective of the factors underlying the age-related alterations on gait, several authors have associated fast-walking with an increased risk of falling (4, 7–9).

In general, healthy older adults are more susceptible to fall in outdoors activities (10), where walking at a faster pace can be a sporadic practice among this population. According to England and Granata (11), fast-walking may influence a successful locomotion by a combination of several mechanisms, as the ability to control movement could be disrupted by the effects of fast-walking on gait kinematics and other clinical correlates of stable walking. Studies involving fast-walking activity and its association with risk of falls are crucial for understanding the strategies that may be involved in falls' prevention. However, most of the research examining the effects of fast-walking and its association with risk of falling (4, 7–9) were conducted after exposing the subjects to increased speed, neglecting changes in gait characteristics during the task. Thus, evaluating the effects of fast-walking activity over time on gait parameters may highlight potential threats that may arise while walking at a faster pace.

An individual's gait strategy can be represented by their temporospatial parameters. Therefore, assessment of the gait parameters, namely fluctuations in temporospatial gait characteristics, may provide additional insight into the motor control of gait (12). In addition, as the coordination pattern between adjacent joint angles reflects a characteristic of the motor control of organizing adjacent structures in terms of timing and position to execute a movement (13), the intra-limb coordination was analyzed to display the impact of fast-walking on the coordinative synergism among the lower-limb angles. Thus, the present study was conducted to determine the impact of walking at a faster pace on temporospatial parameters and lower-limb joint kinematics in young and old adults during the activity.

MATERIALS AND METHODS

Subjects

The participants were 27 young (26.6 ± 6.0 years) and 23 older adults (71.0 ± 5.6 years), the minimum age was 21 and 65 years for the groups of younger and older adults, respectively. Older participants were recruited from local community centers and younger adults from the local student population. Before the session, they were all screened to ensure eligibility. The exclusion criteria included any orthopedical, musculoskeletal, or cardiovascular constraints that might impair normal locomotion. All participants provided written informed consent using procedures approved by the Ethics Committee of the Faculty of Sport from the University of Porto, process number 10-2014.

Procedures

Kinematic data were captured (100 Hz) using an 8-camera motion capture system (Qualisys, QTM). Reflective markers were placed on the anterior–posterior and posterior–superior iliac spines, bilaterally on the greater trochanter, medial and lateral femoral condyles, medial and lateral malleoli, end of the second toes, fifth metatarsal head, and calcanei. These markers were used to define the segments included in the biomechanical model (14). A standing calibration trial was recorded prior to the beginning of the task. Data were then processed using Visual 3D (C-motion, Rockville, MD, USA). Older participants wore a safety harness attached to the ceiling for safety.

Protocol

All participants completed a familiarization session on a treadmill (AMTI Inc., MA, USA) walking at their preferred walking speed for 5 min. After that, the treadmill speed was increased by 0.5 km/h every 30 s until the participants reached the speed where they reached 70% of their age-predicted maximal heart rate (HR, 220 minus age in years). The participants were instructed to walk at this intensity for 20 min or until their self-assessed exhaustion. Two examiners were accompanying closely the participant during the task. HR was measured continuously during the test with a Polar HR monitor (2010 Polar Electro Oy, FI-90440 Kempele, Finland) to ensure subjects were walking at the required intensity. In addition, perceived exertion was assessed using a modified Borg 10-point scale (15). The relative speed was kept the same for each of the participants, and constant throughout the test. During the protocol, a variation of 10% of the target HR was permitted. The participants would be asked to stop the protocol if any of the following clinical indications were met: voluntary cessation, symptoms of cardiovascular discomfort, pulmonary discomfort, or the exertion reached 90% of their maximum HR, as recommended on ACSM's guidelines for submaximal tests (16).

Dominant limb marker trajectories were collected during 30 s every minute until the end of the activity. The dominant limb was defined as the limb with which they would kick a football. Five equally distributed periods were later analyzed using Visual 3D (C-motion Inc., Rockville, MD, USA). The marker trajectories were filtered using a fourth-order low-pass Butterworth filter with a 12 Hz cut-off frequency. Gait cycle was defined by consecutive heel strikes of the dominant foot. Lower-limb angles were assigned with three rotational degrees of freedom and calculated using an XYZ Cardan sequence of rotations, which are equivalent to flexion/extension–abduction/adduction–axial rotation, respectively. Hip flexion, knee flexion, and dorsiflexion were displayed as positive displacement; whereas, hip extension, knee extension, and plantarflexion were displayed as a negative displacement.

The following parameters were assessed: sagittal angles of the hip, knee, and ankle at heel strike and toe off, cadence (number of steps per minute), stride length (distance between two successive right heel strikes), stride time (duration in seconds of a stride), step width (medio-lateral distance between heel position during heel strike of the left and right limbs). Sagittal joint angles at the ankle, knee and hip for each individual were time normalized to 100% of the gait cycle. Hip–knee–ankle sagittal angle plots were used as visual representatives of intra-limb joint coordination.

The relative position between the adjacent joints was displayed along the gait cycle for the first and last stage of the protocol. Mean and SD of all kinematic data from approximately 30 strides were calculated on an individual level and were then averaged across participants for each group at every stage. Gait variability was assessed using SD for the angular kinematic data, and coefficient of variation $CV = \frac{SD}{Mean} \times 100\%$ for all temporospatial parameters.

Data Analysis

Student's *t*-test was used to identify between-group differences in fast-walking task-speed and demographics. Analyses of differences within- and between-group were assessed by repeated measures ANOVA. If the assumption of sphericity was failed, a Greenhouse–Geisser correction was used. All statistical procedures were performed using SPSS 25 (IBM, NY, USA) and a significance level of 0.05 was used.

TABLE 1 | Characteristics of study's participants.

Characteristics	Young adults (*n* = 27)	Old adults (*n* = 23)
Age (years)*	26.6 ± 6.0	71.1 ± 5.6
Height (m)*	1.72 ± 0.11	1.63 ± 0.10
Body mass (kg)	68.0 ± 15.5	69.9 ± 10.2
Fast-walking speed (m/s)*	1.91 ± 0.20	1.22 ± 0.31

Values are displayed as mean ± SD.
**Significant difference (p < 0.05) between age-groups using independent sample t-tests.*

RESULTS

Young and older adults achieved 70% at their maximum HR at significantly different velocities ($P = 0.01$). Old adults were not different from young adults in body mass but were shorter in height than the younger counterpart. Descriptive characteristics can be seen in **Table 1**.

Since gait strategies are directly influenced by the walking speed, both groups had different cadence, stride length, stride time, and step-width mean values. During the activity, both age-groups showed slight, but significant increase of stride length. Young and old adults kept the mean values of the step-width throughout the protocol. The stride time increased only for the group of older adults. Levels of variability (assessed by the coefficient of variation) were higher in the elderly group for the stride length and the stride time (see **Figure 1**). In both age-groups, statistically significant main effects of time were found only for the step-width coefficient of variation ($P = 0.03$).

Between-group comparisons of joint angular kinematics showed differences for the mean values for the ankle, knee (at heel strike), and hip (at toe off). Significant effects of time were found for the ankle and hip at toe off for the older group. For the younger group, only the ankle angle at heel strike changed over time. Older adults had higher lower-limb angular variability at heel strike for the ankle and knee than the younger adults. No time effects were found for the lower-limb joint angle's variability. Time and group differences of the sagittal angles at the heel strike and toe off are presented in **Table 2**, and can be seen in **Figure 2**.

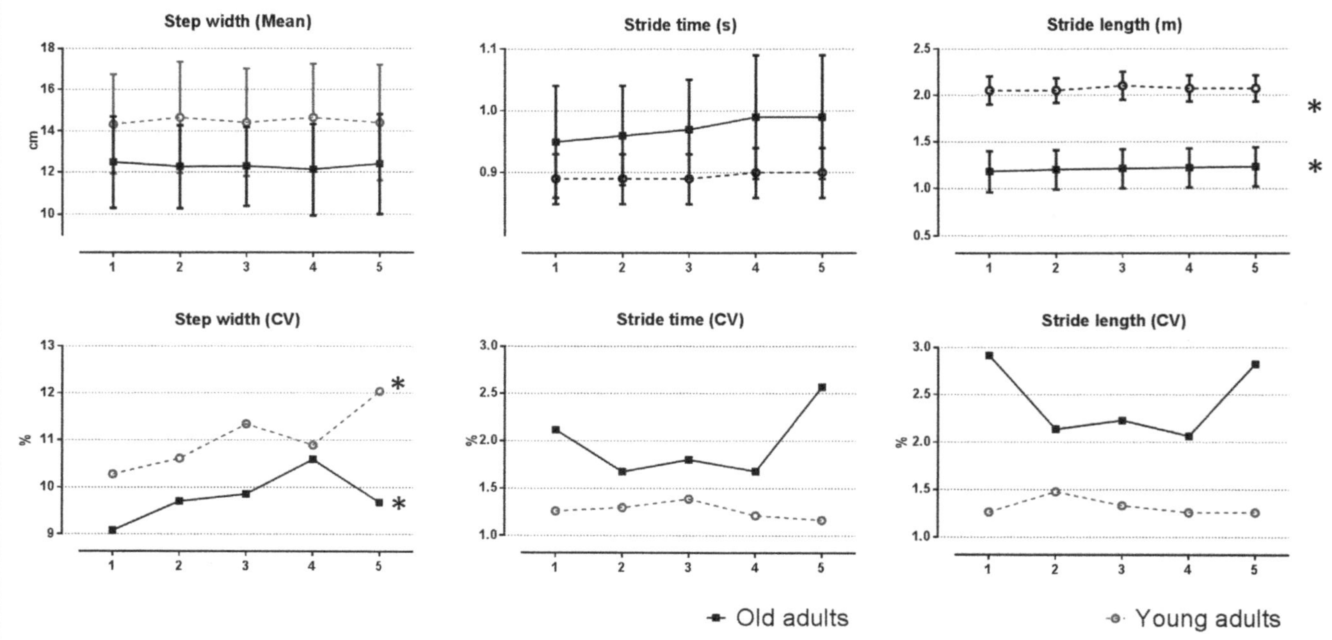

FIGURE 1 | Temporospatial parameters during fast-walking activity at the top. The mean and SD for each subject were subsequently averaged across subjects within the age-group. At the bottom, differences in the coefficient of variation revealed the differences in temporospatial variability along the task. *Indicates statistically significant time effect.

TABLE 2 | Means and SDs for gait variables across all the time points during fast-walking activity.

Variable	Group	Time points					*P* ANOVA		
		T1	T2	T3	T4	T5	Group	Time	Interaction
Temporospatial parameters									
Cadence	OA	**61.4 ± 0.8**	**62.2 ± 0.9**	**61.3 ± 0.8**	**60.2 ± 0.9**	**58.2 ± 0.9**	**0.001**	**0.004**	0.518
	YA	**65.4 ± 0.8**	**63.8 ± 0.9**	**63.2 ± 0.8**	**62.2 ± 0.8**	**61.2 ± 0.7**			
Stride time (s)	OA	**0.95 ± 0.09**	**0.96 ± 0.08**	**0.97 ± 0.08**	**0.99 ± 0.10**	**0.99 ± 0.10**	**0.022**	**0.001**	**0.020**
	YA	0.89 ± 0.04	0.89 ± 0.04	0.89 ± 0.04	0.90 ± 0.04	0.90 ± 0.04			
Step width (cm)	OA	12.5 ± 2.2	12.2 ± 2.0	12.2 ± 1.9	12.1 ± 2.2	12.2 ± 2.4	**0.002**	0.613	0.226
	YA	14.3 ± 2.4	14.6 ± 2.7	14.4 ± 2.6	14.6 ± 2.6	14.1 ± 2.3			
Stride length (m)	OA	**1.18 ± 0.22**	**1.2 ± 0.21**	**1.21 ± 0.21**	**1.22 ± 0.21**	**1.23 ± 0.21**	**0.001**	**0.001**	0.172
	YA	**2.05 ± 0.15**	**2.05 ± 0.13**	**2.1 ± 0.15**	**2.07 ± 14**	**2.07 ± 0.14**			
Stride length (CV)	OA	2.9 ± 2.6	2.1 ± 1.3	2.2 ± 1.3	2.1 ± 1.2	2.9 ± 3.3	**0.012**	0.341	0.174
	YA	1.3 ± 0.4	1.5 ± 1.0	1.3 ± 0.7	1.3 ± 0.3	1.3 ± 0.3			
Stride time (CV)	OA	2.1 ± 1.8	1.7 ± 0.8	1.8 ± 1.2	1.7 ± 0.9	2.5 ± 1.4	**0.007**	0.377	0.178
	YA	1.2 ± 0.4	1.3 ± 0.5	1.4 ± 1.0	1.2 ± 0.4	1.2 ± 0.3			
Step width (CV)	OA	9.6 ± 3.2	10.1 ± 3.6	10.4 ± 2.9	11.2 ± 3.8	11.6 ± 7.9	0.319	**0.031**	0.402
	YA	11.5 ± 8.0	11.9 ± 8.7	12.6 ± 8.9	12.2 ± 8.5	13.2 ± 10.2			
Angular kinematics									
				Differences in the mean values along the activity					
Ankle angular position at HS	OA	−2.9 ± 5.5	−2.9 ± 5.0	−2.9 ± 4.6	−3.4 ± 4.8	−3.4 ± 5.0	**0.001**	**0.032**	**0.034**
	YA	**3.5 ± 4.0**	**2.6 ± 5.0**	**1.3 ± 4.6**	**1.7 ± 4.0**	**1.9 ± 4.2**			
Ankle angular position at TO	OA	**−9.8 ± 6.0**	**−11.4 ± 6.4**	**−11.9 ± 6.4**	**−11.8 ± 7.0**	**−12 ± 6.5**	**0.001**	**0.021**	**0.041**
	YA	−20.9 ± 10	−20.1 ± 11	−21.4 ± 10	−21.3 ± 10	−21.4 ± 10			
Knee angular position at HS	OA	4.0 ± 6.0	3.6 ± 6.6	2.9 ± 6.9	2.2 ± 6.5	1.7 ± 7.0	**0.001**	0.126	0.101
	YA	−3.0 ± 3.4	−2.3 ± 3.4	−2.3 ± 3.2	−2.3 ± 3.4	−2.1 ± 3.2			
Knee angular position at TO	OA	40.1 ± 6.7	40.8 ± 6.4	40.4 ± 6.5	40.4 ± 7.1	40.4 ± 7.2	0.127	0.548	0.374
	YA	37.1 ± 4.0	38.4 ± 4.1	38.0 ± 4.5	38.3 ± 4.4	38.4 ± 4.1			
Hip angle position at HS	OA	35. 1 ± 7.6	35.9 ± 9.3	35.3 ± 9.4	35.1 ± 8.9	32.9 ± 10.8	0.103	0.279	0.246
	YA	31.4 ± 5.8	31.9 ± 6.2	31.4 ± 6.6	31.4 ± 6.0	31.7 ± 6.1			
Hip angle position at TO	OA	**2.8 ± 9.9**	**2.7 ± 9.5**	**1.9 ± 9.8**	**1.4 ± 9.1**	**0.8 ± 9.4**	**0.00**	**0.017**	0.032
	YA	−8.4 ± 6.8	−7.1 ± 7.3	−7.4 ± 6.9	−9.0 ± 7.1	−8.1 ± 6.4			
				Differences in the SD along the activity					
Ankle angular position at HS	OA	1.5 ± 0.8	1.4 ± 0.7	1.3 ± 0.9	1.5 ± 1.2	1.5 ± 1.2	**0.013**	0.657	0.706
	YA	0.9 ± 03	1.1 ± 0.9	1.0 ± 0.4	1.0 ± 0.4	1.2 ± 0.7			
Ankle angular position at TO	OA	1.8 ± 0.9	1.6 ± 0.8	1.4 ± 0.7	1.6 = ± 0.7	1.6 ± 0.3	0.946	0.562	0.089
	YA	1.5 ± 0.5	1.7 ± 0.8	1.7 ± 0.6	1.6 ± 0.9	1.5 ± 0.5			
Knee angular position at HS	OA	2.4 ± 1.3	2.1 ± 1.1	2.1 ± 1.3	2.4 ± 2.3	2.4 ± 2.0	**0.012**	0.939	0.326
	YA	1.2 ± 0.7	1.7 ± 1.2	1.7 ± 1.2	1.5 ± 1.0	1.5 ± 1.0			
Knee angular position at TO	OA	2.1 ± 0.7	2.1 ± 1.1	2 ± 1.1	2.1 ± 1.0	2.1 = 1.[illegible]	0.159	0.533	0.684
	YA	1.8 ± 0.7	2.2 ± 2.0	1.7 ± 0.6	1.8 ± 0.9	1.7 ± 0.6			
Hip angle position at HS	OA	3.2 ± 3.8	1.5 ± 0.9	2.0 ± 1.5	2.9 ± 3.4	2.0 ± 2.8	0.078	0.303	**0.005**
	YA	0.9 ± 0.3	1.7 ± 1.9	1.7 ± 1.1	1.8 ± 1.1	1.8 ± 1.4			
Hip angle position at TO	OA	2.5 ± 1.6	2.2 ± 1.4	2.4 ± 2.0	2.6 ± 2.1	2.5 ± 2.4	0.667	0.344	0.366
	YA	1.6 ± 0.8	2.9 ± 4.4	2.1 ± 1.5	2.0 ± 2.1	2.5 ± 2.1			

Values are presented as mean ± SD, bold indicates $p < 0.05$. OA, old adults; YA, young adults; CV, coefficient of variation; HS, heel strike; TO, toe off.

The intra-limb trajectories representing the coordination among adjacent angles were displayed for the first (blue line) and last stage (red line) of the protocol, as can be seen in **Figure 3**. For both age-groups, visual inspection of the trajectories revealed that the differences between the intra-limb trajectories were more evident during the swing phase, especially for the old group.

DISCUSSION

The objective of this study was to explore the continuous acute effect of a sustained fast-walking along the activity on the gait parameters in healthy young and old adults. We searched for supplementary information regarding potential risks induced by

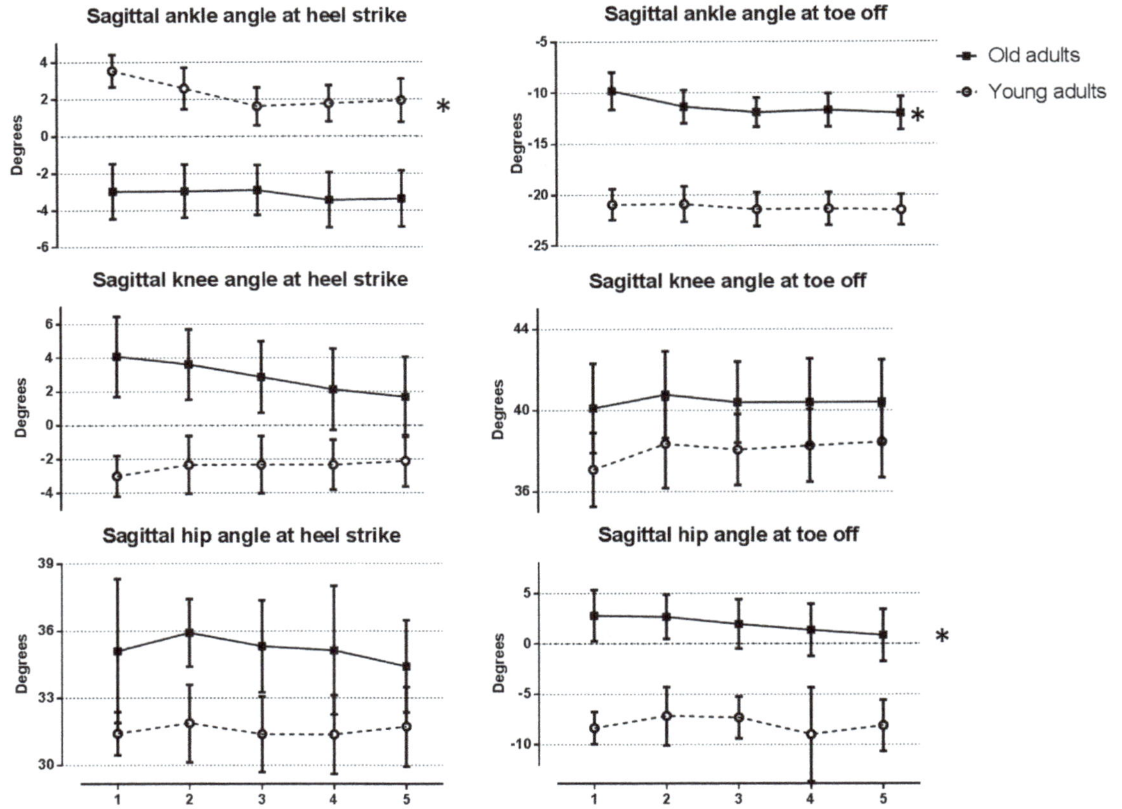

FIGURE 2 | Angular displacements for the hip, knee, and ankle at heel strike and toe off in young and old adults during the five time points along the fast-walking activity. *Indicates statistically significant time effect. The mean and SD for each subject were subsequently averaged across subjects within the age-group.

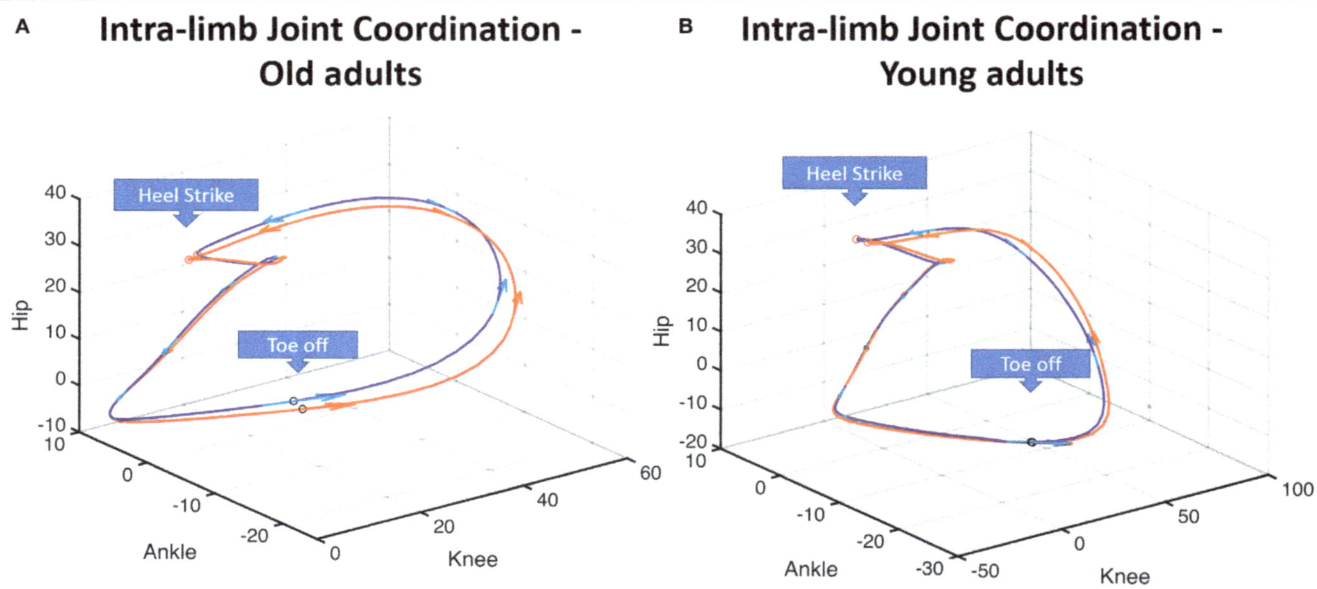

FIGURE 3 | Illustration of hip angle–ankle angle–knee angle intra-limb coordination patterns for the old adults **(A)** and the young adults **(B)**. Blue line represents the relative hip-knee-ankle position averaged for the group for the first stage; red line represents the relative hip-knee-ankle position averaged for the group for the fifth/last stage. These two stages are displayed to highlight the differences induced by the activity. Arrows indicate the direction of the gait.

a more demanding activity than walking at a freely chosen speed as in daily life activities.

Along the activity, both age-groups changed their gait strategy by having fewer, but longer strides. Even though such strategy may minimize the energy cost of walking (17), it may also increase the risk of injury at the knee (18). Stride length and stride time variability were greater in old adults when compared to young participants herein. Similar findings were reported by Kang and Dingwell (19). Literature regarding age-related differences in gait variability (defined here as fluctuations in temporospatial gait characteristics) and its relationship with walking speed are contradictory. Because older adults typically walk slower, increased gait variability in healthy older adults was considered to be related to their slow walking speed. However, previous studies have suggested that age-related changes in variability rather than be a manifestation of walking speed is more likely to reflect an underlying impairment of the motor system (19–21). With respect to changes in temporospatial variability, the most relevant finding here was the effect of fast-walking on step-width variability in both age-groups. Increased step-width variability has been suggested to be a necessary adaptation to maintain lateral stability. The control of lateral foot displacement is regulated by somatosensory, visual, and vestibular input (22). Such an increase in step-width variability may be explained by the reduction of sensory information induced by the activity (23), which is congruent with the negative effects found on postural control and balance induced by a similar walking protocol of previous studies (24, 25). Thus, during fast-walking, for both groups, the increased step-width variability could be a signal of incipient lateral instability, and loss of balance (26, 27). In addition, previous studies have associated the increment in step-width variability to increased risk of falls in old adults (2, 28).

Fast-walking resulted in significant changes on the lower-limb kinematics of both age-groups. Toward the end of the practice, older adults were initiating the swing phase with additional ankle plantarflexion, and a less extended hip while no changes were observed at the knee. Thus, the necessary adjustments that may have taken place for weight acceptance and body propulsion during the activity were restricted to the hip and ankle joints in old adults. A reduction in hip extension may imply a functional tightness that would be preventing the hip to fully extend at the toe-off (29). The increased ankle plantarflexion seems to be a compensatory mechanism to the reduction in hip extension since they managed to keep and even increase the stride length (30). These findings suggest that the relative contribution of the ankle plantarflexion for propelling the body forward has increased during the activity. Meanwhile, young adults manifested early signs of muscle fatigue, as we can see through their progressive reduction of the ankle dorsiflexion at landing (31). Old adults displayed higher variability for the ankle and knee angular position at heel contact, but levels of kinematic variability did not change throughout the protocol. However, in the present study, analyses regarding variability of angular kinematics were restricted to two events of the gait cycle. Further study on progressive effects of fast-walking activity should assess kinematical variability throughout the gait cycle to provide a complete understanding of the effects of fast-walking.

As we could observe from the intra-limb coordination trajectories, both groups displayed different patterns along the gait cycle. In interpreting this finding, one must consider that this difference may be associated with differences in the walking speed between groups and not exclusively to the age-related differences in walking pattern. The intra-limb joint coordination reflects a characteristic of the motor control of organizing adjacent structures in terms of timing and position to execute a movement (13, 32–34). Several studies have studied this outcome to obtain complementary information into gait control across different neuromuscular disorders (32, 34, 35). Changes in the state of intra-limb joint coordination may emerge due to alteration on any component of the motor system, as those caused by fatigue (33), or yet, alterations on muscle co-activation (34). The shift between the first and the fifth (last) intra-limb coordination trajectories reflect the effect of the activity on the related positions among the joint angles throughout the gait cycle and was more evident during the swing phase. Differences in the coordination among the lower-limb adjacent joints may influence the swing foot trajectory (36), which, in turn, may affect gait parameters related to the risk of falls by tripping and slipping.

Some limitations of this study were the absence of kinetic analyses and the use of a treadmill, which may decrease gait variability (37). However, the use of a treadmill allowed us to analyze continuous gait cycles. To the best of our knowledge, this study was the first to describe alterations on gait during sustained faster pace walking. Our findings revealed that old adults progressively changed their kinematics at hip and ankle during the task. Meanwhile, young adults showed incipient signs of fatigue at the ankle joint. Both age-groups changed their gait strategy by reducing cadence and increasing stride length and increased the variability of step-width. Walking at faster pace had no effect on angular kinematics variability assessed at the heel strike and toe off. However, further analyses should verify the effect of fast-walking throughout the gait cycle. In addition, the differences found in intra-limb coordination trajectories revealed that changes were more prominent during the swing phase. Which, in turn, reveals that the changes were phase dependent within the gait cycle. When walking at their typical pace, healthy active elderly subjects with increased step-width variability have more chances to fall (2, 28). Lower-limb kinematics during walking are strictly associated with the safe performance of two important events during the swing phase of gait, the minimum toe clearance, and the heel contact velocity (36, 38). Both gait events are directly linked to the risk of falls by tripping, and slipping, respectively (3, 36). Therefore, the changes induced after a certain period walking faster than usual, shown here, may compromise the quality of gait increasing the risk of falls. Future work should investigate kinematic changes throughout the gait cycle, particularly at the swing phase. The findings reported herein are important for addressing potential risks associated with walking at a faster pace.

AUTHOR CONTRIBUTIONS

CO, principal author, is responsible for the concept, design and intellectual content of the work, data process analysis, and interpretation. EV contributed with the intellectual content of the work, drafting ideas and reviewed analysis, and the final version. FS contributed with the data acquisition, drafting the work, and final revision. JV-B substantially contributed to the analysis and interpretation of the data and critically improved the content of the work. All the authors approved the final version of the manuscript, and declare to have no conflict of interest associated with this work, as well declare to be accountable for all aspects of it.

FUNDING

This publication was made by possible by Grant number 1637-13-4 by coordination for the improvement of higher education personnel within the Ministry of Education Brazil.

REFERENCES

1. WHO. *Global Health and Ageing. NIH 2011 Contract No.: Publication no. 11-7737.* Washington, DC: National Institute on Aging, National Institutes of Health (2011).
2. Maki BE. Gait changes in older adults: predictors of falls or indicators of fear? *J Am Geriatr Soc* (1997) 45(3):313–20. doi:10.1111/j.1532-5415.1997.tb00946.x
3. Lockhart TE, Woldstad JC, Smith JL. Effects of age-related gait changes on the biomechanics of slips and falls. *Ergonomics* (2003) 46(12):1136–60. doi:10.1080/0014013031000139491
4. Kang HG, Dingwell JB. Effects of walking speed, strength and range of motion on gait stability in healthy older adults. *J Biomech* (2008) 41(14):2899–905. doi:10.1016/j.jbiomech.2008.08.002
5. Faulkner JA, Larkin LM, Claflin DR, Brooks SV. Age-related changes in the structure and function of skeletal muscles. *Clin Exp Pharmacol Physiol* (2007) 34(11):1091–6. doi:10.1111/j.1440-1681.2007.04752.x
6. Prince F, Corriveau H, Hébert R, Winter DA. Gait in the elderly. *Gait Posture* (1997) 5(2):128–35. doi:10.1016/S0966-6362(97)01118-1
7. Fan Y, Li Z, Han S, Lv C, Zhang B. The influence of gait speed on the stability of walking among the elderly. *Gait Posture* (2016) 47:31–6. doi:10.1016/j.gaitpost.2016.02.018
8. Callisaya ML, Blizzard L, Schmidt MD, Martin KL, McGinley JL, Sanders LM, et al. Gait, gait variability and the risk of multiple incident falls in older people: a population-based study. *Age Ageing* (2011) 40:481–7. doi:10.1093/ageing/afr055
9. Nagano H, James L, Sparrow WA, Begg RK. Effects of walking-induced fatigue on gait function and tripping risks in older adults. *J Neuroeng Rehabil* (2014) 11:155. doi:10.1186/1743-0003-11-155
10. Li W, Keegan TH, Sternfeld B, Sidney S, Quesenberry CP Jr, Kelsey JL. Outdoor falls among middle-aged and older adults: a neglected public health problem. *Am J Public Health* (2006) 96(7):1192–200. doi:10.2105/AJPH.2005.083055
11. England SA, Granata KP. The influence of gait speed on local dynamic stability of walking. *Gait Posture* (2007) 25(2):172–8. doi:10.1016/j.gaitpost.2006.03.003
12. Hamacher D, Singh N, Van Dieen J, Heller M, Taylor W. Kinematic measures for assessing gait stability in elderly individuals: a systematic review. *J R Soc Interface* (2011) 8(65):1682–98. doi:10.1098/rsif.2011.0416
13. Shumway-Cook A, Woollacott MH. *Controle Motor: teoria e aplicações práticas.* São Paulo: Manole (2003).
14. Cappozzo A, Catani F, Della Croce U, Leardini A. Position and orientation in space of bones during movement: anatomical frame definition and determination. *Clin Biomech* (1995) 10(4):171–8. doi:10.1016/0268-0033(95)91394-T
15. Borg GA. Psychophysical bases of perceived exertion. *Med Sci Sports Exerc* (1982) 14(5):377–81. doi:10.1249/00005768-198205000-00012
16. Medicine ACoS. *ACSM's Guidelines for Exercise Testing and Prescription.* 9th ed. Baltimore: Lippincott Williams & Wilkins (2014).
17. Kuo AD. A simple model of bipedal walking predicts the preferred speed-step length relationship. *J Biomech Eng* (2001) 123(3):264–9. doi:10.1115/1.1372322
18. Ardestani MM, Ferrigno C, Moazen M, Wimmer MA. From normal to fast walking: impact of cadence and stride length on lower extremity joint moments. *Gait Posture* (2016) 46:118–25. doi:10.1016/j.gaitpost.2016.02.005
19. Kang HG, Dingwell JB. Separating the effects of age and walking speed on gait variability. *Gait Posture* (2008) 27(4):572–7. doi:10.1016/j.gaitpost.2007.07.009
20. Ko SU, Hausdorff JM, Ferrucci L. Age-associated differences in the gait pattern changes of older adults during fast-speed and fatigue conditions: results from the Baltimore longitudinal study of ageing. *Age Ageing* (2010) 39(6):688–94. doi:10.1093/ageing/afq113
21. Hausdorff JM. Gait dynamics, fractals and falls: finding meaning in the stride-to-stride fluctuations of human walking. *Hum Mov Sci* (2007) 26(4):555–89. doi:10.1016/j.humov.2007.05.003
22. Bauby CE, Kuo AD. Active control of lateral balance in human walking. *J Biomech* (2000) 33(11):1433–40. doi:10.1016/S0021-9290(00)00101-9
23. Paillard T. Effects of general and local fatigue on postural control: a review. *Neurosci Biobehav Rev* (2012) 36(1):162–76. doi:10.1016/j.neubiorev.2011.05.009
24. Derave W, Tombeux N, Cottyn J, Pannier J-L, De Clercq D. Treadmill exercise negatively affects visual contribution to static postural stability. *Int J Sports Med* (2002) 23(01):44–9. doi:10.1055/s-2002-19374
25. Ghasemi A, Taghizade G, Gharegozli K. Comparing the effect of speedy and endurance walking on postural control and the time for returning to baseline after walking in patients with chronic stroke and healthy subjects. *J Mod Rehabil* (2016) 10(1):1–6.
26. Gabell A, Nayak U. The effect of age on variability in gait. *J Gerontol* (1984) 39(6):662–6. doi:10.1093/geronj/39.6.662
27. Brach JS, Berlin JE, VanSwearingen JM, Newman AB, Studenski SA. Too much or too little step width variability is associated with a fall history in older persons who walk at or near normal gait speed. *J Neuroeng Rehabil* (2005) 2:21. doi:10.1186/1743-0003-2-21
28. Toebes MJP, Hoozemans MJM, Furrer R, Dekker J, van Dieën JH. Local dynamic stability and variability of gait are associated with fall history in elderly subjects. *Gait Posture* (2012) 36(3):527–31. doi:10.1016/j.gaitpost.2012.05.016
29. Lee LW, Kerrigan DC, Della Croce U. Dynamic implications of hip flexion contractures1. *Am J Phys Med Rehabil* (1997) 76(6):502–8. doi:10.1097/00002060-199711000-00013
30. JudgeRoy JO, Davis B, Õunpuu S. Step length reductions in advanced age: the role of ankle and hip kinetics. *J Gerontol A* (1996) 51(6):M303–12. doi:10.1093/gerona/51A.6.M303
31. Parijat P, Lockhart TE. Effects of lower extremity muscle fatigue on the outcomes of slip-induced falls. *Ergonomics* (2008) 51(12):1873–84. doi:10.1080/00140130802567087
32. Shafizadeh M, Watson PJ, Mohammadi B. Intra-limb coordination in gait pattern in healthy people and multiple sclerosis patients. *Clin Kinesiol* (2013) 67(3):32–8.
33. Ferber R, Pohl MB. Changes in joint coupling and variability during walking following tibialis posterior muscle fatigue. *J Foot Ankle Res* (2011) 4(1):6. doi:10.1186/1757-1146-4-6
34. Daly JJ, Roenigk K, Cheng R, Ruff RL. Abnormal leg muscle latencies and relationship to dyscoordination and walking disability after stroke. *Rehabil Res Prac* (2010) 2011:313980. doi:10.1155/2011/313980
35. Awai L, Curt A. Intralimb coordination as a sensitive indicator of motor-control impairment after spinal cord injury. *Front Hum Neurosci* (2014) 8:148. doi:10.3389/fnhum.2014.00148
36. Winter DA. Foot trajectory in human gait: a precise and multifactorial motor control task. *Phys Ther* (1992) 72(1):45–53. doi:10.1093/ptj/72.1.45
37. Dingwell JB, Cavanagh PR. Increased variability of continuous overground walking in neuropathic patients is only indirectly related to sensory loss. *Gait Posture* (2001) 14(1):1–10. doi:10.1016/S0966-6362(01)00101-1
38. Moyer BE, Chambers AJ, Redfern MS, Cham R. Gait parameters as predictors of slip severity in younger and older adults. *Ergonomics* (2006) 49(4):329–43. doi:10.1080/00140130500478553

21

Uremic Myopathy: Is Oxidative Stress Implicated in Muscle Dysfunction in Uremia?

*Antonia Kaltsatou[1], Giorgos K. Sakkas[1,2], Konstantina P. Poulianiti[1], Yiannis Koutedakis[1], Konstantinos Tepetes[3], Grigorios Christodoulidis[3], Ioannis Stefanidis[4] and Christina Karatzaferi[1]**

[1] Department of Physical Education and Sport Sciences (DPESS), School of Physical Education (PE), University of Thessaly, Trikala, Greece, [2] Institute for Research and Technology-Centre for Research and Technology Hellas, Trikala, Greece, [3] Department of Surgery, Faculty of Medicine, University of Thessaly, Larissa, Greece, [4] Department of Nephrology, Faculty of Medicine, University of Thessaly, Larissa, Greece

Edited by:
Brian McDonagh,
University of Liverpool, UK

Reviewed by:
Laszlo Csernoch,
University of Debrecen, Hungary
David Sheehan,
University College Cork, Ireland
Brian McDonagh,
University of Liverpool, UK

***Correspondence:**
Christina Karatzaferi,
Muscle Physiology and Mechanics Group, Department of Physical Education and Sport Sciences (DPESS), School of Physical Education (PE), University of Thessaly, Tmima Epistimis Fysikis Agogis kai Athlitismou - Panepistimio Thessalias, Karyes 42100, Trikala, Thessaly, Greece
ck@pe.uth.gr

Renal failure is accompanied by progressive muscle weakness and premature fatigue, in part linked to hypokinesis and in part to uremic toxicity. These changes are associated with various detrimental biochemical and morphological alterations. All of these pathological parameters are collectively termed uremic myopathy. Various interventions while helpful can't fully remedy the pathological phenotype. Complex mechanisms that stimulate muscle dysfunction in uremia have been proposed, and oxidative stress could be implicated. Skeletal muscles continuously produce reactive oxygen species (ROS) and reactive nitrogen species (RNS) at rest and more so during contraction. The aim of this mini review is to provide an update on recent advances in our understanding of how ROS and RNS generation might contribute to muscle dysfunction in uremia. Thus, a systematic review was conducted searching PubMed and Scopus by using the Cochrane and PRISMA guidelines. While few studies met our criteria their findings are discussed making reference to other available literature data. Oxidative stress can direct muscle cells into a catabolic state and chronic exposure to it leads to wasting. Moreover, redox disturbances can significantly affect force production *per se*. We conclude that oxidative stress can be in part responsible for some aspects of uremic myopathy. Further research is needed to discern clear mechanisms and to help efforts to counteract muscle weakness and exercise intolerance in uremic patients.

Keywords: oxidative stress, uremia, muscle dysfunction, uremic myopathy, premature fatigue, muscle weakness

Introduction

Among the clinical entities affecting thousands of patients, chronic kidney disease (CKD) is a silent epidemic expected to influence more than 50% of the Americans born today (Grams et al., 2013) and approximately 40% of the population in Europe (Zoccali et al., 2010). Muscular weakness, muscle wasting, limited endurance, exercise intolerance, and fatigue are components of the functional and morphological abnormalities collectively termed uremic myopathy, which often also includes uremic cardiomyopathy (Campistol, 2002). While the pathogenesis of uremic myopathy is not clear, it is thought that an interplay of uremic toxicity and hypokinesis guide these abnormalities in patients with CKD and especially in end-stage renal disease (ESRD) patients undergoing hemodialysis (HD) therapy. Observations of a significant correlation between glomerular filtration rate (GFR) and exercise tolerance (e.g., Clyne et al., 1987, 1994) led to studies revealing the very low activity levels and poor functional capacity of renal patients (Kouidi et al., 1998; Johansen et al., 2003; Sakkas et al., 2003a). Moreover, various groups turned their attention to exercise and other interventions to remedy or halt muscle deterioration in pre-dialysis (e.g., Clyne et al., 1991) and dialysis patients (e.g., Sakkas et al., 2003b; Johansen et al., 2006). Despite the evident improvements in exercise capacity and muscle morphology (Sakkas et al., 2003b, 2008a), in increasing muscle mass with steroid supplementation (Topp et al., 2003), in improving sleep and overall quality of life (Sakkas et al., 2008c) it appears that interventions so far cannot restore muscle functionality in ESRD patients to the level of age-matched healthy sedentary individuals (Sakkas et al., 2003b, 2008a; Giannaki et al., 2011).

Components of Uremic Myopathy

Loss of skeletal muscle strength in renal patients, contributes to easy fatigability, and can be linked to loss of muscle fibers and atrophy of the remaining fibers (Porter et al., 1995; Sakkas et al., 2003a). In cross-sectional studies, comparing age-matched controls and end-stage patients, atrophy and loss of type IIα and IIx fibers, reduced muscle fiber capillarization and peripheral activation (Sakkas et al., 2003a), and a significant decrease in the mean diameter of both fiber types (Crowe et al., 2007) has been observed. However, not all functional consequences can be attributed to atrophy. Interventions to improve muscle mass indicate that there is a functional deficit in the existing muscle mass. Dialysis patients present with rapid and large accumulation of inorganic phosphate during submaximal exercise, lower oxidative potential, larger phosphocreatine reduction with slower recovery but also with evidence of central activation failure, all these factors contributing to early and excess fatigue (Johansen et al., 2005). Abnormal mitochondria respiratory capacity, is also a factor responsible for easily fatigability in CKD patients, as mitochondrial morphology is disturbed in patients with CKD (Kouidi et al., 1998), while alterations in respiratory chain proteins likely enhance reactive oxygen species (ROS) production which has been seen in a rat uremia model (Yazdi et al., 2013).

CKD patients, especially the end-stage ones, lead a very sedentary lifestyle. Morphological abnormalities however have been observed in both locomotory and non-locomotory muscles (Sakkas et al., 2003a) thus not all of the dysfunction can be attributed to inactivity.

Biochemical and nutritional changes occurring through the progression of CKD can stimulate protein losses and can contribute to the development of muscle wasting. This has grave significance as catabolic conditions increase the risk of morbidity and mortality (Griffiths, 1996; Gordon et al., 2007).

Pro-dialysis and dialysis patients face increasing dietary restrictions. Malnutrition is associated with hypoalbuminemia, which is inversely correlated with mortality in uremic patients (Lowrie and Lew, 1990), and it is also used as a marker of depleted protein stores (Carrero et al., 2008).

Metabolic acidosis, which is commonly associated with CKD, stimulates the breakdown of muscle proteins resulting in loss of muscle mass (Hu et al., 2013). Furthermore, the observation that insulin resistance, is common in patients with CKD, suggests that impaired insulin signaling could also contribute to protein losses (Sakkas et al., 2008b; Zhang et al., 2009). Moreover, CKD is associated with an increase in circulating levels of inflammatory cytokines. Specifically, levels of circulating IL-6, TNF-α, serum amyloid A, and C-reactive protein are increased in patients with CKD (Zhang et al., 2009, 2011; Cheung et al., 2010). Notably, it is contested that in well-dialyzed patients, circulating proinflammatory markers are the main cause for hypoalbuminemia rather than malnutrition (Kaysen et al., 2004). The possibility of an accelerated protein degradation in CKD mediated by the ubiquitin-proteasome system (UPS) (Wang and Mitch, 2013) should also be considered.

Apart from a compounded or accelerated muscle loss, a reduction in the ability to anabolize muscle could be an issue in CKD. Still, interventions with nandrolone decanoate were successful in increasing muscle mass, albeit without improving muscle strength (Topp et al., 2003), pointing to an available anabolic response. However, there are suggestions that CKD may dampen the function of satellite cells. Zhang et al. (2010) using a mouse model of CKD reported a delayed regeneration of damaged muscle and reductions in MyoD protein and the myogenin expression, indicating a decreased satellite cell proliferation and differentiation (Zhang et al., 2010).

To compound the above, in dialyzed patients, the HD procedure *per se* stimulates protein degradation and reduced protein synthesis with the effect persisting for 2 h following dialysis (Ikizler et al., 2002). Thus, while blunting of anabolic responses can't be excluded, a multitude of factors can promote protein loss, especially in the end-stage patients.

Is there a Role for Oxidative Stress in Uremic Muscle Dysfunction?

Oxidative stress promotes catabolic state and accelerates muscle atrophy (Moylan and Reid, 2007). But it can also affect contractility of the available muscle and sarcomeric protein expression.

Many studies have found that oxidative stress can cause long-term effects and acute effects (Lamb and Westerblad, 2011) on contractility. Long-term effects include altered gene and protein expression or damages in lipids and proteins that are irreversible, while acute effects are reversible. The decrease in Ca^{2+} sensitivity which contributes to muscle fatigue is considered as an acute effect of oxidative stress (Lamb and Westerblad, 2011).

A key mechanism that has been proposed to explain the ROS contribution in muscle fatigue is the reduced myofibrillar Ca^{2+} sensitivity and/or sarcoplasmic reticulum Ca^{2+} release (Allen et al., 2008). Moreover, an increase in NO during fatigue in fast twitch muscle fibers contribute in decreased myofibrillar Ca^{2+} sensitivity (Lamb and Westerblad, 2011). However, in slow-twitch fibers NO donors, did not affect myofibrillar Ca^{2+} sensitivity (Spencer and Posterino, 2009). Also, a study by Reardon and Allen (2009), showed that iron can increase ROS production at high temperature in the skeletal muscle cells, accelerating muscle fatigue.

Moreover, ROS generation can acutely affect contractile function and disturbs structural transition within the actomyosin complex which is crucial for force generation. Exposure to low or high concentrations of peroxide (5 or 50 mM) reduces maximum force and velocity of contraction, with the high peroxide resulting in irreversible loss of calcium regulation of force mediated by oxidation of methionines in the heavy and essential light chains (Prochniewicz et al., 2008a). More elegant work from same group, examining structural dynamics of actin and myosin pointed to an effect of oxidation on weak-to-strong structural transition and by using site-directed mutagenesis of *Dictyostelium* (*Dicty*) myosin II oxidation, a redistribution of existing structural states of the actin-binding cleft was implicated (Prochniewicz et al., 2008b; Klein et al., 2011). Alterations in myosin heavy chain expression in uremic animals have also been reported (Taes et al., 2004).

Many studies have observed increased levels of oxidative stress biomarkers in blood samples of CKD patients (Samouilidou and Grapsa, 2003; Filiopoulos et al., 2009). In the literature, there are sufficient studies with different technical approaches in which the activity and role of ROS and reactive nitrogen species (RNS) in skeletal muscle has been studied using both *in vivo* and *in vitro* methods in a variety of contexts (Powers et al., 2011). Thus, based on recent advances in our understanding of how ROS and RNS affect muscle function, this mini-review aimed to examine if oxidative stress can contribute to muscle dysfunction in ESRD.

Methods

A systematic review was conducted searching PubMed and Scopus by using the Cochrane and PRISMA guidelines. A comprehensive literature search was conducted from September 2014 until November 2014. We used PubMed, ScienceDirect and Scopus or Google Scholar to search for studies that investigated the relationship among (i) oxidative stress and uremic myopathy in humans, and (ii) markers of oxidative stress in the skeletal muscle of uremic patients on HD. Eligibility of the studies based on titles, abstracts and full-text articles was determined by two reviewers. Studies were selected using inclusion and exclusion criteria. We included only those studies that met the following criteria: they assessed oxidative stress markers in the skeletal muscle of patients on HD; they used human biopsies; they addressed randomized control trials, controlled trials, or clinical trials designed to evaluate oxidative stress in skeletal muscle in uremic patients on HD therapy; they were written in English.

Results and Discussion

Only three studies have examined the oxidative damage in human skeletal muscle of uremic patients on HD (**Table 1**). Their findings are discussed with reference to renal human blood findings and/or animal muscle findings either models of CKD or models of other conditions.

Lim et al. (2002a) found increased malondialdehyde (MDA) and protein carbonyls (PC) levels reflecting extensive oxidative damage to total protein content and lipids, in muscle suggested by the authors to be due to increased levels of inflammatory cytokines and to increased protein degradation. Increased levels of lipid peroxidation in blood samples of CKD patients during HD treatment has also been found elsewhere (Varan et al., 2010) and could enhance the susceptibility of LDL oxidation which is a major contributor in the genesis of atherosclerosis. The above observations, together with animal findings in the role of carbonyl stress in vascular injury (Chen et al., 2013) concur to a role of protein oxidation in long-term vascular damage which could impact overall vessel functionality and thus striated muscle's bioenergetics and function.

The same group also reported increased mitochondrial protein and lipid oxidative damage in skeletal muscle of uremic patients compared to age-matched controls (Lim et al., 2002b). The authors also reported mitochondrial DNA mutations, and overall oxidative damage to total cellular DNA, supporting a notion of attenuating regenerative and bioenergetics capacities of the skeletal muscles of renal patients. Also, mitochondrial DNA deletions have been observed in the skeletal muscle of ESRD patients similar with these found in the skeletal muscle of elderly subjects due to oxidative damage which probably contribute to the impaired mitochondrial energy metabolism that characterizes uremic patients (Lim et al., 2000).

It is considered that mitochondrial membranes are more likely to develop oxidative damage due to the relatively high amounts of lipid containing polyunsaturated fatty acids that they possess (Laganiere and Yu, 1993) and this would explain their increased oxidative damage. Given that mitochondria are considered the predominant source of ROS in muscle fibers (Davies et al., 1982; McArdle et al., 2001; Jackson, 2009), due to the elevated oxygen consumption that occurs with increased mitochondrial activity, especially during exercise (Powers et al., 2011) it is conceivable that damage to the mitochondria membrane might further compound their function as a ROS source causing more leaking. Moreover, it has been suggested that mitochondrial ROS leaking depends on fiber type both at resting basal respiration and at an increased respiration (as in exercise). In an animal saponin-treated muscle study of mitochondrial respiration, type IIb skeletal muscle fibers showed significantly higher free radical leaking compared to type IIa and I fibers at basal respiration (Anderson and Neufer, 2006).

If indeed the ROS load in the late stages renal skeletal muscle is high, that might in part explain the higher susceptibility of type II fibers to atrophy observed in end stage patients, where not only generalized muscle atrophy was observed but more prominent atrophy was seen in type II (especially IIx) vs type I fibers either in non-locomotory (Sakkas et al., 2003a) or locomotory muscle samples. Furthermore, on the possible role of the mitochondrial dysfunction in renal muscle atrophy it should be noted that de-innervation studies show that denervated muscle mitochondria release fatty acid hydro peroxides, mediated by calcium dependent phospholipase A_2 (Bhattacharya et al., 2009). Such observations together with observations of an increased sensitivity of human aged mitochondria to apoptosis (Gouspillou et al., 2014), and the findings of Lim et al. (2002b) reviewed above, can collectively substantiate an important role

TABLE 1 | Summary results of the studies meeting the criteria of the present systematic review.

References	Total glutathione nmol/mg protein	GSS Gnmol/mg protein	SOD U/mg protein	MDA nmol/mg protein	CAT U/mg protein	PC nmol /mg of protein	Thiols nmol/mg protein
MARKERS OF OXIDATIVE STRESS IN MUSCLE TISSUE OF UREMIC PATIENTS							
Lim et al., 2002a	–	–	–	0.065 ± 0.009↑	–	3.78 ± −0.14↑	–
Lim et al., 2002b	–	–	–	23.76 ± 6.06↑	–	24.9 ± 4.00↑	–
Crowe et al., 2007	≈ 24↑	≈ 2.6	≈ 20	≈ 0.28↓	≈ 11↓	–	≈ 79
MARKERS OF OXIDATIVE STRESS IN MUSCLE TISSUE OF HEALTHY CONTROLS							
Lim et al., 2002a	–	–	–	0.043 ± 0.005	–	2.97 ± −0.28	–
Lim et al., 2002b	–	–	–	7.67 ± 0.95	–	3.78 ± 0.14	–
Crowe et al., 2007	≈ 5	≈ 3.3	≈ 27	≈ 0.52	≈ 34	–	≈ 60

GSH, glutathione; GSSG, oxidized glutathione; SOD, superoxide dismutase; MDA, malondialdehyde; CAT, catalase; PC, protein carbonyl; Thiols, protein thiol content. Arrows indicate statistically significant differences reported by authors.

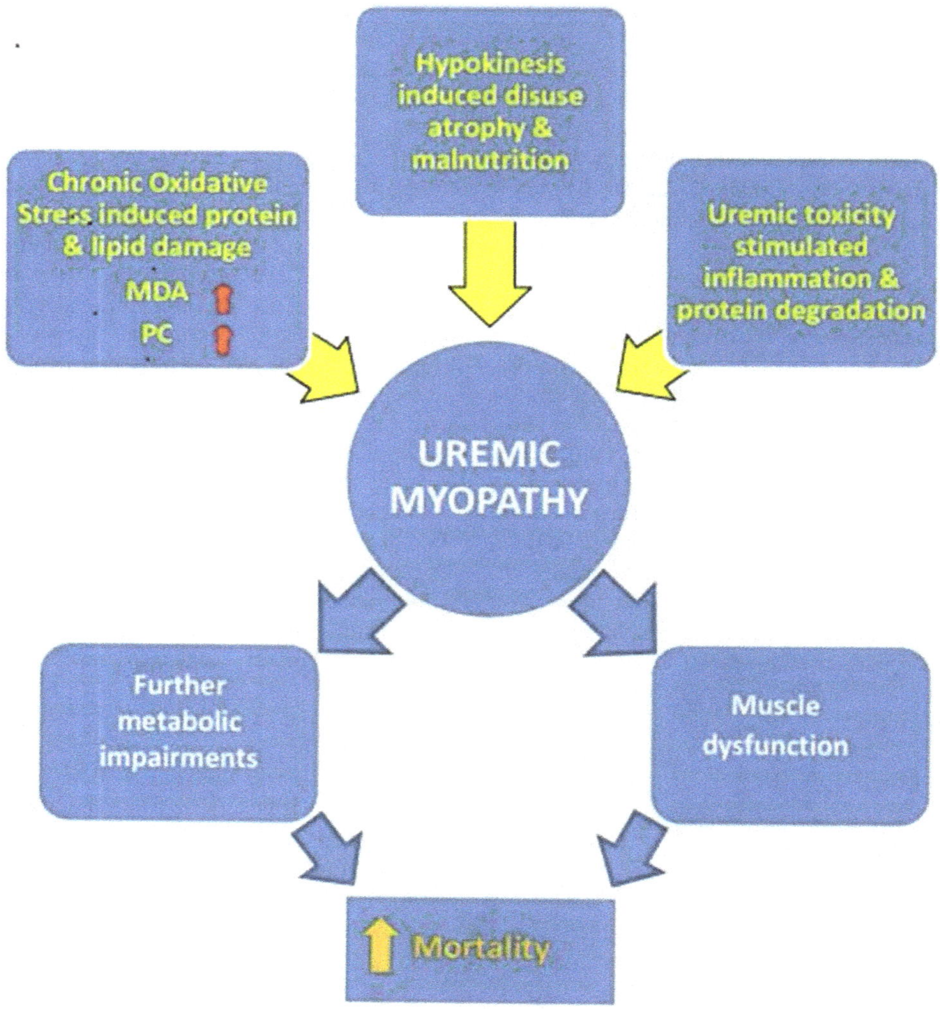

FIGURE 1 | The multifactorial nature of uremic myopathy. Many specific disease-related but also lifestyle factors (e.g., physical inactivity) contribute to the pathological muscle state. Exactly when one factor reaches critical importance cannot be surmised so far. The results of this systematic mini review do point to oxidative stress as a contributor to the development of uremic myopathy. MDA, malondialdehyde; PC, protein carbonyls.

for mitochondrial dysfunction, in the pathogenesis of uremic myopathy.

In contrast to the findings of Lim et al. and Crowe et al. (2007), reported decreased MDA content, increased total glutathione and no change in protein thiols content, superoxide dismutase (SOD), oxidized glutathione (GSSG) and catalase activity and concluded that there is no evident connection between oxidative stress and muscle atrophy in uremia. However, if one considers the age difference in the subjects of the conflicting studies one cannot discount the possibility that the much younger subjects, which also had spent less time on dialysis, of the Crowe et al. study had better preserved mitochondrial status. Adaptation of various antioxidant mechanisms can also explain some of the above differences. It should also be noted that in transgenic mice studies, the model overexpressing phospholipid hydroperoxide glutathione peroxidase, Gpx4-Tg (which is associated with mitochondrial and other membranes) protected against denervation atrophy and not the manganese superoxide dismutase (Sod2-Tg) or copper-zinc superoxide dismutase (Sod1-Tg) models, suggesting that the release of fatty acid hydroperoxides from mitochondria may be a more important factor in denervation-induced atrophy than superoxide and hydrogen peroxide (Bhattacharya et al., 2009).

The above discourse further highlights the difficulty faced by researchers in renal patient studies. Many confounding factors such as years in dialysis, nutrition, physical activity levels, level of treatment, and comorbidities can affect muscle status and accelerate or decelerate disease and aging effects (**Figure 1**).

Conclusions

CKD has a high and increasing prevalence not only in the old retirees but also in the middle-aged Europeans (Zoccali et al., 2010). Skeletal muscle dysfunction is a ubiquitous finding in CKD patients on advanced stages of the disease. The impact is grave as the statistics are implacable. Muscle loss and weakness contribute to the high morbidity and mortality of these patients, especially at the end-stage renal failure. Many specific disease-related but also lifestyle factors (such as physical inactivity) can be seen as contributors to the pathological muscle state. Exactly when one factor reaches critical importance cannot be surmised so far. The few studies meeting our search criteria while not agreeing, do point to a possibly important role for oxidative stress in uremic myopathy. It is not known if hypothesized oxidative stress mediated effects on muscle function are more of an acute or a chronic nature. *In vitro* studies however show clearly that oxidative stress does have a role whether via chronic, protein and other modifications or acute contractility effects. If anything the three studies and the peripheral literature highlight the need for a systematic study of the disease mechanisms affecting skeletal muscle performance in renal disease.

As long as great unknowns remain on the mechanisms and modulation of uremic myopathy, which leads to debilitation and premature death, progress in the management of this new epidemic is the least slowed down. We suggest that more muscle research, human and animal, should be done on pro-dialysis stages including work on the role of oxidative stress. This would allow researchers to decipher early changes, and perhaps identify susceptible individuals for accelerated muscle loss, before moving into the end-stage situation which on its own has detrimental effects on muscle status.

Acknowledgments

This work has been co-financed by the European Union (European Social Fund—ESF) and Greek national funds through the Operational Program "Educational and Lifelong Learning" of the National Strategic Reference Framework (NSRF)—Research Funding Program: Thales (MuscleFun Project-MIS 377260) Investing in knowledge society through the European Social Fund.

References

Allen, D. G., Lamb, G. D., and Westerblad, H. (2008). Skeletal muscle fatigue: cellular mechanisms. *Physiol. Rev.* 88, 287–332. doi: 10.1152/physrev.00015.2007

Anderson, E. J., and Neufer, P. D. (2006). Type II skeletal myofibers possess unique properties that potentiate mitochondrial H(2)O(2) generation. *Am. J. Physiol. Cell Physiol.* 290, C844–C851. doi: 10.1152/ajpcell.00402.2005

Bhattacharya, A., Muller, F. L., Liu, Y., Sabia, M., Liang, H., Song, W., et al. (2009). Denervation induces cytosolic phospholipase A2-mediated fatty acid hydroperoxide generation by muscle mitochondria. *J. Biol. Chem.* 284, 46–55. doi: 10.1074/jbc.M806311200

Campistol, J. M. (2002). Uremic myopathy. *Kidney Int.* 62, 1901–1913. doi: 10.1046/j.1523-1755.2002.00614.x

Carrero, J. J., Chmielewski, M., Axelsson, J., Snaedal, S., Heimburger, O., Barany, P., et al. (2008). Muscle atrophy, inflammation and clinical outcome in incident and prevalent dialysis patients. *Clin. Nutr.* 27, 557–564. doi: 10.1016/j.clnu.2008.04.007

Chen, X., Mori, T., Guo, Q., Hu, C., Ohsaki, Y., Yoneki, Y., et al. (2013). Carbonyl stress induces hypertension and cardio-renal vascular injury in Dahl salt-sensitive rats. *Hypertens. Res.* 36, 361–367. doi: 10.1038/hr.2012.204

Cheung, W. W., Paik, K. H., and Mak, R. H. (2010). Inflammation and cachexia in chronic kidney disease. *Pediatr. Nephrol.* 25, 711–724. doi: 10.1007/s00467-009-1427-z

Clyne, N., Ekholm, J., Jogestrand, T., Lins, L. E., and Pehrsson, S. K. (1991). Effects of exercise training in predialytic uremic patients. *Nephron* 59, 84–89. doi: 10.1159/000186524

Clyne, N., Jogestrand, T., Lins, L. E., and Pehrsson, S. K. (1994). Progressive decline in renal function induces a gradual decrease in total hemoglobin and exercise capacity. *Nephron* 67, 322–326. doi: 10.1159/000187987

Clyne, N., Jogestrand, T., Lins, L. E., Pehrsson, S. K., and Ekelund, L. G. (1987). Factors limiting physical working capacity in predialytic uraemic patients. *Acta Med. Scand.* 222, 183–190. doi: 10.1111/j.0954-6820.1987.tb10657.x

Crowe, A. V., McArdle, A., McArdle, F., Pattwell, D. M., Bell, G. M., Kemp, G. J., et al. (2007). Markers of oxidative stress in the skeletal muscle of patients on haemodialysis. *Nephrol. Dial. Transplant.* 22, 1177–1183. doi: 10.1093/ndt/gfl721

Davies, K. J., Quintanilha, A. T., Brooks, G. A., and Packer, L. (1982). Free radicals and tissue damage produced by exercise. *Biochem. Biophys. Res. Commun.* 107, 1198–1205. doi: 10.1016/S0006-291X(82)80124-1

Filiopoulos, V., Hadjiyannakos, D., Takouli, L., Metaxaki, P., Sideris, V., and Vlassopoulos, D. (2009). Inflammation and oxidative stress in end-stage renal disease patients treated with hemodialysis or peritoneal dialysis. *Int. J. Artif. Organs* 32, 872–882.

Giannaki, C. D., Stefanidis, I., Karatzaferi, C., Liakos, N., Roka, V., Ntente, I., et al. (2011). The effect of prolonged intradialytic exercise in hemodialysis efficiency indices. *ASAIO J.* 57, 213–218. doi: 10.1097/MAT.0b013e318215dc9e

Gordon, P. L., Sakkas, G. K., Doyle, J. W., Shubert, T., and Johansen, K. L. (2007). Relationship between vitamin D and muscle size and strength in patients on hemodialysis. *J. Ren. Nutr.* 17, 397–407. doi: 10.1053/j.jrn.2007.06.001

Gouspillou, G., Bourdel-Marchasson, I., Rouland, R., Calmettes, G., Biran, M., Deschodt-Arsac, V., et al. (2014). Mitochondrial energetics is impaired *in vivo* in aged skeletal muscle. *Aging Cell* 13, 39–48. doi: 10.1111/acel.12147

Grams, M. E., Chow, E. K. H., Segev, D. L., and Coresh, J. (2013). Lifetime Incidence of CKD Stages 3-5 in the United States. *Am. J. Kidney Dis.* 62, 245–252. doi: 10.1053/j.ajkd.2013.03.009

Griffiths, R. D. (1996). Muscle mass, survival, and the elderly ICU patient. *Nutrition* 12, 456–458. doi: 10.1016/S0899-9007(96)00141-4

Hu, W. T., Shelnutt, M., Wilson, A., Yarab, N., Kelly, C., Grossman, M., et al. (2013). Behavior Matters-Cognitive Predictors of Survival in Amyotrophic Lateral Sclerosis. *PLoS ONE* 8:e57584. doi: 10.1371/journal.pone.0057584

Ikizler, T. A., Pupim, L. B., Brouillette, J. R., Levenhagen, D. K., Farmer, K., Hakim, R. M., et al. (2002). Hemodialysis stimulates muscle and whole body protein loss and alters substrate oxidation. *Am. J. Physiol. Endocrinol. Metab.* 282, E107–E116.

Jackson, M. J. (2009). Redox regulation of adaptive responses in skeletal muscle to contractile activity. *Free Radic. Biol. Med.* 47, 1267–1275. doi: 10.1016/j.freeradbiomed.2009.09.005

Johansen, K. L., Doyle, J., Sakkas, G. K., and Kent-Braun, J. A. (2005). Neural and metabolic mechanisms of excessive muscle fatigue in maintenance hemodialysis patients. *Am. J. Physiol. Regul. Integr. Comp. Physiol.* 289, R805–R813. doi: 10.1152/ajpregu.00187.2005

Johansen, K. L., Painter, P. L., Sakkas, G. K., Gordon, P., Doyle, J., and Shubert, T. (2006). Effects of resistance exercise training and nandrolone decanoate on body composition and muscle function among patients who receive hemodialysis: a randomized, controlled trial. *J. Am. Soc. Nephrol.* 17, 2307–2314. doi: 10.1681/ASN.2006010034

Johansen, K. L., Shubert, T., Doyle, J., Soher, B., Sakkas, G. K., and Kent-Braun, J. A. (2003). Muscle atrophy in patients receiving hemodialysis: effects on muscle strength, muscle quality, and physical function. *Kidney Int.* 63, 291–297. doi: 10.1046/j.1523-1755.2003.00704.x

Kaysen, G. A., Dubin, J. A., Muller, H. G., Rosales, L., Levin, N. W., and Mitch, W. E. (2004). Inflammation and reduced albumin synthesis associated with stable decline in serum albumin in hemodialysis patients. *Kidney Int.* 65, 1408–1415. doi: 10.1111/j.1523-1755.2004.00520.x

Klein, J. C., Moen, R. J., Smith, E. A., Titus, M. A., and Thomas, D. D. (2011). Structural and functional impact of site-directed methionine oxidation in myosin. *Biochemistry* 50, 10318–10327. doi: 10.1021/bi201279u

Kouidi, E., Albani, M., Natsis, K., Megalopoulos, A., Gigis, P., Guiba-Tziampiri, O., et al. (1998). The effects of exercise training on muscle atrophy in haemodialysis patients. *Nephrol. Dial. Transplant.* 13, 685–699. doi: 10.1093/ndt/13.3.685

Laganiere, S., and Yu, B. P. (1993). Modulation of membrane phospholipid fatty acid composition by age and food restriction. *Gerontology* 39, 7–18. doi: 10.1159/000213509

Lamb, G. D., and Westerblad, H. (2011). Acute effects of reactive oxygen and nitrogen species on the contractile function of skeletal muscle. *J. Physiol.* 589, 2119–2127. doi: 10.1113/jphysiol.2010.199059

Lim, P. S., Cheng, Y. M., and Wei, Y. H. (2000). Large-scale mitochondrial DNA deletions in skeletal muscle of patients with end-stage renal disease. *Free Radic. Biol. Med.* 29, 454–463. doi: 10.1016/S0891-5849(00)00334-8

Lim, P. S., Cheng, Y. M., and Wei, Y. H. (2002a). Increase in oxidative damage to lipids and proteins in skeletal muscle of uremic patients. *Free Radic. Res.* 36, 295–301. doi: 10.1080/10715760290019318

Lim, P. S., Ma, Y. S., Cheng, Y. M., Chai, H., Lee, C. F., Chen, T. L., et al. (2002b). Mitochondrial DNA mutations and oxidative damage in skeletal muscle of patients with chronic uremia. *J. Biomed. Sci.* 9, 549–560. doi: 10.1007/BF02254982

Lowrie, E. G., and Lew, N. L. (1990). Death risk in hemodialysis patients: the predictive value of commonly measured variables and an evaluation of death rate differences between facilities. *Am. J. Kidney Dis.* 15, 458–482. doi: 10.1016/S0272-6386(12)70364-5

McArdle, A., Pattwell, D., Vasilaki, A., Griffiths, R. D., and Jackson, M. J. (2001). Contractile activity-induced oxidative stress: cellular origin and adaptive responses. *Am. J. Physiol. Cell Physiol.* 280, C621–C627.

Moylan, J. S., and Reid, M. B. (2007). Oxidative stress, chronic disease, and muscle wasting. *Muscle Nerve* 35, 411–429. doi: 10.1002/mus.20743

Porter, M. M., Vandervoort, A. A., and Lexell, J. (1995). Aging of human muscle: structure, function and adaptability. *Scand. J. Med. Sci. Sports* 5, 129–142. doi: 10.1111/j.1600-0838.1995.tb00026.x

Powers, S. K., Ji, L. L., Kavazis, A. N., and Jackson, M. J. (2011). Reactive oxygen species: impact on skeletal muscle. *Compr. Physiol.* 1, 941–969. doi: 10.1002/cphy.c100054

Prochniewicz, E., Lowe, D. A., Spakowicz, D. J., Higgins, L., O'conor, K., Thompson, L. V., et al. (2008a). Functional, structural, and chemical changes in myosin associated with hydrogen peroxide treatment of skeletal muscle fibers. *Am. J. Physiol. Cell Physiol.* 294, C613–C626. doi: 10.1152/ajpcell.00232.2007

Prochniewicz, E., Spakowicz, D., and Thomas, D. D. (2008b). Changes in actin structural transitions associated with oxidative inhibition of muscle contraction. *Biochemistry* 47, 11811–11817. doi: 10.1021/bi801080x

Reardon, T. F., and Allen, D. G. (2009). Time to fatigue is increased in mouse muscle at 37 degrees C; the role of iron and reactive oxygen species. *J. Physiol.* 587, 4705–4716. doi: 10.1113/jphysiol.2009.173005

Sakkas, G. K., Ball, D., Mercer, T. H., Sargeant, A. J., Tolfrey, K., and Naish, P. F. (2003a). Atrophy of non-locomotor muscle in patients with end-stage renal failure. *Nephrol. Dial. Transplant.* 18, 2074–2081. doi: 10.1093/ndt/gfg325

Sakkas, G. K., Hadjigeorgiou, G. M., Karatzaferi, C., Maridaki, M. D., Giannaki, C. D., Mertens, P. R., et al. (2008a). Intradialytic aerobic exercise training ameliorates symptoms of restless legs syndrome and improves functional capacity in patients on hemodialysis. *ASAIO J.* 54, 185–190. doi: 10.1097/MAT.0b013e3181641b07

Sakkas, G. K., Karatzaferi, C., Zintzaras, E., Giannaki, C. D., Liakopoulos, V., Lavdas, E., et al. (2008b). Liver fat, visceral adiposity, and sleep disturbances contribute to the development of insulin resistance and glucose intolerance in nondiabetic dialysis patients. *Am. J. Physiol. Regul. Integr. Comp. Physiol.* 295, R1721–R1729. doi: 10.1152/ajpregu.00935.2007

Sakkas, G. K., Liakopoulos, V., Karatzaferi, C., and Stefanidis, I. (2008c). Sleep quality and dialysis efficacy affect functional capacity in patients receiving haemodialysis therapy. *Nephrol. Dial. Transplant.* 23, 2703–2704. doi: 10.1093/ndt/gfn048

Sakkas, G. K., Sargeant, A. J., Mercer, T. H., Ball, D., Koufaki, P., Karatzaferi, C., et al. (2003b). Changes in muscle morphology in dialysis patients after 6 months of aerobic exercise training. *Nephrol. Dial. Transplant.* 18, 1854–1861. doi: 10.1093/ndt/gfg237

Samouilidou, E., and Grapsa, E. (2003). Effect of dialysis on plasma total antioxidant capacity and lipid peroxidation products in patients with end-stage renal failure. *Blood Purif.* 21, 209–212. doi: 10.1159/000070691

Spencer, T., and Posterino, G. S. (2009). Sequential effects of GSNO and H2O2 on the Ca2+ sensitivity of the contractile apparatus of fast- and slow-twitch skeletal muscle fibers from the rat. *Am. J. Physiol. Cell Physiol.* 296, C1015–C1023. doi: 10.1152/ajpcell.00251.2008

Taes, Y. E. C., Speeckaert, M., Bauwens, E., De Buyzere, M. R., Libbrecht, J., Lameire, N. H., et al. (2004). Effect of dietary creatine on skeletal muscle myosin heavy chain isoform expression in an animal model of uremia. *Nephron Exp. Nephrol.* 96, E103–E110. doi: 10.1159/000077376

Topp, K. S., Painter, P. L., Walcott, S., Krasnoff, J. B., Adey, D., Sakkas, G. K., et al. (2003). Alterations in skeletal muscle structure are minimized with steroid withdrawal after renal transplantation. *Transplantation* 76, 667–673. doi: 10.1097/01.TP.0000076096.45542.1B

Varan, H. I., Dursun, B., Dursun, E., Ozben, T., and Suleymanlar, G. (2010). Acute effects of hemodialysis on oxidative stress parameters in chronic uremic patients: comparison of two dialysis membranes. *Int. J. Nephrol. Renovasc. Dis.* 3, 39–45.

Wang, X. H., and Mitch, W. E. (2013). Muscle wasting from kidney failure-a model for catabolic conditions. *Int. J. Biochem. Cell Biol.* 45, 2230–2238. doi: 10.1016/j.biocel.2013.06.027

Yazdi, P. G., Moradi, H., Yang, J. Y., Wang, P. H., and Vaziri, N. D. (2013). Skeletal muscle mitochondrial depletion and dysfunction in chronic kidney disease. *Int. J. Clin. Exp. Med.* 6, 532–539.

Zhang, L., Du, J., Hu, Z., Han, G., Delafontaine, P., Garcia, G., et al. (2009). IL-6 and serum amyloid A synergy mediates angiotensin II-induced muscle wasting. *J. Am. Soc. Nephrol.* 20, 604–612. doi: 10.1681/ASN.2008060628

Zhang, L., Rajan, V., Lin, E., Hu, Z., Han, H. Q., Zhou, X., et al. (2011). Pharmacological inhibition of myostatin suppresses systemic inflammation and muscle atrophy in mice with chronic kidney disease. *FASEB J.* 25, 1653–1663. doi: 10.1096/fj.10-176917

Zhang, L., Wang, X. H., Wang, H., Du, J., and Mitch, W. E. (2010). Satellite cell dysfunction and impaired IGF-1 signaling cause CKD-induced muscle atrophy. *J. Am. Soc. Nephrol.* 21, 419–427. doi: 10.1681/ASN.2009060571

Zoccali, C., Kramer, A., and Jager, K. J. (2010). Epidemiology of CKD in Europe: an uncertain scenario. *Nephrol. Dial. Transplant.* 25, 1731–1733. doi: 10.1093/ndt/gfq250

Permissions

All chapters in this book were first published in AADM & RRSMAE, by Frontiers; hereby published with permission under the Creative Commons Attribution License or equivalent. Every chapter published in this book has been scrutinized by our experts. Their significance has been extensively debated. The topics covered herein carry significant findings which will fuel the growth of the discipline. They may even be implemented as practical applications or may be referred to as a beginning point for another development.

The contributors of this book come from diverse backgrounds, making this book a truly international effort. This book will bring forth new frontiers with its revolutionizing research information and detailed analysis of the nascent developments around the world.

We would like to thank all the contributing authors for lending their expertise to make the book truly unique. They have played a crucial role in the development of this book. Without their invaluable contributions this book wouldn't have been possible. They have made vital efforts to compile up to date information on the varied aspects of this subject to make this book a valuable addition to the collection of many professionals and students.

This book was conceptualized with the vision of imparting up-to-date information and advanced data in this field. To ensure the same, a matchless editorial board was set up. Every individual on the board went through rigorous rounds of assessment to prove their worth. After which they invested a large part of their time researching and compiling the most relevant data for our readers.

The editorial board has been involved in producing this book since its inception. They have spent rigorous hours researching and exploring the diverse topics which have resulted in the successful publishing of this book. They have passed on their knowledge of decades through this book. To expedite this challenging task, the publisher supported the team at every step. A small team of assistant editors was also appointed to further simplify the editing procedure and attain best results for the readers.

Apart from the editorial board, the designing team has also invested a significant amount of their time in understanding the subject and creating the most relevant covers. They scrutinized every image to scout for the most suitable representation of the subject and create an appropriate cover for the book.

The publishing team has been an ardent support to the editorial, designing and production team. Their endless efforts to recruit the best for this project, has resulted in the accomplishment of this book. They are a veteran in the field of academics and their pool of knowledge is as vast as their experience in printing. Their expertise and guidance has proved useful at every step. Their uncompromising quality standards have made this book an exceptional effort. Their encouragement from time to time has been an inspiration for everyone.

The publisher and the editorial board hope that this book will prove to be a valuable piece of knowledge for researchers, students, practitioners and scholars across the globe.

List of Contributors

Marianne A. Andersen, Holti Kellezi, Steve Risis, Sara G. Vienberg and Jonas T. Treebak
Section of Integrative Physiology, The Novo Nordisk Foundation Center for Basic Metabolic Research, University of Copenhagen, Copenhagen, Denmark

Josef Brandauer
Section of Integrative Physiology, The Novo Nordisk Foundation Center for Basic Metabolic Research, University of Copenhagen, Copenhagen, Denmark
Department of Health Sciences, Gettysburg College, Gettysburg, PA, USA

Christian Frøsig
Section of Molecular Physiology, Department of Nutrition, Exercise and Sports, The August Krogh Centre, University of Copenhagen, Copenhagen, Denmark

Marios Kyriazis
ELPIS Foundation for Indefinite Lifespans, Larnaca, Cyprus

Elisavet Kiourti
University of Cyprus, Nicosia, Cyprus

Pedro Pita Barros
Nova Healthcare Initiative Research, Nova School of Business and Economics, Universidade Nova de Lisboa, Lisbon, Portugal

Judite Gonçalves
Nova Healthcare Initiative Research, Nova School of Business and Economics, Universidade Nova de Lisboa, Lisbon, Portugal
School of Business and Management, Queen Mary University of London, London, United Kingdom

Maria Isabel Gomes, Miguel Fonseca
Center for Mathematics and Applications, Faculty of Sciences and Technology, Universidade Nova de Lisboa, Lisbon, Portugal

Maria-Amália Botelho and Tomás Teodoro
Chronic Diseases Research Center, Nova Medical School, Universidade Nova de Lisboa, Lisbon, Portugal

Maria Teresa Tomás and Beatriz Fernandes
Escola Superior de Tecnologia da Saúde de Lisboa (ESTeSL), Instituto Politécnico de Lisboa, Lisboa, Portugal

Alejandro Galán-Mercant
Health Science Department, Jaén University, Jaén, Spain

Elvis Alvarez Carnero
Translational Research Institute for Metabolism and Diabetes, Florida Hospital, Orlando, FL, United States

Genaro Barrientos and Jorge Hidalgo
Physiology and Biophysics Program, Institute of Biomedical Sciences, School of Medicine, University of Chile, Santiago, Chile

Paola Llanos
Institute for Research in Dental Sciences, Faculty of Dentistry, University of Chile, Santiago, Chile

Pura Bolaños and Carlo Caputo
Centre of Biophysics and Biochemistry, Venezuelan Institute for Scientific Research, Caracas, Venezuela

Alexander Riquelme
Biomedical Neuroscience Institute, School of Medicine, University of Chile, Santiago, Chile

Gina Sánchez
Biomedical Neuroscience Institute, School of Medicine, University of Chile, Santiago, Chile
Pathophysiology Program, Institute of Biomedical Sciences, School of Medicine, University of Chile, Santiago, Chile
Center for Molecular Studies of the Cell, School of Medicine, University of Chile, Santiago, Chile

Cecilia Hidalgo
Physiology and Biophysics Program, Institute of Biomedical Sciences, School of Medicine, University of Chile, Santiago, Chile
Biomedical Neuroscience Institute, School of Medicine, University of Chile, Santiago, Chile
Center for Molecular Studies of the Cell, School of Medicine, University of Chile, Santiago, Chile

Andrew F. G. Quest
Center for Molecular Studies of the Cell, School of Medicine, University of Chile, Santiago, Chile
Laboratory of Cell Communication, Program in Cell and Molecular Biology, Institute of Biomedical Sciences, School of Medicine, University of Chile, Santiago, Chile
Advanced Center for Chronic Diseases and Network for Metabolic Stress Signaling, University of Chile, Santiago, Chile

Edward P. Debold
Department of Kinesiology, University of Massachusetts, Amherst, MA, USA

Natália Duarte and Constança Paúl
Research Unit on Ageing, Instituto de Ciências Biomédicas Abel Salazar (ICBAS), Centro de Investigação em Tecnologias e Serviços de Saúde (CINTESIS), University of Porto, Porto, Portugal

Ana Maria Rodrigues
EpiReumaPt Study Group—Sociedade Portuguesa de Reumatologia, Lisboa, Portugal
EpiDoc Unit—Unidade de Epidemiologia em Doenças Crónicas (CEDOC, NMS/UNL), Unidade de Investigação em Reumatologia, Instituto de Medicina Molecular, Faculdade de Medicina da Universidade de Lisboa, Lisboa, Portugal

Jaime Da Cunha Branco
EpiReumaPt Study Group—Centro de Estudos de Doenças Crónicas (CEDOC) da NOVA Medical School, Universidade Nova de Lisboa (NMS/UNL), Centro Hospitalar Lisboa Ocidental (CHLO-EPE), Sociedade Portuguesa de Reumatologia, Lisbon, Portugal

Helena Canhão
EpiReumaPt Study Group—Centro de Estudos de Doenças Crónicas (CEDOC), EpiDoC Unit, NOVA Medical School, Universidade Nova de Lisboa (NMS/UNL), Escola Nacional de Saúde Publica, Universidade Nova de Lisboa, Sociedade Portuguesa de Reumatologia, Serviço de Reumatologia do Hospital de Santa Maria, Centro Hospitalar Lisboa Norte (CHLN-EPE), Lisboa, Portugal

Susan L. Hughes
Community Health Sciences, School of Public Health, Center for Research on Health and Aging, University of Illinois at Chicago, Chicago, IL, United States

João O. Malva and António F. Ambrósio
Ageing@Coimbra, EIP on AHA Reference Site, Coimbra, Portugal
Faculty of Medicine, Coimbra Institute for Clinical and Biomedical Research (iCBR), and CNC.IBILI, University of Coimbra, Coimbra, Portugal

Manuel T. Veríssimo
Ageing@Coimbra, EIP on AHA Reference Site, Coimbra, Portugal
Faculty of Medicine, Coimbra Institute for Clinical and Biomedical Research (iCBR), and CNC.IBILI, University of Coimbra, Coimbra, Portugal
University of Coimbra Hospital, CHUC, Coimbra, Portugal

Alda Amado
Ageing@Coimbra, EIP on AHA Reference Site, Coimbra, Portugal
Instituto de Segurança Social, Centro Distrital de Coimbra, Coimbra, Portugal

Alexandra Rodrigues
Ageing@Coimbra, EIP on AHA Reference Site, Coimbra, Portugal
Comissão de Coordenação e Desenvolvimento Regional do Centro, Coimbra, Portugal

Vitor Rodrigues
Ageing@Coimbra, EIP on AHA Reference Site, Coimbra, Portugal
Centre of Investigation in Environment, Genetics and Oncobiology (CIMAGO), Faculty of Medicine, University of Coimbra, Coimbra, Portugal

Anabela Mota-Pinto
Ageing@Coimbra, EIP on AHA Reference Site, Coimbra, Portugal
Centre of Investigation in Environment, Genetics and Oncobiology (CIMAGO), Faculty of Medicine, University of Coimbra, Coimbra, Portugal
Faculty of Medicine, General Pathology Institute, University of Coimbra, Coimbra, Portugal

Ana F. Cardoso, Cidalina Abreu and João Apóstolo
Ageing@Coimbra, EIP on AHA Reference Site, Coimbra, Portugal
Centre for Evidence Based Practice, Health Sciences Research Unit: Nursing (UICISA: E), Nursing School of Coimbra, Coimbra, Portugal

Ana M. Teixeira
Ageing@Coimbra, EIP on AHA Reference Site, Coimbra, Portugal
Research Center for Sport and Physical Activity, Faculty of Sport Sciences and Physical Education, University of Coimbra, Coimbra, Portugal

Ana Todo-Bom
Ageing@Coimbra, EIP on AHA Reference Site, Coimbra, Portugal
Faculty of Medicine, General Pathology Institute, University of Coimbra, Coimbra, Portugal
University of Coimbra Hospital, CHUC, Coimbra, Portugal

António Devesa
Ageing@Coimbra, EIP on AHA Reference Site, Coimbra, Portugal
Municipality of Coimbra, Coimbra, Portugal

António L. Cunha
Ageing@Coimbra, EIP on AHA Reference Site, Coimbra, Portugal
Pedro Nunes Institute, Laboratory of Automatics and Systems, Coimbra, Portugal

Bárbara Gomes
Ageing@Coimbra, EIP on AHA Reference Site, Coimbra, Portugal
Faculty of Medicine, Coimbra Institute for Clinical and Biomedical Research (iCBR), and CNC.IBILI, University of Coimbra, Coimbra, Portugal
King's College London, Cicely Saunders Institute of Palliative Care, Policy and Rehabilitation, London, United Kingdom

Carina Dantas
Ageing@Coimbra, EIP on AHA Reference Site, Coimbra, Portugal
Caritas Coimbra, Coimbra, Portugal

Isabel Santana
University of Coimbra Hospital, CHUC, Coimbra, Portugal
Ageing@Coimbra, EIP on AHA Reference Site, Coimbra, Portugal
Center for Neuroscience and Cell Biology (CNC), University of Coimbra, Coimbra, Portugal

Jean Bousquet
Contre les Maladies Chroniques pour un VIeilissement Active (MACVIA) en France en EIP on AHA Reference Site, Montpellier, France

Lúcia Santos
Ageing@Coimbra, EIP on AHA Reference Site, Coimbra, Portugal
Portuguese Pharmaceutical Society - Center Region Branch, Coimbra, Portugal

Lúcio Meneses de Almeida
Ageing@Coimbra, EIP on AHA Reference Site, Coimbra, Portugal
Regional Health Authority, ARS Centro, Coimbra, Portugal

Maddalena Illario
Division for Health Innovation, Campania Region and Federico II University Hospital Naples (R&D and DISMET), Naples, Italy

Rafaela Veríssimo
Centro Hospitalar de Gaia/Espinho, Gaia, Portugal

Sára Sándor and Enikő Kubinyi
Department of Ethology, Eötvös Loránd University, Budapest, Hungary

Rónán O'Caoimh
Clinical Sciences Institute, National University of Ireland, Galway, Galway, Ireland
National Clinical Programme for Older People, Royal College of Physicians of Ireland, Dublin, Ireland

Siobhán Kennelly
National Clinical Programme for Older People, Royal College of Physicians of Ireland, Dublin, Ireland
Department of Medicine for the Elderly, Connolly Hospital, Blanchardstown, Dublin, Ireland

Diamuid O'Shea
National Clinical Programme for Older People, Royal College of Physicians of Ireland, Dublin, Ireland
Department of Geriatric Medicine, St Vincent's University Hospital, Dublin, Ireland

Sara Palermo and Massimo Bartoli
Department of Psychology, University of Turin, Turin, Italy

Martina Amanzio
European Innovation Partnership on Active and Healthy Ageing, Brussels, Belgium
Department of Psychology, University of Turin, Turin, Italy

Milena Zucca Elisa Rubino and Innocenzo Rainero
Department of Neuroscience "Rita Levi Montalcini", University of Turin, Turin, Italy

Rosalba Rosato
Department of Psychology, University of Turin, Turin, Italy
Unit of Cancer Epidemiology, "Città della Salute e della Scienza" Hospital and CPO Piemonte, Turin, Italy

Daniela Leotta
Neurology Division, Martini Hospital, Turin, Italy

Lília Jorge, Nádia Canário and Hugo Quental
Coimbra Institute for Biomedical Imaging and Translational Research (CIBIT), University of Coimbra, Coimbra, Portugal
Institute for Nuclear Sciences Applied to Health (ICNAS), University of Coimbra, Coimbra, Portugal

Rui Bernardes and Miguel Castelo-Branco
Coimbra Institute for Biomedical Imaging and Translational Research (CIBIT), University of Coimbra, Coimbra, Portugal
Institute for Nuclear Sciences Applied to Health (ICNAS), University of Coimbra, Coimbra, Portugal
Faculty of Medicine, University of Coimbra, Coimbra, Portugal

Giuseppe Liotta, Ercole Vellone and Leonardo Palombi
Department of Biomedicine and Prevention, University of Rome "Tor Vergata", Rome, Italy

Helena Canhao and Rute Dinis Sousa
CEDOC, EpiDoC Unit, NOVA Medical School, Nova University of Lisbon, Lisbon, Portugal

Fabian Cenko
Catholic University "Our Lady of Good Counsel", Tirana, Albania

Rita Cutini
Sociology, University for Foreigners "Dante Alighieri", Reggio Calabria, Italy

Maddalena Illario
UOD Health Innovation, Campania Region, Naples, Italy

Przemyslaw Kardas
Department of Family Medicine, Medical University of Lodz, Lodz, Poland

Andrea Poscia
Institute of Hygiene, University of Sacred Heart, Rome, Italy

Maria Cristina Marazzi
LUMSA University, Rome, Italy

Simone G. Fernandes
Escola Nacional de Saúde Pública, Universidade Nova de Lisboa, Lisbon, Portugal

Ana M. Rodrigues Maria J. Gregório, Rute Dinis de Sousa and Sara Dias
CEDOC, EpiDoc Unit - Unidade de Epidemiologia em Doenças Crónicas, NOVA Medical School, Universidade Nova de Lisboa, Lisbon, Portugal

Helena Canhão
Escola Nacional de Saúde Pública, Universidade Nova de Lisboa, Lisbon, Portugal
CEDOC, EpiDoc Unit - Unidade de Epidemiologia em Doenças Crónicas, NOVA Medical School, Universidade Nova de Lisboa, Lisbon, Portugal

Carla Nunes
Escola Nacional de Saúde Pública, Universidade Nova de Lisboa, Lisbon, Portugal
Centro de Investigação em Saúde Pública, Escola Nacional de Saúde Pública, Universidade Nova de Lisboa, Lisbon, Portugal

Osvaldo Santos
Instituto de Medicina Preventiva e Saúde Pública, Faculdade de Medicina, Universidade de Lisboa, Lisbon, Portugal
Instituto de Saúde Ambiental, Faculdade de Medicina, Universidade de Lisboa, Lisbon, Portuga

Daniela Bakula and Morten Scheibye-Knudsen
Department of Cellular and Molecular Medicine, Center for Healthy Aging, University of Copenhagen, Copenhagen, Denmark

Philip Lewis and Ken D. O'Halloran
Department of Physiology, School of Medicine, University College Cork, Cork, Ireland

David Sheehan
School of Biochemistry and Cell Biology, University College Cork, Cork, Ireland

Renata Soares and Ana Varela Coelho
Instituto de Tecnologia Química e Biológica António Xavier, New University of Lisbon, Lisbon, Portugal

Maria Ana Pego
Unidade de Investigação e Desenvolvimento em Enfermagem, Escola Superior de Enfermagem de Lisboa, Lisbon, Portugal

Carla Nunes
Centro de Investigação em Saúde Pública, Escola Nacional de Saúde Pública, Universidade Nova de Lisboa, Lisbon, Portugal
Escola Nacional de Saúde Pública, Universidade Nova de Lisboa, Lisbon, Portugal

Michael P. Wiggs
Department of Applied Physiology and Kinesiology, Center for Exercise Science, University of Florida, Gainesville, FL, USA

Rute Dinis de Sousa
Chronic Diseases Research Center (CEDOC), EpiDoC Unit, NOVA Medical School, Universidade Nova de Lisboa (NMS/UNL), Lisbon, Portugal
EpiSaúde - Associa*ção* Científica, *Évora*, Portugal

Ana Maria Rodrigues
Chronic Diseases Research Center (CEDOC), EpiDoC Unit, NOVA Medical School, Universidade Nova de Lisboa (NMS/UNL), Lisbon, Portugal
EpiSaúde - Associa*ção* Científica, *Évora*, Portugal
Sociedade Portuguesa de Reumatologia, Lisbon, Portugal
Rheumatology Research Unit, Instituto de Medicina Molecular, Lisbon, Portugal

Maria João Gregório
Chronic Diseases Research Center (CEDOC), EpiDoC Unit, NOVA Medical School, Universidade Nova de Lisboa (NMS/UNL), Lisbon, Portugal
EpiSaúde - Associa*ção* Científica, *Évora*, Portugal
Faculdade de Ciências da Nutrição e Alimentação da Universidade do Porto, Porto, Portugal

Jaime Da Cunha Branco
Chronic Diseases Research Center (CEDOC), EpiDoC Unit, NOVA Medical School, Universidade Nova de Lisboa (NMS/UNL), Lisbon, Portugal
EpiSaúde - Associa*ção* Científica, *Évora*, Portugal
Sociedade Portuguesa de Reumatologia, Lisbon, Portugal
Serviço de Reumatologia do Hospital Egas Moniz - Centro Hospitalar Lisboa Ocidental (CHLO-E.P.E.), Lisbon, Portugal

Maria João Gouveia
Promoting Human Potential Research Group, ISPA - Instituto Universitário, Lisbon, Portugal

Helena Canhão
Chronic Diseases Research Center (CEDOC), EpiDoC Unit, NOVA Medical School, Universidade Nova de Lisboa (NMS/UNL), Lisbon, Portugal
EpiSaúde - Associa*ção* Científica, *Évora*, Portugal
Sociedade Portuguesa de Reumatologia, Lisbon, Portugal
Escola Nacional de Saúde Publica, Universidade Nova de Lisboa, Lisbon, Portugal

Sara Simões Dias
Chronic Diseases Research Center (CEDOC), EpiDoC Unit, NOVA Medical School, Universidade Nova de Lisboa (NMS/UNL), Lisbon, Portugal
EpiSaúde - Associa*ção* Científica, *Évora*, Portugal
Escola Superior de Saúde do Instituto Politécnico de Leiria, Leiria, Portugal

Camila Fonseca Oliveira, Filipa Manuel Machado Sousa and João Paulo Vilas-Boas
Center of Research, Education, Innovation and Intervention in Sport (CIFI2D), Faculty of Sport, University of Porto, Porto, Portugal
Porto Biomechanics Laboratory (LABIOMEP), University of Porto, Porto, Portugal

Edgar Ramos Vieira
Department of Physical Therapy, Florida International University, Miami, FL, United States

Konstantina P. Poulianiti, Yiannis Koutedakis and Christina Karatzaferi
Department of Physical Education and Sport Sciences (DPESS), School of Physical Education (PE), University of Thessaly, Trikala, Greece

Sakkas
Department of Physical Education and Sport Sciences (DPESS), School of Physical Education (PE), University of Thessaly, Trikala, Greece
Institute for Research and Technology-Centre for Research and Technology Hellas, Trikala, Greece

Konstantinos Tepetes and Grigorios Christodoulidis
Department of Surgery, Faculty of Medicine, University of Thessaly, Larissa, Greece

Ioannis Stefanidis
Department of Nephrology, Faculty of Medicine, University of Thessaly, Larissa, Greece

Index